Intermittent High Intensity Exercise

Other titles from E & FN Spon

Sport and Physical Activity
Moving towards excellence
L. Almond and T. Williams

Physiology of Sports
T. Reilly, N. Secher, P. Snell and C. Williams

Exercise
Benefits, limits and adaptations
D. Macleod, R. Maughan, M. Nimmo, T. Reilly and C. Williams

Drugs in Sport
D.R. Mottram

Science and Football
T. Reilly, A. Lees, K. Davids and W.J. Murphy

Writing Successfully in Science
M. O'Connor

For more information about these and other titles published by us, please contact:
The Promotion Department, E & FN Spon, 2–6 Boundary Row, London
SE1 8HN. Telephone: 071 522 9966.

Intermittent High Intensity Exercise

Preparation, stresses and damage limitation

Edited by

D.A.D. Macleod

St John's Hospital at Howden, West Lothian

R.J. Maughan

Dept of Occupational and Environmental Medicine
Aberdeen University, Aberdeen

C. Williams

Dept of Physical Education
Loughborough University, Loughborough

C.R. Madeley

Dept of Virology
The Royal Victoria Infirmary, Newcastle upon Tyne

J.C.M. Sharp

Communicable Diseases (Scotland) Unit
Ruchill Hospital, Glasgow

R.W. Nutton

Princess Margaret Rose Hospital, Edinburgh

E & FN SPON

An Imprint of Chapman & Hall

London · Glasgow · New York · Tokyo · Melbourne · Madras

Published by E & FN Spon, an imprint of Chapman & Hall, 2–6 Boundary Row, London SE1 8HN

Chapman & Hall, 2–6 Boundary Row, London SE1 8HN, UK

Blackie Academic & Professional, Wester Cleddens Road, Bishopbriggs, Glasgow G64 2NZ, UK

Chapman & Hall Inc., 29 West 35th Street, New York, NY10001, USA

Chapman & Hall Japan, Thomson Publishing Japan, Hirakawacho Nemoto Building, 6F, 1–7–11 Hirakawa-cho, Chiyoda-ku, Tokyo 102, Japan

Chapman & Hall Australia, Thomas Nelson Australia, 102 Dodds Street, South Melbourne, Victoria 3205, Australia

Chapman & Hall India, R. Seshadri, 32 Second Main Road, CIT East, Madras 600 035, India

First edition 1993

© 1993 D.A.D. Macleod, R.J. Maughan, C. Williams, C.R. Madeley, J.C.M. Sharp and R.W. Nutton.

ISBN 0 419 17860 0

A catalogue record for this book is available from the British Library

Library of Congress Cataloging-in-Publication data available

Contents

Sports Medicine Congress 1991 Editorial Board and Speakers

Editorial Board

Macleod, Mr D.A.D. (Convenor), St John's Hospital at Howden, Livingston, West Lothian EH54 6PP

Graham, Mr J., Dept of Orthopaedics, Western Infirmary, Glasgow G11 6NT

Madeley, Professor C.R., Dept of Virology, The Royal Victoria Infirmary, Queen Victoria Road, Newcastle upon Tyne NE1 4LP

Maughan, Dr R.J., Dept of Occupational & Environmental Medicine, Aberdeen University, Foresterhill Hospitals, Aberdeen

Nutton, Mr R.W., Princess Margaret Rose Hospital, Frogston Road West, Edinburgh EH10 7ED

Sharp, Dr J.C.M., Communicable Diseases (Scotland) Unit, Ruchill Hospital, Glasgow G20 9NB

Williams, Professor C., Dept of Physical Education, Sports Science & Recreation Management, Loughborough University, Ashby Road, Loughborough LE11 3TU

Conference Speakers

Adams, Dr I., St James' Hospital, Leeds

Anderson, Dr T., Cleveland Clinic Foundation, 9500 Euclid Avenue, Cleveland, Ohio 44195–5027, USA

Armstrong, Dr R.B., Muscle Biology Laboratory, University of Georgia, Athens, Georgia 30602, USA

Banatvala, Professor J.E., Dept of Virology, United Medical and Dental Schools of Guy's and St Thomas' Hospitals, London SE1 7EH

Bangsbo, Dr J., Human Physiology Dept, August Krogh Institute, University of Copenhagen, 13 Universitetsparken, DK-2100

Organizing Committee

Chairman   Mr Donald A.D. Macleod

EXECUTIVE COMMITTEE

Dr J.C.M. Sharp
Dr B. Slawson
Dr E. Lloyd
Mr D. Bolton
Dr S. Hillis
Mr G. McLatchie
Mr D. McLean

ACADEMIC COMMITTEE

Prof. C. Willliams
Dr R.J. Maughan
Prof. C.R. Madeley
Mr J. Graham
Prof. T. Reilly
Mr R. Nutton

Additional advice on the programme was received from:

Dr I. Todd
Mr P. Edmond
Prof. P. Radford
Mr M. Macnicol
Mr P. Scott
Mr T. McGlashan

Foreword

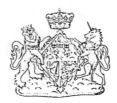

BUCKINGHAM PALACE

The International Rugby Football Board and the Scottish Rugby Union are to be congratulated on organizing a Sports Medicine Congress to coincide with the second Rugby World Cup.

Sports Medicine has been recognized over the last 10 years to be an increasingly important speciality and this has been reflected by the support and interest given to the Congress by the Royal College of Physicians and Royal College of Surgeons of Edinburgh.

The programme of the Congress reflected a wide range of interests involved with sport, ranging from the scientific aspects of preparing an athlete for top class performance, the stresses of performing at the top levels in contact sport and clinical aspects of illness and injury occurring during sport. The quality and range of material presented at the Congress deserves a wide audience and I hope the publication of the proceedings will act as a stimulus to science and medicine to continue their endeavours promoting fitness and ensuring that sportsmen and women have every opportunity to achieve their full potential without coming to any harm.

Introduction

The International Rugby Football Board decided to capitalize on the opportunities afforded by the 1991 Rugby World Cup by promoting three Congresses which were held during the Tournament:

Coaching, organized by the Rugby Football Union, 15–18 October;
Sports Medicine, organized by the Scottish Rugby Union, 23–25 October;
Referees, organized by the Welsh Rugby Union, 27–30 October.

Each Congress was encouraged to submit proposals for consideration by the International Rugby Football Board to help ensure safe and enjoyable rugby at all levels of the game throughout the forty-six National Rugby Football Unions in membership with the Board.

The International Rugby Football Board would like to record their appreciation to the speakers and participants at the Sports Medicine Congress for the wide range and quality of the academic presentations, which were associated with ample opportunity for discussion. The Board is particularly pleased that the Proceedings of the Congress have been published, ensuring that the papers presented will reach a wide international audience.

The International Rugby Football Board are most grateful to the Scottish Rugby Union and the Sports Medicine Congress Committees for their considerable efforts in organizing a stimulating and enjoyable Congress.

Dr I.R. Vanderfield O.B.E.
Chairman
International Rugby Football Board

The Scottish Rugby Union was delighted to accept the invitation from the International Rugby Football Board to organize a Sports Medicine Congress at the time of the semi-final of the Rugby World Cup, played at Murrayfield, Edinburgh. The Congress was held in conjunction with a meeting of the Medical Advisory Committee of the International Rugby Football Board.

The Congress consisted of two parallel Conferences. A scientific meeting entitled 'The Biology of Intermittent, High Intensity Exercise' was held at the Royal College of Surgeons of Edinburgh and covered aspects of preparation for performance including nutrition, response to stress and damage limitation. The theme of damage limitation was continued at the meeting held at the Royal College of Physicians of Edinburgh, which dealt with the epidemiology of injury, clinical aspects of injuries in contact sports, preparation and prevention of injuries, looking at the surface on which a sport is played and the boot, and biorhythms and assessment of fitness.

The Scottish Rugby Union was honoured to welcome their patron, Her Royal Highness the Princess Royal, to the Congress and are most grateful to Her Royal Highness for allowing her remarks at the Congress to be included in the Proceedings and for writing the Foreword. Her Royal Highness is a great supporter of Scottish Rugby, in addition to her many wide-ranging interests in sport and her commitments to the International Olympic Commission.

The International Rugby Football Board and the Scottish Rugby Union are most grateful for the support they received from the Royal College of Surgeons of Edinburgh, The Royal College of Physicians of Edinburgh and the Lothian Regional Council. The Executive Committee organizing the Congress received tremendous help from the staff of the Scottish Rugby Union. In particular we would like to record our appreciation to Mr Adam Robson, Scottish Regional Director of the Rugby World Cup, Mrs Rona Stevenson, Miss Ann Turner, Mrs Margit Tilley, Mr Hugh Penman, Mr Ian Hunter and the staff of the Rugby World Cup Ticket Office. The Scottish Rugby Union is especially grateful for the tremendous amount of work undertaken by the editors involved with the publication of the Proceedings of the Congress. Dr Ron Maughan has made a major contribution with standardization of the text. Finally, we would acknowledge the support received from Mr Phillip Read and E & FN Spon Ltd.

Mr D.A.D. Macleod
Chairman
Sports Medicine Congress Committee

PART ONE

Preparation for performance

Introduction   Muscle

Rugby football is one of the most demanding of all the multiple-sprint sports. It involves periods of support running interspersed with brief periods of sprinting and frequent strength-sapping body contacts. Therefore, players have to have the combined fitness of sprinters and endurance runners as well as the strength and agility to cope successfully with repeated tackles and scrummaging. Although match analyses provide some insight into the physical demands of the sport in terms of the distance covered during a game, there is relatively little information on the physiological responses of players to participation. From an analysis of the support running, sprinting, tackling and scrummaging during a game, coaches attempt to design appropriate training pro- grammes for players. Unfortunately, these training programmes are all too often based on little knowledge of the biological response of individuals to different types of exercise and training. Therefore, the aim of this session is to provide reviews of the biological responses and adaptations to different types of exercise as well as to consider the dynamic nature of recovery from exercise. An additional aim is to offer examples of the effective translation of the principles of training into successful practice.

In the first review Professor Henriksson describes the adaptations of skeletal muscle to endurance training and the metabolic mechanisms by which these changes delay the onset of fatigue. Strength is an essential component of fitness for rugby, and in his review of the topic Dr Ira Jacobs explains clearly how skeletal muscle adapts to strength training. He also raises the question of whether or not players can train for both endurance and for strength without compromising either of these two different forms of fitness. Sprint training improves speed and recovery and common experience has shown that the ability to recover quickly improves to a greater extent than absolute speed. The adaptations of skeletal muscle to sprint training is covered by Steve Brooks who draws on the results of several of his studies on this topic to offer explanations for these improvements in performance. How muscle recovers from exhaustive exercise is central to any discussion on adaptations to intermittent exercise of brief duration and maximal intensity. Dr Jens Bangsbo describes the results of the studies which he and his colleagues have completed on the metabolic events taking place during recovery and the influence of prior exercise on subsequent bouts of exercise to exhaustion. These studies provide an insight into the limitations of the recovery process and challenge existing dogma about the link between acidosis and fatigue in skeletal muscle. Rex Hazeldine and David McLean have first-hand experience of translating laboratory generated information about training into practice. They provide sports science support for their respective national rugby teams. Rex Hazeldine offers examples of how training programmes for a national rugby team are designed and implemented according to sound scientific principles. David McLean describes how the essential features of fitness for rugby can be assessed by field tests and as such provides the coach with an accessible method of monitoring the progress of players during their preparation for competition.

We hope that this mixture of reviews of research studies and research-informed practices will give you a better understanding of the biological responses to multiple-sprint sports in general, and to rugby football in particular.

C. Williams

Skeletal muscle adaptations to endurance training

J. Henriksson and R.C. Hickner

Abstract. Skeletal muscle undergoes major adaptations in response to endurance training. It seems quite likely that an increase in mitochondrial density is the most important factor in preserving metabolic homeostasis in the muscle cell during exercise. The resultant increased $ATP/ADP + P_i$ ratio during exercise in trained muscle would inhibit phosphofructokinase and result in less stimulation of glycogen phosphorylase, thereby slowing glycolysis and the accompanying glycogen depletion and lactate production. In addition, the increased fat oxidation in trained skeletal muscle plays a major role in the sparing of muscle glycogen. The above mentioned adaptations are accompanied by the increased capillarization in trained skeletal muscle and, after several years of endurance training, by fibre type transformations from fasttwitch to slow-twitch. The increased insulin action in skeletal muscle of individuals regularly involved in endurance training demonstrates the importance of consistent exercise if insulin action is to be improved in pathological states such as obesity or if exercise is to protect against the development of insulin resistance with ageing. Many of the above mentioned adaptations are well described, while others have yet to be fully elucidated. In this paper, we give a brief overview of several of these adaptations to endurance training in skeletal muscle.

Keywords: Endurance training, fibre-type, capillarization, insulin sensitivity, insulin responsiveness, mitochondria, oxidative capacity.

Introduction

Endurance training induces marked adaptive changes in several structural components and metabolic variables in the engaged skeletal muscles. These adaptive changes allow for the muscle to maintain contraction force in times of increased demand. Among the observed changes with different training regimens are those involving the muscle's content of metabolic enzymes, the sensitivity to hormones and the composition of the contracting filaments. Other adaptations affect membrane transport processes and the muscular capillary network. The adaptive changes in metabolic enzymes and capillaries are particularly well described consequences of endurance training and both these factors are likely to be important determinants for an individual's physical working capacity. The enhanced muscle glucose transport and insulin sensitivity represents another major effect of exercise and training on muscle metabolism. It is the adaptive changes in the above mentioned variables that we will focus on in the following pages.

Estimation of skeletal muscle metabolic capacity

The muscle biopsy procedure, whereby small (10-100 mg) muscle pieces can be sampled, may be combined with sensitive biochemical techniques to permit estimation of the capacity of different metabolic pathways in human muscle. Today, biochemical measurements can be done even at the single fibre level. Enzymes which are commonly measured as indicators of the capacity of their respective metabolic pathways are listed here. **Glycolysis:** phosphofructokinase (PFK), lactate dehydrogenase (LDH). **Fatty acid oxidation:** 3 -hydroxyacylCoA dehydrogenase (HAD). **Citric acid cycle:** citrate synthase (CS), succinate dehydrogenase (SDH). **Respiratory chain:** cytochrome c oxidase.

Skeletal muscle adaptation to endurance training

Enzymatic changes

An illustration of the effects of endurance training on human muscle enzymatic capacity is the observed differences between endurance athletes and untrained individuals (Fig. 1). With regard to oxidative enzymes (i.e. enzymes of fatty acid oxidation, the citric acid cycle and the respiratory chain), the values are approximately 3-fold higher in the trained thigh muscle of the athletes than in the thigh muscle of untrained individuals. With total inactivity, the oxidative enzyme contents decrease to 70-75% of the "untrained level". The maximal range of oxidative enzyme content in the human thigh muscle is therefore approximately 4-fold, but it may be supposed that a very long training time would be required for an individual to cover this whole range. A comparison with chronically stimulated rabbit muscle (used here as an example of the maximal attainable response in oxidative capacity) reveals that muscles of endurance athletes have approximately 40% lower levels of oxidative enzymes than these chronically stimulated muscles (Fig. 1). The difference with respect to fat oxidation enzymes is somewhat higher. Ignoring possible differences between the rabbit and man, these results indicate that the trained muscles of our best endurance athletes have an oxidative capacity that is half to two thirds of the theoretically attainable maximal level.

Information is available from a large number of more applied investigations in which different research groups have studied the effects of 2-3 months of training on the oxidative enzyme content of leg or arm muscles. These studies have usually involved bouts of 30-60 minutes of exercise at intensities corresponding to 70-80% of VO_2max, 3-5 times per week. With a group of previously untrained individuals, the general finding is an approximately 40-50% increase in the content of oxidative enzymes in the trained muscle (Fig. 2). This increase occurs gradually over 6-8 weeks, with the most rapid change taking place during the first three weeks of training (see Saltin & Gollnick, 1983).

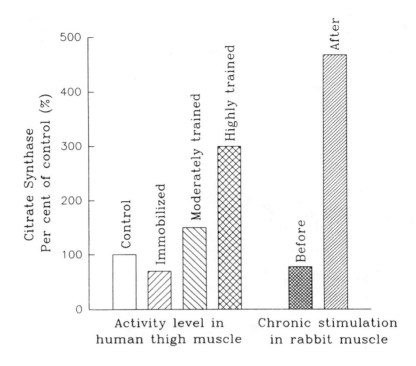

Fig. 1 The influence of the physical fitness level on skeletal muscle oxidative capacity, measured as the content of citrate synthase. Muscle tissue from normal sedentary individual (controls) has been compared to muscle subjected to encasement in plaster after injury (immobilized) or to 2-3 months of moderate endurance training as well as to values recorded in top class cyclists and long-distance runners (highly trained). As a further comparison, the corresponding values from the rabbit anterior tibial muscle before and after 3-5 weeks of chronic electrical stimulation are indicated to the right. (The human data have generously been placed at our disposal by Dr. Eva Jansson, Dept. of Clinical Physiology, Karolinska Hospital, Stockholm; the results regarding chronic stimulation are from Henriksson et al, 1986).

Should one train longer or more intensely?

A question of practical importance is the intensity and duration of training needed to obtain optimal results with respect to enzyme adaptation. For an untrained person, some increase in the muscle content of oxidative enzymes can

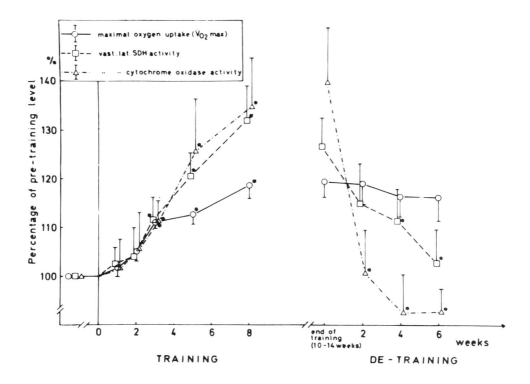

Fig. 2 The effect of endurance training on the content of oxidative enzymes in human skeletal muscle. A group of previously untrained subjects trained for 10-14 weeks on bicycle ergometers (40 min/day, 4 days/week; the rate of work corresponded to 80% of the maximal oxygen uptake) and was subsequently studied for 6 weeks after cessation of training. Thigh muscle biopsy samples were analyzed for the oxidative enzymes SDH (succinate dehydrogenase of the citric acid cycle) and cytochrome c oxidase (the last enzyme of the respiratory chain). In addition, the subjects' maximal oxygen uptake was determined during bicycling using the Douglas bag technique. It is noteworthy that, in the post-training period, the whole-body VO₂max is maintained significantly longer than the muscle oxidative enzyme content. (Modified from Henriksson & Reitman, 1977).

be obtained by fairly light running (jogging), but the enzyme adaptation becomes much more marked if the training intensity is increased to work rates demanding 70-80% of the individual's VO₂max. Dudley and colleagues (Dudley et al, 1982) subjected rats to training in the form of treadmill running 5 days per week for two months at varying speeds and daily training durations. The rats trained at six different running speeds, demanding approximately 60%, 70%, 80%, 95%, 105% and 115% of their maximal oxygen uptake. At the two highest speeds, the exercise was performed intermittently. For each speed, the muscle enzyme adaptation increased with the duration of the daily exercise, but no additional training effect was noted when the daily duration exceeded 45-60 minutes. At the two highest speeds, the rats could only tolerate exercise for 30 and 15 minutes daily, but this was sufficient for marked training effects to occur. The initial period of the daily exercise bout gave the highest training effect per unit of training time, with successively smaller effects for the following periods. In a previous study by Fitts et al (1975), rats trained 10, 30, 60, or 120 min/day on a motor-driven treadmill and displayed progressively larger increases in the gastrocnemius muscle oxidative capacity with increasing exercise duration. Beyond 120 minutes there were no further increases.

Fibre-type recruitment patterns in the rat

In the study by Dudley et al (1982), the training response differed markedly between the fibre types, likely due to differences in fibre-type related recruitment patterns. For a training effect to occur in the fast-glycolytic fibres (type 2b), the exercise intensity had to require at least 80% of the rat's VO_2max. Higher running speeds gave successively better training effects in this fibre type. On the contrary, for the fast-oxidative-glycolytic fibre type (2a), the training effect increased with increasing speeds up to an intensity (speed) demanding 80% of VO_2max. Higher running speeds did not result in an enhanced training effect. The slow-twitch fibre type (type 1) responded in yet another fashion. In this fibre type, the training effect increased up to a running speed demanding 80% of the VO_2max. Paradoxically, higher speeds than this resulted in a decreased training effect.

Fibre-type recruitment patterns in man

The referred data on the rat clearly illustrate that knowledge of the fibre type recruitment pattern during exercise is essential when trying to predict the effects of different training regimens. For humans, quite detailed information is available on cycle ergometer exercise at different rates of work. It has been shown that, as in the rat, the slow-twitch (type 1) muscle fibres are the first to be activated and are kept activated even at higher exercise intensities. With increasing rates of work there is a recruitment of the fast-twitch motor units, type 2a followed by type 2b. It is believed that fibres (motor units) of all types are recruited at exercise intensities demanding more than 80-85% of the VO_2max. However, very strenuous exercise is probably required to activate maximally all the type 2b motor units in a given muscle (for references, see Saltin & Gollnick, 1983).

It may be concluded that, for a large training effect per unit of training time, it is advisable to use high training intensities. With very heavy exercise, the duration of the exercise bouts may be insufficient, however, for an optimal training effect. The rat study by Dudley and colleagues, referred to above, gives some hints about the optimal balance between the intensity and duration of training but there is still insufficient human data available.

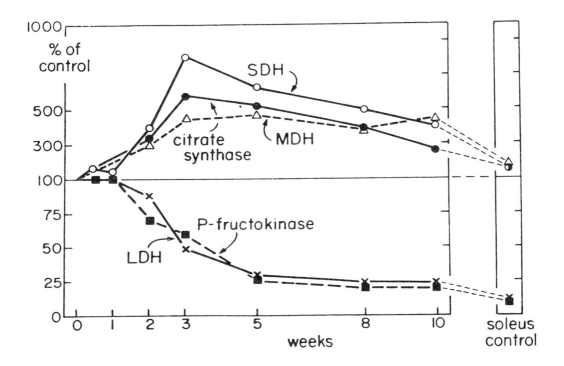

Fig. 3 Enzyme changes induced by chronic electrical muscle stimulation. The rabbit anterior tibial muscle was stimulated at 10 impulses per second, 24 hours a day, for 3 days to 10 weeks. The figure depicts changes in 3 oxidative and 2 glycolytic enzymes. SDH (succinate dehydrogenase), citrate synthase and MDH (malate dehydrogenase) are enzymes in the citric acid cycle, LDH (lactate dehydrogenase) and P-fructokinase (6-phosphofructokinase) are involved in glycolysis. The value for unstimulated control muscles has been set at 100%. To the right, enzyme levels are given for the slow-twitch soleus muscle in unstimulated control rabbits; thus illustrating that, as a result of the chronic stimulation, the originally fast-twitch anterior tibial muscle acquires a clearly higher oxidative enzyme content than a normal slow-twitch muscle. (From Henriksson et al, 1986).

Endurance training: glycolytic enzymes, capillarization and fibre types

The muscle cell's content of glycolytic enzymes is not, or only marginally, affected by endurance training programs of 2-6 months in duration. The content of glycolytic enzymes is normally low in the skeletal muscles of endurance athletes, but this finding is entirely explained by the large percentage of slow-twitch fibres (which have only half of the glycolytic enzyme content of fast-twitch fibres) in their muscles. The mean glycolytic enzyme level of athletes' slow-twitch or fast-twitch muscle fibres has thus been found to be normal, or even slightly enhanced (Chi et al, 1983; Essen-Gustavsson and Henriksson, 1984). This finding is in accord with what has been observed during chronic stimulation (see above), when there is a complete fibre type transformation from fast-twitch glycolytic (type 2b) to slow-twitch (type 1) fibres. In this situation the glycolytic enzyme content of the muscle is decreased to 20% of the initial level (Fig. 3,4), a decrease which reflects the large difference in glycolytic potential between fast-twitch glycolytic and slow-twitch fibres in the rabbit (Chi et al, 1986). It therefore seems as if the type of muscle fibre, based on its composition of myofibrillar proteins, is a strong determinant of its content of glycolytic enzymes, while a change in training status is the main determinant of the muscles oxidative enzyme content.

Skeletal muscle capillarization in man is rapidly enhanced with endurance training, with two months of training at high submaximal exercise intensities being sufficient to increase the total number, and number per mm^2, of muscle capillaries by 50% and 20%, respectively (Fig. 5; Andersen and Henriksson, 1977a, see also Brodal et al, 1977). The difference between endurance athletes and untrained individuals with respect to the capillary count per muscle fibre (leg muscles) has been found to be 2-3-fold (Saltin and Gollnick, 1983). There is a lack of information about to what extent capillary neoformation is dependent upon training intensity and duration. It is known, however, that less intense training regimens often result in oxidative enzyme increases without any change in capillarization.

When stains for myofibrillar ATPase have been used as the basis for fibre type classification, most longitudinal studies in man have failed to demonstrate an interconversion of fibre types (i.e. fast-twitch to slow-twitch) in response to endurance training. The stable nature of a muscle's fibre type composition is further illustrated by the results of chronic stimulation studies in rabbits, where quite long periods of chronic stimulation are required for the complete replacement of fast-twitch by slow-twitch fibres. The fibre type changes are also the first to revert to normal when stimulation is discontinued (Brown et al, 1989). On the basis of these findings, the high percentage of slow-twitch (type 1) fibres in endurance athletes and the opposite finding in sprinters have therefore been ascribed to genetic factors (Komi et al, 1976). Endurance training is known, however, to lead to a complete type transformation within the fast-twitch (type 2) fibres from type 2b to type 2a (Andersen and Henriksson, 1977b; Jansson and Kaijser, 1977).

The concept that endurance training does not change the relative occurrence of fast- and slow-twitch fibres has been challenged in recent years. It has been

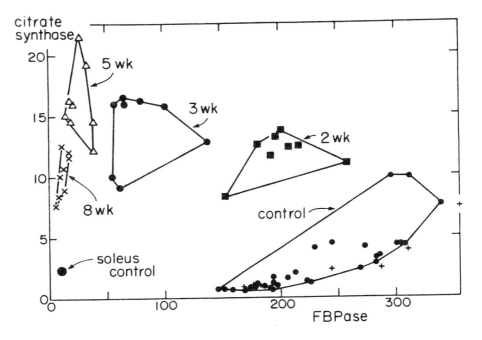

Fig. 4 Enzyme changes in single skeletal muscle fibres induced by chronic electrical muscle stimulation. The anterior tibial muscle of the rabbit was stimulated as described in the text to figure 3. Single fibres were isolated by microdissection from muscles stimulated for different periods of time (2,3,5 and 8 weeks respectively) as well as from unstimulated control muscles. Citrate synthase is a member of the citric acid cycle, and was therefore used as a measure of the fibre's oxidative capacity, while fructose bisphosphatase catalyses the reversal of the phosphofructokinase reaction in glycolysis, and was used as a measure of glycolytic capacity. The average value for fibres in the control slow-twitch soleus muscle is included for reference (for explanation see the text to figure 3). All fibres in a normal unstimulated (control) muscle have a high content of glycolytic enzymes, whereas the content of oxidative enzymes varies 10-fold. The chronic stimulation induces a high oxidative capacity in all fibres, whereas the glycolytic capacity decreases to low levels. Figures are moles (CS) or millimoles (FBPase) per kg dry weight per hour at 20°C. Each symbol (except soleus control) denotes one individual fibre. (From Chi et al, 1986).

shown, for example, that 1) endurance training of long duration leads to the appearance of fibres intermediate between fast- and slow-twitch, 2) the muscles of the dominant leg in different types of athletes, such as badminton players, contain a significantly increased percentage of slow-twitch fibres, and 3) in several studies of detraining the percentage of fast-twitch muscle fibres increases. In

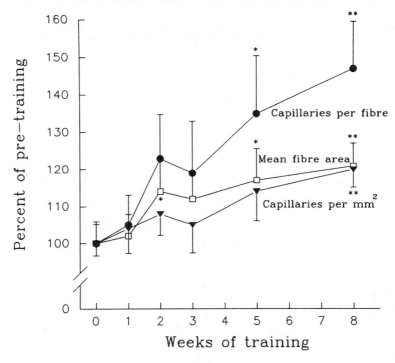

Fig. 5 The effect of 2 months of endurance training (identical with that described in figure 2) on capillary formation in the human thigh muscle. Muscle biopsies were histochemically stained for capillaries, which appear as dark spots in a muscle cross-section (amylase-PAS method). The number of capillaries per fibre was calculated in each muscle cross-section as the number of cross-sected capillaries divided by the number of cross-sected muscle fibres. * ($p < 0.05$) and ** ($p < 0.01$) denote significant differences from pre-training values. (Modified from Andersen & Henriksson, 1977a).

accord with these results, Bauman et al (1987) demonstrated the appearance with training of fast-twitch fibres containing a mixed pattern of fast and slow myofibrillar protein isoforms. It is therefore reasonable to conclude that extensive endurance training will result in an enhanced percentage of slow-twitch fibres. The extent to which this might occur still remains to be demonstrated (for a detailed discussion, see Schantz, 1986).

An increase in the oxidative capacity of a muscle, induced by two months of endurance training, is lost in 4-6 weeks if the training is stopped (Fig. 2). This loss of muscle oxidative enzymes occurs faster than the decrease in muscle capillarization (Schantz et al, 1983) and in the whole-body peak oxygen uptake attained during bicycling (Fig. 2). Interestingly, the oxidative capacity of the fast-

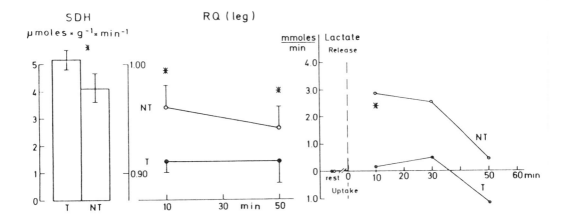

Fig. 6 The metabolic significance of the training-induced adaptation of human skeletal muscle. A group of subjects underwent one-leg endurance training on the bicycle ergometer during 6 weeks. With one well-trained leg (T) (the level of succinate dehydrogenase (SDH) being 25% higher than in the nontrained leg (NT), left figure), the subjects performed two-leg bicycle ergometer exercise at 70% of the VO_2max, in which both legs performed identically. Arterial and venous catheterization made possible measurements of the oxygen uptake (VO_2) and the carbon dioxide production (VCO_2) of both legs separately. The VCO_2/VO_2 ratio, known as the respiratory quotient (RQ), indicates the relative contributions of carbohydrate and fat to the

oxidative metabolism; an RQ of 1.0 indicating oxidation of carbohydrate only and an RQ of 0.7 indicating oxidation of fat only. The middle figure thus indicates a higher level of fat oxidation in the trained leg than for the untrained one. Accompanying the greater use of carbohydrates in the untrained leg, there is a larger formation and release of lactate (see figure to the right). In the trained leg, the lactate release is low, with a tendency towards an uptake of lactate from the blood at the end of exercise. (n=6, mean ±SEM) (Modified from Henriksson, 1977).

twitch fibres in well trained subjects remains elevated throughout a 12-week period of detraining, suggesting that changes had occurred with training in the normal impulse pattern of fast motorneurons in the spinal cord (Chi et al, 1983).

Mediators of enzymatic adaptation to training

The cellular content of a certain enzyme is the result of a balance between synthesis and degradation, of which a change in the synthesis rate of enzyme proteins is the most important factor in explaining enzymatic changes resulting from chronic stimulation or training (Booth and Holloszy, 1977; Pette, 1984; Williams et al, 1986). An interesting area of research now is to explore the biochemical mechanisms underlying the altered rate of enzyme synthesis. That is, how is the information transferred to the genes that there is a need for an increased amount of oxidative enzymes in the muscle cell? Suggested mediators include: decreases in the concentration of adenosine triphosphate (ATP) or other high-energy phosphate compounds; a decreased oxygen tension; an increased sympatho-adrenal stimulation of the muscle cell; substances released from the motor nerve; and calcium-induced diacylglycerol release with subsequent activation of protein kinase C.

Metabolic significance of the training-induced adaptation of skeletal muscle

Endurance training and glycogen depletion rates

Many authors have confirmed a close association between muscle glycogen depletion and fatigue (for references, see Karlsson and Saltin, 1971; Sherman and Costill, 1984). Preservation of glycogen stores during exercise is therefore of great importance. As illustrated in Fig. 6, during two-leg exercise following one-leg training there was a significantly smaller release of lactate from the trained leg than from the untrained one, and a significantly larger percentage of the energy output in the trained leg stemmed from fat combustion. In the following, a review will be given of the large number of studies showing that at the same absolute exercise intensity (and possibly even at the same relative intensity (% of VO$_2$max),

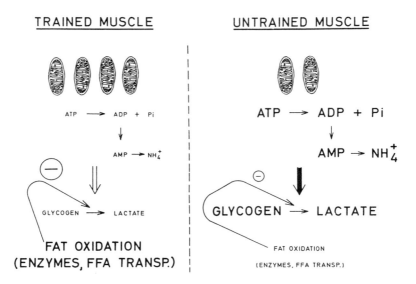

Fig. 7 A hypothetical biochemical mechanism for the increased reliance on fat metabolism, the lower rate of lactate formation and sparing of muscle glycogen during exercise in trained muscle. The increased content of oxidative enzymes (i.e. citric acid cycle and fat oxidation enzymes and respiratory chain components) in trained skeletal muscle is explained to a large extent by a larger mitochondrial volume (volume fraction), indicated above schematically with mitochondrial symbols. Suppose that, in the untrained muscle, there are only half as many enzyme molecules of the citric acid cycle and half as many components of the respiratory chain as in the trained muscle (which is a reasonable assumption, see Fig. 4). It follows that, at a given rate of oxygen uptake, each mitochondrial unit has to be activated twice as much in the untrained muscle as in the trained one. An important component of this activation is the increased levels of the degradation products of ATP (e.g. ADP), which are the result of muscle contractions. These levels must thus be stabilized at a higher level in the untrained muscle than in the trained muscle. However, these ATP degradation products are also powerful stimulators of the glycolytic pathway, which would result in a greater lactate release and carbohydrate oxidation. The higher fat oxidation rate in trained than in untrained muscle is mainly due to the higher content of enzymes of fatty acid transport and oxidation. In addition, this leads to a more pronounced inhibition of glycolysis in the trained muscle. In concert, these factors lead to sparing of glycogen during exercise in trained skeletal muscle (After Holloszy and Booth, 1976).

trained individuals rely more on fat as an energy substrate than untrained ones, thereby reducing reliance on carbohydrate stores. This is the case despite the fact that, at a given rate of work, the plasma level of free fatty acids is either similar or lower in endurance-trained subjects.

Increased oxidative capacity

Glycogen depletion has consistently been found to be reduced during prolonged exercise in trained individuals as compared to untrained individuals working at the same absolute oxygen consumption (Fitts et al, 1975), although findings at the same relative exercise intensity are not as conclusive (Jansson and Kaijser, 1987; Hermansen et al, 1967; Saltin and Karlsson, 1971a). The cause of the decreased muscle glycogen utilization upon initiation of exercise is not clear, but it has been found by Constable et al (1987) to be accompanied by smaller increases in inorganic phosphate (Pi), AMP and estimated free ADP concentrations in trained muscles than in untrained muscles during electrically induced contractions. The trained muscles furthermore display smaller decreases in ATP and phosphocreatine concentrations. The observed changes have been suggested to be consequences of the adaptive increase in muscle mitochondria, leading to an increased oxidative capacity in muscle (see below and Fig. 7 for hypothetical mechanisms). These authors furthermore suggested that reduced levels of Pi in trained muscle might play a role in the decreased initial burst of glycolysis. This hypothesis was supported by Jansson and Kaijser (1987) and Green et al (1990), who found that training exerts its greatest effect in reducing glycogen degradation early in exercise. Green et al (1990) were also able to show that this effect occurs in both fast- and slow-twitch fibres.

Utilization of blood-derived glucose

In addition to a decreased utilization of muscle glycogen, the carbohydrate-sparing effect of training also involves a decreased utilization of blood-derived glucose. In the study by Coggan et al (1990), this accounted for approximately one half of the total decrease in carbohydrate oxidation following training during the final 30 min of a 2-hour cycle ergometer exercise session at 60% of the pre-training VO_2max. These results were supported by Jansson and Kaijser, (1987), who suggested that an increased blood glucose extraction by the legs of untrained subjects was secondary to their low muscle glycogen concentration during the later stages of the exercise session. This is in accord with Essen et al (1977) and Gollnick et al (1981), who found an inverse relationship between blood glucose extraction and muscle glycogen concentration.

Lactate formation

It is well documented that endurance trained individuals have lower blood lactate levels than untrained individuals during exercise at both the same absolute exercise intensity (Bang, 1936; Ekblom et al, 1968; Hurley et al, 1986) and the same relative exercise intensity (% of VO_2max) (Jansson and Kaijser, 1987; Hermansen et al, 1967; Saltin and Karlsson, 1971b). This is likely to be attributable to a decreased rate of lactate formation in trained muscles (Jansson and Kaijser, 1987), although it cannot be ruled out that there is an increased lactate clearance in endurance-trained individuals. The enzyme isoforms of lactate dehydrogenase (LDH) are also known to shift to favour the LDH1 2 (heart) isoforms over the LDH4 5 (muscle) isoforms following endurance training (Karlsson et al, 1975), increasing lactate conversion to pyruvate. In addition, the increased capacity of the malate-aspartate shuttle system for the transport of NADH electrons from the cytosol into the mitochondria likely contributes to the lowered lactate production in response to training (Schantz et al, 1986).

Free fatty acid utilization

It is evident that trained individuals rely more on fat as an energy substrate than untrained ones. The source of this increased fat supply has been debated, however, since the plasma levels of free fatty acids are often lower in endurance-trained subjects (see Holloszy, 1988). The suggestion that muscle triglycerides may supply the substrate for this increased fat oxidation is supported by findings of an increased muscle triglyceride utilization in the trained state when individuals exercise at both the same absolute (Hurley et al, 1986), and relative (Jansson and Kaijser, 1987), intensity. However, resting intramuscular triglyceride stores have not been conclusively found to be higher in trained than in untrained muscle (Morgan et al, 1969; Howald et al, 1985; Hurley et al, 1986).

Mechanisms of increased fat oxidation

There are many mechanisms which may lead to a greater fatty acid utilization in the trained state. The increased mitochondrial density and the increased content of mitochondrial enzymes in aerobically trained muscle are accompanied by increases in the enzymes involved in activation, transfer into the mitochondria and B-oxidation of fatty acids (Holloszy and Booth, 1976; Saltin and Gollnick, 1983; Mole et al, 1971). Paulussen and Veerkamp (1990) have presented evidence that this adaptation may include increases in the low molecular weight cytosolic fatty acid binding proteins, which may play an important role in the intracellular transport and targeting of fatty acids. At a given exercise intensity, these adaptations in skeletal muscle would permit the rate of fatty acid oxidation to be higher in the trained than in the untrained muscle, even in the presence of a lower intracellular fatty acid concentration in the trained state. Included in this response may also be a change in the activity of regulatory molecules, as a 36% decrease in Malonyl-CoA (an inhibitor of carnitine acyltransferase I activity) has been noted during 30 minutes of treadmill exercise in rats (Winder et al, 1989). This would lead to an increased oxidation of fatty acids. Whether Malonyl-CoA is reduced in trained individuals is, however, not known at present. Beta-receptor mechanisms, which have been found to regulate skeletal muscle triglyceride hydrolysis

(Stankiewicz-Choroszucha and Gorski, 1978), as well as possible training-induced increases in hormone-sensitive lipase, the enzyme which hydrolyses intracellular triglycerides into fatty acids (Oscai et al, 1990), may also play a role here.

Another potential source of free fatty acids for skeletal muscle is the hydrolysis of intravascular triglycerides, catalysed by the enzyme lipoprotein lipase (LPL), which is located on the intraluminal surface of the capillaries. There is still conflicting evidence, however, as to whether (Svedenhag et al, 1983; Nikkila et al, 1978) or not (Stubbe et al, 1983) this enzyme is increased by endurance training. LPL is known to be activated following a single bout of exercise (Lithell et al, 1981) and it is possible that the resulting variability may mask possible effects of training.

Yki-Jarvinen et al (1991) recently presented evidence of a feedback mechanism which serves to maintain a certain rate of cellular fatty acid oxidation under conditions of changing inflow of plasma free fatty acids. This mechanism is supposed to involve stimulation of LPL at times of lowered intracellular free fatty acid concentration, resulting from either insufficient hormone-sensitive lipase activity or lowered plasma free fatty acid concentrations. Whether such mechanisms explain the increased fat reliance in endurance-trained muscle remains to be demonstrated.

Muscle glucose uptake and insulin action

Although it is a well-established fact that an acute exercise bout leads to an increase in muscle glucose uptake (Nesher et al, 1985; Wallberg-Henriksson et al, 1988; Cartee et al, 1989) the question of whether training produces an additional effect has been debated.

Contraction-stimulated glucose transport

There is very little information available regarding possible training effects here, but a recent investigation by Coggan et al (1990) suggested that endurance training may in fact reduce glucose transport during submaximal exercise in man. However, in a recent study using the perfused hindquarter, Ploug et al (1990) found an increased contraction-stimulated glucose-transport rate with training, but only in slow-twitch fibres. This effect, which could not be ascribed to an influence of the last training session, was paralleled by signs of an increased abundance of glucose transporter proteins. As it is impossible to eliminate all insulin from the environment in the in vivo situation, it will be difficult to come to any definitive conclusion in this area.

Insulin-mediated glucose disposal and glucose tolerance

The fact that training can increase insulin-mediated glucose disposal at submaximal insulin concentrations has been demonstrated in a number of studies

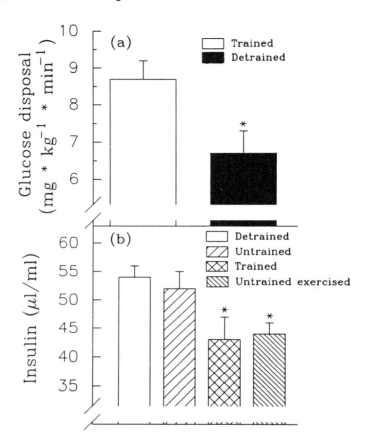

Fig. 8 Effects of exercise and inactivity on insulin sensitivity.
(a) Nine well-trained individuals were studied with the hyperinsulinaemic, euglycaemic clamp procedure in the trained exercising state (16 h after the last exercise bout) and again after 10 days of physical inactivity. Insulin sensitivity is estimated from the whole-body glucose disposal rate at a submaximal plasma insulin concentration (78ul/ml)(mean±SEM). (From King et al, 1988).
(b) Insulin sensitivity (the insulin concentration eliciting 50% of maximal insulin-mediated glucose disposal) was measured in 7 trained individuals in the habitual state 15 h after the last training bout; and 5 days after the last training session (detrained). In addition, seven untrained subjects were studied at rest and after 60 min of bicycle exercise at 150 watts (mean±SEM). (Hyperinsulinaemic euglycaemic clamp experiments from Mikines et al, 1989a; Mikines et al, 1989b).

(Ploug et al, 1990; Mikines et al, 1989a; King et al, 1987). However, most of this effect is likely to be mediated by short-term effects of the last exercise bouts. Many investigators have demonstrated a reduction of glucose disposal at submaximal insulin concentrations, to levels found in untrained subjects, following 3-10 days of inactivity in previously trained subjects (see Fig. 8) (Mikines et al, 1989b; King et al, 1988; Rogers et al, 1990). Thus, the enhanced glucose uptake at submaximal insulin concentrations in trained individuals is likely not a true training-induced adaptation, but merely an effect of the last exercise bout.

Results with respect to insulin responsiveness

Findings regarding insulin responsiveness, or the response to a maximally stimulating dose of insulin, are much less conclusive. Several studies have shown that endurance training results in an increased insulin responsiveness in skeletal muscle (Mikines et al, 1989a; Rodnick et al, 1990; James et al, 1985), consistent with findings of increased muscle content of glucose transporters. However, King et al (1987, 1988) found no difference in insulin responsiveness between trained and untrained subjects, as well as no decrease in responsiveness following 10 days of detraining in previously trained subjects. The question of whether endurance training actually results in a long-term adaptation with respect to insulin responsiveness must therefore still be left open.

Whether increases in insulin sensitivity and responsiveness represent a long--term adaptation or are just the result of consistently performing a single bout of exercise cannot yet be determined. This question may be purely academic, however, and the results demonstrate the importance of regularly performed exercise to protect against the development of insulin resistance, e.g. with ageing, or to improve insulin action in such pathological states as obesity and type II diabetes. This increased insulin action with training also likely enhances glycogen replenishment rates following exercise sessions; although it may be noted here that not all types of exercise are associated with increased insulin action, as one bout of eccentric exercise has been found to be associated with insulin resistance (Ploug et al, 1990; Kirwan et al, 1991).

Summary

It seems quite likely that an increase in mitochondrial density preserves metabolic homeostasis in the muscle cell. The resultant increased ATP/ADP + Pi ratio during exercise in trained muscle would inhibit phosphofructokinase and result in less stimulation of glycogen phosphorylase, thereby slowing glycolysis and the accompanying glycogen depletion and lactate production. In addition, the increased fat oxidation in trained skeletal muscle plays a major role in the sparing of muscle glycogen (Holloszy and Coyle, 1984). The above mentioned adaptations are accompanied by the increased capillarization in trained skeletal muscle, which provides a longer mean transit time for the oxygen and substrate exchange between blood and tissue. After several years of endurance training, fibre type transformations from fast-twitch to slow-twitch (Schantz, 1986), which would serve to increase the overall muscle oxidative capacity and possibly also reduce energy expenditure, would be expected to further positively influence the endurance capacity of the muscle. The increased insulin action in skeletal muscle of individuals regularly involved in endurance training demonstrates the importance of consistent exercise if insulin action is to be improved in pathological states such as obesity or if exercise is to protect against the development of insulin resistance with ageing. However, the described training-induced adaptations in skeletal muscle must be considered in the light of adaptations in all other organs and organ systems of the body in order to obtain an accurate picture of how endurance training may influence the metabolic homeostasis of the organism as a whole.

Acknowledgements

Jan Henriksson's own cited work was supported by grants from the Swedish Medical Research Council, the Karolinska Institute, the Research Council of the Swedish Sports Federation and the National Institutes of Health (U.S.A.). The authors wish to express their appreciation to Meg Hickner for her help in the preparation of this manuscript.

References

Andersen P and Henriksson J. (1977) Capillary supply of the quadriceps femoris muscle of man: adaptive response to exercise. J Physiol, **270**, 677-690.

Andersen P and Henriksson J. (1977) Training induced changes in the subgroups of human type II skeletal muscle fibres. Acta Physiol Scand, **99**, 123-125.

Bang O. (1936) The lactate content of the blood during and after muscular exercise in man. Scand Arch Physiol, **74** (suppl 10), 51-82.

Baumann H, Jaggi M, Soland F, Howald H and Schaub MC. (1987) Exercise training induces transitions of myosin isoform subunits within histochemically typed human muscle fibres. Pflugers Arch, **409**, 349-360.

Booth FW, and Holloszy JO. (1977) Cytochrome c turnover in rat skeletal muscles. J Biol Chem, **252**, 416-419.

Brodal P, Ingjer F and Hermansen L. (1977) Capillary supply of skeletal muscle fibres in untrained and endurance-trained men. Am J Physiol, **232**, H705-H712.

Brown JMC, Henriksson J and Salmons S. (1989) Restoration of fast muscle characteristics following cessation of chronic stimulation: physiological, histochemical and metabolic changes during slow-to-fast transformation. Proc Roy Soc (London) Ser B, **235**, 321-346.

Cartee GD, Young DA, Sleeper MD, Zierath J, Wallberg-Henriksson H and Holloszy JO. (1989) Prolonged increase in insulin-stimulated glucose transport in muscle after exercise. Am J Physiol, **256**, E494-E499.

Chi MM-Y, Hintz CS, Coyle EF, Martin III WH, Ivy JL, Nemeth PM, Holloszy JO and Lowry OH. (1983) Effects of detraining on enzymes of energy metabolism in individual human muscle fibres. Am J Physiol, **244**, C276-C287.

Chi MM-Y, Hintz CS, Henriksson J, Salmons S, Hellendahl RP, Park JL, Nemeth PM and Lowry OH. (1986) Chronic stimulation of mammalian muscle: enzyme changes in individual fibres. Am J Physiol, **251**, C633-C642.

Coggan AR, Kohrt WM, Spina RJ, Bier DM and Holloszy JO. (1990) Endurance training decreases plasma glucose turnover and oxidation during moderate-intensity exercise in men. J Appl Physiol, **68**, 990-996.

Constable SH, Favier RJ, McLane JA, Fell RD, Chen M and Holloszy JO. (1987) Energy metabolism in contracting rat skeletal muscle: adaptation to exercise training. Am J Physiol, **253**, C316-C322.

Dudley GA, Abraham WM and Terjung RJ. (1982) Influence of exercise intensity and duration on biochemical adaptations in skeletal muscle. J Appl Physiol, **53**, 844-850.

Ekblom B, Astrand P-O, Saltin B, Stenberg J and Wallstrom B. (1968) Effect of training on circulatory response to exercise. J Appl Physiol, **24**, 518-528.

Essen B, Hagenfeldt L and Kaijser L. (1977) Utilization of blood-borne and intramuscular substrates during continuous and intermittent exercise in man. J Physiol, **265**, 489-506.

Essen-Gustavsson B and Henriksson J. (1984) Enzyme levels in pools of microdissected human muscle fibres of identified type. Adaptive response to exercise. Acta Physiol Scand, **120**, 505-515.

Fitts RH, Booth FW, Winder WW and Holloszy JO. (1975) Skeletal muscle respiratory capacity, endurance, and glycogen utilization. Am J Physiol, **228**, 1029-1033.

Gollnick PD, Pernow B, Essen B, Jansson E and Saltin B. (1981) Availability of glycogen and plasma FFA for substrate utilization in leg muscle of man during exercise. Clin Physiol, **1**, 27-42.

Green HJ, Smith D, Murphy P and Fraser I. (1990) Training-induced alterations in muscle glycogen utilization in fibre-specific types during prolonged exercise. Can J Physiol Pharmacol, **68**, 1372-1376.

Henriksson J. (1977) Training induced adaptation of skeletal muscle and metabolism during submaximal exercise. J Physiol, **270**, 661-675.

Henriksson J, Chi MM-Y, Hintz CS, Young DA, Kaiser KK, Salmons S and Lowry OH. (1986) Chronic stimulation of mammalian muscle: changes in enzymes of six metabolic pathways. Am J Physiol, **251**, C614-C632.

Henriksson J and Reitman JS. (1977) Time course of changes in human skeletal muscle succinate dehydrogenase and cytochrome oxidase activities and maximal oxygen uptake with physical activity and inactivity. Acta Physiol Scand, **99**, 91-97.

Hermansen L, Hultman E and Saltin B. (1967) Muscle glycogen during prolonged severe exercise. Acta Physiol Scand, **71**, 129-139.

Holloszy JO. (1988) Metabolic consequences of endurance exercise training, in Exercise, Nutrition and Energy Metabolism (eds ES Horton and RL Terjung), Macmillan, New York, pp. ll6-131.

Holloszy JO and Booth FW. (1976) Biochemical adaptations to endurance exercise in muscle. Ann Rev Physiol, **38**, 273-291.

Holloszy JO and Coyle EF. (1984) Adaptations of skeletal muscle to endurance exercise and their metabolic consequences. J Appl Physiol, **56**, 831-838.

Howald H, Hoppeler H, Claassen H, Mathieu O and Straub R. (1985) Influences of endurance training on the ultrastructural composition of the different muscle fiber types in humans. Pflugers Arch, **403**, 369-376.

Hurley BF, Nemeth PM, Martin III WH, Hagberg JM, Dalsky GP and Holloszy JO. (1986) Muscle triglyceride utilization during exercise: effect of training. J Appl Physiol, **60**, 562-567.

James DE, Kraegen EW and Chisholm DL. (1985) Effect of exercise training on in vivo insulin action in individual tissues of the rat. J Clin Invest, **23**, SllO.

Jansson E and Kaijser L. (1977) Muscle adaptation to extreme endurance training in man. Acta

Physiol Scand, **100**, 315-324.

Jansson E and Kaijser L. (1987) Substrate utilization and enzymes in skeletal muscle of extremely endurance-trained men. J Appl Physiol, **62**, 999-1005.

Karlsson J and Saltin B (1971) Diet, muscle glycogen, and endurance performance. J Appl Physiol, **31**, 203-206.

Karlsson J, Sjodin B, Thorstensson A, Hulten B and Frith K. (1975) LDH isozymes in skeletal muscles of endurance and strength trained athletes. Acta Physiol Scand, **93**, 150-156.

King DS, Dalsky GP, Clutter WE, Young DA, Staten MA, Cryer PE and Holloszy JO. (1988) Effects of exercise and lack of exercise on insulin sensitivity and responsiveness. J Appl Physiol, **64**, 1942-1946.

King DS, Dalsky GP, Staten MA, Clutter WE, Van Houten DR and Holloszy JO. (1987) Insulin action and secretion in endurance-trained and untrained humans. J Appl Physiol, **63**, 2247-2252.

Kirwan JP, Hickner RC, Yarasheski KE, Wiethop BV, Kohrt WM and Holloszy JO. (1991) Eccentric exercise causes transient insulin resistance in young subjects. Med Sci Sports Exerc, **23**, S110.

Komi PV, Viitasalo JT, Havu M, Thorstensson A and Karlsson J. (1976) Physiological and structural performance capacity: effect of heredity, in International Series of Biomechanics (ed PV Komi), University Park Press, Baltimore, pp. 118-123.

Lithell H, Cedermark M, Froberg J, Tesch P and Karlsson J. (1981) Increase of lipoprotein-lipase activity in skeletal muscle during heavy exercise relation to epinephrine excretion. Metabolism, **30**, 1130-1138.

Mikines KJ, Sonne B, Farrell PA, Tronier B and Galbo H. (1989) Effect of training on the dose-response relationship for insulin action in men. J Appl Physiol, **66**, 695-703.

Mikines KJ, Sonne B, Tronier B and Galbo H. (1989) Effects of acute exercise and detraining on insulin action in trained men. J Appl Physiol, **66**, 704-711.

Mole PA, Oscai LB and Holloszy JO. (1971) Adaptation of muscle to exercise. Increase in levels of palmityl CoA synthetase, carnitine palmityltransferase, and palmityl CoA dehydrogenase, and in the capacity to oxidize fatty acids. J Clin Invest, **50**, 2323-2330.

Morgan TE, Short FA and Cobb LA. (1969) Effect of long-term exercise on skeletal muscle lipid composition. Am J Physiol, **216**, 82-86.

Nesher R, Karl IE and Kipnis DM. (1985) Dissociation of effects of insulin and contraction on glucose transport in rat epitrochlearis muscle. Am J Physiol, **249**, C226-C232.

Nikkila EA, Taskinen M-R, Rehunen S and Harkonen M (1978) Lipoprotein lipase activity in adipose tissue and skeletal muscle of runners: relation to serum lipoproteins. Metabolism, **27**, 1661-1671.

Oscai LB, Essig DA and Palmer WK. (1990) Lipase regulation of muscle triglyceride hydrolysis. J Appl Physiol, **69**, 1571-1577.

Paulussen RJA and Veerkamp JH. (1990) Intracellular fatty-acid-binding proteins. Characteristics and function, in Subcellular Biochemistry: intracellular transfer of lipid molecules (ed HJ Hilderson), Plenum Press, New York, pp. 175-226.

Pette D. (1984) Activity-induced fast to slow transitions in mammalian muscle. Med Sci Sports Exerc, **16**, 517-528.

Ploug T, Stallknecht BM, Pedersen O, Kahn BB, Ohkuwa T, Vinten J and Galbo H. (1990) Effect of endurance training on glucose transport capacity and glucose transporter expression in rat skeletal muscle. Am J Physiol, **259**, E778-E786.

Rodnick KJ, Reaven GM, Azhar S, Goodman MN and Mondon CE. (1990) Effects of insulin on carbohydrate and protein metabolism in voluntary running rats. Am J Physiol, **259**, E706-E714.

Rogers MA, King DS, Hagberg JM, Ehsani AA and Holloszy JO. (1990) Effect of 10 days of physical inactivity on glucose tolerance in master athletes. J Appl Physiol, **68**, 1833-1837.

Saltin B and Gollnick PD. (1983) Skeletal muscle adaptability: significance for metabolism and performance, in Handbook of Physiology: Skeletal Muscle (eds LD Peachy, RH Adrian and SR Geiger), Am Physiol Soc, Bethesda, MD, pp. 555-631.

Saltin B and Karlsson J. (1971) Muscle glycogen utilization during work of different intensities, in Muscle Metabolism During Exercise (eds B Pernow and B Saltin), Plenum, New York, pp. 289-299.

Saltin B and Karlsson J. (1971) Muscle ATP, CP, and lactate during exercise after physical conditioning, in Muscle Metabolism During Exercise (eds B Pernow and B Saltin), Plenum, New York, pp. 395-399.

Schantz P. (1986) Plasticity of human skeletal muscle. Acta Physiol Scand, 128 (suppl 558), 1-62.

Schantz P, Henriksson J and Jansson E. (1983) Adaptation of human skeletal muscle to endurance training of long duration. Clin Physiol, 3, 141-151.

Schantz P, Sjoberg B and Svedenhag J. (1986) Malate-aspartate and alphaglycerophosphate shuttle enzyme levels in human skeletal muscle: methodological considerations and effect of endurance training. Acta Physiol Scand, 128, 397-407.

Sherman WM and Costill DL. (1984) The marathon: dietary manipulation to optimize performance. Am J Sports Med, 12, 44-51.

Stankiewicz-Choroszucha B and Gorski J. (1978) Effect of beta-adrenergic blockade on intramuscular triglyceride mobilization during exercise. Experientia, 34, 357-358.

Stubbe I, Hansson P, Gustafson A and Nilsson-Ehle P. (1983) Plasma lipoproteins and lipolytic enzymes activities during endurance training in sedentary men: changes in high-density lipoprotein subfractions and composition. Metabolism, 32, 1120-1128.

Svedenhag J, Lithell H, Juhlin-Dannfelt, A and Henriksson J. (1983) Increase in skeletal muscle lipoprotein lipase following endurance training in man. Atherosclerosis, 49, 203-207.

Wallberg-Henriksson H, Constable SH, Young DA and Holloszy JO. (1988) Glucose transport into rat skeletal muscle: interaction between exercise and insulin. J Appl Physiol, 65, 909-913.

Williams RS, Salmons S, Newsholme EA, Kaufman RE and Mellor J. (1986) Regulation of nuclear and mitochondrial expression by contractile activity in skeletal muscle. J Biol Chem, 261, 376-380.

Winder WW, Arogyasami J, Barton RJ, Elayan IM and Vehrs PR. (1989) Muscle malonyl-CoA decreases during exercise. J Appl Physiol, 67, 2230-2233.

Yki-Jarvinen H, Puhakainen I, Saloranta C, Groop L and Taskinen M-R. (1991) Demonstration of a novel feedback mechanism between FFA oxidation from intracellular and intravascular sources. Am J Physiol, 260, E680-E689.

Adaptations to strength training

I. Jacobs

Abstract. This article will focus on more recent findings concerning some selected skeletal muscle cell responses to acute stimuli in the form of a strength training session, as well as the morphological and neuromuscular adaptations to specific types of strength training sessions. In addition, a brief review of recent literature documenting the effects of combining strength and endurance training will also be presented.

Keywords: Body builders, hyperplasia, hypertrophy, metabolism, muscle, strength training

Introduction

The qualitative and quantitative aspects of adaptations to aerobic/endurance training have been, and continue to be, the focus of much research. The effect of intensity, duration and frequency of the endurance training stimulus, as well as genetic predisposition for specific physiologic adaptations, on the extent of adaptations is well elucidated. Such is not the case for adaptations to strength training. The reader is referred elsewhere for an excellent general review of what is known about strength training methodologies, and applications (Fleck and Kraemer, 1987).

This article will focus on more recent findings concerning some selected skeletal muscle cell responses to acute stimuli in the form of a strength training session, as well as the morphological and neuromuscular adaptations to specific types of strength training sessions. In addition, a brief review of recent literature documenting the effects of combining strength and endurance training will also be presented.

Muscle metabolism during an acute strength training workout

Tesch et al (1986) described the changes in selected muscle metabolites in nine body builders who had performed a leg training session typically used to strength train the quadriceps. The workout consisted of five sets of each of the following exercises: front squats, rear squats, sitting leg press, sitting leg extensions. Each set consisted of 6-10 repetitions, lasted about 30 s, and 60 s of rest intervened between sets and different exercises. Muscle biopsies were taken from the vastus lateralis before the first exercise and immediately after the 30 min workout. There were increased concentrations of intracellular glucose, glycolytic intermediates and lactate, and significant decreases in glycogen concentration, creatine phosphate and ATP. The results suggest that the metabolic pathways of anaerobic glycogenolysis and high energy phosphate hydrolysis receive a significant stimulus from such a strength training session.

In further support of the relative importance of anaerobic glycogenolysis in transducing energy to skeletal muscle, lactate dehydrogenase activity is higher in strength trained athletes than untrained subjects, and mitochondrial enzyme activities are lower in strength trained athletes (Tesch et al, 1989). An indication of the repeated utilization of endogenous intramuscular ATP stores is reflected in the increased myokinase activity (catalyzing the condensation of two ADP molecules for the regeneration of ATP) in the strength trained subjects, but only in their type II (fast twitch) muscle fibres (Tesch et al, 1989).

The absolute change in muscle glycogen and lactate concentration during a routine strength training exercise, sitting leg extensions, seems to be more a function of the total amount of mechanical work performed by the muscle than the intensity of the muscular contractions (Robergs et al, 1991). This conclusion was based on a comparison of metabolite changes between a trial when the resistance was set at 70% of the maximal resistance that could be overcome one time (70% 1 RM) and a trial when resistance was set at 35% 1 RM. In the latter lighter intensity trial the number of repetitions was greater than in the former trial so that total work was equal between trials. Thus, even though the rate of glycogen breakdown was slower in the 35% 1 RM trial, the absolute change in muscle glycogen concentration was similar. Such a finding contrasts with the overriding influence of relative exercise intensity on the rate of glycogenolysis during exercise of a primarily aerobic nature (Saltin and Karlsson, 1971).

Training effects

Although total work performed during strength training may dictate the extent of glycogenolysis (as discussed above), the extent of changes in muscular strength are a function of the relative strength exerted during training, the number of muscle contractions performed per training session, the frequency of training, the speed of muscular contraction, the type of muscle contraction (e.g. eccentric, concentric, isometric, isoinertial, isokinetic) and perhaps the rest interval between sets. It is these factors that can be manipulated in various fashions in order to achieve specific and varying goals in strength training. Unfortunately, most of the mixing and matching has yet to be scientifically validated. The reader is referred to Atha (1982) and Hakkinen (1989) for reviews of what little research there is devoted to these aspects.

Strength vs. explosive power training

It is accepted that in novices to strength training the rapid increases in strength that occur during the first 2-4 weeks of training can be largely attributed to neural factors, i.e. to "learning" to maximally recruit and exploit the motor units available in the musculature. This conclusion is based on the repeated observation that the maximum integrated electromyographic activity of the trained musculature increases significantly without any measurable hypertrophy of the muscles (Moritani and DeVries, 1979; Hakkinen and Komi, 1983; Sale, 1987). Hypertrophy of individual muscle fibres is detectable in biopsy samples after about 8 weeks of training (Hakkinen, 1989).

Appropriate manipulation of strength training methods will determine whether the resultant training effects improve primarily muscular strength or the ability to generate strength more rapidly, i.e. to increase maximal muscular power. For example, heavy resistance training of the leg extensors using classical barbell squat exercises will induce large increases in maximal force which will be associated with both significant increases in "neural activation of the trained muscles" (Hakkinen and Komi, 1986) and hypertrophy of the muscle fibres (Hakkinen, 1989). This type of training does not cause extensive changes in the rate of force development, i.e. muscular power.

These adaptations contrast with explosive power-type training of the legs consisting of the performance of various types of vertical jumps (Hakkinen and Komi, 1986). Such training induced much smaller increases in maximal strength and slower changes in muscle fibre hypertrophy, but had a much greater effect on the rate of force development than did the classical strength training.

Hypertrophy and hyperplasia

The strength training methods employed by body builders result in dramatic muscular enlargement. As a result body builders have been employed frequently as subjects in order to evaluate the effects of several years of this specific form of strength training, just as the endurance runner has been used as a model of the effects of several years of aerobic training. For example, the cross-sectional area of the elbow flexors, determined with computed tomography, is at least 50% greater in male body builders than in untrained subjects (Sale et al, 1987). Some studies suggest that such muscular enlargement is proportional to, and can be explained by, the more hypertrophied mean cross-sectional area of the muscle fibres comprising the musculature of body builders (Schantz et al, 1981; MacDougall et al, 1984; Sale et al, 1987). In particular, it has been recently pointed out that elite body builders are characterized by not only hypertrophied average muscle fibre areas, but a particularly selective and exaggerated hypertrophy of the type II (fast twitch) muscle fibres (Alway et al, 1989; Bell and Jacobs, 1990). At least one study has suggested that the propensity for strength improvement is also directly related to the proportion of type II fibres comprising the trained musculature (Dons et al, 1979).

In contrast, other investigators have calculated the number of muscle fibres comprising a muscle and found that the muscular enlargement in body builders cannot be totally explained by a larger mean fibre area; they suggest that a larger number of muscle fibres in body builders, attributed either to training or genetic endowment, may also be responsible for their dramatic increases in muscle volume (Alway et al, 1989; Tesch and Larsson, 1982).

"Electrophysiological signs of muscle fibre hyperplasia" were reported by Larsson and Tesch (1986). They reported that in contrast with great differences in limb circumferences between body builders and control subjects, the muscle fibre areas, analyzed in biopsy samples from the vastus lateralis of body builders, were similar. They interpreted this as meaning that there must have been a greater number of muscle fibres in the body builders. They found support for this hypothesis in their observation of abnormally high numbers of muscle fibres associated with a single motor unit in the body builders.

Compatibility of strength and aerobic training

The vast majority of team sports, particularly ball games, have components of the game which demand not only strength but also cardiorespiratory fitness. The compatibility of simultaneously engaging in strength and cardiorespiratory training has been the focus of increasing research activity in recent years (Bell et al, 1988; Dudley and Djamil, 1985; Sale et al, 1990a, 1990b). This research was stimulated by the work of Hickson (1980). He reported that the rate of improvement in strength was impaired in subjects who engaged in concurrent strength and endurance training, particularly in the last 5 weeks of a 10-week training programme, when compared to the improvement rate in subjects who engaged only in strength training. This finding was supported by Dudley and Djamil (1985) who, using a similar approach, reported that the improvement rate in peak isokinetic muscular torque generation was impaired in the concurrent training group, but only during relatively fast muscle contractions. Since subjects can vary widely in their trainability, such cross-sectional studies comparing the responses to different training programmes are confounded by a certain lack of experimental control, which can be partially addressed with intrasubject designs.

Such control was attempted by Sale et al (1990b) who had their subjects train one leg with a single mode of training (either strength or endurance) while the other leg performed both strength and endurance training. Although confounded by potential neurological and endocrinological adaptations that might affect both legs, this study concluded that concurrent training did not interfere with the development of either muscular strength or maximal aerobic power.

All related studies have reported significant strength and endurance training effects in the subjects engaged in concurrent strength and endurance training. What is arguable is whether the rate of adaptation to training is impaired by concurrent training. Yet even in those studies that have found statistically significant impairments in adapting to concurrent training, the extent of the impairments are relatively minor (Dudley and Djamil, 1985) or could be equally well explained by overtraining due to the volume and intensity of training required to elicit both strength and endurance training effects (Dudley and Fleck, 1987; Hickson, 1980).

This author's conclusion, therefore, is that the main limiting factor to inducing simultaneous adaptations to strength and endurance training is not physiologic but rather the time required to engage in the training and to give the body sufficient time to recover between training sessions. Accepting that premise, more research should be devoted to strategies to exploit the available training time optimally, as in Bell et al (1988, 1991) and Sale et al (1990a).

References

Alway S, Grumbt WH, Gonyea WJ and Stray-Gundersen J. (1989) Contrasts in muscle and myofibers of elite male and female bodybuilders. J Appl Physiol, **67**, 24-31.

Atha J. (1982) Strengthening muscle, in Exercise and Sport Sciences Reviews, Volume 9 (ed. D Miller), The Franklin Institute, Chicago, pp. 1-73.

Bell DG and Jacobs I. (1990) Muscle fibre area, fibre type and capillarization in male and female body builders. Can J Sport Sci, **15**, 115-119.

Bell G, Petersen S, Quinney AH and Wenger H. (1988) Sequencing of endurance and high velocity strength training. Can J Sport Sci, **13**, 214-219.

Bell G, Petersen SR, Wessel J, Bagnall K and Quinney HA. (1991) Adaptations to endurance and low velocity resistance training performed in a sequence. Can J Sport Sci, **16**, 186-192.

Dons B, Bollerup K, Bonde-Petersen F and Hancke S. (1979) The effect of weight-lifting exercise related to muscle fiber composition and muscle cross-sectional area in humans. Eur J Appl Physiol, **40**, 95-106.

Dudley GA and Djamil R. (1985) Incompatibility of endurance and strength-training modes of exercise. J Appl Physiol, **59**, 1446-1451.

Dudley GA and Fleck SJ. (1987) Strength and endurance training: Are they mutually exclusive? Sports Med, **4**, 79-85.

Fleck SJ and Kraemer WJ. (1987) Designing Resistance Training Programs. Human Kinetics Books, Champaign, IL.

Hakkinen K. (1989) Neuromuscular and hormonal adaptations during strength training. J Sports Med, **29**, 9-26.

Hakkinen K and Komi PV. (1983) Electromyographic changes during strength training and detraining. Med Sci Sports Exercise, **15**, 455-460.

Hakkinen K and Komi PV. (1986) Training-induced changes in neuromuscular performance under voluntary and reflex conditions. Eur J Appl Physiol, **55**, 147-155.

Hickson RC. (1980) Interference of strength development by simultaneously training for strength and endurance. Eur J Appl Physiol, **45**, 255-269.

Larsson L and Tesch PA. (1986) Motor unit fibre density in extremely hypertrophied skeletal muscles in man. Eur J Appl Physiol, **55**, 130-136.

MacDougall JD, Sale DG, Alway SE and Sutton JR. (1984) Muscle fiber number in biceps brachii in bodybuilders and control subjects. J Appl Physiol, **57**, 1399-1403.

Moritani T and DeVries H. (1979) Neural factors versus hypertrophy in the time course of muscle strength gain. Amer J Physical Med, **58**, 115-130.

Robergs RA, Pearson DR, Costill DL, Fink WJ, Pascoe DD, Benedict MA, Lambert CP and Zachweija JJ. (1991) Muscle glycogenolysis during differing intensities of weight-resistance exercise. J Appl Physiol, 70, 1700-1706.

Sale DG. (1987) Influence of exercise and training on motor unit activation, in Exercise and Sport Sciences Reviews, Volume 15, (ed. K Pandolf), MacMillan Publishing Company, New York, pp. 95-151.

Sale DG, Jacobs I, MacDougall JD and Garner S. (1990) Comparison of two regimens of concurrent strength and endurance training. Med Sci Sports Exercise, 22, 348-356.

Sale DG, MacDougall JD, Alway SE and Sutton JR. (1987) Voluntary strength and muscle characteristics in untrained men and women and male bodybuilders. J Appl Physiol, 62,1786-1793.

Sale DG, MacDougall JD, Jacobs I and Garner S. (1990) Interaction between concurrent strength and endurance training. J Appl Physiol, 68, 260-270.

Saltin B and Karlsson J. (1971) Muscle glycogen utilization during work of different intensities, in Muscle Metabolism During Exercise, (ed. B Pernow and B Saltin), Plenum Press, New York, pp. 289-299.

Schantz P, Randall-Fox E, Norgen P and Tyden A. (1981) The relationship between the mean muscle fibre area and the muscle cross-sectional area of the thigh in subjects with large differences in thigh girth. Acta Physiol Scand, 113, 537-539.

Tesch PA, Colliander EB and Kaiser P. (1986) Muscle metabolism during intense, heavy-resistance exercise. Eur J Appl Physiol, 55, 362-366.

Tesch PA and Larsson L. (1982) Muscle hypertrophy in bodybuilders. Eur J Appl Physiol, 49, 301-306.

Tesch PA, Thorsson A and Essen-Gustavsson B. (1989) Enzyme activities of FT and ST muscle fibers in heavy-resistance trained athletes. J Appl Physiol, 67, 83-87.

Metabolic responses to sprint training

S. Brooks, M.E. Nevill, G. Gaitanos and C. Williams

Abstract. The metabolic responses to training are dependent on the nature of the training stimulus and with sprint training this stimulus can be characterised as periods of brief maximal exercise. The primary feature of brief maximal exercise is the fatigue that occurs where decreases in power output of 50% are seen with 30s of exercise; most investigations of adaptations with training have centred on the metabolic causes of fatigue and the possible modifications of this process. This paper reviews the reported matabolic adaptations to sprint training with regard to those factors that determine the performance of muscle during sprinting.

Keywords: Exercise, training, fatigue, anaerobic metabolism, oxygen uptake.

Introduction

The stimulus for the adaptations seen in response to training is overload and the nature of the adaptations are determined by the intensity and duration of this overload. Whilst many of the adaptations to endurance training have been elucidated the extent and nature of those to sprint training are less dear. Of the studies that have been published, the nature of the training and the type of sprint exercise studied have been many and varied. In the determination of performance single exercise bouts or, if the pattern of exercise has been modelled on that seen during team games (e.g. rugby), brief repetitive periods of maximal exercise separated by intervals of rest have been used. For the purposes of this paper a definition of sprinting as brief maximal exercise has been adopted with the implications that the exercise period is of brief duration, typically less than 30s, and that the exercise is maximal for each subject with no distribution of effort during the exercise period. The intensity of such exercise is well in excess of that required to elicit 100% of VO_2 max and will challenge the processes of anaerobic ATP resynthesis. In this paper a short review of the results of previous studies into the adaptations that occur with sprint training are presented incorporating the results from our recent studies.

Performance

The majority of studies have shown that a period of sprint training results in an improvement in sprint performance (see Table 1). The development of specific and sensitive laboratory models of sprint exercise (e.g. Bar-Or, 1978; Lakomy, 1987) have enabled the nature of the changes in performance with training to be more fully described and have made some comparisons between published work possible. However given the multipicity of methods used to assess performance it is difficult to extract a unified description of the specific changes in performance with training although three trends are apparent, an inaease in maximum power output, an increase in the work done during a brief exercise bout and an increase in exercise duration at high intensities. The changes in the performance of a 30s sprint test with training using a non-motorised treadmill are shown in Fig 1. The most marked adaptation is an increase in the maximum power attained during the sprint test of 12% and an increase in the total work done during the test of 6% (the sensitivity of this test to the training status of the subjects is illustrated in Fig. 1 by the inclusion of the results from an endurance training study). This improvement in performance corresponded to a mean decrease in the time taken to compete a 200m sprint of 1.5s. These changes are of a similar magnitude to those seen with eight weeks of sprint training where peak power (8% increase, Wootton, 1984) or torque (26% increase, Sharp et al, 1946) have been reported . As the power output at the end of the sprint was similar before and after training the fatigue during the test ([peak power - end power]/peak power x 100) was increased by training from 50% to 61%. This finding suggests that sprint training increases fatigue however the result is a consequence of the exercise model used as can be demonstrated when a different exercise model is employed. Using a modified Wingate test protocol the work done

Table 1. The changes in sprint performance and VO$_2$ max reported with sprint training

Performance	VO$_2$max	Reference
Increase	No change	Aitken et al, 1989
Increase	Increase	Bell & Wenger, 1988
No change	Increase	Fox et al, 1977
Increase	No change	Houston & Thomson, 1977
Increase	Increase	Nevill et al, 1989
Increase	No change	Medbo & Burgers, 1990
Increase	Increase	Sharp et al, 1986
Increase	Increase	Simoneau et al, 1987
Increase	No change	Thorstensson et al, 1975
Increase	No change	Wootton, 1984

in 6s was determined before and after eight weeks of sprint training and in the training group was increased by 8%. When the time taken to complete the pre-training work for ten repetitive bouts was measured there was a 12% decrease in the time taken to perform the tenth bout with training (see Fig. 2). This study demonstrated that training had decreased fatigue. Using a multiple sprint protocol (Brooks et al, 1990) the results of a recent study have confirmed that training decreased the fatigue with repetitive exercise bouts and also increased the maximum power output. Overall, the main change in performance with sprint training is an increase in the power output during the initial period of exercise which can also be expressed as an increase in the work done during this period.

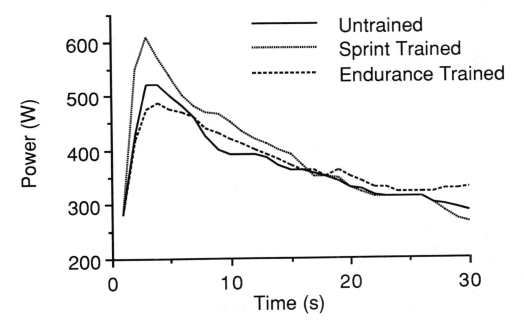

Fig. 1 The changes in performance of a 30s sprint after 8 weeks of sprint training and 10 weeks of endurance training (adapted from Nevill et al, 1989 and Brooks et al, 1984).

Adaptation

The challenge with any training study is to relate the change in performance to the adaptations in physiological systems that permit or enable the improvement in performance. In sprint training where the predominant change in performance

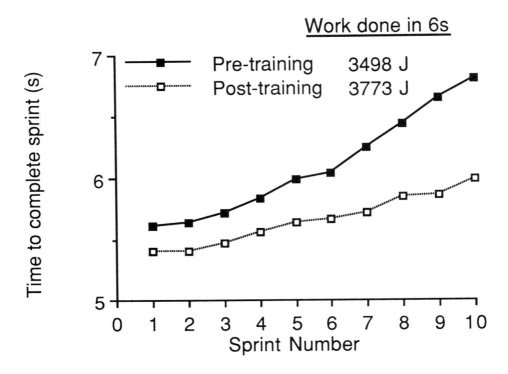

Fig. 2 The times taken to complete 10 repetitions of the same absolute work load on a cycle ergometer before and after 8 weeks of sprint training.

is an increase in power output during the initial period of exercise there are a range of possible mechanisms operating at the level of each individual fibre, at the muscle group and at the whole body level which could account for the improvement in performance. What is not clear is whether the maximum power output is itself limited by the same processes that produce the resultant fatigue. If the factors that influence maximum power and fatigue are different and a dissociation between the effects of intramuscular pH on force and endurance has been demonstrated by Sahlin and Ren (1989) then a complete description of adaptations to sprint training will involve more than one of the factors discussed here.

The determinants of muscle tension are shown in Table 2 and the possible contribution of these factors to the improvements in sprint performance will be considered.

Table 2   The determinants of muscle tension (after Vander et al, 1990).

SINGLE FIBRE

Action-potential frequency	
Fibre length	
Fibre diameter	Hypertrophy
Fatigue	E-C coupling
	ATP
	pH
	Others

WHOLE MUSCLE

Number of active motor units	Recruitment
	Fibre type

Number of active fibres per motor unit NM transmission

Single fibre

Action-potential frequency
   The relationship between the action-potential frequency and the tension developed by individual fibres has been well established from the twitch response to an individual stimulus to a fully fused tetanus. In the longer term, the influence of the patterns of innervation on gene expression and hence fibre type will also occur and slow to fast fibre type transformations have been demonstrated in animal experiments (Gorza et al, 1988)

Fibre length
   The fibre length at the onset of contraction and hence the range of movement of the active muscles are assumed to be the same before and after training.

Fibre diameter
   An increase in the contractile units per fibre (hypertrophy) will result in an increase in the tension developed. In a study by Wootton (1984) an extensive assessment of leg muscle volume changes with eight weeks of sprint training found no evidence of any change although Aitken et al (1989) have reported

increases in the cross-sectional areas of type I and type II fibres with 6 weeks of high intensity training. In the 30s sprint study of Nevill et al (1989) there was a tendency for an increase in the maximum voluntary contraction of the quadriceps group with training (7%) and significant increases (12%) have been reported with training periods of similar duration (Thorstensson et al, 1975). However on the evidence of body weight no consistent changes in muscle volume are seen.

Fatigue

Excitation-contraction coupling

A role for e-c coupling failure in fatigue has been proposed by Vollestad and Sjersted (1988). Whilst the disruption by high intensity exercise of e-c coupling and specifically sarcoplasmic reticulum function has been demonstrated by Byrd et al (1989) in the horse, the possibility of changes with training remains unexplored although alterations have been inferred by Troup et al (1986) to explain some of the changes in muscle function with sprint training in rats.

ATP resynthesis
a.   Substrate and energy stores

One explanation for the increase in power output seen with training could be an increase in the muscle stores of ATP and PCr. The results from six studies are shown in Table 3. No consistent increase in the storage of ATP or PCr is apparent in these experiments. It is of interest that chronically low levels of muscle PCr have profound effects on muscle enzymes and fibre type in rats (Shoubridge et al, 1985). If a similar response occurs in humans, this suggests one possible factor in initiating changes in muscle with sprint training. In three experiments where the muscle glycogen content was investigated there was a trend towards an increase in the stores with training. The importance of the size of glycogen stores is unclear as with sprinting fatigue occurs before any significant depletion of glycogen is apparent and with repetitive maximal contractions low muscle glycogen does not impair performance (Symonds and Jacobs, 1989).

b.   Oxidative metabolism

The results from previous sprint training studies (see Table 1) are equally divided amongst those that reported increases in VO_2 max values with training and those that found no changes. The VO_2 max value per se is not a determinant of sprint performance and increases in VO_2 max values with training do not result in increases in peak power outputs (Brooks et al, 1984). The aerobic contribution to 30s of maximal exercise has been estimated by Kavanagh and Jacobs (1988) as 18.5% which compares to the estimate of 21.5% before and 19.6% after training in the 30s sprint study. of Nevill at al (1989). In this study the excess post-exercise oxygen consumption was increased by 18% after training (see Fig. 3) an increase that was not accompanied by a rise in muscle myoglobin (Jacobs et al,

Table 3. The changes in resting muscle ATP, PCr and glycogen in response to a period of sprint training (mmol kg⁻¹ dry wt)

ATP	PCr	Glycogen	Reference
-0.7	- 8.0	+96.3	Boobis et al, 1983
+3.7	+ 3.4	-	Houston & Thomson, 1977
-2.8	- 0.9	+30.4	Nevill et al, 1989
+1.2	-10.3	_	Sharp et al, 1986
+1.3	+ 2.2	+30.0	Unpublished

1987). Medbo et al (1988) have proposed that the accumulated oxygen deficit during maximal exercise of short duration is a method of assessing anaerobic capacity and that this deficit increases with training (Medbo and Burgers, 1990). In a recent study using a multiple sprint protocol of 10 x 6s sprints separated by 30s of rest, a strong correlation between the oxygen uptake during the whole exercise period (6 min) and the work done was found (r = 0.90). However no good correlation was found between the increase in the work done and the increase in oxygen uptake after training (r = 0.21).The importance and magnitude of oxygen uptake during recovery has been demonstrated by Gaitanos (1990) who occluded the blood supply to the legs during 30s of recovery between successive 6s sprints and found a 25% reduction in oxygen uptake but a 55% reduction in the power output by the time of the tenth repetition. The basis of excess post-exercise oxygen consumption has been reviewed by Gaesser and Brooks (1984) and many of the factors they associated with the increase are affected by sprinting e.g. with 30s of sprinting muscle temperatuire is increased by over 2°C (Allsop et al, 1990) and plasma catecholamines are increased over four fold (Cheetham et al, 1986). Thus the increase in post-exercise oxygen consumption may be due to the larger perturbation of homeostasis associated with the enhanced performance post-training.

c. Anaerobic metabolism

The measurement from which inferences are drawn concerning the amount of anaerobic glycolytic activity is blood lactate. However no consistent results of training on the exercise-induced increase in blood lactate have been reported. Of the ten studies referred to in Table 1 four reported increased post-exercise blood lactate concentrations after training whilst three reported no change or a decrease.

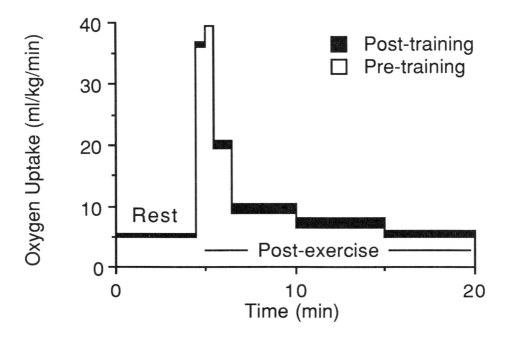

Fig. 3 The changes in oxygen uptake before, during and after a 30s sprint with weeks of sprint training (adapted from Nevill et al, 1989).

The unreliability of blood lactate concentration as an indicator of glycolysis has been demonstrated in the experiments of Nevill et al (1989) where despite an increase of 8% in the work done after training there was no increase in post-exercise blood lactate despite an increase in muscle lactate of 20%. The use of the muscle biopsy technique allows a more detailed investigation of muscle metabolism to be made and allows for the estimation of ATP resynthesis during exercise based on the concentrations of muscle metabolites as described by Sahlin (1978) and Hultman and Sjoholm (1983). Studies by Boobis et al (1983) and Nevill et al (1989) have demonstrated that the rates of glycogenolysis exceed the rates of glycolysis both before and after training (i.e. glycogen breakdown is not a limiting factor) and that the major adaptation associated with the improvement in performance seen after training was an increase in the ATP resynthesis from anaerobic glycolysis. The contribution of the estimated ATP resynthesis from anaerobic sources is shown in Fig. 4 where the total anaerobic ATP resynthesis increased by 14% whilst the estimated contribution from anaerobic glycolysis increased by 20%. A survey of sprint training studies reveals that increases in muscle phosphofructokinase activity, the rate-limiting enzyme in anaerobic glycolysis (Jones et al, 1985), has been reported in five studies (see Table 4). These findings suggest that the increase in power output resulting from sprint training is associated with an increase in the capacity of muscle to regenerate ATP by the process of anaerobic glycolysis.

Table 4   The changes in muscle fibre type and increases in enzyme activities with sprint training (PFK phosphofructokinase, CS citrate synthetase, PHOS phosphorylase, LDH lactate dehydrogenase, GAPDH glyceraldehyde phosphate dehydrogenase, MDH malate dehydrogenase, HK hexokinase, HADH 3-hydroxyacyl-CoA dehydrogenase, OGDH oxoglutarate dehydrogenase and MK myokinase).

Fibre Type	Muscle Enzymes	Reference
FOG	-	Aitken et al, 1989
No change	PFK	Fournier et al, 1982
No change	-	Houston & Thomson, 1977
FOG	PFK.CS	Jacobs et al, 1987
-	PHOS, PFK, LDH, GAPDH, MDH	Roberts et al, 1982
-	PFK	Sharp et al, 1986
-	PFK, HK, LDH, MDH, HADH, OGDH	Simoneau et al, 1987
No change	MK, Mg^{++}ATP'ase	Thorstensson et al, 1975

pH
   The reported changes in muscle buffering with training are shown in Table 5. There is little evidence for major increases in muscle physio-chemical buffering as determined by titration however when buffering is calculated based on post-

exercise muscle pH and lactate content buffering capacity is seen to rise with training. The two components of buffering not determined by the titration method are the contributions of bicarbonate and transmembrane ion fluxes. The maximum

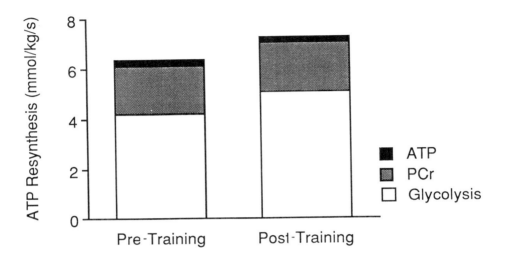

Fig. 4 The contributions to anaerobic ATP resynthesis during a 30s sprint before and after training (adapted from Nevill et al, 1989).

contribution to buffering of bicarbonate has been estimated by Sahlin et al (1978) as 10 Slykes which would appear to be insufficient to account for the increases in calculated buffering capacity seen with training. The other component is transmembrane fluxes and it is interesting to note that in the study by Nevill et al (1989) the post exercise muscle physiochemical component of buffering and the post-exercise muscle pH were the same before and after training even though the post-exercise muscle lactate content was 20% higher after training, as this increase in muscle lactate was not accompanied by an increase in blood lactate the transmembrane flux of hydrogen ions would appear to provide an explanation of these results. A recent experiment by Sahlin and Ren (1989) has shown a differential effect of muscle pH on force generation and endurance which suggests that there is more than one consequence of an increase in muscle hydrogen ion concentration.

Table 5   The effects of sprint training on muscle buffering (muscle buffering as Slykes, mmol[H^+]kg^{-1} wet wt pH^{-1})

Pre-Training		Post-Training	MethodReference
49.9	57.8	Titration	Bell and Wenger, 1988
36.5	37.7	Titration	Mannion et al, 1990
67.6	71.2	Titration	Nevill et al, 1989
87.9	126.7	Calculation	Nevill et al, 1989
44.7	61.0	Calculation	Sharp et al, 1986

Other causes

The possible biochemical causes of fatigue have been reviewed recently by Roberts and Smith (1989) however the effects of sprint training on many of the postulated causes remain to be investigated.

Whole Muscle

Number of active motor units

a. Recruitment

The depletion of muscle PCr in response to exercise pre- and post-training is shown in Table 6. If more muscle fibres are recruited after training then, given the limitations of sampling imposed by the biopsy technique, a larger decrease in muscle PCr would result. The change in PCr depletion with exercise after training shows no consistent pattern and in consequence no evidence for a greater recruitment of muscle fibres post-training. The interaction of sensory systems and the central control of motor activity and recruitment is not well understood. However anecdotal evidence, if not personal experience, suggests that sprint training can modify some of the central responses to high intensity exercise. An

example is the nausea often experienced after acute exposure a response which passes with training. Exercise-induced increases in the pain threshold have been demonstrated (Droste et al, 1991) and may be associated with plasma B-endorphin concentrations. Whilst a relationship between plasma B-endorphin concentrations and performance has been reported for sprint exercise (Brooks et al, 1988) possible adaptations to training remain unknown although an
increased B-endorphin response to exercise has been reported with physical conditioning (Carr et al, 1981)

Table 6   The changes in muscle PCr in response to exercise before and after training (PCr in mmol kg^{-1} dry wt).

Pre-training	Post-training	Reference
61.6	57.6	Boobis et al, 1983
56.0	57.5	Nevill et al, 1989
39.8	41.3	Sharp et al, 1986
54.5	50.6	Unpublished

b. Fibre type
Given the short duration of most sprint training studies any significant changes in the fibre type population may be hard to detect. Of the five studies presented in Table 4, only two reported a change in fibre type and the responses to training remain equivocal.

Number of active fibres per motor unit
The failure of neuromuscular transmission in mammalian preparations at high frequencies has been demonstrated by Krnjevic and Miledi (1959). However at the frequencies of innervation seen in man little evidence for neuromuscular transmission failure exists as Bigland-Ritchie et al (1982) have demonstrated with maximum voluntary contractions.

Conclusions

These results show that the major improvement in performance after sprint training can be expressed as an increase in power output during the initial period of exercise. Associated with this improvement in performance is an increase in the energy supply from anaerobic glycolysis possibly secondary to an improvement in muscle buffering. These changes are also associated with an increased oxygen uptake postexercise. In consequence of the paucity of information on adaptations to sprint training several questions remain unanswered. Recent experiments have cast light on two areas that require further investigation, the differences in the response to exercise (and training) of the three main fibre types (Park et al, 1987) and the nature of the signal that initiates the adaptation in muscle in response to training although some possibilities for other modes of training have been reviewed by Booth and Thompson (1991).

References

Aitken JC, Bennet WM, Thompson J. (1989) The effects of high intensity training upon respiratory gas exchanges during fixed term maximal incremental exercise in man. Eur J Appl Physiol, **58**, 717-721.

Allsop P, Cheetham M, Brooks S, Hall GM, Williams C. (1990) Continuous intramuscular pH measurement during the recovery from brief, maximal exercise in man. Eur J Appl Physiol, **59**, 465-470.

Bar-Or O. (1978) A new anaerobic capacity test- characteristics and applications. Proceedings of the 21st World Congress of Sports Medicine, Brasilia, pp. 1-27.

Bell GJ, Wenger HA. (1988) The effect of one-legged sprint training on intramuscular pH and nonbicarbonate buffering capacity. Eur J Appl Physiol, **58**, 158-164.

Bigland-Ritchie B, Kakula CB, Lippold OCJ, Woods JJ. (1982) The absence of neuromuscular transmission failure in sustained maximal voluntary contractions. J Physiol, **330**, 265-278.

Boobis LH, Williams C, Wootton SA. (1983) Influence of trainng on muscle metabolism during brief maximal exercise in man. J Physiol, **342**, 36-37P.

Booth FW, Thompson DB. (1991) Molecular and cellular adaptations of muscle in response to exercise: perspectives of various models. Physiol Rev, **71**, 541-585.

Brooks S, Burrin J, Cheetham ME, Hall GM, Yeo T, Williams C. (1988) The responses of the catecholamines and B-endorphin to brief maximal exercise in man. Eur J Appl Physiol, **57**, 230-234.

Brooks S, Cheetham M, Williams C. (1984) Endurance training and the catecholamine response to brief maximal exercise in man. J Physiol, **361**, 81P.

Brooks S, Nevill ME, Meleagros L, Lakomy HKA, Hall GM, Bloom SR, Williams C. (1990) The hormonal responses to repetitive brief maximal exercise in humans. Eur J Appl Physiol, **60**, 144-148.

Byrd SK, McCutcheon LJ, Hodgson DR, Gollnick PD. (1989) Altered sarcoplasmic reticulum function after high-intensity exercise. J Appl Physiol, **67**, 2072-2077.

Carr DB, Bullen BA, Skrinar GS, Arnold MA, Rosenblatt M, Beitins IZ, Martin JB, McArthur JW. (1981) Physical conditioning facilitates the exercise-induced secretion of B-endorphin and B-lipotropin in women. New Eng J Med, **305**, 560-563.

Cheetham ME, Boobis LH, Brooks S, Williams C. (1986) Human muscle metabolism during sprint running. J Appl Physiol, **61**, 54-60.

Droste C, Greenlee MW, Schreck M, Roskamm H. (1991) Experimental pain thresholds and plasma beta-endorphin levels during exercise. Med Sci Sports Exerc, **23**, 334-342.

Fournier M, Ricci J, Taylor AW, Ferguson RJ, Montpetit RR, Chaitman BR. (1982) Skeletal muscle adaptation in adolescent boys: sprint and endurance training and detraining. Med Sci Sports

Exerc, **14**, 453-456.

Fox EL, Bartels RL, Klinzing J, Ragg K. (1977) Metabolic responses to interval training programs of high and low power output. Med Sci Sport, **9**, 191-196.

Gaesser GA, Brooks GA. (1984) Metabolic basis of excess post-exercise oxygen consumption: a review. Med Sci Sports Exerc, **16**, 29-43.

Gaitanos GC. (1990) Human muscle metabolism during intermittent maximal exercise. PhD thesis, Loughborough University, UK.

Gorza L, Gundersen K, Lomo T, Schiaffino S, Westgaard RH. (1988) Slow-to-fast transformation of denervated soleus muscles by chronic high-frequency stimulation in the rat. J Physiol, **402**, 627-649.

Houston ME, Thomson JA. (1977) The responses of endurance-adapted adults to intense anaerobic training. Eur J Appl Physiol, **36**, 207-213.

Hultman E, Sjoholm H. (1983) Energy metabolism and contraction force of human skeletal muscle in situ during electrical stimulation. J Physiol, **345**, 525-532.

Jacobs I, Esbjornsson M, Sylven C, Holm I, Jansson E. (1987) Sprint training effects on muscle myoglobin, enzymes, fibre types and blood lactate. Med Sci Sports Exerc, **19**, 368-374.

Jones NL, McCartney N, Graham T, Spriet LL, Kowalchuk JM, Heigenhauser JF, Sutton JR. (1985) Muscle performance and metabolism in maximal isokinetic cycling at slow and fast speeds. J Appl Physiol, **59**, 132-136.

Kavanagh MF, Jacobs I. (1988) Breath-by-breath oxygen consumption during performance of the wingate test. Can J Spt Sci, **13**, 91-93.

Krnjevic K, Miledi R. (1959) Presynaptic failure of neuromuscular propogation in rats. J Physiol, **149**, 1-22.

Lakomy HKA. (1987) The use of a non-motorised treadmill for analysing sprint performance. Ergonomics, **31**, 627-637.

Medbo JI, Burgers S. (1990) Effect of training on the anaerobic capacity. Med Sci Sports Exerc, **22**, 501-507.

Medbo JI, Mohn A-C, Tabata I, Bahr R, Vaage O, Sejersted OM. (1988) Anaerobic capacity determined by maximal accumulated O_2 deficit. J Appl Physiol, **64**, 50-60.

Nevill ME, Boobis LH, Brooks S, Williams C. (1989) Effect of training on muscle metabolism during treadmill sprinting. J Appl Physiol, **67**, 2376-2382.

Park JH, Brown RL, Park CR, McCully K, Cohn M, Haselgrove J, Chance B. (1987) Functional pools of oxidative and glycolytic fibres in human muscle observed by [31]p magnetic resonance spectroscopy during exercise. Proc Natl Acad Sci, USA, **84**, 8976-8980.

Roberts AD, Billeter R, Howald H. (1982) Anaerobic muscle enzyme changes after interval training. Int J Sports Med, **3**, 18-21.

Roberts D, Smith DJ. (1989) Biochemical aspects of peripheral muscle fatigue. Sports Medicine, **7**, 125-138.

Sahlin K. (1978) Intracellular pH and energy metabolism in skeletal muscle of man. Acta Physiol Scand Suppl, 455, 33-56.

Sahlin K, Alvestrand A, Brandt R, Hultman E. (1978) Intracellular pH and bicarbonate concentrations in human muscle during recovery from exercise. J Appl Physiol, **45**, 474-480.

Sahlin K, Ren JM. (1989) Relationship of contraction capacity to metabolic changes during recovery from a fatiguing contraction. J Appl Physiol, **67**, 648-654.

Sharp RL, Costill DL, Fink WJ, King DS. (1986) Effects of eight weeks bicycle ergometer sprint training on human muscle buffer capacity. Int J Sports Med, **7**, 13-17.

Shoubridge EA, Challiss RAJ, Hayes DJ, Radda GK. (1985) Biochemical adaptation in the skeletal muscle of rats depleted of creatine with the substrate analogue B-guanidinopropionic acid. Biochem J, **232**, 125-131.

Simoneau J-A, Lortie G, Boulay MR, Marcotte M, Thibault M-C, Bouchard C. (1987) Effects of two high-intensity intermittent training programs interspaced by detraining on human skeletal muscle and performance. Eur J Appl Physiol, **56**, 516-521.

Symons JD, Jacobs I. (1989) High-intensity exercise performance is not impared by low intramuscular glycogen. Med Sci Sports Exerc, 21, 550-557.

Thorstensson A, Sjodin B, Karlsson J. (1975) Enzyme activities and muscle strength after "sprint training" in man. Acta Physiol Scand, 94, 313-318.

Troup JP, Metzger JM, Fitts RH. (1986) Effect of high-intensity exercise training on functional capacity of limb skeletal muscle. J Appl Physiol, 60, 1743-1751.

Vander AJ, Sherman JH, Luciano DS. (1990) Human Physiology: the mechanisms of body function. McGraw-Hill, New York, pp. 309.

Vollestad NK, Sejersted OM. (1988) Biochemical correlates of fatigue. Eur J Appl Physiol, 57, 336-347.

Wootton SA. (1984) The influence of diet and training on the metabolic responses to maximal exercise in man. PhD Thesis Loughborough University, UK.

Recovery of muscle from exercise - its importance for subsequent performance

J. Bangsbo and B. Saltin

Abstract. The present paper evaluates the relative roles of various substrates used by muscles following intense exercise, and their consequences for subsequent exercise. Most of the lactate that accumulates in the active skeletal muscle is released to the blood, and the role of loctate for muscle glyconeogenesis appears to be minor. Instead glucose extracted from the blood and muscle glycolytic intermediates seem to be the most important substrates for carbohydrate mmetabolism during recovery. As the O_2 debt is much higher than can be accounted for by the resynthesis of glycogen, CP and ATP, it appears that other energy-demanding processes occur during recovery from intense exercise. Part of this could be linked to the metabolic use of intramuscular triacylglycerol. Active recovery appears to elevate the muscle lactate removal rate. Previous intense exercise reduces performane time and the lactate production rate during subsequent intense exercise even with one hour between the exercises. It appears that these effects are caused by factors other than elevated lactate and lowered pH.

Keywords: Muscle glyconeogenesis, carbohydarte metabolism, fat metabolism, O_2 debt, active recovery, lactate production, fatigue.

Introduction

Repetitive high intensity exercise is performed in many sports. As the final outcome in these sports might be influenced by the athletes' ability to perform maximally at a given time, it is of great importance that the athlete recovers from an intense exercise bout as rapidly as possible. This capacity can be improved by training, but for optimal training efficiency there is a need for knowledge of skeletal muscle recovery processes after intense exercise and their importance for metabolism and performance during a subsequent exercise bout.

During intense exercise, anaerobic energy results from the splitting of endogenous energy-rich phosphagens (i.e. intra-muscular stores of adenosinetriphosphate (ATP) and creatinephosphate (CP)) and from glycolysis which leads to lactate production (Hultman and Sjoholm, 1983; Boobis, 1987). During the subsequent recovery period muscle CP and ATP are resynthesized in a rapid (about 70% of rest after 1-2 min) and a slow phase (Sahlin et al, 1979). It is well-known that muscle lactate removal processes are slower, but the fate of the accumulated lactate is not well-established Hermansen and Vaage, 1978; Bonen et al, 1990). Lactate can leave the muscle, as well as being metabolized within the muscle. One possibility would be that lactate is a substrate for intramuscular glyconeogenesis, which in turn contributes to oxygen repayment (oxygen debt) in recovery from intense exercise.

Low intensity exercise accelerates lactate removal from the blood (Hermansen and Stensvold, 1972; Dood et al, 1984), but the influence of such exercise on muscle lactate concentration is unclear, as is the role of elevated muscle lactate and the concomitant increase in acidity for the development of fatigue (for references see Mainwood and Renaud, 1985). Within the sports community, it is well-accepted that lactate accumulation is the cause of perceived fatigue during high intensity exercise. However, based on several recent investigations, the exclusive role of lactate and pH may not be that obvious (Sahlin and Henriksson, 1984; Sjogaard et al, 1985; Juel et al, 1990). In studies where intense exercise was repeated, it was observed that performance deteriorated, and muscle glycogenolytic rate and lactate accumulation decreased considerably (Wotton and Williams, 1983; McCartney et al, 1986; Spriet et al, 1989: Gaitainos et al, 1991). However, in these studies lactate release to the blood was not measured, and muscle aerobic metabolism was not quantified. As well the continuous decrease in work output during the exercise made it difficult to relate the metabolic changes to development of force.

The present experiments evaluated the metabolism during both passive and active recovery from intense exercise. Furthermore, the effect of previous exercise on anaerobic energy production and performance during subsequent exercise was evaluated. The exercise model chosen was the one-legged knee-extensor exercise (Fig. 1), which enables precise and quantitative metabolic evaluation, as well as the establishment of relationships between these metabolic events and exercise performance (Bangsbo et al, 1990). Another advantage with one-legged exercise is that different interventions can be applied to the subjects two limbs, which allow for more direct comparison. Particular details related to the problems discussed can be found elsewhere (Bangsbo et al, 1991a,b,c).

Methods

Protocols

The subjects exercised in a supine position with the knee-extensors of one limb (Fig. 1).

In experiment I (long recovery) seven male subjects performed exhaustive exercise at a supramaximal work load (mean: 65 W, range: 52--79 W) and then rested for 1 h. Another six male subjects exercised at a mean power output of 67 W (range: 54-78 W) until exhaustion (EX1), which was followed by 1 h of recovery before they repeated the exhaustive exercise at the same work rate (EX2).

In experiment II (short recovery) six male subjects exercised at a supramaximal work rate (mean: 59 W; range: 52--72 W) to exhaustion (EX1). This was followed by: 1) 10 min of recovery, 2) intense intermittent exercise (7 x 15 s exercise (90 W) and 15 s recovery) and 3) a 2.5 min recovery period. Then, the exhaustive

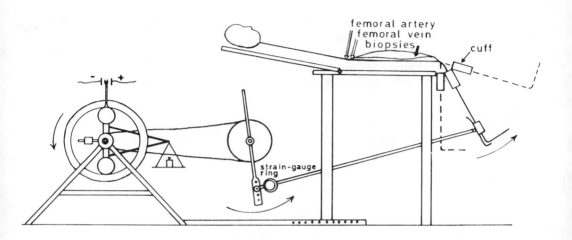

Fig. 1 Schematic graph of the exercise ergometer. The ankle is attached to the crank of a Krogh bicycle ergometer via an aluminimum bar. The exercise consists of kicking the lower part of one leg "upwards". The repositioning of the leg is completely passive (i.e. gravity and momentum of the wheel).

exercise was repeated at the same power output (EX2). During all recovery periods the leg either rested (Passive-P) or performed low intensity exercise (Active-A). After a rest period of 1 h the other leg carried out the same exercise protocol, but with the opposite pattern of activity during the recovery periods. The choice of legs was randomized.

Measurements

A muscle biopsy was taken from m. vastus lateralis of the active muscle prior to and immediately after each exhaustive exercise bout, and biopsies were also taken 3 and 10 min after EX1 in the first part of experiment I and in experiment II. Muscle samples were analysed for total water, lactate, glycogen, CP, ATP, adenosinediphosphate (ADP), adenosinemonophosphate (AMP), :idenosinemonophosphate (IMP) and pH. Furthermore, muscle glucose, glucose-1-phosphate (G-1-P), glucose-6-phosphate (G-6-P) and fructose-6-phosphate (F-6-P) were determined in muscle samples taken in the first part of experiment I. Catheters were placed in the femoral veins of the exercising legs and in one femoral artery. Measurements of leg blood flow and arterial-venous difference for oxygen, lactate, glucose, FFA, glycerol and potassium (K^+) were performed before and regularly during the supramaximal exercises and during the recovery periods after EX1. As to details about the methods and calculations of leg oxygen uptake, substrate exchange, muscle lactate production, and leg oxygen deficit, which has been shown to express the total leg anaerobic energy production, the reader is referred to earlier publications (Bangsbo et al, 1990; Bangsho et al, 1991a).

Statistics
Differences between values were determined by the Wilcoxon ranking test for paired data (Siegel, 1965) and a significance level of 0.05 was used.

Results

At the end of EX1 in experiment I (long recovery), muscle lactate (27.1 mmol-kg^{-1} w.w.) decreased to 14.5, 6.7 and 3.0 mmol kg^{-1} w.w. after 3, 10, and 60 min of recovery, respectively. Total reduction in muscle lactate was equivalent to 26.2 mmol kg^{-1} w.w. The net leg lactate efflux of 15.7 mmol min^{-1} at exhaustion decreased rapidly to 8.3 and 2.5 mmol min^{-1} after 1 and 5 min, respectively. However, it was still above 0.5 mmol min^{-1} after 10 min and it was slightly higher ($p<0.05$) than the pre-exercise value after 20 min, and remained so during the rest of the recovery period. The total net lactate release of the first 3 min, next 7 min, and last 50 min of recovery could account for 71, 66 and 95% of the muscle lactate which disappeared during the recovery periods. Thus, less than one-third of the muscle lactate which disappeared was metabolized within the muscle (Fig. 2).

Effect of active recovery
In experiment II (short recovery) muscle lactate was 23 mmol-kg^{-1} w.w. at the end of EX1 for both legs, and it decreased to 11.2 and 13.4 mmol-kg^{-1} w.w. during the first 3 min of recovery for the P-and A-leg, respectively, and further to 4.4 and 3.2 mmol kg^{-1} w.w. during the next 7 min. The latter two values were significantly different ($p<0.05$). For the A-leg blood flow during recovery was higher ($p<0.05$) than for the P-leg, being 3.68 and 2.94 l min^{-1} for the first 3 min, respectively, and 3.00 and 1.74 l min^{-1} during the next 7 min (Fig. 3). However,

no difference in lactate release was observed (Fig. 3) and, thus, the total release for the P-leg (37.3 mmol) was the same as for the A-leg (41.6 mmol). For both legs the total net release could account for about 60% of the total net muscle lactate removal, which was 19.9 (P-leg) and 21.5 (A-leg) mmol kg^{-1} w.w. (Fig. 2).

Muscle glycogen, glycolytic intermediates and glucose uptake

Muscle glycogen increased from 93.7 to 108.8 mmol kg^{-1} w.w. during the 1 h of recovery in experiment I, corresponding to a net glycogen rebuilding of 14.5 mmol kg^{-1} w.w. Immediately after EX1 muscle glucose, G-1-P, G-6-P and F-6-P was 1.76, 0.04, 1.42 and 0.19 mmol kg^{-1} w.w., respectively, and they decreased to 0.33, 0.01, 0.15 and 0.03 mmol kg^{-1} w.w., respectively, during 1 h of recovery. The glucose uptake was 0.5-0.9 mmol min^{-1} during the first 10 min of recovery and remained at approximately 0.2 mmol min^{-1} during rest of recovery. The total net leg glucose uptake by the thigh was 18.2 mmol, which could account for about 45% of the glycogen synthesis during 1 h of recovery.

Active recovery

The muscle glycogen at the end of EX1 in experiment II was 99.3 mmol kg^{-1} w.w., and it was 110.4 (P-leg) and 90.6 (A-leg) mmol kg^{-1} w.w. after 10 min resulting in no significant changes during the 10 min recovery period. The glucose uptake at the end of the EX1 bouts (0.3 mmol min^{-1}) increased to about 0.7 (P-leg) and 1.0 (A-leg) mmol min^{-1} after 0.75 min of recovery. Thereafter it remained constant for the A-leg and it was 1.1 mmol min^{-1} after 10 min, which was higher (p<0.05) than the uptake by the P-leg (0.1 mmol min^{-1}) The total net uptake of glucose was 6.65 (P-leg) and 9.82 mmol (A-leg) (p<0.05).

O_2 debt

In experiment I leg VO_2 at the end of exercise was 0.61 l min^{-1} and decreased rapidly to 0.11 and 0.03 l min^{-1} respectively. In the remaining part of recovery the decline in leg VO_2 was moderate, and 60 min elapsed before it returned to resting level (0.02 l min^{-1}). The leg O_2 debt (VO_2 - pre-exercise VO_2) was 0.42 (0-3 min), 0.21 (3-10 min) and 0.89 (10-60 min) l and totalled 1.51 l during 1 h of recovery (Fig. 4). The pulmonary O_2 debt was 4.51 l for the entire 60 min.

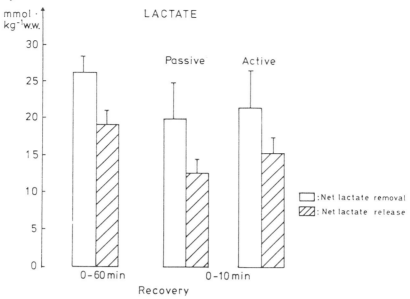

Fig. 2 Net decrease in muscle lactate (open columns) and net release of lactate (filled columns) during 1 h of recovery in Experiment I (0-60 min) and during 10 min of passive and active recovery in experiment II (0-10 min) (data from Bangsbo et al, 1991a,c).

The ATP concentration decreased to 4.2 ± 0.5 mmol kg^{-1} w.w. during EX1, and increased to 5.5 ± 0.2 mmol kg^{-1} w.w. after 10 min (Table 1). The CP concentration increased from 7.6 mmol kg^{-1} w.w. at the end of EX1 to 12.5, 17.1 and 19.6 mmol.kg^{-1} w.w. during the first 3, next 7 and last 50 min of recovery, respectively (Table 1). The net resynthesis of ATP and CP could account for 25 and 5% of the O_2 debt during 0-10 and 10-60 min of recovery, respectively (Fig. 4).

Active recovery

In experiment II the leg VO_2 during recovery was higher in the A-leg than the P-leg. After 0.8 min of recovery it was 0.30 (A-leg) and 0.12 (P-leg) l min^{-1} . Thereafter VO_2 remained constant for the A-leg, while it decreased for the P-leg, being 0.26 (A-leg) and 0.02 (P-leg) l min^{-1} after 10 min of recovery. The latter

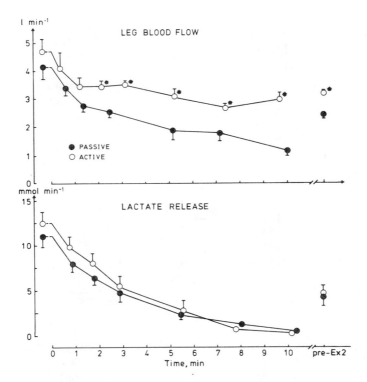

Fig. 3 Leg blood flow (upper) and lactate release (lower) during 10 min of passive (filled symbols) and active (open symbols) recovery (data from Bangsbo et al, 1991c). *: Significant ($p<0.05$) difference between passive and active recovery.

values were higher ($p<0.05$) than the VO_2 during the 10 W exercise prior to the intense exercise (0.20 l min^{-1}) and than the resting VO_2 (0.02 l min $^{-1}$), respectively. The total leg oxygen debt for the P-leg of 0.44 l was lower ($p<0.05$) compared to the oxygen debt (leg VO_2 - leg VO_2 at 10W) for the A-leg (0.75 l) (Fig. 4).

The muscle concentrations of ATP at the end of EX1 (5.0 mmol kg $^{-1}$ w.w.) increased during 10 min of recovery to the resting level for the P-leg (6.1 mmol

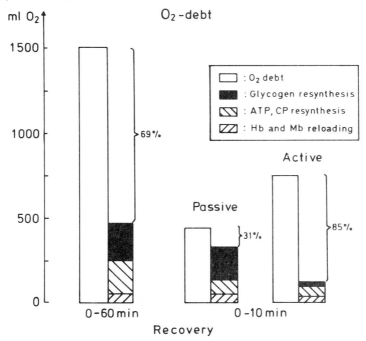

Fig. 4 Oxygen debt and estimated reloading of Hb and Mb ( ), energy demand of resynthesis of ATP and CP ( ) and glycogen ( ) in the quadriceps muscle during 1 h of recovery in Experiment I (0-60 min) and during 10 min of passive and active recovery in Experiment II (0-10 min) (data from Bangsbo et al, 1991a,c).

kg^{-1} w.w.), but not for the A-leg (5.4 mmol kg^{-1} w.w.) (Table 1). The muscle CP concentration was 3.6 mmol kg^{-1} w.w. at the end of EX1, and increased rapidly during recovery for both legs, being similar to the resting level after 10 min (Table 1). The net rebuilding of ATP and CP could account for 19 and 8% of the O_2 debt for the P- and A-leg, respectively (Fig. 4).

Energy production and performance of subsequent exercise

In experiment I the exhaustive exercise was repeated after 1 h of recovery and time to exhaustion in EX2 was reduced ($p < -0.05$) to 91% of EX1 (2.87 min). The decrease of muscle glycogen in EX2 was 22.5 mmol kg^{-1} w.w. or 13% less than during EX1, but the mean glycogen utilization rate was about 10 mmol kg^{-1} w.w. min^{-1} for both EX1 and EX2. Lactate production was reduced by 39% in EX2 ($p < 0.05$) (Fig. 5).

This was reflected in a reduced lactate production rate duringEX2, which amounted to 6.7 as compared to 10.1 mmol kg^{-1} w.w. min during EX1 ($p < 0.05$).

The oxygen deficit was lowered from 0.88 (EX1) to 0.82 (EX2) l O_2 Eq min^{-1}, but ATP and CP utilization, and the accumulation of ADP, AMP and IMP was similar for the two exercise bouts. The increase in leg oxygen uptake was also similar for EX1 and EX2, but the total oxygen uptake was 14% lower (p<0.05) for EX2 due to the shorter exercise time. The K$^+$ release during EX2 was similar to that occurring during EX1, with no difference between EX1 and EX2 in neither arterial (4.91 and 4.95 mmol l^{-1}, respectively) nor venous plasma K$^+$ concentration (5.85 and 5.71 mmol l^{-1}, respectively) at exhaustion.

Table 1   Muscle CP and ATP concentrations (mmol kg^{-1} w.w.) in recovery from EX1 in Experiment I (Exp. I) and II (Exp. II) with either passive (P) or active (A) recovery

Recovery, min	0	3	10	60
CP				
Exp. I	7.06 ±0.5	12.5 ±2.1	17.1 ±2.1	19.6 ±1.0
Exp. II - P	3.6 ±0.4	14.2 ±1.3	20.7 ±1.1	
Exp. II - A	3.6 ±0.4	16.8 ±0.9	18.3 ±1.3	
ATP				
Exp. I	4.21 ±0.51	4.92 ±0.49	5.48 ±0.22	5.68 ±0.42
Exp. II - P	5.06 ±0.63	4.55 ±0.42	6.06 ±0.45	
Exp. II - A	5.06 ±0.63	5.07 ±0.53	5.42 ±0.55	

Active recovery

In experiment II the recovery period was reduced to 16 min and during the last part of this period seven bouts of very intense exercise were performed. Thus, muscle lactate was elevated prior to EX2 and more so for the P-leg than for the A-leg (13.1 and 9.9 mmol kg^{-1} w.w., respectively), and muscle pH for the P-leg (6.85) and A-leg (6.84) prior to EX2 was lower (p<0.05) than before EX1 (7.04). Also muscle glycogen was lower prior to EX2 (94.1 (P-leg) and 97.2 (A-leg) mmol kg^{-1} w.w.) compared to EX1 (133.5 mmol-kg^{-1} w.w.).

The metabolic responses during EX2 were more extreme than those described above for the EX2 after 1 h recovery. For the P-leg the time to exhaustion for EX2-P was reduced by 45 s or 20% compared to EX1 (3.73 min), hence twice as much as in experiment I. The reduction for the A-leg was 13% or slightly less than for the P-leg. The muscle glycogen utilization during EX2 was depressed compared with EX1, and the reduction amounted to 6.6 (P-leg) and 3.4 (A-leg) mmol kg^{-1} w.w. or 26 and 13%. Lactate production during EX2 was reduced compared to EX1 by 18.7 (P-leg) and 16.5 (A-leg) mmol kg^{-1} w.w. or 55 and 52%, which values were greater than those observed in experiment I (Fig. 5).

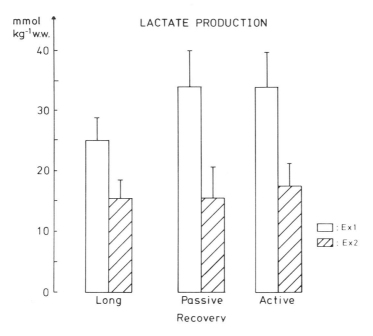

Fig. 5   Muscle lactate production during EX1 and EX2 performed after 1 h of recovery in Experiment I or after intermittent exercise with either passive or active recovery in experiment II (data from Bangsbo et al, 1991a,b,c).

The oxygen deficit for the P-leg was 22% lower ($p>0.05$) during EX2 as a result of the shorter exercise time, while the difference of 28% ($p<0.05$) for the A-leg primarily was an effect of the elevated leg VO_2 at the start of EX2. Actual changes in CP and ATP during EX1 and EX2 were similar and the same accumulation of ADP, AMP and IMP occurred at the end of EX1 and EX2 (Table 2).

For the A-leg the total oxygen uptake was the same for EX1 (1.67 l) and EX2 (1.59 l), while for the P-leg the oxygen uptake during EX2 was 9% lower ($p>0.05$) compared to EX1 as a result of the shorter exercise time. At exhaustion following the EX2 bouts muscle pH was 6.77 for both the P- and A-leg, which tended to be higher ($p<0.1$) than at the end of EX1 (6 73).

The total K^+ release during EX1 of 5.1 (P-leg) and 5.2 (A-leg) mmol tended ($p<0.1$) to be higher than the release during EX2 (3.9 and 3.0 mmol) as a result of the difference in exercise time. The arterial-venous K^+ difference at exhaustion was the same for EX1 and EX2, as were the femoral venous plasma concentrations similar for both the P-leg (6.15 (EX1) and 5.93 (EX2) mmol l^{-1}) and the A-leg, (6.05 (EX1) and 5.93 (EX2) mmol l^{-1}).

Discussion

Lactate removal and glycogen synthesis

More than two-thirds of the lactate that accumulated in muscle during intense exercise was released to the blood during 1 h of recovery in experiment I. The relative release was similar during the first two periods (0-3 and 3-10) and higher during the last 50 min, when blood flow was lower, indicating that blood flow is not crucial for the lactate efflux to blood. This was supported by the finding of a similar release whether the leg performed passive or active recovery, when the blood flow was elevated. The large release of lactate results in less than one-third of the accumulated lactate at exhaustion was available for metabolism within the muscle. Some of this lactate might have been converted to glycogen (glyconeogenesis), but the question is how much?

The amount of carbohydrate for oxidation was calculated from leg VO_2 and leg RQ, and it corresponded to 11 mmol lactate (pyruvate) during the 1 h of recovery. It appears that the majority of the carbohydrate oxidized was lactate, since the carbohydrate oxidation primarily occurred during the first 10 min, when there is the greatest potential to form pyruvate from lactate due to the high concentration of the latter. This notion is supported by Bendall and Taylor's (1970) finding that the glycogen synthesis equalled the lactate available for glyconeogenesis, when the latter was calculated based on the assumption that lactate was the only substrate for carbohydrate oxidation. Thus, if lactate was the substrate for the entire carbohydrate oxidation, at the most 13% of the accumulated lactate was used for glyconeogenesis (Fig. 6). Part of this could have been converted to alanine, but this route seems not quantitatively important (Felig & Wahren, 1974; Bangsbo et al, 1991a). Similar findings were obtained during 10 min of recovery in Experiment II, with no difference between active and passive recovery.

The lactate removed within the muscle could account for 19% of the total carbohydrate metabolism during 1 h of recovery (Fig. 7). The question is, what was the substrate for the remaining carbohydrate turnover? The magnitude of the glucose nptake equalled a carbohydrate metabolism of 18.2 mmol (37% of total) or 45% of the glycogen resynthesis, if all the glucose was converted to glycogen. The remaining substrate for the carbohydrate utilization might have been the glycolytic intermediates, which accumulated during exercise and declined during recovery. These are quantitatively large enough to account for a major part of the remaining carbohydrate metabolism (Fig. 7). These findings are in agreement with results from in vitro studies showing that glucose was the dominant substrate for glycogen synthesis in recovery (Shiota et al, 1986; Bonen et al, 1990).

Table 2 Muscle CP and nucleotide concentrations (mmol kg^{-1} w.w.) before (PRE) and after (POST) the exhaustive exercise bouts (EX1 and EX2) in experiment II.

	Passive			Active	
	EX1		EX2		EX2	
PRE	POST	PRE	POST	PRE	POST
CP 19.75	3.63	15.46	3.32	16.40	3.11
±0.43	±0.36	±1.81	±2.76	±2.26	±1.29
ATP 6.15	5.06	4.90*	3.99*	4.96*	3.57*
±0.42	±0.63	±0.65	±0.72	±0.53	±0.60
ADP 0.69	0.70	0.59	0.61	0.61	0.66
±0.07	±0.04	±0.09	±0.11	±0.07	±0.10
AMP 0.02	0.05	0.10*	0.12*	0.04	0.15*
±0.00	±0.02	±0.02	±0.03	±0.01	±0.03
IMP <0.01	0.42	0.38*	0.51	0.13	0.83
	±0.14	±0.16	±0.21	±0.09	±0.35

Means ±SE are given.   *: Significant difference (p<0.05) between EX1 and EX2.

However, they are not in accordance with studies by Astrand et al (1986) and Hermansen & Vaage (1977), who estimated that more than 44 and 75%, respectively, of the lactate present in the muscle at the end of exercise could have supported glycogen synthesis. It is difficult to compare the results of the present study with those of Astrand et al, (1986) since they used an indirect estimation. The deviation from the findings of Hermansen and Vaage (1977) was related to a markedly lower leg blood flow in their study. They used plethysmography blood flow determinations of the calf after bicycle exercise in the calculation of lactate release, and glucose uptake from the limb after treadmill exercise. Thus, it is likely that the latter values were underestimated and the role of lactate for glyconeogenesis was overestimated in their study.

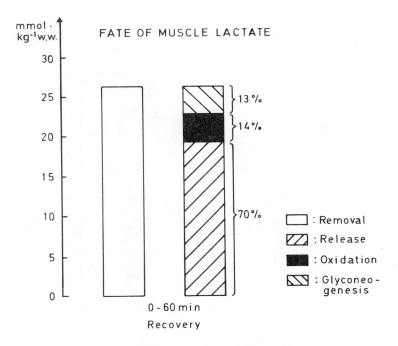

Fig. 6   Fate of intramuscular lactate accumulated at the end of EX1 during 1 h of recovery in Experiment I (data from Bangsbo et al, 1991a).

Oxygen debt

During 60 min of recovery the whole body O_2 debt was 4.5 l of which the leg accounted for one-third or 1.5 l, and during 10 min of recovery it was 0.48 l for the P-leg and higher for the A-leg (0.75 l). Part of the O_2 debt could be attributed to reloading of Hb and Mb, resynthesis of ATP, CP and glycogen, but these could only account for minor fractions of the O_2 debt during the recovery periods (Fig. 4). It is unclear what causes the remaining elevation of VO_2 after exercise.

At early recovery, energy needed for the restoration of ionic homeostasis may to some extent have increased the oxygen expenditure. During the remaining part

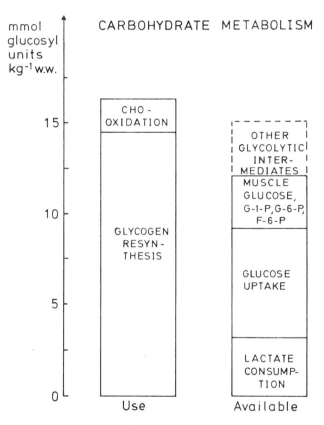

Fig. 7   Carbohydrate metabolism (left) and available carbohydrates (right), including data of some glycolytic intermediates obtained from other studies (dotted bar), during 1 h of recovery in Experiment I (data from Bangsbo et al, 1991a).

of recovery the extra energy consumption may be linked with fat turnover. The finding of a large net release of glycerol and a minor net uptake of FFA from the blood suggest that triacylglycerol (TG), either intramuscular or blood borne, is the major substrate for fat oxidation during recovery (Fig. 8). Then, part of the higher VO_2 after exercise might have been related to high activity of the TG-fatty acid substrate cycle which in turn has been shown to be energy demanding e.g. the net cost of one turn of the triacylglycerol-fatty acid substrate cycle is eight molecules of ATP (Brooks et al, 1983; Wolfe & Peters, 1987). This notion was supported by the finding of a higher O_2 debt during active compared to passive recovery, since total fat oxidation most likely was elevated during active recovery. Increased post-exercise catecholamine concentrations and elevated temperature have been suggested to cause elevation in muscle metabolic rate (Maehlum et al, 1986). However, they are unlikely explanations in the present study as the changes in these variables are small during knee-extensor exercise, and both variables returned to control level within 20 min of recovery.

Performance and anaerobic energy production during subsequent exercise

In experiment II performance of EX2 was reduced. The question is, to what extent was this caused by elevated lactate and acidity prior to this exercise? It appears not to be very dramatic, since the same responses were also observed, although not to the same extent, after 1 h of recovery even though muscle and blood lactate was almost back to resting level. Furthermore, in the latter experiment muscle lactate concentration at the end of EX2 was significantly lower compared to EX1. The findings of large variation between subjects of muscle lactate and pH at exhaustion, and that muscle pH tended to be higher at the end of the second exercise bouts in experiment II, although muscle pH was lowered prior to these exercises, indicates further that muscle pH is not crucial for development of fatigue. In accordance with these findings are data from Sahlin and Ren (1989) showing that despite a persistently high muscle lactate (probably lowered muscle pH), contraction force was completely restored 2 min after intensive isometric muscle contractions. Thus, it appears that other factors caused fatigue and impaired performance in the second exercise bouts. Lack of available ATP does not appear to be among these, since in every case muscle ATP at exhaustion was only slightly lower than the level prior to exercise (less than 20%). This conclusion was supported by a lower anaerobic energy production during the second exercise bout after the active recovery when the initial oxygen uptake was elevated compared to the EX2-P. Thus, the exercise was terminated before the anaerobic capacity was utilized. It appears that the elements responsible for the development of fatigue are retarding cross-bridge cycling and, thus, concomitant usage of ATP, which leads to a gradual decrease in muscle tension development and ultimately to exhaustion. The same reduction in ATP concentration in each exercise bout indicates that ATP utilization is tightly matched by its rate of resynthesis.

Another site for failure of the excitation-contracting coupling (EC) would be an inhibition of the propagation of the action potential (AP) due to ion disturbances over the sarcolemma (Sjogaard, 1991). During the exhaustive exercise K_+ was released in similar amounts during the different interventions. The absolute value for its loss was rather small due to the short exercise times. More importantly, however, was the finding of identical femoral venous K_+ concentrations at exhaustion, as these reflect the interstitial K^+ concentration of the muscle. The question, however, is whether a venous K^+ concentration of 6 mM is high enough

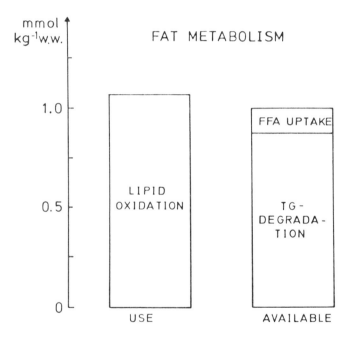

Fig. 8   Total fat oxidation calculated from leg RQ and VO_2 (left) and available FFA (right) determined from net FFA uptake and net glycerol release (TG degradation) during 1 h of recovery in Experiment I (data from Bangsbo et al, 1991a).

to slow the AP and possibly block its propagation into the T tubuli.

The neural activation of the muscle may also be reduced during an exhaustive exercise bout. A central nervous (cortical) origin is unlikely. A more plausible explanation would be inhibition at the spinal level. Garland and McComas (1990) have recently demonstrated reflex inhibition occurring during fatiguing exercise of the soleus muscle. The question to be raised in relation to the present experiment is: What could activate such a reflex? It is tempting to suggest certain metabolites or ions accumulatlng in the interstitium of active muscle, triggering sensory receptors of group III and IV nerve fibres. Again, K^+ as well as H^+ could be the compounds. The scheme which may prevail is that this sensory input causes inhibition of spinal motor nerves. This is likely a gradual phenomenon, and can at first be overcome by the drive from the motor cortex as new motor units are activated. A point is reached, however, where the reflex inhibition causes a reduction in spinal motor activity output, adding to the inability of the muscle to reach target force and maintain kicking rate. Characteristically, this failure to produce sufficient force recovers very rapidly. This is not to say that it is possible to perform at the same exercise intensity for long periods, but after some 20-60 s of rest, the exercise can be continued at the same intensity for a brief time (Sahlin and Ren, 1989). This could be related to the quick normalization of the K^+ which occurs upon termination of the exercise. The time course for a change is quite different from that of H^+ (Fig. 9), which suggests that K^+ rather than H^+ would be the critical factor, or a compound which is as quickly restored to normal level as K^+.

Performance during the second exercise bout after the active recovery was less impaired than exercise followed by passive recovery. Based on the discussion above and the fact that the same muscle pH was observed prior to the two exercise bouts, lower muscle lactate prior to EX2-A cannot explain the difference in performance. Other factors involved in the development of muscle fatigue must have been influenced by the low intensity exercise.

The intense intermittent exercise prior to the second exercise bouts also resulted in a lowering of the glycogenolytic rate and lactate production rate during the subsequently intense exercise, which was not influenced by the low intensity activities during the recovery periods. The question remains as to what causes these effects. The lowered muscle glycogen concentration is an unlikely candidate, since it has been demonstrated that glycogenolytic and glycolytic rates during short term intense exercise are independent of initial muscle glycogen concentration above 30 mmol kg^{-1} w.w. (Bangsbo et al, 1991d). The lowered pH prior to the second exercise bout could be a possibility, as it has been shown in vitro that elevated H^+ in the muscle inhibits phosphorylase and PFK activities, both of which being considered the key regulating enzymes of the glycogenolytic and glycolytic rates, respectively (Danforth, 1965; Chasiotis, 1983). However, it is questionable whether the reduction in pH was large enough to inhibit these enzymes in vivo. Recent studies on the allosteric regulation of PFK within the physiological range have shown that the effect of pH is negated as long as pH is above 6.6 (Dobson et al, 1986; Spriet et al, 1987), and the lactate production rate was also significantly reduced even after 1 h of recovery. Thus, it appears that the elevated H^+ concentration is not the only explanation for the reduction in glycolytic rate.

There were no indications, however, that other crucial factors are changed. Alteration of ATP (decrease), ADP, AMP and IMP (increase) were similar for all exercise bouts, and would appear to cause the same degree of activation. However, it cannot be excluded that the ratio between bound and unbound is changed from

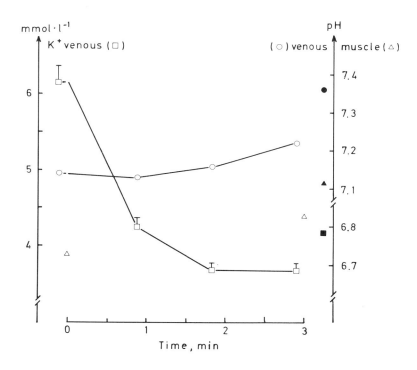

Fig. 9   Changes in femoral venous K^+ and pH during the first 3 min of recovery after exhaustive knee-extensor exercise. The filled symbols to the right depict pre-exercise values (data from Bangsbo et al, 1991b).

EX1 to EX2. A higher binding of ADP, AMP and IMP during EX2 would lower the stimulating effect on PFK, and thus, rate of glycolysis. Cytosolic citrate has been proposed to stimulate the fructose-1, 6-diphosphatase activity and to be an inhibitor of PFK activity, and it has been shown that muscle citrate was elevated during intense intermittent exercise (Parmeggiani et al, 1963; Fu and Kemp, 1973; Essen, 1978). Thus, elevated citrate concentrations prior to the EX2 bouts in the present experiments might have inhibited the glycolysis particularly at the initial phase of exercise. This is supported by a lower efflux of lactate even after 45 s despite a higher muscle lactate concentration before EX2 in experiment II, indicating retardation of glycolysis from the start of exercise. However, the rate of oxidation during exercise was similar in all experiments, which suggests that supply of acetyl-CoA from b-oxidation or decarboxylation of pyruvate was not enhanced during the EX2 bouts. Furthermore, although oxygen uptake prior to EX2 was higher for the active leg compared to the passive leg, and perhaps higher muscle citrate concentrations were obtained, the same reduction of the glycolytic rate occurred during EX2 for the two legs. Thus, it is questionable if elevated cytosolic citrate concentration was the cause of the lowered glycolytic activity during EX2.

Summary

More than two-thirds of the lactate that accumulated in the muscle during the intense exercise was released to the blood, and a maximum of 27% was converted to glycogen. Low intensity exercise during recovery elevated muscle lactate removal, but not lactate release to the blood. Glucose absorbed from the blood stream and muscle glycolytic intermediates accumulated during the exercise were the dominant substrates for glycogen synthesis. Furthermore, intramuscular/bloodborne TG appeared to be the major source of fat oxidation during recovery, and energy turnover related to the fat-metabolism might account for a significant part of the O_2 debt in recovery after exercise.

Previous intense exercise had definite effects on subsequent short term intense exercise, resulting in a lowering of lactate production and performance. These effects appear not to be directly related to elevated muscle lactate and H^+ concentrations.

Acknowledgement

The study was supported by grants from Team Danmark and Danish Natural Science Foundation (11-7776).

References

Astrand P-0, Hultman E, Juhlin-Danfelt A and Reynolds G. (1986) Disposal of lactate during and after strenuous exercise. Journal of Applied Physiology 61, 338-343.

Bangsbo J, Gollnick PD, Graham TE, Juel C, Kiens B, Mizuno M and Saltin B. (1990) Anaerobic energy production & O_2 deficit - debt relationship during exhaustive exercise in humans. J Physiol, **422**, 539-559.

Bangsbo J, Gollnick PD, Graham TE and Saltin B. (1991) Substrates for muscle glycogen synthesis in recovery from intense exercise in man. J Physiol, **434**, 423-440.

Bangsbo J, Graham T, Johansen L, Strange S and Saltin B. (1991b) Elevated muscle acidity and energy production during exhaustive exercise in man. J Physiol, submitted.

Bangsbo J, Johansen L, Graham TE and Saltin B. (1991c) Lactate efflux from skeletal muscle in man. J Appl Physiol, submitted.

Bangsbo J, Graham TE, Kiens B and Saltin B. (1991d) Elevated muscle glycogen and anaerobic energy production during exhaustive exercise in man. J Physiol, submitted.

Bendall JR and Taylor A. (1970) The Meyerhof quotient and the synthesis of glycogen from lactate in frog and rabbit muscle. Biochem J, **118**, 887-893.

Bonen A, McDermott JC and Tan MH. (1990) Glycogenesis and glyconeogenesis in skeletal muscle: effects of pH and hormones. Am J Physiol, **21**, E693-E700.

Boobis LH. (1987) Metabolic aspects of fatigue during sprinting. in "Exercise, Benefits, Limits and Adaptations" (eds. Macleod D, Maughan R, Nimmo M, Reilly T and Williams C). E & FN Spon, London/New York, pp. 116-143.

Brooks BJ, Arch JRS and Newsholme EA. (1983) Effect of some hormones on the rate of the triacylglycerol/fatty acid substrate cycle in adipose tissue of the mouse :in vivo. Biosci Rep, **3**, 263-267.

Chasiotis D. (1983) The regulation of glycogen phosphorylase and glycogen breakdown in human skeletal muscle. Acta Physiol Scand Suppl, **518**, 1-68.

Danforth WH. (1965) Activation of glycolytic pathway in muscle. In "Control of energy metabolism" (eds. Chance B, Estrabrook BW, Williamson JR). New York, Academic press, pp. 287-297.

Dobson GP, Yamamoto E and Hochachka PW. (1986) Phosphofructokinase control in muscle: Nature and reversal of pH-dependent ATP inhibition. Am J Physiol, **250**, R71-76.

Dodds S, Powers SK, Callender T and Brooks E. (1984) Blood lactate disappearance at various intensities of recovery exercise. J Appl Physiol, **57**, 1462-1465.

Essen B. (1978) Studies on the regulation of metabolism in human skeletal muscle using intermittent exercise as an experimental model. Acta Physiol Scand Suppl, **454**, 1-32.

Felig P and Wahren J. (1974) Amino acids metabolism in exercising man. J Clin Invest, **50**, 2703-2714.

Fu JY and Kemp RG. (1973) Activation of muscle fructose 1,6 diphosphatase by creatine and citrate. J Biol Chem, **248**, 1124-1125.

Gaitanos GC. (1990) Human muscle metabolism during intermittent maximal exercise. PhD thesis. Loughborough University, 1990.

Garland SJ. and McComas AJ. (1990) Reflex inhibition of human soleus muscle during fatigue. J Physiol, **429**, 17-27.

Hermansen L and Stendsvold I. (1972) Production and removal of lactate during exercise in man. Acta Physiol Scand, **86**, 191-201.

Hermansen L and Vaage O (1977) Lactate disappearance and glycogen synthesis in human muscle after maximal exercise. Am J Physiol, **233**, E422-E429.

Hultman E and Sjoholm H. (1983) Substrate availability. In "Biochemistry of Exercise" (eds. Knuttgen HC, Vogel JA and Poortmans J). Champeign IL. Human Kinetics, pp. 63-75.

Juel C, Bangsbo J and Saltin B. (1990) Lactate and potassium fluxes from skeletal muscle during intense dynamic knee-extensor exercise in man. Acta Physiol Scand, **140**, 147-159.

Mainwood GW and Renaud JM. (1985) The effect of acid-base balance on fatigue of skeletal muscle. Can J Physiol Pharmacol, **63**, 403-416.

McCartney N, Spriet LL, Heigenhauser JF, Kowalchuk JM, Sutton JR and Jones NL (1986) Muscle power and metabolism in maximal intermittent exercise. J Appl Physiol, **60**, 1164-1169.

Maehlum S, Grandmontagne M, Newsholme EA and Sejersted O. (1986) Magnitude and duration of excess post-exercise oxygen consumption in healthy young subjects. Metabolism, **35**, 425-429.

Parmeggiani A and Bowman RH. (1963) Regulation of phosphofructokinase activity by citrate in normal and diabetic muscle. Biochem Biophys Res Comm, **12**, 268-273.

Sahlin K, Harris RC and Hultman E. (1979) Resynthesis of creatine phosphate in human muscle after exercise in relation to intramuscular pH and availability of oxygen. Scand J Invest, **39**, 551-558.

Sahlin K and Henrikson J. (1984) Buffer capacity and lactate accumulation in skeletal muscle of trained and untrained men. Acta Physiol Scand, **122**, 331-339.

Sahlin K and Ren JM. (1989) Relationship of contraction capacity changes during recovery from a fatiguing contraction. J Appl Physiol, **67**, 648-654.

Shiota M, Golden S and Katz J. (1984) Lactate metabolism in the perfused rat hindlimb. Biochem J, **222**, 281-292.

Siegel S. (1965) Nomparametric Statistics for the behavioral Sciences. McGraw-Hill, New York, 1965.

Sjogaard G, Adams RP and Saltin B. (1985) Water and ion shifts in skeletal muscle of humans with intense dynamic knee extension. Am J Physiol, **248**, R190-196.

Sjogaard G. (1990) Exercise induced muscle fatigue: the significance of potassium. Acta Physiol Scand, **140** (Suppl 593), 1-63.

Spriet LL, Soderlund K, Bergstrom M and Hultman E. (1987) Skeletal muscle glycogenolysis, glycolysis and pH during electrical stimulation in men. J Appl Physiol, **62**, 616-621.

Spriet LL Lindinger MI, McKelvie S, Heigenhauser GJF and Jones NL. (1989) Muscle glycogenolysis and H_+ concentration during maximal intermittent cycling. J Appl Physiol, **66**, 8-13.

Wolfe RR and Peters EJ. (1987) Lipolytic response to glucose infusion in human subjects. Am J Physio, **252**, E218-E223.

Wotton and Williams C. (1983) The influence of recovery duration on repeated maximal sprints. In "Biochemistry of Exercise" (eds. Knuttgen HC, Vogel JA and Poortmans J) Champeign IL: Human Kinetics.

Preparation for performance

R.J. Hazeldine and D.J. Holmyard

Abstract. This consideration of preparation for performance is based on work carried out with the England Rugby Union squad. Successful Rugby Football at international level requires a high level of physical fitness. The structuring and implementation of the preparation programme covers three main areas of interest: planning and periodisation of training; monitoring of fitness levels and interpretation of results. A year long periodised training schedule was devised leading to the 1991 Five Nations Championship. Testing was administered at 2-3 month intervals. The parameters assessed on each player (nine forwards, nine backs) were height, weight, body fat percentage, maximum oxygen uptake, speed and anaerobic capacity. A student t-test revealed significant differences between the individuals in the different player units. The forwards were taller [$p > 0.05$] and heavier [$p < 0.01$] than the backs. For the whole group a one-way analysis of variance revealed a significant fall in percentage body fat [$p < 0.001$] and a significant increase in predicted maximum oxygen uptake [$p < 0.001$] during the monitoring period. There was a significant reduction in 30m sprint time for the whole group with the fastest mean time in January 1991 [4.34 ± 0.16] and [3.90 ± 0.10s] for sub-groups of forwards and backs respectively. There were no significant changes in mean anaerobic capacity as predicted from a high intensity shuttle run test. The results demonstrated that international rugby union players in this squad experienced significant improvements in body composition, aerobic power and speed but no significant changes in anaerobic power during the training programme. The integration of fitness testing and monitoring with the devising and structuring of the training schedules proved effective in that it enabled more precise, individualistic training to be presented and provided evaluation of the effectiveness of the training methods prescribed.

Keywords: Training; Fitness; Periodisation; Rugby Union

Introduction

This consideration of preparation for performance will be based on Rugby Football in general and the England Rugby Squad in particular. Rugby Football at International level requires a high level of physical fitness. The essence of rugby is the ability to sustain high levels of skill at high speed over the full eighty minutes of the game. The aim of any preparation programme is to make this possible. Fitness, in effect, is the background against which skill can be achieved and maintained within the game. The core of fitness lies in endurance, the ability to sustain high quality effort and produce whatever skills and techniques a player possesses over the whole game. The crisis-point in many games is towards the end of the first half and more often towards the end of the second half when fatigue begins to dull vision, errors begin to occur, tackles are missed. Endurance fitness enables players to retain the quality of their play in these crucial periods. Of course, endurance is not the only element. Running speed is also critical, as rugby is essentially a running game. Similarly, strength, particularly upper body strength, is essential, and leg power. Rugby is also a multi-sprint activity, with intervals of work and rest, which requires large bursts of energy over short periods of time and the need to recover quickly.

Fitness training for rugby football involves an endless search for the link between training and performance. The starting point is an evaluation of the fitness requirements of rugby and in order to clarify the various components which affect fitness for the game it is useful to develop a model of physical fitness for rugby football. This enables the fitness elements which make up the training programme to be identified. This evaluation is then developed into firstly **match demands:** for example in the 1991 Wales v England game there were 132 sequences of play of which 98 lasted from 0-14 seconds. Secondly, the **positional requirements** appreciating that rugby of all games incorporates the most marked inter-positional differences in fitness requirements. Thirdly, the player profile which incorporates the individual needs of the player.

The structuring and implementation of the fitness preparation programme covers three main areas of interest:

1. Planning and periodisation of training involving the sub-division of the training year into macro, meso and micro-cycles taking into account Club league matches, Divisional matches and the performance peaks required for International matches.
2. Monitoring of fitness levels involving the regular implementation of a battery of valid and reliable tests.
3. Interpretation of the results to players and coaches with the prescription of individualised training programmes.

Planning and periodisation of training

At the outset planning is based on a simple cycle of training which includes preparation, competition and recuperation. Training is planned on a year-long cyclical process, but one which is also part of a long-term progression of training. The structure has to meet the particular training and match requirements of a team. An example of this is the England squad's training schedule for the 1991 Five Nations Championship. The training plan which was illustrated in the form of a colour-coded chart, given to each player, was periodised into training cycles with particular goals and fitness objectives within each macro-cycle. The plan shows the time-scale in weeks; the international, divisional and club commitments of the players; the squad training and fitness testing sessions; the macro-cycles and meso-cycles specifying the area of fitness to be developed; the micro-cycle specifying the details of each training session which would be prescribed after each testing session; the changes in volume of training and the timing and loadings to achieve peak levels of fitness. The training plan attempts to show how all these factors need to be considered and successfully integrated into a total fitness training schedule.

Monitoring of fitness levels

Physical and physiological parameters can be measured at various stages of the training programme in order to monitor the training-induced changes in the player's fitness. For the England Rugby squad testing was administered at 2-3 month intervals to monitor fitness levels, provide a fitness profile for each player and to assist with the planning of training programmes based on a player's strengths and weaknesses. For reasons of convenience, the tests had to be conducted in a field environment at National Squad training.

The parameters assessed on each player were height, weight, body fat percentage, maximum oxygen uptake, flexibility, speed and anaerobic capacity.

Standard measurements of weight and height were taken for each player. Body fat was measured at four sites (biceps, triceps, subscapular, iliac crest. The percentage of body fat was calculated according to the procedures of Durnin and Womersley (1974) and lean body mass was calculated from body weight and absolute body fat. A 20m progressive shuttle run test (Ramsbottom, Brewer and Williams, 1988) was used to determine indirectly each player's maximum oxygen uptake.

For flexibility a Sit and Reach test according to Wells and Dillon (1952) was used in addition to a modified test performed on each leg separately. Speed was assessed from 15m and 30m sprints conducted from a standing start one metre behind an electronic beam. Timing began once the first beam was broken and stopped when the player crossed the beam of the finish line.

Muscular endurance was assessed through two field tests:

1. Paced push-ups: an extended push-up procedure was performed to a series of bleeps on an audio cassette at the rate of 50 b.p.m. On the first bleep the arms were flexed so that the chest touched a tester's clenched fist placed immediately below the chest, and at the next bleep the arms were back in the extended position. As many repetitions as possible maintaining the dictated pace were required.

2. <u>Paced trunk curls</u>: the procedure involves the player on his back with bent legs, feet supported, arms folded across the chest and to a series of bleeps on an audio cassette at 50 b.p.m., the player sat up to touch the elbows to thighs on the first bleep, then back to touch shoulders to the floor on the next bleep. As many repetitions as possible maintaining the dictated pace were required.

Leg power was measured using a jump meter which was fixed round the waist with the end of the cord attached to a rubber mat. With any necessary arm swings the player bent at the knees and drove vertically upwards from the mat. The height of the vertical jump was recorded on the meter.

A 20m high intensity shuttle run test (Ramsbottom, Hazeldine, Nevill and Williams, 1990) was used to indirectly estimate maximal accumulated oxygen deficit which was used as an indicator of anaerobic capacity. This test was based on laboratory work designed to estimate maximal accumulated oxygen deficit during treadmill running. Initially oxygen demand during supramaximal exercise (i.e. during exercise designed to engage the anaerobic energy system maximally) was calculated from the individual relationship between oxygen demand and running speed established during submaximal exercise (Hermansen and Medbo, 1984; Medbo et al, 1988). In order to establish maximal values for oxygen deficit the subjects exercised at 120% of their respective maximal oxygen uptake values to voluntary exhaustion. The accumulated oxygen demand was taken as the product of the O_2 demand and the duration of the exercise. The accumulated oxygen uptake was the product of the total exercise time and the measured O_2 during exercise. The accumulated oxygen deficit was the difference between the accumulated oxygen demand and the accumulated oxygen uptake (Medbo et al, 1988).

In developing the high intensity shuttle run test subjects performed two field tests. The first test was the 20m progressive shuttle run test which indirectly predicted maximum oxygen uptake and determined the maximal "aerobic" running speed. From the results of this test subjects were asked to perform "sprint" shuttle runs at a speed equivalent to 120% of their maximal aerobic running speed. The performance criterion was the total number of 20m shuttles the subject performed at the respective level and this was used as a determination of their anaerobic capacity.

During the monitoring period 18 players from the England Rugby Squad were studied for selected anthropometric and physiological characteristics on five occasions at 2-3 month intervals. The players were sub-divided into positional categories: 9 forwards (2 Props, 2 Hookers, 2 Locks, 3 Backrow) and 9 backs (2 Scrum Halves, 2 Flyhalves, 1 Centre, 3 Wings, 1 Fullback). The players were assessed in January 1990 (mid-season), April 1990 (end of season), June 1990 (early off season), September 1990 (pre-season) and January 1991 (mid-season). The players followed a training programme designed to achieve peak levels of fitness in January 1991 for the Five Nations Championship. Each macro-cycle of training contained particular objectives based on increases in the major fitness components of endurance, strength, power, speed and flexibility. At each stage the training schedules were outlined in detail. The players were required to complete on average five sessions of one to one-and-a-half hours per week. This volume of training was increased at particular phases in the schedule.

A one-way analysis of variance was used to examine changes in the means of the whole group of players (n=18) over the five testing sessions, whilst a students' t-test was used to assess differences in the means of forwards and backs at any one session.

There have been several studies which have reported the physiological and anthropometric characteristics of Rugby Union players (Williams et al, 1973; Bell, 1980; Maud, 1983; Maud & Schultz, 1984; Cheetham et al, 1987; Ueno et al, 1987; Rigg and Reilly, 1987). In studies which have compared between playing positions, interpositional differences have been recorded between the forwards and backs. Differences between playing positions have been demonstrated to be more pronounced at higher playing levels.

In this squad of players the forwards were older, taller (p<0.05) and heavier (p<0.01) than the backs. There was a significant fall in percentage body fat for the whole group during the monitoring period (p<O.OOl).

The sub-group of forwards had a higher percentage body fat than the backs on all occasions except at the June testing session eg 13.3±1.9 and 11.4±1.5% for forwards and backs respectively in January 1991.

There was a significant increase in predicted maximum oxygen uptake for the whole group during the monitoring period (p<0.001). The values are somewhat higher, particularly towards the end of the assessment period, than those that have previously been predicted (Bell, 1980; Maud and Schultz, 1984) or directly measured (Ueno et al, 1987) for Rugby Union players.

There was a significant reduction in 30m sprint time for the whole group during the monitoring period with the fastest mean time in January 1991 (4.34±0.16 and 3.90±0.10s) for the sub-groups of forwards and backs respectively. On all testing occasions the sub-group of backs was significantly faster than the forwards over 30m (p<0.01).

There were no significant changes overall in the mean predicted maximal accumulated oxvgen deficit for the whole group throughout the monitoring period. The predicted mean MAOD of the forwards and backs was not significantly different except in January 1991, when the backs had a significantly higher value than the forwards (p<0.05),

The results demonstrated that international rugby union players in this squad experienced significant improvements in body composition, aerobic power and speed but no significant changes in anaerobic power during the training programme. The monitoring also demonstrated that there are positional differences in the anthropometric and physiological characteristics of International players. The most pronounced of these differences between backs and forwards being in weight, body fat percentage and speed. Predicted aerobic power and anaerobic capacity did not distinguish well between backs and forwards.

Interpretation of results and prescription of training

The test results were used to monitor changes in fitness status, identify player strengths and weaknesses and plan individual training programmes based on the player's fitness profile linked to the training objectives identified for the current stage of training within the overall plan.

Results of the tests were added to previous results and presented on a spreadsheet which was given to the player together with a summary sheet of mean results by position and for the whole squad. Each player received an individual report with advice and guidance for the next phase of training designed to meet his particular needs and positional requirements.

Conclusions

The integration of fitness testing and monitoring with the devising and structuring of the training schedules proved a strong feature of the work. It enabled more precise, individualistic training to be presented and provided ongoing evaluation of the effectiveness of the training methods and schedules prescribed. There became greater player awareness and understanding of the principles and body of knowledge underlying fitness training and its effects. The increase in fitness levels was accompanied by a decrease in injury and subsequent treatment. It is suggested that the approach helped to optimise the player's playing potential and performance and could have been a factor in the successful outcome of the recent Five Nations championship.

References

Bangsbo J and Mizuno M. (1987) Morphological and metabolic alterations in soccer players with detraining and their relation to performance. In T Reilly, A Lees, K Davids and WJ Murphy (Eds), Proceedings of The First World Congress of Science and Football, pp. 114-124, London, E & FN Spon.

Bell W. (1979) Body Composition of Rugby Union Football Players, Br J Sports Med, 13, 19-23.

Bell W. (1980) Body composition and maximal aerobic power of rugby union forwards. J Sports Med Phys Fit, 20, 447-451 .

Brewer J. (1990) Changes in selected physiological characteristics on an English first division soccer squad during a league season. J Sports Sci, 8, 76-77.

heetham ME, Hazeldine RJ, Robinson A and Williams C. (1987) Power output of rugby forwards during maximal treadmill sprinting. In T Reilly, A Lees, K Davids and WJ Murphy (Eds),

Proceedings of The First World Congress of Science and Football, (pp. 206-210), London, E & FN Spon.

Durnin and Womersley J. (1974) Body fat assessment from total-body density and its estimation from skinfold thickness measurements on 481 men and women aged 16 to 72 years. Br J Nutr, 32, 169-179

Hazeldine R, McDonald K, Williams C. (1982) An evaluation of the physical fitness of university rugby football players. J Sports Sc, 1, 138.

Hermansen L and Medbo JI. (1984) The relative significance of aerobic and anaerobic processes during maximal exercise of short duration. Physiological Chemistry of Training and Detraining, Medicine and Sports Science (Ed P Marconnet, J Poortmans, and L Hermansen). Basel, Karger, Vol 17, 56-67.

Holmyard D, Cheetham M, Lakomy H and Williams C. (1988) Effect on recovery Duration on Performance during Multiple Treadmill Sprints. Proceedings of the First World Congress of Science and Football, 13, 134-142.

Maud PJ. (1983) Physiological and anthropometric parameters that describe a rugby team. Br J Sports Med, 17, 16-23.

Maud PJ and Schultz BB. (1984) The US National rugby team: A physiological and anthropometric assessment. Physician Sports Med, 12, 86-99.

Medbo JI, Mohn AC, Tabata I, Bahr R, Vaage D and Sejersted O. (1988) Anaerobic capacity determined by maximal accumulated deficit. J Appl Physiol, 64, 50-60.

Ramsbottom R, Brewer J and Williams C. (1988) A progressive shuttle run test to estimate maximal oxygen uptake. Br J Sports Med, 22, 141-144.

Ramsbottom R, Hazeldine R, Nevill A and Williams C. (1990) Shuttle run performance and maximal accumulated oxygen deficit. J Sports Sci, 8, 292.

Rigg P and Reilly T. (1987) A fitness profile and anthropometric analysis of first and second class rugby union players. In T Reilly, A Lees, K Davids and WJ Murphy (Eds), Proceedings of the First World Congress of Science and Football.

Ueno Y, Watai E, and Ishii K. (1987) Aerobic and anaerobic power of rugby football players. In T Reilly, A Lees, K Davids and WJ Murphy. (Eds), Proceedings of the First World Congress of Science and Football, (pp. 201-205), London, E & FN Spon.

Wells K, and Dillon E. (1952) The sit and reach test - a test of back and leg flexibility, Res Q, 23, 115-118.

Williams C, Reid R and Coutts R. (1973) Observations on the aerobic power of university rugby players and professional soccer players. Br J Sports Med, 7, 390-391.

Williams C. (1987) Short term high intensity activity Exercise: benefits, limitations and adaptations (Eds D Macleod, RJ Maughan, M Nimmo, T Reilly and C Williams). E & FN Spon Publishers, London, 59-60.

Field testing in rugby union football

D.A. McLean

Abstract. Two field tests have been developed for use by coaches to assess the effectiveness of conditioning programmes for rugby. The 85% maximimum 100 m shuttle run test was developed using athletic training principles and information gained from a time-motion analysis of international rugby. It is predominantly an anaerobic test. A complementary functional field test is described which includes acceleration, speed, agility, rugby skills and drop off in performance. This test has been shown to be reliable, discriminative and sensitive to change.

Keywords: Rugby Union, Field Testing, Fitness, VO_2 max.

Introduction

Traditionally fitness testing has been laboratory based. The laboratory has much to offer the exercise physiologist and sports scientist when the purpose of exercise testing is to investigate the mechanisms underlying performance. If the purpose of fitness testing is to provide feedback to players and coaches about individual and squad fitness levels then the sophistication of the laboratory is not essential.

In Rugby Union, there is very little time available for fitness testing because coaches perceive that monitoring erodes valuable time which is required for skills practice. This is inspite of the fact there is general acceptance that training programmes need to be monitored if standards of fitness are to improve.

To facilitate the use of fitness assessment in the development of rugby, testing should fulfil the following criteria by being:

1   inexpensive
2   easy to set up
3   short in duration
4   able to test many players simultaneously
5   focussed on specific fitness components of the game
6   reliable and valid
7   sensitive to change.

One option which exists is field testing. Field testing is generally ignored because of problems of standardisation, however, in comparison with laboratory testing it can have greater external validity.

The reputation of field testing has been enhanced by the development of the 20 m shuttle run test by Leger et al (1988). It is a maximal test which identifies maximum oxygen uptake (VO_2max) and is a test of intermediate endurance. It fulfils many of the criteria that coaches require of a fitness test but it is debatable if the 20 m shuttle run test fulfils criteria 5 and 7.

The ideal range of values of VO_2 max has not been identified for rugby. Levels quoted in the literature have been barely higher than the average for the population. Scotland Rugby Team won the Grand Slam in 1990 with a mean VO_2 max of 52 ml kg^{-1} min^{-1} which is well below that quoted for soccer (Ekblom, 1986).

The traditional view of conditioning for sport is to ensure that a player can gain as much energy as possible from aerobic sources. This avoids the muscle cell becoming acidic which is one major precursor of fatigue. Rugby is not a steady state sport and demands conditioning which will facilitate anaerobic metabolism. There is no doubt that oxidative metabolism has a role to play in recovery from high intensity work (Mazzeo et al, 1982) but the fact that a team can be successful at the highest level with a moderate aerobic capacity suggests that this component of fitness, although relevant, is not a priority for development or testing.

Another important consideration is the sensitivity of the test. The variable being measured must change by a significant amount as fitness changes otherwise the effect of training programmes cannot be judged.

The lack of sensitivity of VO_2 max in mature athletes is well documented (Astrand and Rodahl, 1986). Results from the Scotland Squad confirm this (Fig 1). The May figure was at the conclusion of a successful conditioning programme before touring New Zealand in 1990.

The 20 m shuttle run test does provide a model for tests to be developed to measure other components of fitness specific to the game. This plus information from time-motion analysis of rugby have been used to develop two field tests, an 85% maximum 100 m shuttle run test and a functional field test.

The 85% maximum 100m shuttle run test

This is designed to be largely anaerobic thus should reflect athletic training principles for anaerobic work (Dick, 1980). These are that the run should be over--distance and the running pace should be greater than 85% of maximum.

Time motion analysis of the 1990 Five Nations Championship (McLean, in press) showed that when the ball was in play those in close pursuit of the ball ran at average speeds ranging from 5-8 m s^{-1} over distances of up to 80 m. This pace was faster than steady state pace for the Scots of 4.2-4.7 m s^{-1} which supports the view that rugby is largely anaerobic. The most frequent work rest ratios (W:RRs) were in a range of 1:1-1.9. Therefore the test is structured as follows:

the distance is 100m since it is over distance and coincides with the length of a standard rugby pitch,

the pace should be greater than 85% of maximum,

the running should be intermittent with a W:RR within the range 1:1-1.9.

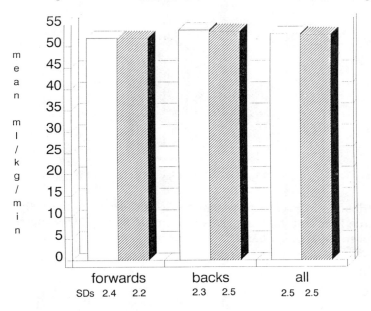

Fig 1. Maximum oxygen uptake of the Scottish international squad (n=23) in January 1990 (open bars) and May 1990 (filled bars).

The protocol includes timing players over two 50 m sprints. The faster time is used to place the player in a category which ensures a minimum of 85% of their maximum pace for the 100m shuttle run. A distribution of players by pace is shown in Figure 2.

The players run 100m in time to an audio signal which breaks the time for the run into four equal parts. Every 25 m is marked to ensure the players maintain a steady pace. Between each run a recovery of 20 seconds is given. When the player fails to complete two consecutive runs he is withdrawn and the number of repetitions minus one is recorded.

Audio tapes have been made to time runs of 17, 16, 15, and 14 seconds duration which is adequate to cope with any level of rugby union. Figure 3 compares the squad before and after the pre-tour training in 1990. It shows a

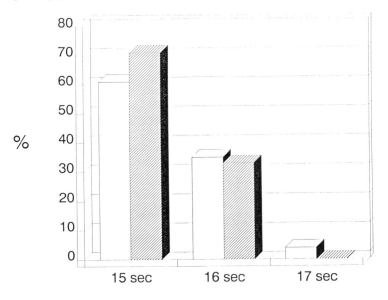

Fig 2. Distribution by pace of players in the Scottish squad in the 100m 85% max Shuttle Run Test. Measurements were made in May 1990 (open bars) and October 1991 (filled bars).

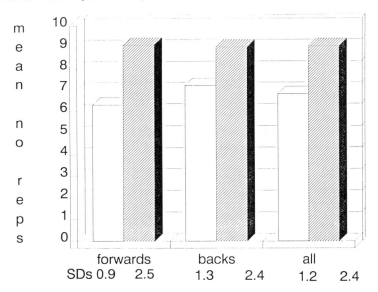

Fig 3. Performance of the Scottish squad in the 100m 85% max Shuttle Run Test in January 1990 (open bars) and May 1990 (filled bars): $p=0.00001$.

significant difference which is in contrast to the 20 m shuttle run test the results of which are in Figure 1. This difference was replicated in August and October of 1991 prior to the Rugby World Cup (p=0.001) and shows the test to be sensitive to change.

The 85% max. test fulfils the seven criteria outlined above with one exception. It has not been compared to a gold standard anaerobic test.

Reliability is at risk because it is a field test, however, strategies exist to reduce error to a minimum. The speed of the cassette player should be checked. Weather and ground conditions should be recorded and flexibility must be exercised in selecting dates for testing to ensure conditions are similar. The dates chosen should also ensure that the players have not played or undergone a vigorous training session the day before. Any test results will improve due to learning thus the results of the first test should be disregarded.

The aspects of acceleration, change of direction, agility, body contact and skills of passing the ball have not been accounted for. These have been included in the second field test.

Functional Field Test (FFT) for Rugby

Nettleton and Briggs (1980) modified and validated a functional field test for soccer developed by Zelenka et al. It was shown to be a better predictor of performance in the sport than other indirect measures such as VO_2 max. It is likely that FFTs achieve this because their structure and content closely relate to the type of effort and skill patterns that a player is called upon to produce in the game. The FFT for rugby which is currently under developement follows the principles and conditions included by Nettleton and Briggs.

The current version (Mark 2) is illustrated and described in Figure 4, Diagram 1a and b. The area of the pitch between the two 10 m lines was chosen so that the amount of measurement required to set up the test would be kept to a minimum.

The distance run is approximately 99 m. The course is run twice with a 45 second recovery to enable drop-off in performance to be identified. Penalty points are recorded for errors in the skill elements.

The original format (Mark 1) involved a course of approximately 110m. The recovery period was 2 minutes. The reasons for altering the test will be made clear from the results of the pilot study (vide infra).

The pilot was used to test reliability, the effect of learning, the effect of rest period on drop off, the ability of the test to discriminate between different ability levels of players, and sensitivity to change.

Measurement error was assessed by timing eight subjects on two occasions 6 days apart. The mean of the differences was 0.154 seconds and the standard deviation 0.53. Thus the practical application of this is that for a coach to be 95%

Functional Field Test

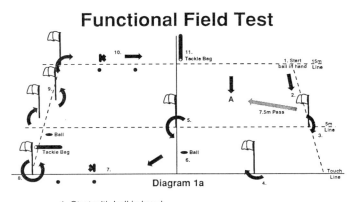

Diagram 1a

1. Start with ball in hand
2. Run and pass right
3.4.5. Continue round 3 flags
6. Dive and win ball on ground
7. Drive man and crash pad 2m and post ball
8. Run round the flag, jump the tackle bag and pick up the ball
9. Slalom round flags
10. As number 7

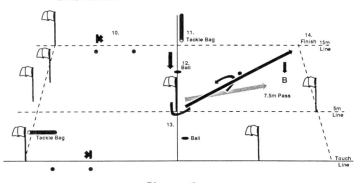

Diagram 1b

11. Tackle tackle bag
12. Run, pick up the ball, run and pass left to the receiver at B
13. Run round flag and run along the diagonal to the centre of the square. Turn back to touch the flag at 13 then run the diagonal to the finish at 14

Fig 4. Illustration of the functional field test. See text for further details.

confident that a player's performance has changed his time would need to change by more than 1.2 seconds.

There is a learning effect but it appears to stabilise quickly (Figure 5).

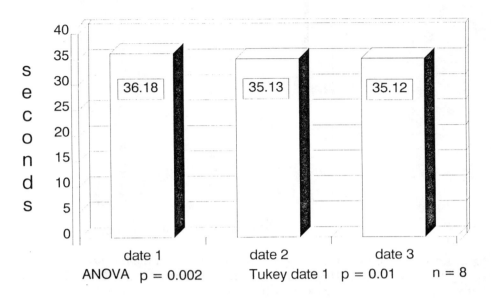

Fig 5. Learning effect in the functional field test.

The effect of duration of recovery on drop-off is shown in Figure 6. The 45 second recovery would be required to ensure a drop-off larger than the error in measurement referred to above. Although the drop-off using 2 minutes recovery was an average of 0.36 seconds this was significant (p=0.013, n= 60). The number of errors is significantly greater in the second run (p<0.01) which in spite of the small drop-off suggests that fatigue may have had an effect.

To examine the discriminative ability of the test twenty players (10 forwards and 10 backs) from each of three populations (Internationalists, First, and Second Division) were included. A two-way analysis of variance was used.

Forwards were slower than backs irrespective of group p<0.01). There was no difference among the groups for time on the first run, however, the Second Division were slower in the second run (p<0.05). They were the only group to show a significant drop-off in the second run (p=0.0003). There was no difference in the number of errors made between forwards and backs. The Internationalists made the fewest errors (p=0.05).

A general finding which distiguishes between the three groups of players is that

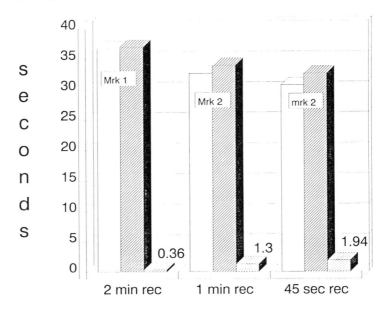

Fig 6. Effect of recovery on the drop-off in performance in the functional field test Mrk 1 and Mrk 2. Time 1 is shown in open bars and time 2 in filled bars: the drop off in performance is indicated in the cross-hatched bars

Second Division players show the greatest variability of measurement and Internationalists the least. (This apparent trend is not great enough to threaten homogeneity of variance). The inability of the time on the first run to discriminate among the three groups caused the FFT to be altered. The number of turns was reduced in the first slalom (Fig 4. Diagram 1a nos. 3,4,5) to try to ensure that flat running speed would have a greater effect. This change has resulted in the average running speed for the test increasing from 3.05 to 3.42 m sec^{-1}.Recent use of the newly structured test has shown that it is sensitive to change (Figure 7). The ability of the FFT to discriminate between players of different ability is being compared to the discriminative ability of other fitness tests.

Conclusion

A great deal of information can be gained about a whole squad in a short time by using field tests. This may be used to evaluate conditioning programmes provided every effort is made to achieve standardisation, and that the limitations of field testing are taken into account when interpreting the results. Experience in using these tests indicates that they help to motivate players and build team spirit.

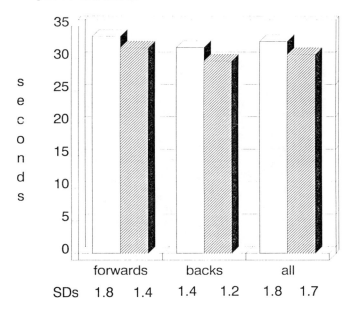

Fig 7. Comparison over time by the Scottish squad on the first run of a functional field test in August 1991 (open bars) and October 1991 (filled bars).

References

Astrand P and Rodahl K. (1986) Textbook of Work Physiology Physiological Basis of Exercise. 3rd Ed, McGraw-Hill International, New York.

Dick FW. (1980) Sports Training Principles. London Lepus Books.

Ekblom B. (1986) Applied Physiology of Soccer. Sports Med, 3, 50-60.

Leger LA, Mercier D, Gadouray C and Lambert J. (1988) A maximal multistage 20 m shuttle run test for aerobic fitness. J Sport Sci, 6, 93-101.

McLean DA. (In press) Analysis of the physical demands of International Rugby Union. J Sports Sci

Mazzeo RS, Brooks GA, Budinger TF and Schoeller DA. (1982) Pulse injection [13] C tracer studies of lactate metabolism in humans during rest and two levels of exercise, Biomed Mass Spec, 9, 310-314.

Nettleton B and Briggs CA. (1980) The development of specific function tests as a measure of performance. J Sports Med 20, 47-54.

Introduction Nutrition

At the highest level of sport, the participants are highly trained and well motivated, in addition to being genetically predisposed to success in their chosen event. The difference between winning and losing is generally small, and every potential advantage, however small in itself, is eagerly sought. It is not surprising, therefore, that sportsmen have explored and exploited dietary strategies that offer the prospect of easy rewards. Some of these dietary practices have evolved by a long process of trial and error, and have been substantiated by scientific investigation. Often, however, there is no justification for the practices which athletes follow, and in some cases these may even be harmful.

Correct nutrition will not make the average individual into an elite athlete, but, where other things are equal, it will make the difference between finishing on the winning side or the losing one. Although attention is often focussed on the diet in the immediate pre-competition period, good nutrition during the training phase may be more important by allowing hard training to be sustained over a long period. In this section, the authors have reviewed different aspects of sports nutrition, and offer practical suggestions, based on scientific evidence, as to how the diet might be optimized to allow peak performance to be achieved.

Dr Eddie Coyle has reviewed the evidence regarding the effects of diets on intermittent high intensity exercise: this type of exercise is typical of most team ball games, including hockey and soccer in addition to rugby football. There is no doubt that performance is improved by consumption of an appropriate diet and is impaired by a diet that is inadequate. In this context, an appropriate diet is one that is high in carbohydrate, allowing the muscles to store large amounts of glycogen which they can then use as a fuel during competition or during training. Dr Fred Brouns has examined some of the problems that confront athletes when they try to replace energy and water losses during competition. Replacement is limited by the functional capacity of the gastro-intestinal tract, and attempts to exceed this will result in problems.

The search for a short cut to success has led athletes to explore nutritional and pharmacological factors that can enhance performance. Dr Mel Williams has examined the evidence regarding the effectiveness of some of the supplements that are currently used by athletes, and also highlighted the dangerous side-effects associated with some of these.

Efforts to improve the diet of athletes demand an understanding of the nutritional principles on which successful performance is based, but also require information regarding the current dietary habits of athletes. If the diet is already optimal, intervention is not warranted, but identification of dietary problems allows these to be corrected. Lisa Piearce has collected data on the dietary habits of football and rugby players, and has analysed these in the light of current recommendations. Finally, Dr Bente Kiens has considered how the nutritional information collected in laboratory studies can be translated into practical advice for men and women engaged in sport. This requires a knowledge of what foods and what dietary strategies can provide the necessary nutrients in appropriate amounts.

The papers in this section show that good nutrition can make a major contribution to successful performance. They also reveal that current dietary habits among athletes are not always ideal, and that both nutritional awareness and knowledge need to be improved.

R.J. Maughan

Nutrition and diet in sport - an introduction

R.J. Maughan

Astract. Correct nutrition can make the difference between winning and losing in competitive sport. Without an adequate dietary intake, the athlete cannot sustain high intensity training on a daily basis. The training diet must aim to meet the increased energy demands of exercise, unless the athlete is attempting to reduce body fat content. If the carbohydrate intake is inadequate, training intensity must be reduced, resulting in a decreased effectiveness of the training programme. If the athlete consumes sufficient food to meet the increased energy requirements, it is likely that the need for protein, vitamins and minerals will be met without recourse to supplements. Performance in endurance exercise and in multiple sprint events is impaired if the body's carbohydrate stores are inadequate, and sufficient rest must be allowed and sufficient carbohydrate consumed to ensure that the muscle glycogen stores are fully repleted before competition. During exercise carbohydrate-containing drinks can serve to supply additional substrate for the muscles and also to offset the effects of dehydration. The type and amount of drink consumed will depend on individual circumstances.

Keywords: Nutrition, glycogen, fatigue, dehydration, protein, electrolytes, rehydration.

Introduction

All sporting events involve some degree of muscular exercise, both during the preparation or training phase and during competition. These activities will increase the rate of energy expenditure and may alter the body's nutritional requirements. Performance will be impaired if the diet is inadequate, although the concept of dietary inadequacy may be quite different for the athlete compared with the sedentary individual. Conversely, performance may be improved by dietary manipulation, but we still have an incomplete understanding of how best to control diet to optimise sports performance. This is true at all levels of competition, and at the highest level, where competitors are predisposed to success by genetic endowment and have undergone the most rigorous training, nutritional intervention may make the difference between success and failure. It is not surprising therefore that sportsmen generally are concerned about their diet, although this concern is not always matched by a knowledge of basic nutrition. Some of the dietary practices followed by athletes in pursuit of success are sound, but others have no beneficial effect and may even be harmful. As in other areas of nutrition, these ideas are often encouraged by those who stand to gain financially from sales of dietary supplements.

Two distinct aspects must be considered; the first is the diet in training, which must be consumed on a daily basis for a large part of the year, and the second is the diet in the immediate pre-competition period and during competition itself. Considering the range of activities encompassed by the term sport and the variation in the characteristics of the individuals taking part, it is not surprising that the nutritional requirements vary.

Diet for training

The primary need for the diet of the athlete in training is to meet the additional nutrient requirement imposed by the training load. In sports involving prolonged strenuous exercise on a regular basis, participation has a significant effect on energy balance. Metabolic rate during running or cycling, for example, may be 15-20 times the resting rate, and such levels of activity may be sustained for several hours by trained athletes (Astrand and Rodahl, 1986). There is some evidence to suggest that the metabolic rate may remain elevated for at least 12 and possibly up to 24 hours if the exercise is prolonged and close to the maximum intensity that can be sustained (Maehlum et al, 1986); this has been disputed, and it is unlikely that metabolic rate remains elevated for long periods after more moderate exercise (Garrow, 1986).

If body weight and performance levels are to be maintained, the high rate of energy expenditure must be matched by a high energy intake. Available data for most athletes suggest that they are in energy balance within the limits of the techniques used for measuring intake and expenditure. This is to be expected as a chronic deficit in energy intake would lead to a progressive loss of body mass. However, data for women engaged in sports where a low body weight, and especially a low body fat content, are important, including events such as gymnastics, distance running and ballet, consistently show a lower than expected energy intake (Parizkova, 1985). There is no obvious physiological explanation for this finding other than methodological errors in the calculation of energy intake and expenditure, but it seems odd that these should apply specifically to this group of athletes. Many of these women do, however, have a very low body fat content: a body fat content of less than 10% is not uncommon in female long distance runners (Wilmore, 1982). Secondary amenorrhoea, possibly related more to the training regimen than to the low body fat content, is common in these women, but is usually reversed when training stops.

Athletes engaged in strength and power events have traditionally been concerned with achieving a high dietary protein intake in the belief that this is necessary for muscle hypertrophy. In a survey of American college athletes, 98% believed that a high protein diet would improve performance (Grandjean et al, 1981). While it is undoubtedly true that a diet deficient in protein will lead to loss of muscle tissue, there is no evidence to support the idea that excess dietary protein will drive the system in favour of protein synthesis. Excess protein will simply be used as a substrate for oxidative metabolism, either directly or as a precursor of glucose, and the excess nitrogen will be lost in the urine.

Exercise, whether it is long distance running or weight training, will cause an increased protein oxidation compared with the resting state. Although the contribution of protein oxidation to energy production during the exercise period may decrease to about 5% of the total energy requirement, compared with about 10-15% (i.e. the normal fraction of protein in the diet) at rest, the absolute rate of protein degradation is increased during exercise (Dohm, 1986).

This leads to an increase in the minimum daily protein requirement, but this will be met if a normal mixed diet, adequate to meet the increased energy expenditure, is consumed. In spite of this, however, many athletes ingest large quantities of protein-containing foods and expensive protein supplements; daily protein intakes of up to 400 grams are not unknown in some sports (Darden and Schendel, 1971). Disposal of the excess nitrogen is theoretically a problem if renal function is compromised, but there does not appear to be any evidence that excessive protein intake among athletes is in any way damaging to health.

The energy requirements of training are largely met by oxidation of fat and carbohydrate. The higher the intensity of exercise, the greater the reliance on carbohydrate as a fuel: at an exercise intensity corresponding to about 50% of an individual's maximum oxygen uptake (VO_2max), approximately two thirds of the total energy requirement is met by fat oxidation, with carbohydrate oxidation supplying about one third. If the exercise intensity is increased to about 75% of VO_2max, the total energy expenditure is increased, and carbohydrate is now the major fuel. If carbohydrate is not available, or is available in only a limited amount, the intensity of the exercise must be reduced to a level where the energy requirement can be met by fat oxidation.

The primary need, therefore, is for the carbohydrate intake to be sufficient to enable the training load to be sustained at the high level necessary to produce a response. During each strenuous training session, substantial depletion of the glycogen stores in the exercising muscles and in the liver takes place. If this carbohydrate reserve is not replenished before the next training session, training intensity must be reduced, leading to corresponding decrements in the training response (Costill and Miller, 1980). Any athlete training hard on a daily basis can readily observe this; if a low carbohydrate diet, consisting mostly of fat and protein, is consumed after a day's training, it will be difficult to repeat the same training load on the following day.

Feeding a high-fat, low-carbohydrate diet for prolonged periods has been shown to increase the capacity of muscle to oxidise fat and hence improve endurance capacity in the rat, but may not be effective in man (Phinney et al, 1983); similarly short term fasting increases endurance capacity in the rat (Dohm et al, 1983), but results in a decreased exercise tolerance in man (Loy et al, 1986). The training diet, therefore should be high in carbohydrate, preferably with a large proportion in the form of complex carbohydrates rather than simple sugars; this suggestion conforms with the recommendations of NACNE that carbohydrates provide 50% of dietary energy intake (NACNE, 1983). Costill et al (1971) showed that a high carbohydrate diet (70% of energy intake as carbohydrate) enabled runners who were training for 2h per day to maintain muscle glycogen levels, whereas if the carbohydrate content was only 40%, a progressive fall in muscle glycogen content was observed. A dietary carbohydrate intake of 500-600g was necessary to ensure adequate glycogen resynthesis. These high levels of intake are difficult to achieve without consuming large amounts of simple sugars: most athletes find that they can only satisfy the requirement for carbohydrate by eating confectionery and sweet snacks between, or even instead of, meals.

With regular strenuous training, there must be an increased total intake to balance the increased energy expenditure. Provided that a reasonably normal diet is consumed, this will supply more than adequate amounts of protein, minerals, vitamins and other dietary requirements. There is no good evidence to suggest that specific supplementation with any of these dietary components is necessary or that it will improve performance (Williams, 1985). A diet which may be inadequate in micronutrient content for a sedentary individual consuming 4MJ per day, may meet the requirements of an athlete taking 12-15 MJ/day. Indeed without resorting to sweets, snacks and so-called "junk food", such a high intake may be difficult to achieve.

The only exceptions to the generalisation about dietary supplements may be iron and, in the case of very active women, calcium. Highly trained endurance athletes commonly have low circulating haemoglobin levels, although total red cell mass may be elevated due to an increased blood volume. This may be considered to be an adaptation to the trained state, but hard training may result in an increased iron requirement and exercise tolerance is impaired in the presence of anaemia (Clement and Sawchuk, 1984). Low serum folate and serum ferritin levels are not associated with impaired performance, however, and correction of these deficiencies does not influence indices of fitness in trained athletes (Matter et al, 1987).

Moderate exercise has been reported to increase bone mineral density in women (Pocock et al, 1986), but hard training may reduce circulating oestrogen levels and hence accelerate bone loss (Drinkwater et al, 1984). For these athletes, an adequate calcium intake should be ensured, although calcium supplements themselves will not reverse bone loss while oestrogen levels remain low.

Diet for competition

There is no doubt that the ability to perform prolonged exercise can be substantiaily modified by dietary intake in the pre-competition period. The competitive period can conveniently be divided into two phases - the few days prior to the competition, and competition day itself.

Dietary manipulation to increase muscle glycogen content in the few days prior to exercise has been extensively recommended for endurance athletes following observations that these procedures were effective in increasing endurance capacity in cycle ergometer exercise lasting about 1½-2h. The suggested procedure was to deplete muscle glycogen by prolonged exercise about one week prior to competition and to prevent resynthesis by consuming a low-carbohydrate diet for 2-3 days before changing to a high-carbohydrate diet for the last 3 days during which little or no exercise was performed. This procedure can double the muscle glycogen content and is effective in increasing cycling performance, measured as the time for which a given workload can be sustained (Bergstrom et al, 1967).

In a race situation such as in marathon running or cycling, however, the aim is to cover a given distance in the shortest possible time, and there have been no definitive studies showing that comparable improvements in racing performance can be achieved by the same means. Karlsson and Saltin (1971) showed that performance in a 30km running race was improved by 7.5 min when muscle glycogen stores were artificially elevated prior to competition: these runners were able to maintain their speed for longer and slowed down less in the closing stages of the race when glycogen levels were high. Brewer et al (1988) found that treadmill running time to exhaustion at 70% of VO_2 max was improved by a high-carbohydrate diet fed in the 3-day period between two such exhausting runs. There seems little doubt that increased dietary carbohydrate intake in the few days prior to a race is likely to lead to improved performance (Costill and Miller, 1980; Costill, 1988) but some reservations have been expressed (Brotherhood, 1984) as many runners complain of fatigue and muscle discomfort associated with a high carbohydrate intake.

There is now a considerable amount of evidence that it is not necessary to include the low-carbohydrate glycogen depletion phase of the diet for endurance athletes. All that is necessary is to reduce the training load over the last 5 or 6 days before competition and to simultaneously increase the dietary carbohydrate intake. This avoids many of the problems associated with the more extreme forms of the diet. Although an increased pre competition muscle glycogen content is undoubtedly beneficial, there is a faster rate of muscle glycogen utilisation when the glycogen content itself is increased, thus nullifying some of the advantage gained (Jansson, 1980; Richter and Galbo, 1986). Caffeine ingestion has been shown to promote fat mobilisation thus sparing muscle glycogen (Costill et al, 1978), but is not effective for everyone and caffeine in large doses may have an unwanted diuretic effect. It has also been reported that the stimulatory effect of caffeine on fat mobilisation and oxidation is not observed if a high carbohydrate diet is consumed in the pre-exercise period (Weir et al, 1987).

Consumption of a high carbohydrate diet in the days prior to competition may also benefit competitors in games such as rugby, soccer or hockey, although it appears not to be usual for these players to pay attention to this aspect of their diet. Saltin and Karlsson (1986) showed that players starting a soccer game with low muscle glycogen content did less running, and much less running at high speed, than those players who began the game with a normal muscle glycogen content. It is common for players to have one game in midweek as well as one at the weekend, and it is likely that full restoration of the muscle glycogen content will not occur between games unless a conscious effort is made to achieve a high carbohydrate intake (Jacobs et al, 1982).

Although this glycogen-loading procedure is generally restricted to use by athletes engaged in endurance events, there is some evidence that the muscle glycogen content may influence performance in events lasting only a few minutes (Maughan and Poole, 1981). A high muscle glycogen content may be particularly important when repeated sprints at near maximum speed have to be made. Short term high-intensity exercise can also be improved by ingestion of alkaline salts prior to exercise to enhance the buffering of the protons produced by anaerobic glycolysis (Heigenhauser and Jones, 1991). There is scope for nutritional intervention during exercise only when the duration of events is sufficient to allow absorption of drinks or foods ingested and where the rules of the sport permit. The primary aims must be to ingest a source of energy, usually in the form of carbohydrate, and fluid for replacement of water lost as sweat. High rates of sweat secretion are necessary during hard exercise in order to limit the rise in body temperature which would otherwise occur. If the exercise is prolonged, this leads to progressive dehydration and loss of electrolytes. At very high sweat rates, much of the sweat secreted is not evaporated, but simply drips from the skin. This water loss is not effective in cooling the body, and increases the risk of dehydration without benefit to the runner.

The rate of sweat secretion is proportional to the rate of heat production and depends also on climatic factors. In a marathon race, the faster runners generally lose sweat at a higher rate than the slower runners, but they are active for a shorter period of time, so total sweat loss is unrelated to finishing time (Maughan, 1985). It is also apparent that the rate of sweat secretion varies considerably between individuals, even when other factors such as exercise intensity and ambient temperature are constant; the reasons for this inter-individual variability are not clearly understood. Marathon runners in the same race and with the same fluid intake may lose from as little as 1% to as much as 6% of body weight during a race (Whiting et al, 1984). At high ambient temperatures, runners may lose 8% of body weight in a race, equivalent to about 5-6l of water for a 70 kg individual (Costill et al, 1970). Fluid losses corresponding to as little as 2% of body weight can impair the ability to exercise (Saltin, 1964). The reduction in plasma volume may be particularly important, as there is a requirement for a high blood flow to the skin to promote heat loss, while blood flow to the working muscles must be maintained to provide an adequate supply of oxygen and substrates. Fatigue towards the end of a prolonged event may thus result as much from the effects of dehydration as from substrate depletion.

Along with the water secreted as sweat are a variety of electrolytes and organic molecules. The electrolytes are present in varying concentrations, which bear some relationship to their concentration in plasma, but sweat composition varies widely between individuals and also varies at different times within the same individual. The total electrolyte content of sweat is less than that of plasma, so large sweat losses tend to concentrate the plasma. Although sweat potassium content may be high, large amounts of potassium are added to the plasma from liver, muscle and red cells during hard exercise, and plasma concentrations of most if not all of the major electrolytes rise during prolonged exercise. This suggests that it is not necessary, nor perhaps even advisable, to attempt to replace the electrolytes lost in sweat during exercise.

The belief that a relationship exists between electrolyte loss and muscle cramp, although often advanced, has not been proved (Maughan, 1986b). Absorption of water from gut, however, is promoted by the presence of sodium and actively transported sugars. If the glucose content of drinks is high, more glucose will be absorbed, but the rate of water uptake will be decreased; at very high concentrations, secretion of water will occur, even as glucose absorption is taking place. As a compromise, therefore, drinks should generally contain relatively small amounts of glucose (about 30-80 g/l) together with small amounts of electrolytes, particularly sodium. Fluid replacement in events such as marathon running may be more of a problem for the faster runners, as the time available for replacement is less, and the higher exercise intensity tends to reduce the availability of ingested fluids. A report by Noakes et al (1985) suggests that it is possible for slow competitors in ultramarathon races to develop water intoxication as a result of excessive intake, but marathon runners should generally aim to drink as much as is possible during the race, particularly on hot days.

The composition of drinks to be taken during exercise should be chosen to suit individual circumstances. During exercise in the cold, fluid replacement may not be necessary as sweat rates will be low, but there is still a need to supply additional glucose to the exercising muscles. In this situation, more concentrated glucose drinks are to be preferred. These will supply more glucose thus sparing the limited glycogen stores in the muscles and liver without overloading the body with fluid. It may also be worth remembering that there is a need for drinks to be palatable; athletes are understandably reluctant to consume large amounts of unpleasant-tasting drinks. The taste mechanisms appears to change with exercise; strong flavours should be avoided although many people find an increased preference for slightly salty tasting drinks.

The amount and frequency of drinks in many sporting situations is governed by the rules of the event. In the laboratory, where no such restrictions are imposed, large volumes can be given so long as the composition is such as to allow rapid emptying from the stomach. During bicycle or treadmill exercise, it is possible to drink 150-200ml every 10-15 minutes; over prolonged periods: this can allow replacement at close to the rate of sweat loss for many individuals. In many sports there is little provision for fluid replacement: participants in games such as football or hockey can lose large amounts of fluid, but replacement is possible only at the half-time interval. Until very recently the opportunities for drinking during long road races were severely restricted, but the rules have now been relaxed to allow more frequent intake.

Once exercise has begun, drinks should be taken at the earliest opportunity. The subjective sensation of thirst is not an adequate guide to the need to drink, and competitors should be encouraged to drink freely. One point often neglected is the need to practice drinking during training to become accustomed to the sensation of exercising with fluid in the stomach. Marathon runners in particular seldom drink during training so it is perhaps not surprising that they often encounter problems with fluid intake in competition. In any situation, but especially where intake during the event is restricted, the athlete must be fully hydrated before competition begins. This can be achieved by ensuring a high fluid intake in the last few days before competition; a useful check is to ensure that the urine is pale in colour. In the last 10-30 minutes prior to competition it is advisable to drink up to 500ml of fluid; drinking earlier than this may cause problems with the need to urinate during the event, but once exercise has begun blood flow to the kidney is decreased resulting in little urine formation.

In the post exercise period, replacement of fluid and electrolytes can usually be achieved through the normal dietary intake. If there is a need to ensure adequate replacement for subsequent competition, extra fluids should be taken and additional salt (sodium chloride) might usefully be added to food. Consuming fluids with a relatively high sodium content will maintain the osmotic drive to thirst, thus helping to ensure an adequate intake, and will also increase the fraction of the ingested fluid which is retained (Nadel et al, 1990). The other major electrolytes, particularly potassium, magnesium and calcium, are present in abundance in fruit and fruit juices, and although these are not advisable for consumption during exercise on account of their high osmolality, they may be appropriate in the post-exercise period. Supplements are not normally necessary.

References

Astrand P-O, Rodahl K. (1986) Textbook of Work Physiology. 3rd Ed. New York, McGraw Hill.

Bergstrom J, Hermansen L, Hultman E, Saltin B. (1967) Diet, muscle glycogen and physical performance. Acta Physiol Scand, 71, 140-150.

Brewer J, Williams C, Patton A. (1988) The influence of high carbohydrate diets on endurance running performance. Eur J Appl Physiol, 57, 698-706.

Clement DB, Sawchuk LL. (1984) Iron status and sports performance. Sports Med, 1, 65-70.

Costill D. (1988) Carbohydrates for exercise; dietary demands and optimum performance. Int J Sports Med, 9, 1-18.

Costill DL, Miller JM. (1980) Nutrition for endurance sport: Carbohydrate and fluid balance. Int J Sports Med, 1, 2-14.

Costill DL, Kammer WF, Fisher A. (1970) Fluid ingestion during distance running. Arch Environ Health, **21**, 520-525.

Costill DL, Dalsky GP, Fink WJ. (1978) Effects of caffeine ingestion on metabolism and exercise performance. Med Sci Sports Ex, **10**, 155-158.

Darden E, Schendel HE. (1971) Dietary protein and muscle building. Scholastic Coach, **40**, 70-76.

Dohm GL. (1986) Protein as a fuel for endurance exercise. Ex Sport Sci Rev, **14**, 143-173.

Dohm GL, Tapscott EB, Borakat HA, Kasperek GJ. (1983) Influence of fasting in rats on glycogen depletion during exercise. J Appl Physiol, **55**, 830-833.

Drinkwater BL, Nelson K, Chesnut CH, Bremner WJ, Skainholtz S, Southworth MB. (1984) Bone mineral content of amenorrheic and eumenorrheic athletes. New Engl J Med, **311**, 277-281.

Garrow JS. (1986) Effect of exercise on obesity. Acta Med Scand, Suppl 711, 67-73.

Grandjean AC, Hursh LM, Maguire WC, Hanley DF. (1981) Nutrition knowledge and practices of college athletes. Med Sci Sports Ex, **13**, 82.

Heigenhauser GJF, Jones NL. (1991) Bicarbonate loading. In: Lamb DR, Williams MH (eds) Ergogenics enhancement of performance in exercise and sport. Brown & Benchmark, pp. 183-207

Jacobs I, Westlin N, Karlsson J, Rasmusson M, Houghton B. (1982) Muscle glycogen and elite soccer players. Eur J Appl Physiol, **48**, 297-302.

Jansson E. (1980) Diet and muscle metabolism in man. Acta Physiol Scand, Suppl 487, 1-24.

Karlsson J, Saltin B. (1971) Diet, muscle glycogen, and endurance performance. J Appl Physiol, **31**, 203-206.

Loy SF, Conlee RK, Winder WW, Nelson AG, Arnall DA, Fisher AG. (1986) Effects of a 24-hour fast on cycling endurance time at two different intensities. J Appl Physiol, **61**, 654-659.

Maehlum S, Grandmontagne M, Newsholme EA, Sejersted OM. (1986) Magnitude and duration of excess postexercise oxygen consumption in healthy young adults. Metabolism, **35**, 425-429.

Matter M, Stittfall T, Graves J, Myburgh K, Adams B, Jacobs P, Noakes TD. (1987) The effect of iron and folate therapy on maximal exercise performance in female marathon runners with iron and folate deficiency. Clin Sci, **72**, 415-422.

Maughan RJ. (1985) Thermoregulation and fluid balance in marathon competition at low ambient temperature. Int J Sports Med, **6**, 15-19.

Maughan RJ. (1986) Exercise-induced muscle cramp; a prospective biochemical study in marathon runners. J Sports Sci, **4**, 31-34.

Maughan RJ, Poole DC. (1981) The effects of a glycogen loading regimen on the capacity to perform anaerobic exercise. Eur J Appl Physiol, **46**, 211-221.

Maughan RJ, Fenn CE, Gleeson M, Leiper JB. (1987) Metabolic and circulating responses to the ingestion of glucose polymer and glucose/electrolyte solutions during exercise in man. Eur J Appl Physiol, **56**, 356-362.

Nadel ER, Mack GW, Nose H. (1990) Influence of fluid replacement beverages on body fluid homeostasis during exercise and recovery. In: Gisolfi CV, Lamb DR, (eds.) Perspectives in exercise science and sports medicine. Volume 3: Fluid homeostasis during exercise. Carmel, Benchmark. 181-205.

National Advisory Committee on Nutrition Education. (1983) Proposals for nutritional guidelines for health education in Britain. Health Education Council.

Noakes TD, Goodwin N, Rayner BL, Branken T, Taylor RKN. (1985) Water intoxication: a possible complication during endurance exercise. Med Sci Sports Ex, **17**, 370-375

Parizkova J. (1985) Adaptation of functional capacity and exercise. In: Blaxter K, Waterlow JC, (eds.) Nutritional adaptation in man. London: John Libbey, pp. 127-138.

Phinney SD, Bistrian BR, Evans WJ, Cervino E, Blackburn GL. (1983) The human metabolic response to chronic ketosis without caloric restrictions: preservation of submaximal exercise capability with reduced carbohydrate oxidation. Metabolism, **32**, 769-776.

Pocock NA, Eisman IA, Yeates MG, Sambrook PN, Eberl S. (1986) Physical fitness is a major determinant of femoral neck and lumber spine bone mineral density. J Clin Invest, **78**, 618-621.

Richter E, Galbo H. (1986) High glycogen levels enhance glycogen breakdown in isolated contracting skeletal muscle. J Appl Physiol, **61**, 827-831.

Saltin B. (1964) Aerobic work capacity and circulation at exercise in man. Acta Physiol Scand, 62 Suppl 230, 1-52.

Saltin B, J Karlsson. Die Ernährung des Sportlers. In: Zentrale Themen der Sportmedizin. Ed W Hollman. 3rd Ed. Springer-Verlag, Berlin, pp. 245-260.

Weir J, Noakes TD, Myburgh K, Adams B. (1987) A high carbohydrate diet negates the metabolic effects of caffeine during exercise. Med Sci Sports Ex, **19**, 100-105.

Whiting PH, Maughan RJ, Miller JDB. (1984) Dehydration and serum biochemical changes in runners. Eur J Appl Physiol, **52**, 183-187.

Wilkes D, Gledhill N, Smyth R. (1983) Effect of induced metabolic alkalosis on 800m racing time. Med Sci Sports Ex, **15**, 277-280.

Williams MH. (1985) Nutritional aspects of human physical and athletic performance. Springfield, Charles C Thomas.

Wilmore JH. (1982) The female athlete: Physique, body composition and physiological profile. Aust J Sports Sci, **2**, 2-9.

Effects of diet on intermittent high intensity exercise

E. F. Coyle

Abstract. Athletes who participate in sports such as rugby can experience severe muscle glycogen depletion during play of less than one hour duration. These athletes are advised to drink solutions during the game which provide them with 30-60 grams per hour of carbohydrate and up to 1 liter per hour of fluid. When diet between games is optimal, at least 20 hours are required to fully recover muscle glycogen stores. In reality, athletes are not always able to consume an optimal diet, in which case recovery of muscle glycogen may take two or more days. To speed recovery, carbohydrate intake after exhaustive exercise should average 50 grams per 2 hours of mostly moderate or high glycemic index foods. The aim should be to ingest a total of about 600 grams in 24 hours. Carbohydrate intake should not be avoided during the 4 hour period before exercise and in fact it is best to eat at least 200 grams during this time. When diet is not carefully planned according to these guidelines, athletes tend to consume too little carbohydrate because they become satiated with high fat in their diet, and they go through periods of the day when recivery of glycogen stores is suboptimal and thus precious time is wasted.

Keywords: Recovery, muscle glycogen, carbohydrate, diet, exercise.

Introduction

Attention to the importance of a proper diet for optimal athletic training and competition is often focused upon the endurance athlete's (i.e. runners, cyclists, crosscountry skiers) need for an adequate amount of dietary carbohydrate. Indeed, these endurance athletes typically exercise continuously at moderately high intensities (i.e. 70-85% maximum oxygen uptake) for periods of two hours or more. As a result they often experience fatigue due to depletion of their bodily carbohydrate stores (i.e. muscle glycogen, liver glycogen and blood glucose concentration). These observations in endurance athletes are sometimes interpreted to imply that in order to experience bodily carbohydrate depletion a person must exercise continuously and for long durations. This is clearly not the case! In fact, athletes who participate in sports such as rugby, soccer and ice hockey, which require them to repeatedly perform intermittent exercise, often at the highest intensity they can maintain for long sprints, may experience severe muscle glycogen depletion during play of less than one hour duration. Unlike most endurance athletes, rugby, soccer and hockey players sometimes compete with insufficient time between games for optimal recovery. As discussed in this chapter, it takes at least 20 hours to fully resynthesize muscle glycogen after intense exercise under ideal conditions when an athlete is given the proper type and amount of carbohydrate to eat at the appropriate times after exercise. In reality, athletes are not always able to consume an optimal diet, in which case recovery of muscle glycogen may require two or more days. The methods for increasing carbohydrate consumption to cope with heavy training and competition will be discussed.

Simple description of continuous exercise

Exercise which is performed continuously can be simply described by the given intensity of exercise and the duration over which it is performed. Total work accomplished is the product of these two factors. Table 1 describes the energy demands of running continuously at intensities ranging from jogging at 50% of maximum oxygen uptake (VO_2max) to sprinting at maximum velocities. This example predicts the responses of a well-trained player who has a VO_2max of 4.5 liters/min (i.e. 65 ml/kg/min for a 70 kg person) and who has good speed and thus can run 100 meters in 11.5 seconds. If this athlete ran continuously at a velocity of about 4 meters/sec (i.e. approximately 75% VO_2max) fatigue would occur after 2-3 hours due to a depletion of muscle glycogen and a lowering of blood glucose concentration. If exercise were continued after this point, this athlete would have to slow to a jog (i.e. 50% VO_2max or about 2.7 meters/sec). That is the pace which could be maintained continuously while relying solely on fat as the source of oxidative energy.

Energy demands of high intensity exercise

The energy demands of playing games involving intermittent exercise can vary tremendously depending upon differences in the intensity and duration of the sprinting and the rest period between sprints. Players of course know this and therefore they pace themselves accordingly. It is possible for a player to become totally exhausted after only a short period of play. Additionally, players must attempt to maintain their energy reserves above the minimum required for sprinting repeatedly toward the end of their play. These considerations are largely determined by the rate at which muscle lactic acid is produced as a result of muscle glycogenolysis as well as the availability of glycogen and blood glucose as substrate for these processes.

Table 1 lists the approximate energy demands when this exemplary athlete runs at speeds which allow him to cover 100 meters in varying amounts of time. In this chapter, we consider this athlete to be sprinting when running velocity equals or exceeds 6.7 meters/sec which translates into running 100 meters in 15 sec or faster. A pace of 15 sec/100 meters (i.e. 125% VO_2max) could be maintained for approximately 800 meters (i.e. 2 min) whereas a pace of 12.5 sec/100 meters (150% VO_2max) could be maintained for approximately 400 meters (i.e. 50 sec). In both cases the athlete would be forced to stop exercise due to lactic acid accumulation in muscle and partial recovery would require 5-20 min. In game situations, the athlete would obviously not attempt to sprint for durations approaching 1 min. In fact, the athlete should not sprint for longer than 100 meters at speeds of 15 sec/100 meter or faster without allowing adequate rest.

Table 1. Running speeds for an exemplary well-trained player.

Intensity	Velocity (meters/sec)	Time for 100 meters (sec)	% of maximal sprinting velocity	Duration Possible
175% VO_2max*	8.7	11.5	100%	20 sec
150% VO_2max	8.0	12.5	92%	50 sec
125% VO_2max	6.7	15	75%	2 min
100% VO_2max	5.3	18.7	61%	8 min
75% VO_2max	4.0	25	46%	150 min
50% VO_2max	2.7	37.5	30%	>360 min
25% VO_2max	1.3	75	15%	very long

This individual possesses a VO_2max of 4.5 liters/min and weighs 70 kg.
* This value is an approximation, which may be higher.

Description of intermittent sprinting

With intense intermittent exercise, however, description of the energy demands and the degree of fatigue experienced due to lactic acid accumulation and glycogen depletion requires careful consideration of several factors. Namely, 1) the intensity or velocity of running; 2) the duration; 3) the time allowed for recovery as well as the exercise intensity during recovery; and finally 4) the number of times these work recovery cycles are repeated. Most competitive games require athletes to perform intermittent sprinting at speeds between 75-100% of maximum sprinting velocity (i.e. 125-175% VO_2max).

Figure 1 describes the responses to intermittent sprinting at only 75% maximum sprinting velocity (i.e. 125% VO_2max) in an exemplary player who, after sprinting for a given duration, allows himself to recover by jogging for a duration twice as long as the sprint. Therefore, the work-recovery time ratio is 1:2. This example was modelled after the report of Astrand et al. (1960) and includes unpublished data as well as some assumptions by the author. Even at this modest sprinting velocity and despite the recovery period, a player must attempt to limit the duration of sprints. When sprinting intermittently for 100 meters in 15 sec and then jogging (i.e. 25% VO_2max) for 30 sec, this athlete would experience only a small increase in blood lactic acid levels and exercise could be maintained for at least 1 hour with only moderate muscle glycogen depletion. When the duration of sprinting at 75% of maximum sprinting velocity is limited to 10-15 seconds, the exercising muscles appear capable of meeting the energy requirements without excessive stimulation of glycogenolysis, provided the recovery period is adequate. However, when the intermittent exercise involves sprinting for 200 meters in 30 seconds and jogging for 60 sec, the athlete will experience moderate fatigue and an increase in blood lactic acid concentration, as well as a more marked lowering of muscle glycogen concentration after 1 hour of play. If the athlete chose to sprint intermittently for durations of 60 seconds with 120 seconds of jogging recovery, total exhaustion would be experienced within about 20 min, despite the fact that the sprints were performed at only 75% of maximal sprinting velocity (i.e. 125% VO_2max). As shown in Figure 1, lactic acid would increase progressively due to these long sprints, reaching levels which prevent muscular contraction after the 6th or 7th interval. After another 20 min of jogging recovery, this athlete could attempt to perform another set of 6 or 7 sprints of 60 sec duration, with the same result, total exhaustion. However, it is likely that muscle glycogen would become depleted during this period.

Intermittent sprinting can cause even greater rates of lactic acid formation and glycogen depletion when it is performed at maximal sprinting speeds and with shorter durations of recovery. In fact, intermittent high intensity exercise is probably the most effective method for producing glycogen depletion. This can occur despite the fact that the running distance may only amount to 5 km if the sprinting is performed at close to top speed and for durations of 1 minute or longer forcing the athlete to stop running due to lactic acid accumulation in muscle.

Muscle glycogen depletion during games

Figure 2 describes the muscle glycogen patterns in soccer players before, at half-time, and after the game (Karlsson, 1969). By half-time, muscle glycogen was fairly low, whereas it was depleted after the game in all players. Those who had

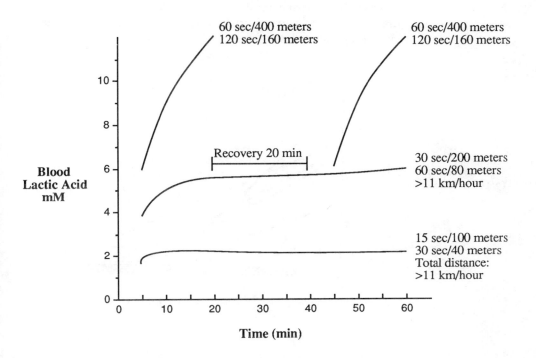

Work-Recovery Time Ratio 1:2

Fig. 1   Responses of an exemplary well trained player to intermittent sprinting at 75% maximal sprinting velocity for durations of l5 sec, 30 sec and 60 sec. After each sprint, the athlete would recover by jogging (i.e. 25% VO₂max) for a duration which is twice as long as the work period (i.e. 30 sec or 60 sec or 120 sec). Therefore the work recovery ratio is 1:2. In all cases the average velocity of both the sprint and the jog would be 186 meters/min and if completed 11 km would be covered in 1 hour. However, when the athlete sprints for 60 sec, with 120 sec of recovery, total exhaustion would be experienced in 20 min due to lactic acid accumulation in muscle. If after 20 min of jogging recovery the athlete attempted to continue intermittent 60 sec sprints, it is likely that fatigue would again develop, this time with possible glycogen depletion. These data were modelled after the report of Astrand et al (1960) and include some unpublished observations and assumptions.

the lowest muscle glycogen concentration at half-time played the second half with the slowest speed and shortest running distances. Of interest in Figure 2 is the observation that some players began the game with very little muscle glycogen. Jacobs et al (1982) have also reported muscle glycogen to be very low after a soccer game, and that it remained below normal levels 2 days after the game, probably due to carbohydrate-poor diets.

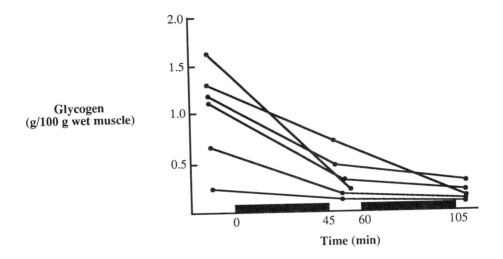

Fig. 2   Muscle glycogen concentration before, at half-time and after a soccer game. From Karlsson 1969.

Carbohydrate feedings during a game

Muckle (1973) reported that glucose feedings improved team performance as measured by the number of goals scored, especially in the second half of play. Additionally, Kirkendall et al (1988) showed that carbohydrate feeding during a game increased the total distance run as well as the amount run at top velocities. Simard et al (1988) found that hockey players fed carbohydrate during a game skated 10% more distance during a game and at 4% greater speeds compared to other players who drank flavored water (i.e. a placebo). These observations of improved performance as a result of carbohydrate feeding during intermittent exercise agrees with the observation that carbohydrate ingestion during continuous cycling or running delays fatigue by 30-60 min when exercising at 70% VO_2max (Coggan and Coyle, 1991). The optimal rate of carbohydrate ingestion during continuous exercise is generally 30-60 grams per hour. Whether it is different during intermittent exercise has not been determined. Unlike continuous exercise at 70% VO$_2$max, it is possible that carbohydrate ingestion during intermittent exercise can be used to synthesize glycogen during the periods of rest and jogging (Brouns et al, 1989; Constable et al, 1984; Kuipers et al, 1987).

Does carbohydrate ingestion compromise fluid replacement and cardiovascular function ?

Several investigations have compared the influence of drinking tap water or carbohydrate-electrolyte solutions on core temperature and heart rate during prolonged exercise (Candas et al, 1986; Costill et al, 1970; Davis et al, 1988; Murray et al, 1987; Owen et al, 1986). These experiments have demonstrated that carbohydrate-electrolyte solutions of up to 8-10% carbohydrate are equally as effective as water in attenuating hyperthermia and heart rate during prolonged exercise. Ingestion of approximately 30-60 grams of carbohydrate (i.e. glucose, sucrose, or starch) during each hour of the game and another 60 grams at half-time will generally be sufficient. Since the average rate of gastric emptying and intestinal absorption exceeds 1 liter/h for water and solutions containing up to 8% carbohydrate, exercising players can be supplemented with both carbohydrate and fluids at relatively high rates (over 60 grams/h of carbohydrate and 1 liter/h of fluid). Therefore, when sweat rate is not very high (i.e. less than 1 liter/ h), the addition of carbohydrate to fluids, and vice versa, does not prevent adequate supplementation of each, especially if large volumes are consumed to keep the stomach somewhat full and thus increase gastric emptying.

Muscle glycogen resynthesis after exercise

The restoration of muscle glycogen after heavy training or competition quite often dictates the time needed to recover between bouts of intense intermittent exercise. Muscle glycogen is resynthesized to normally high levels at a rate of only about 5 mmoles/kg muscle/hour, which corresponds to a rate of about 5% per hour. Therefore, approximately 20 hours are required to recover muscle glycogen stores. A longer time will be necessary if the diet is not optimal. The important dietary factors to consider are 1) the rate of carbohydrate ingestion, 2) carbohydrate type, and 3) timing of carbohydrate ingestion after exercise.

Rate of carbohydrate ingestion

Blom et al (1987) and Ivy et al (1988b) reported that glycogen synthesis increased from 2% per hour (i.e. 2 mmoles/kg/hour) when 25 grams of high glycemic carbohydrates were ingested every 2 hours to 5-6% per hour (i.e. 5-6 mmoles/kg/hour) when 50 grams was ingested every 2 hours. However, they did not observe muscle glycogen synthesis to increase to more than 5-6% per hour (i.e. 5-6 mmoles/kg/hour) even when 100, 112 or 225 grams were ingested every 2 hours. This suggests that the muscle glycogen synthesis is near optimal (5-7 mmoles/kg/hour) when at least 50 grams of glucose is ingested every 2 hours. This forms the basis for the recommendation that the amount and type of food to be eaten after exercise for near optimal muscle glycogen resynthesis should be that which promotes glucose entry into the blood and the systemic circulation at a rate of at least 50 grams every two hours. This goal can be achieved by considering both the glycemic index, which reflects the rate at which our food is absorbed into the blood and/or converted to glucose, and the amount of carbohydrate ingested. Tables 2-4 present the portions of various foods which contain 50 grams of carbohydrate. It should be realized that these recommendations are based on a person who weighs 70 kg. In general, however, it is recommended that a person eat at least 0.7 gram of carbohydrate per kg of body weight every two hours.

Carbohydrate type and glycogen resynthesis

As discussed, the rate of glycogen synthesis after exercise and ingestion of glucose, or food with a high glycemic index (Table 2), is 5-6% per hour (i.e. 5-6 mmoles/kg/h) (Blom et al, 1987; Ivy et al, 1988a; Ivy et al, 1988b; Reed et al, 1989). When sucrose is ingested, it is hydrolyzed to equal amounts of glucose and fructose. Its ingestion elicits a similar rate of glycogen synthesis as glucose ingestion, despite the fact that the glycemic index of sucrose is less than that of glucose (Blom et al, 1987; Jenkins et al, 1988), which classifies it as having a moderate to high glycemic index (Tables 2 and 3). However, fructose ingestion alone promotes muscle glycogen to be resynthesized at only 3% per hour (i.e. 3 mmoles/kg/hour) because of its low glycemic index (20-30% of that of glucose; Table 3) (Blom et al, 1987; Jenkins et al, 1988) probably because of the relatively slow rate with which the liver converts fructose to glucose. Concerning simple sugars, it appears that glucose and sucrose, which possess high and moderate glycemic indexes, are equally effective in the partial restoration of muscle glycogen during the 4-6 hour period after exercise, yet fructose is only one-half as effective due to a low glycemic index.

A limited amount of information is available about the rates of glycogen synthesis elicited by eating common foods containing various starches and sugars. When the type of carbohydrate ingested elicits a high or moderate glycemic index

(Tables 2 and 3), it makes little difference if the carbohydrate is in liquid or solid form (Keizer et al, 1986; Reed et al, 1989). Little data exists as to the extent to which carbohydrate foods with a low glycemic index (Table 4) promote muscle glycogen resynthesis, yet it appears that glycogen resynthesis from low glycemic foods is suboptimal during the first few hours after exercise, but not during the 6-24 hour period after exercise (Kiens et al, 1990).

Comparison of simple sugars and complex carbohydrates

Carbohydrates are often classified as being simple sugars (i.e. glucose, fructose or sucrose) or complex carbohydrates, (i.e. bread, potatoes, rice, beans etc). For the most part, all ingested carbohydrate must be digested to glucose before it can be used for energy or stored as glycogen. Therefore, as far as their energy potential, simple and complex carbohydrates are no different. Carbohydrates can be functionally classified according to the extent to which they increase blood glucose concentration (i.e. glycemic index).

The glycemic index is generally determined by the rate at which the ingested carbohydrate is made available to intestinal enzymes for hydrolysis and intestinal absorption (O'Dea et al, 1980). This is a function of the gastric emptying time and the physical availability of the sugar or starch to hydrolytic enzymes. The latter is influenced by cooking which alters the integrity of the starch granule (Wursch et al, 1988) and the degree of gelatinization (O'Dea et al, 1980). It is a misconception to think that the glycemic index is simply a function of whether the carbohydrate is complex (i.e. starch) or a simple sugar. Some starchy foods produce glycemic responses which are identical to that of glucose (i.e. baked potato, maltodextrins) (Crapo et al, 1977; Guezennec et al, 1989; Thomas et al, 1991). On the other hand, the rise in blood glucose after eating fructose or sucrose is less than that observed for a wide range of starchy complex carbohydrates (e.g. potato, bread, cornflakes) (Jenkins et al, 1988). These points are summarized in Tables 2, 3 and 4 which display various foods classified as having a high, moderate or low glycemic index (Jenkins et al, 1988). The amount of food which contains 50 grams of carbohydrate is also reported so that practical recommendations can be quantified.

Timing of carbohydrate ingestion after exercise

During the first two hours following exercise, the rate of muscle glycogen resynthesis is 7-8% per hour (i.e. 7-8 mmoles/kg/hour), somewhat faster than the normal rate of 5-6% per hour, but certainly not rapid (Ivy et al, 1988b). A recovering athlete should ingest carbohydrate as soon after exercise as is practical. The most important reason for this is to allow more time for resynthesis.

Table 2. Carbohydrate foods with a <u>High</u> <u>Glycemic</u> <u>Index</u> and less than 30% fat.

Food Classification	Food	Amount for 50 grams of carbohydrate
Sugars	Glucose	4.2 Tablespoons or 0.26 cup
	Sucrose*(white granular)	4.2 Tablespoons or 0.26 cup
	(white powdered)	6.6 Tablespoons or 0.42 cup
Syrups/Jelly	Honey	2.8 Tablespoons or 0.18 cup
	Corn Syrup (light)	3.4 Tablespoons or 0.26 cup
	Molasses (medium)	4.2 Tablespoons or 0.25 cup
	Cane & Maple Syrup	3.9 Tablespoons or 0.24 cup
Beverages	6% Sucrose Solution	833 ml or 3.5 cups
	7.5% Maltodextrin & Sugar	666 ml or 2.8 cups
	10% corn syrup-carbonated drink	500 ml or 2.1 cups
	20% maltodextrin solution	250 ml or 1.1 cups
Cereal Products	Bagel	1.6 Bagels (55 g each)
	Bread (white, wholemeal or rye)	3.8 slices, 1 inch, 28g each
	Bread Sticks	6.7 sticks
	Cornflakes	2 cups
Fruit	Raisins	0.41 cup
Vegetable	Potato (baked; medium, 200 g)	1 potato
	Potato (boiled and mashed)	1.5 cups
	Sweet corn* (yellow)	1.2 cups

According to Jenkins et al (1988), high glycemic foods have been classified according to those which have values above 85, with 100 being the glycemic index of bread. * Sucrose and sweet corn have a glycemic index of 86, which is lower than the other high glycemic foods but higher than the moderate glycemic foods. Modified from Food Values of Portions Commonly Used. Jean AT Pennington. Harper & Row Publishers. 15th Ed. New York

Practical recommendations

Athletes are not usually hungry immediately following a game and often prefer to drink fluids rather than to eat solid foods (Keizer et al, 1986). Therefore, Table beverages which contain glucose, sucrose, maltodextrins or corn syrups in concentrations of 6 grams/100 ml or higher should be made available. If preferred, there is no reason an athlete should not eat solid food. However, since appetite is usually suppressed, foods which are more concentrated in carbohydrate and which have a high glycemic index should be available. These foods generally have a relatively small amount of fat, protein and fiber.

When the desire for solid food returns, the athlete should eat enough to ensure that a total of approximately 600 grams (for a 70 kg person) of carbohydrate are eaten within 24 hours. Most of the food chosen should have a moderate or high glycemic index (Tables 2 and 3), although a certain amount of low glycemic carbohydrate is acceptable. The athlete should avoid eating meals which contain less than 70% carbohydrate, and thus have high fat and protein content, especially during the first six hours after exercise because this often suppresses hunger and limits carbohydrate intake. Realistically, due to other daily activities, including sleep, it is usually not possible to eat frequent meals (every 2 hours) which contain at least 70% and 50 grams of carbohydrate. Therefore, when a person must go for an extended period between meals, their last meal should contain enough carbohydrate to suffice for that period (i.e. 50 grams per 2 hours and therefore 150 grams for a 6 hour period or 250 grams for a 10 hour period).

Table 3. Carbohydrate food with a <u>Moderate Glycemic Index</u> and less than 30% fat.

Food Classification	Food	Amount for 50 grams of carbohydrate
Cereal Products	Spaghetti; Macaroni	1.5 cups; cooked
	Noodles	1.4 cups; cooked
	Oatmeal	2.1 cups; cooked
	Whole grain rye bread	3.8 slices- 1 inch
	Rice	1 cup; cooked
Fruit	Grapes (American-slip skin)	3.1 cups
	Grapes (European)	1.8 cups
	Orange (Navel, 140 g)	3.0 oranges
Vegetables	Yams (boiled or baked)	1.3 cups of cubes
	Corn (yellow-boiled)	1.2 cups
Legumes	Baked beans	0.9 cups

Moderate glycemic foods have a rating of 60-85 (see Table 2).

Maximizing muscle glycogen prior to a game

A few days prior to a game, athletes should regulate their diets and training in an attempt to maximize ("super compensate" or "load") muscle

Table 4. Carbohydrate food with a <u>Low Glycemic Index</u> and less than 30% fat (except dairy products).

Food Classification	Food	Amount for 50 grams of carbohydrate
Fruits	Apple (medium, 138 g)	2.4 medium
	Applesauce (sweetened)	1.0 cups
	Dates (dried)	8 dates
	Figs (raw, medium, 50 g)	5 figs
	Grapefruit (medium, 118 g)	2.5 grapefruits
	Peach (raw medium, 90 g)	5 peaches
	Plum (raw medium, 66 g)	5.6 plums
Legumes	Butter beans	1.4 cups
	Kidney beans	1.2 cups
	Chick peas (Garbanzo beans)	1.1 cups
	Green beans	1.7 cups
	Green peas	2.1 cups
	Red lentils	1.2 cups
Dairy Products	Whole cow's milk	1,037 ml or 4.4 cups
	Skim milk	995 ml or 4.2 cups
	Yoghurt (plain custard)	658 ml or 2.8 cups

Low glycemic foods have a rating less than 60 according to Jenkins et al. (1988), where bread has a glycemic index of 100. Modified from Food Values of Portions Commonly Used. Jean A.T. Pennington. Harper & Row Publishers. 15th Ed. New York.

glycogen stores. High preexercise glycogen levels will allow athletes to exercise for longer periods by delaying fatigue. The most practical method (Sherman et al, 1981) of "glycogen loading" involves altering training and diet for 7 days. On days 7, 6, 5, and 4 before competition one should train moderately hard (e.g. 1-2 hours) and consume a moderately low carbohydrate diet (i.e. 350 grams/day). This will make the muscle sufficiently carbohydrate deprived and ready to supercompensate, without making the person sick as sometimes occurs when all carbohydrate is eliminated. During the 3 days prior to competition, training should be tapered (30-60 min/day of low to moderate intensity) and a high carbohydrate diet consumed (i.e. 500-600 grams per day). Such a regimen will increase muscle glycogen stores 20-40 percent or more above normal. This "modified" glycogen loading regimen is as effective as the "classic" regimen (Bergstrom and Hultman, 1966), and more practical since it does not require athletes to attempt to train while consuming a high fat diet.

Pre-Game nutrition

Although it is agreed that athletes should eat sufficient carbohydrate the day before exercise, there is less agreement as to when, how much and what type of carbohydrate should be eaten during the hours before exercise. In an attempt to avoid a decline in blood glucose at the onset of exercise, it is sometimes recommended that carbohydrate meals be eaten 3-4 hours before exercise so as to allow enough time for plasma insulin concentration to return to basal levels so as to prevent a possible decline in blood glucose at the onset of exercise. However, there is no practical reason to recommend that players fast during the 4 hour period before exercise, except if they are too nervous to eat or they feel uncomfortable with some food in their stomach when playing. The decline in blood glucose with the onset of exercise is not problematic (Brouns et al, 1988). Actually, it can be prevented simply by having the subjects exercise slightly more intensely, which probably causes liver glucose output to increase and match blood glucose uptake by muscle (Montain et al, 1991). Additionally, the elevation in carbohydrate oxidation should not cause problems if enough carbohydrate was stored in the body as a result of the meal. Therefore, high and moderate glycemic food should be ingested prior to events which will result in fatigue due to carbohydrate depletion. It is generally recommended that approximately 200-300 grams of carbohydrate be ingested during the 4 hours before exercise. Most importantly, the meals should be low in fat, protein and fibre and they should not cause gastrointestinal discomfort.

Daily high intensity intermittent exercise training requires ample dietary carbohydrate

Athletes who attempt to perform high intensity intermittent exercise day after day will derive greater training-induced improvements in performance over the course of several weeks of training if they ingest a diet very high in carbohydrate. Recently, Simonsen et al (1991) reported that rowers who trained twice daily, which included intermittent exercise of 3-10 min duration at 90% VO_2max, improved time trial performance by 11% over 4 weeks when daily carbohydrate intake averaged 10 grams/kg body weight per day (i.e. 70% of total calories). The rowers on this high carbohydrate diet displayed weekly increases in the average power output during training and concomitant progressive increases in muscle glycogen concentration over the course of the 4 week training period. Another group of rowers ate a diet containing a moderate amount of carbohydrate (i.e. 5 gram/kg body weight per day or 42% of total calories) which is not unlike that of many endurance athletes. During the 4 week training period the subjects consuming a moderate amount of carbohydrate did not display any training-induced increases in time trial performance. Apparently, there was sufficient carbohydrate in the moderate carbohydrate diets (i.e. 5 gram/kg/day) to prevent a progressive reduction of muscle glycogen and a reduced ability to train. Therefore, the moderate amount of dietary carbohydrate in this case was tolerable but certainly not optimal for improving performance. Kirwan et al (1988) have reported that when runners eat only 3.9 gram/kg/day of carbohydrate during a 5 day period of intense training, muscle glycogen concentration declines and running economy deteriorates and as a result the runner experiences greater fatigue. Similar observations have been made in swimmers (Costill et al, 1988).

Diet and performance during short term high intensity exercise

It is clear that athletes who ingest a very low carbohydrate (i.e. only 5% of calories) and thus a high fat and protein diet for the 2-3 days before a game will reduce, by about 20% (i.e. 4.3 min to 3.3 min), the length of time they can exercise continuously at an intensity slightly above VO$_2$max (Maughan and Poole, 1981; Greenhaff et al 1987a, 1987b, 1988). This effect could be due to the fact that a high fat and protein diet causes metabolic acidosis which by itself could impair the ability for high intensity exercise. It is also possible that the reductions in pre-exercise muscle glycogen as a result of this low carbohydrate diet may reduce tolerance for continuous high intensity exercise. Therefore, it is reasonable to recommend that athletes participating in games involving high intensity intermittent exercise avoid high fat and protein diets which are low in carbohydrate during the few days before a game. It is not clear, however, the minimal amount of dietary carbohydrate need to prevent this impairment.

It is clearly advantageous for an athlete to attempt to maximize muscle glycogen stores prior to a game which will demand repeated intermittent sprinting and result in fatigue due to glycogen depletion. However, it is less clear if changes in muscle glycogen concentration alters performance in an athlete who does not sprint long or often enough to experience muscle glycogen depletion (Maughan and Poole, 1981; Greenhaff et al, 1987; Symons and Jacobs, 1989).

References

Astrand I, Astrand PO, Christensen EH et al. (1960) Myohemoglobin as an oxygen store in man. Acta Physiol Scand, **48**, 454.

Bergstrom J, Hultman E. (1966) The effect of exercise on muscle glycogen and electrolytes in normals. Scand J Clin Invest, **18**, 16-20.

Blom PC, Hostmark AT, Vaage O, Vardal KR, Maehlum S. (1987) Effect of different post-exercise sugar diets on the rate of muscle glycogen synthesis. Med Sci Sports Exerc, **19**, 491-

496.

Brouns F, Saris WHM, Beckers E. (1989) Metabolic changes induced by sustained exhaustive cycling and diet manipulation. Int J Sports Med, **10**, S49-S62.

Candas V, Libert JP, Brandenberger G et al. (1986) Hydration during exercise: effects on thermal and cardiovascular adjustments. Eur J Appl Physiol, **55**, 113-122.

Coggan AR, Coyle EF. (1991) Carbohydrate ingestion during prolonged exercise: effects on metabolism and performance. Exercise and Sports Sciences Reviews, **19**, 1-40.

Constable SH, Young JC, Higuchi M, Holloszy JO. (1984) Glycogen resynthesis in leg muscles of rats during exercise. Am J Physiol, **247**, R880-R883.

Costill DL, Kammer WF, Fisher A. (1970) Fluid ingestion during distance running. Arch Environ Health, **21**, 520-525.

Costill DL, Flynn MG, Kirwan JP, Houmard JA, Mitchell JB, Thomas R, Park SH. (1988) Effects of repeated days of intensified training on muscle glycogen and swimming performance. Med Sci Sports Exerc, **20**, 249-254.

Crapo PA, Reaven G, Olefsky J. (1977) Postprandial plasma glucose and insulin responses to different complex carbohydrates. Diabetes, **26**, 1178-1183.

Davis JM, Lamb DR, Pate RR et al. (1988) Carbohydrate-electrolyte drinks: effects on endurance cycling in the heat. Am J Clin Nutr, **48**, 10_23-1030.

Ekblom B. (1986) Applied physiology of soccer. Sports Med, **3**, 50-60.

Essen B, Hagenfeldt L, Kaijser L. (1977) Utilization of blood-borne and intramuscular substrates during continuous and intermittent exercise in man. J Physiol, **265**, 489-506.

Greenhaff PL, Gleeson M, Maughan RJ. (1987a) The effects of dietary manipulation on blood acid-base status and the performance of high intensity exercise. Eur J Appl Physiol, **56**, 331-337.

Greenhaff PL, Gleeson M, Whiting PH, Maughan RJ. (1987b) Dietary composition and acidbase status: limiting factors in the performance of maximal exercise in man? Eur J Appl Physiol, **56**, 444-450.

Greenhaff PL, Gleeson M, Maughan RJ. (1988) Diet-induced metabolic acidosis and the performance of high intensity exercise in man. Eur J Appl Physiol, **57**, 583-590.

Guezennec CY, Satabin P, Duforez F, Merino D, Peronnet F, Koziet J. (1989) Oxidation of corn starch, glucose, and fructose ingested before exercise. Med Sci Sports Exerc, **21**, 45-50.

Ivy JL, Katz AL, Cutler CL, Sherman WM, Coyle EF. (1988a) Muscle glycogen synthesis after exercise: effect of time of carbohydrate ingestion. J Appl Physiol, **65**, 1480-1485.

Ivy JL, Lee MC, Brozinick Jr JT, Reed MJ. (1988b) Muscle glycogen storage after different amounts of carbohydrate ingestion. J Appl Physiol, **65**, 2018-2023.

Jacobs I, Westlin N, Karlsson J et al. (1982) Muscle glycogen and diet in elite soccer players. Eur J Appl Physiol, **48**, 297-302.

Jenkins DJA, Wolever TMS, Buckley G, Lam KY, Giudici S, Kalmusky J, Jenkins AL, Patten RL, Bird J, Wong GS, Josse RG. (1988) Low glycemic index starchy foods in the diabetic diet. Am J Clin Nutr, **48**, 248-254.

Karlsson HG. (1969) Kolhydratomsattning under en fotbolismatch. Report Department of Physiology, reference 6, Karolinska Institute, Stockholm.

Keizer HA, Kuipers H, Van Kranenburg G, and Geurten P. (1986) Influence of liquid and solid meals on muscle glycogen resynthesis, plasma fuel hormone response, and maximal physical working capacity. Int J Sports Med, **8**, 99-104.

Kiens B, Raben AB, Valeur A-K et al. (1990) Benefit of dietary simple carbohydrates on the early postexercise muscle glycogen repletion in male athletes. Med Sci Sports Exerc, **22**, S88.

Kirkendall DT, Foster C, Dean JA, et al. (1988) in Science and Football, (eds T Reilly, A Lees, K Davids and W Murphy), E & FN Spon, London, pp. 33-41.

Kirwan JP, Costill DL, Mitchell JB, Houmard JA, Flynn MG, Fink WJ, Beltz JD. (1988) Carbohydrate balance in competitive runners during successive days of intense training. J Appl Physiol, **65**, 2601-2606.

Kuipers H, Keizer HA, Brouns F, Saris WHM. (1987) Carbohydrate feeding and glycogen synthesis during exercise in man. Pfluegers Arch, 410, 652-656.

Leatt PB, Jacobs I. (1989) Effect of glucose polymer ingestion on glycogen depletion during a soccer match. Can J Sports Sci, 14, 112-116.

Maughan RJ, Poole DC. (1981) The effects of a glycogen-loading regimen on the capacity to perform anaerobic exercise. Eur J Appl Physiol, 46, 211-219.

Montain SJ, Hopper MK, Coggan AR, Coyle EF. (1991) Exercise metabolism at different time intervals following a meal. J Appl Physiol, 70.

Muckle DS. (1973) Glucose syrup ingestion and team performance in soccer. Br J Sports Med, 7, 340-343.

Murray R, Eddy DE, Murray TW et al. (1987) The effects of fluid and carbohydrate feedings during intermittent cycling exercise. Med Sci Sports Exerc, 19, 597-604.

Murray R, Siefert JG, Eddy DE, Paul GL, Halaby GA. (1989a) Carbohydrate feeding and exercise: effect of beverage carbohydrate content. Eur J Appl Physiol, 59, 152-158.

Murray R, Paul GL, Seifert JG, Eddy DE, Halaby GA. (1989b) The effects of glucose, fructose, and sucrose ingestion during exercise. Med Sci Sports Exerc, 21, 275-282.

O'Dea K, Nestel PJ, Antonoff L. (1980) Physical factors influencing postprandial glucose and insulin responses to starch. Am J Clin Nutr, 33, 760-765.

Owen MD, Kregel KC, Wall PT et al. (1986) Effects of ingesting carbohydrate beverages during exercise in the heat. Med Sci Sports Exerc, 18, 568-575.

Reed MJ, Brozinick Jr JT, Lee MC, Ivy JL. (1989) Muscle glycogen storage post exercise: Effect of mode of carbohyrate administration. J Appl Physiol, 66, 720-726.

Sherman WM, Costill DL, Fink WJ, Miller JM. (1981) The effect of exercise and diet manipulation on muscle glycogen and its subsequent utilization during performance. Int J Sports Med, 2, 114-118.

Simard C, Tremblay A, Jobin M. (1988) Effects of carbohydrate intake before and during an ice hockey game on blood and muscle energy substrates. Res Quart Exerc Sport, 59, 144-147.

Simonsen JC, Sherman WM, Lamb DR et al. (1991) Dietary carbohydrate, muscle glycogen, and power output during rowing training. J Appl Physiol, 70, 1500-1505.

Symons JD, Jacobs I. (1989) High-intensity exercise performance is not impaired by low intramuscular glycogen. Med Sci Sports Exerc, 21, 550-557.

Thomas DE, Brotherhood JR, Brand JC. (1991) Carbohydrate feeding before exercise: effect of glycemic index. Int J Sports Med, 12, 180-186.

Wursch P, Del Vedovo S, Koellreutter B. (1986) Cell structure and starch nature as key determinants of the digestion rate of starch in legume. Am J Clin Nutr, 43, 2529.

Effects of exercise on gastrointestinal function: implications for water and substrate provision during exercise

F. Brouns, N.J. Rehrer, E.J. Beckers and W.H.M. Saris

Abstract. Exercise on a full stomach is not well tolerated by athletes when the exercise intensity is moderate to high. The reason for this is that a state of increased sympathetic and decreased parasympathetic activity leads to dramatic changes in gastrointestinal blood flow as well as in motor activity. These changes affect digestion and absorption. Therefore, it is generally advised that exercising athletes ingest foods which are easily digestible, low in dietary fibre, fat and protein content and preferably are liquid or semi-liquid. There are several reasons for athletes to combine water, electrolytes and carbohydrate in beverages taken during exercise. Carbohydrate is known to be one of the most potent nutrients affecting performance and fatigue, and electrolytes together with carbohydrate enhance fluid absorption, as long as the drink is not hypertonic. The present review describes the effects of exercise on the gastrointestinal tract and highlights the aspects which determine optimal nutrient and fluid delivery in the exercising athlete.

Keywords: Gastrointestinal tract, exercise, rehydration, gastric emptying, digestion, intestinal absorption, sports drinks

Introduction

The importance of the gastrointestinal (GI) tract should not be overlooked when considering the factors which determine working capacity. Besides being a source of sometimes unpleasant and debilitating symptoms, the GI tract provides the interface for the assimilation of water and substrates which may become limited during exercise and may therefore impair performance capacity. Knowledge of GI function allows one to supplement during exercise as efficiently as possible. Any choice for supplementation during exercise is based on needs. Several factors, including exercise intensity and duration, ambient temperature and humidity and the availability of supplementation must be taken into account.

In general, supplementation immediately prior to and during exercise is conducted to keep an athlete in fluid balance and in "carbohydrate balance" or more accurately stated, to supply an additional, exogenous, supply of readily available water and oxidisable carbohydrate. Additionally electrolytes are often provided to replace those lost with sweat. To what degree the inclusion of these ingredients is soundly based on scientific evidence and under which circumstances might one expect one or the other ingredient to take priority is the subject of this treatise.

Substrate

The intensity of exercise is important in determining to what degree substrates will be used. At rest, fat oxidation makes up a larger proportion of energetic needs than carbohydrate (CHO). As the intensity of exercise increases the rate of energy utilisation is increased as well as the proportion of energy that is provided by carbohydrate oxidation. CHO is a necessary fuel for high intensity exercise since the rate of release of energy (ie ATP production) is greater than with fat and the amount of oxygen necessary per mole ATP produced is less with the oxidation of CHO than with that of fat. Carbohydrate is found primarily stored in man as glycogen in skeletal muscle and in the liver.

The average total amount of glycogen in man, however, is limited to amounts (~400g) that will, when used totally, provide energy for approximately 90 min at 70 % VO_2max (Newsholme and Leech, 1983). These facts support the contention that carbohydrate supplementation during intensive endurance exercise improves performance. Practical experiments have shown this to be the case. Several reviews have been written recently which cover carbohydrate metabolism during exercise and summarise the findings in relation to performance and the proposed mechanisms affecting performance (Bonen et al, 1989; Coggan and Coyle, 1991; Hargreaves, 1991; Coyle, 1991).

A recent number of well controlled studies have shown that rehydration drinks enriched with CHO (2.5 up to 10%) do maintain normal fluid regulatory functions and additionally delay fatigue/enhance performance because of the CHO substrate supply (Maughan 1991, Table 1).

Water

Water is often forgotten when one speaks of the dietary requirements. Deficiency of water has a much more immediate effect on bodily functions than all other nutrients. The symptoms of water deficiency are apparent with several hours of water deprivation, whereas with other nutrients it is a matter of days or weeks before the lack of intake has a serious, detrimental effect on bodily functions.

During physical exercise, substrates, primarily carbohydrate and fat, are metabolised to provide energy to allow muscles to contract repeatedly. The process of transforming one form of energy to another (chemically bound energy to energy for mechanical work) is never completely efficient. During physical exercise approximately 75% of the energy is lost as heat. The higher the intensity of exercise is the greater the rate of heat production will be (Nadel et al, 1977). Dissipation of heat is increased via increased peripheral circulation and perspiration. As exercise intensity increases the sweat rate also increases (Nadel et al, 1977; Maughan, 1985; Greenhaff and Clough, 1989).

Large fluid losses can result in a decreased plasma volume, stroke volume, circulatory capacity and a resulting decreased capacity to cool via a reduced transport of heat to the periphery. Eventually as dehydration progresses the sweat extraction as well as nutrient delivery and waste product disposal are reduced. Additionally, the body temperature may rise above the range in which enzymatic reactions function optimally, sometimes to levels of risk for health. The ambient conditions (temperature, humidity, wind speed, solar radiation, body size, hydration status prior to exercise, clothing and an individual's unique sweat response), also response may also be down-regulated or curtailed. As a result, oxygen influence the magnitude of the sweat losses. The latter is of importance with respect to the priorities for quantitative fluid and/or carbohydrate supplementation (Brouns 1991c). Sweat losses resulting in dehydration (body weightloss of >2%) will impair physiological functions and may decrease performance. Alternatively, rehydration to offset these effects will minimize these changes and will maintain normal performance capacity (for review see Maughan 1991).

Minerals

Because of the high rate of sweat production that occurs with high intensity exercise (particularly in a warm environment), much attention has been given to the electrolyte losses which may result herewith. Electrolytes, especially sodium, have been included in many sports beverages in quantities designed to replace these losses and to enhance fluid absorption (sodium). Costill (1977) reviewed data from his lab as well as those of others concerning sweat composition and the magnitude of electrolyte losses incurred by trained and untrained subjects subjected to either an exercise-dehydration regimen or simply thermal dehydration. Several points are worth noting here with respect to the magnitude of electrolyte losses during endurance exercise and the rationale for including these minerals in beverages designed to replace these losses.

The concentration of electrolytes (Na^+, K^+, Cl^-, Ca^{2+} and Mg^{2+}) in sweat is highly variable between individuals. The rate of sweating, which varies greatly from one individual to another, influences the composition of the sweat. As sweat rate increases the concentration of Na^+ and Cl^- in the sweat increases while the concentration of K^+ and Mg^{2+} remains unchanged and that of Ca^{2+} decreases. Thus, it is loss of the extra-cellular components Na^+ and Cl^- that may present the greatest possibility for deficit. From the available literature it can be concluded

Table 1. Effect of carbohydrate-electrolyte drinks on performance.

Study	Work	Effect
Murray 1987	4x20 min intermittent endurance work with two in between sprint performances	First in between sprint no differences, second sprint 6%- and 7% carbohydrate (CHO) solution, sign better than water.
Mitchell 1988	8x12 min intermittent endurance work	5%-, 6%-, 7.5% CHO solution, sign better than water.
Davis 1988	120 min endurance work + 30 min break + all out work	6% CHO solution, sign better than water. 2.5% CHO solution, not different from water.
Davis 1988	2 times 60 min work with 2 in between sprint performances + 20 min break + final sprint	Second and third sprint 6% glucose solution, tendency to better performance compared to water.
Murray 1989	3x20 min intermittent endurance work + time trial	6%, 8% and 10% CHO solution, tendency to better performance compared to water.
Murray 1989	88 min endurance work + time trial	6% glucose and 6% sucrose solution, sign better than 6% fructose solution.
Maughan 1989	Endurance work at 70% VO_2 max, until exhaustion	4% isotonic glucose solution, sign better as no fluid or 35% fructose solution.
Coggan 1989	Endurance work at 70% VO_2 max, until exhaustion	With carbohydrate supplement-ation, sign better performance compared to water.
Brouns 1989	Endurance work at 90% Wmax, exhaustion	With carbohydrate supplement-ation, sign better than water.
Williams 1990	30 km running	Sign decrease of blood glucose and running speed with water. Maintenance of speed with 7 % CHO-electrolyte solution.

120

that mineral replacement/ supplementation will not enhance performance but may contribute to adequate daily intakes in some circumstances, especially very prolonged exercise in the heat. Sweat is hypotonic relative to body fluids and becomes more so with training and heat acclimatisation. Because of this an increase in plasma concentrations of electrolytes (and osmolality) may actually occur during exercise, if no fluid to replace the losses is ingested. Exercise induced shifts of water and also of some electrolytes, e.g. from intracellular to extracellular compartments (e.g. K^+) and vice versa (e.g. Mg^{2+}) make the use of plasma concentrations for determining actual status of some electrolytes difficult

Further, a short-term (48-72 h) effect of exercise is to increase plasma volume. Repeated daily exercise bouts bring maintenance of this increase in plasma volume, which in itself will lead to a decreased concentration of plasma proteins and possibly also electrolytes, simply by dilution. Based upon daily electrolyte measurements in several compartments, it is concluded by some authors that the effects of sweat-induced electrolyte losses are partly compensated for by decreased secretion of electrolytes by sweat and urine (Na^+), and that generally the post-exercise extraction from the daily diet is sufficient to prevent a progressive deficit occurring that will influence health or performance. However, post-exercise supply of minerals does not compensate for short term deficits which may occur during long lasting exercise.

Therefore, an exception may be ultraendurance exercise, such as triathlon, during which substantial fluid replacement by ingesting plain water has been observed to induce hyponatremia in some athletes, up to as much as 25% of participants in some races, when exercising in the heat (Noakes, 1985; 1990). Recently hyponatremia has also been observed in a marathon runner (Nelson, 1988). Therefore replacement of sodium along with water is advisable during ultraendurance events. Salt tablets are discouraged, no matter how great the losses, since negative effects on the gastrointestinal tract, including net water secretion into the lumen and possible GI distress, may occur. Based upon a stimulating effect on water absorption in the intestine, the inclusion of Na^+ in a carbohydrate containing beverage is generally warranted (For further details see under: Intestinal absorption). Addition of sodium to rehydration beverages has also been shown to re-establish fluid balance and plasma volume better through water retention when compared with plain water. Additionally fluid regulatory hormones are normalized faster (Nose et al, 1988; Brandenberger et al, 1986; 1989).

Addition of other electrolytes to rehydration drinks for athletic populations, to replace exercise induced losses is acceptable as long as the quantities do not exceed the upper levels reported for losses through whole body sweat (Table 2).

Table 2: Electrolyte content of whole body wash-down sampled sweat deri- ved from 13 studies. Some of these were single experiments. Some were performed during a prolonged period to study influences of acclimation and adaptation. In the latter case multiple samples were obtained. For the major electrolytes the table represents 274 observations made on 123 subjects. (Brouns 1991)

Electrolyte	Cl	Na	K	Ca	Mg
AVERAGE (mmol/l)	28.6	32.7	4.4	1	0.79
S D	13.5	14.7	1.3	0.7	0.6
AVERAGE (mg/l)	1014	752	173	40	19
S D	481	339	52	27	15
RANGE mg/l:	533-1495	413-1091	121-225	(13-67)	(4-34)
Net absorption (%)	100%	1000%	100%	30%	35%
Correction factor:	-	-	-	x3.33	x2.86
Proposed replace- ment range	500-1500	400-1100	120-225	45-225	10-100

From stomach to gut

The alimentary canal provides one long tube that runs through the body from which nutrients are selectively absorbed and to which secretions are added. In this short review general functions of only the stomach and intestines will be covered since these areas are the most important in the assimilation of foodstuffs and liquids in relation to exercise. The stomach is primarily a holding tank for fluids. It also prepares solid foods by churning the ingestate into smaller particles. Gastric secretions are added in this process, most importantly: gastric acid (HCL), which kills many unwanted microorganisms and performs a digestive function. Further pepsinogen, which is transformed into pepsin in the acid environment and which functions to breakdown proteins into peptides and amino acids so that they become available for absorption when delivered to the gut .

Although there is some water (Scholer and Code, 1954) (and electrolyte) flux across the gastric mucosa, and there is net absorption (and metabolism) of alcohol in the gastric mucosa (Caballeria et al, 1989), quantitative absorption of water and most nutrients occurs in the intestine. Thus, the pyloric sphincter (together with the intra-gastric pressure gradient), which closes the intestine off from the stomach, regulates the rate at which nutrients are made available for absorption.

Control of gastric emptying (GE)

The stomach is under regulatory control from the duodenum. Gastric emptying is regulated via neural and hormonal control mechanisms, primarily in response to input from receptors in the duodenum. The presence of nutrients and the characteristics of nutrients in the duodenum are particularly important in regulating GE.

Particle size and osmolality

Particle size is one factor which influences GE. Particles with a size of >2mm normally do not leave the stomach during digestion. For this reason, liquids or homogenised meals empty more quickly than solid meals. Dietary fibre also delays gastric emptying, possibly due to the presence of "particles" which remain intact through the upper portions of the GI tract and their influence on the unstirred water layer in the gut. Increased energy density and osmolality are also negatively related to gastric emptying rate. An increase in macro nutrient density, resulting in an increased energy density and/or osmolality, has been found to be associated with a decreased GE rate of fluids. A theory of osmoreceptors in the duodenum (Hunt and Pathak, 1960) has been developed to explain this effect.

Specific nutrients, glucose

Several specific nutrients are known to exert a strong inhibitory effect on GE. Among these is glucose. In most early studies both glucose content and osmolality increased simultaneously. Thus some of the early results regarding the effect of osmolality on GE may actually be explained by the glucose content which, rather than the osmolality, retarded GE. More recently, studies have been conducted in which glucose and glucose polymer (maltodextrin) solutions of equal concentration have been compared.

Glucose polymer solutions have a lower osmolality than free glucose solutions of similar concentration. In such a manner the influences of osmolality and CHO concentration can be separated. Several studies have been conducted with eucaloric glucose and glucose polymer solutions In some of these studies there was a trend for faster emptying of the polymers but in others there was no difference (Rehrer et al, 1989, 1991; Sole and Noakes, 1989; Fink et al, 1983). However, when total gastric volume has been compared, a significantly greater remaining volume has been observed with a glucose solution (Foster et al, 1980). These differences are explained by the fact that a greater osmolality of gastric contents stimulates gastric secretions (Costill and Saltin, 1974; Sole and Noakes, 1989). The fact that a more concentrated glucose solution empties more slowly than a less concentrated solution means that the rate of fluid provision to the intestines is less with a more concentrated solution. However, the rate of CHO provision is nevertheless greater with a more concentrated solution (Fig. 1). Other nutrients which are known to exert a strong, inhibitory effect on GE are fat and protein (amino acids).

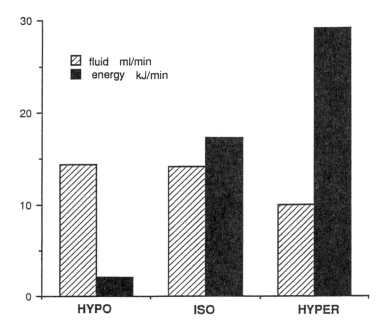

Fig. 1   Comparison of gastric emptying rates of artificially sweetened water (HYPO), a 7% carbohydrate-electrolyte solution (Isostar[R] - ISO) and a hypertonic glucose-polymer solution (Perform [R] - HYPER). The gastric emptying rate of fluid from HYPO and ISO is the same. However ISO delivers substantially more energy (carbohydrate) to the intestine. The fluid delivery of HYPER is smaller than from HYPO and ISO. However, due to the high carbohydrate content HYPER delivers the most carbohydrate to the intestine.

Beverage temperature
    The effects of beverage temperature on gastric emptying are less clear. In the only study concerning beverage temperature conducted during exercise, an increased GE rate was observed with a beverage at 5° C compared to ingestion of the same beverage at 15, 25 or 35° C (Costill and Saltin, 1974). At rest, Sun et al (1988) observed that the initial emptying rates (10 min) of both hot (50° C)

and cold (4° C) orange juice were slower than that of orange juice at body temperature (37° C), but the half-emptying times were not significantly different. McArthur and Feldman (1989) also observed no difference in GE rate of hot (58° C), warm (37° C) or cold (4° C) coffee at rest, when measured at 15, 30 and 60 min after ingestion. From these results it may be concluded that temperature most probably only affects gastric emptying as long as the intragastric temperature differs from body temperature

Volume

The effect of the volume of ingested contents is one of enhanced GE with increasing volume (Hunt and MacDonald, 1954; Marbaix, 1898). This explains why a phased semi-exponential emptying pattern is observed after ingestion of one large bolus (Hunt and Spurrell, 1951). Additionally, with a 7% isotonic carbohydrate solution, the fast phase of emptying seen after ingestion of a single bolus of 600 ml was found to be maintained with repeated drinking (150 ml/20 min) during exercise (Fig. 2; Rehrer et al, 1990). With this knowledge one must question the advice often given to athletes to ingest only small quantities frequently instead of filling the stomach with a larger quantity and refilling it periodically. For a review of the influence of volume on GE see Noakes et al (1991). An upper limit to the stimulatory effect of volume on GE of ~ 600 ml has been suggested by Costill and Saltin (1974). However, Hunt and Spurrell (1951) found increasing rates of emptying with volumes of up to 750 ml. Additionally, Mitchell and Voss (1991) observed increasing emptying rates with an ingestion rate of 23 ml/kg^{-1}/h^{-1}, which resulted in a gastric residue of over 1000 ml. It may be that adaptation to ingestion of large volumes takes place. If so, then this may explain the discrepancy in results.

Effects of exercise and training status on gastric emptying

Training status

When two groups, one trained and competitive in bicycling and the other untrained for all endurance activity, were compared, no differences in the GE rates of varying beverages were observed, at rest or during exercise (Fig. 3 Rehrer et al, 1989).

Type of exercise

No effect of type of exercise (running vs. bicycling) on GE rate has been observed (Rehrer et al, 1990; Houmard et al, 1991). Gastric emptying data with repeated ingestion of a 7% CHO-electrolyte beverage in the same individuals while biking and running at 70% Wmax (maximal workload) were found to be the same (Rehrer, 1990). Large variation in emptying rates is

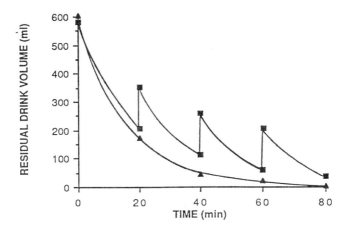

Fig. 2   Gastric emptying rate of one bolus (600 ml) of a 7% carbohydrate--
electrolyte solution (Isostar[R]) or water followed by repeated intakes of
150 ml/20 min. Both studies were performed on the same subjects
during exercise (70% exercise intensity). The comparison shows that a
high rate of gastric emptying can be maintained through repeated
drinking and that virtually no fluid remains in the stomach with intakes
as high as 900 ml/hr.

observed as a result of beverage composition, but no difference is observed as a
result of exercise type. Although the amount of vibration experienced by the body
during running is more than double that experienced during bicycling (Rehrer and
Meijer, 1991), this apparently does not affect GE. This difference in body vibration
may, however, be related to the greater frequency of gastrointestinal symptoms
reported during running versus bicycling (Sullivan, 1987; Rehrer et al, 1990b, for
review see Brouns, 1991) (Fig. 4).

Exercise intensity
    No consistent, significant effect of exercise at $\leq$ 70% VO$_2$ max on GE has been
observed (Fordtran and Saltin, 1967; Costill et al, 1970; Costill and Saltin, 1974;
Feldman and Nixon, 1982; Neufer et al, 1986; Neufer et al, 1989; Rehrer et al,
1989). However, above this intensity a significant decrease in GE

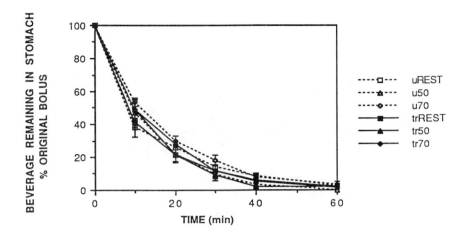

Fig. 3   Comparison of gastric emptying rates of a 7% carbohydrate-electrolyte
solution (Isostar[R]) in trained (tr) and untrained (u) subjects at rest, 50%
of maximal working capacity (50) and 70 % (70). The study shows that
there is no effect of training status or exercise intensity up to 70 % of
maximal working capacity, on gastric emptying rate.

has been observed (Fordtran and Saltin, 1967; Costill and Saltin, 1974; Neufer
et al, 1989; Sole and Noakes, 1989).

Intestinal absorption
    Absorption of glucose is primarily an active process. This active transport is
coupled to the absorption of sodium (Crane, 1962; Curran, 1960; Riklis and
Quastel, 1958; Schedl and Clifton, 1963; Schultz and Zalusky, 1964). This is in
contrast to the absorption of fructose which is not transported actively, but is
transported via sodium independent facilitated diffusion. This results in faster
absorption of glucose than fructose (Fordtran, 1975; Holdsworth and Dawson,
1964). The coupled, active transport of glucose and sodium also results in
enhanced water absorption with dilute glucose, sucrose, glucose polymer and
starch solutions. Several authors have found increased <u>net</u> absorption (subtracting
secretion losses) of water from solutions containing $\leq$ 7% glucose-containing CHO
and sodium which are also hypo- or isotonic (<300 mosm.kg[-1]) above that of plain
water.   Additionally plain water induces a net secretion of electrolytes into the
gastrointestinal lumen (Leiper and Maughan, 1986; Gisolfi

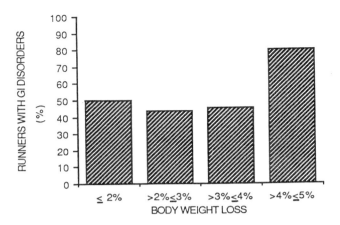

Fig. 4   Frequency of gastrointestinal problems in 44 participants of a marathon. Subjects who lost > 4% of body weight (sweatloss of approximately 2.5 liters) experienced significantly more problems.

et al 1990; Rehrer, 1990). These results are based upon results obtained with triple lumen jejunal perfusion, which measures the net absorption of a perfused, 30 cm segment of the intestine. This technique limits measurement to only a limited section of the intestine, with a constant perfusion rate, which may not represent the rate at which fluids are normally made available to the intestine as a result of variation in gastric emptying. Nevertheless, these results are further supported by clinical data which show that oral rehydration solutions (usually containing ~3-5% glucose and ~30-60 meq. l⁻¹ sodium) improve net water and sodium balance and reduce stool output in patients with dehydrating diarrhoea (for review see Farthing, 1988).   The osmolality of the luminal contents will be increased by ingestion of a strongly hypertonic solution. This will result in net secretion of water into the intestinal lumen, instead of absorption.   Accordingly iso-osmotic solutions remain practically iso-osmotic throughout the absorption period (Miller, 1949; Leiper and Maughan, 1986; Rehrer et al, in press). The inward flux of water into the intestinal lumen, during exercise, may only be transient. However, when extracellular fluid volume has been compromised, this flux may temporarily increase the degree of dehydration.

In light of the effect of increased beverage osmolality on gastric as well as intestinal secretions one does well to keep the osmolality of a beverage in mind when choosing a solution for supplementation during exercise. Particularly when more concentrated solutions (>10% CHO) are consumed an advantage may be found, in this respect, with glucose polymer solutions versus mono- or di-saccharide solutions. The concentration of glucose per se, in addition to the may be found, in this respect, with glucose polymer solutions versus mono- or di-saccharide solutions. The concentration of glucose per se, in addition to the osmolality, influences the net water absorption. Absorption rates, as determined by triple lumen perfusion, of water and two CHO-electrolyte solutions with varying concentrations and osmolality, are depicted in Figure 5. As can be observed, perfusion with an isotonic solution containing 7% CHO, mainly sucrose (Isostar(^{R})), resulted in a significantly greater water absorption than with plain water. A hypertonic 17% glucose solution (1223 mosm.kg^{-1}) resulted in net water secretion. In contrast, a 17% maltodextrin solution (Perform(^{R})) which had an osmolality similar to that of the 4.5% solution (313 mosm.kg^{-1}) resulted in net water absorption, but the rate of absorption was significantly less than that of the 4.5% solution. The more concentrated carbohydrate solutions however, induced the greatest carbohydrate absorption at the cost of reduced water absorption (Fig. 5).

Dehydration

Gisolfi et al (1977) were the first to note that gastrointestinal distress occured specifically in an athlete exercising in the heat. In a survey among marathon runners a higher frequency of gastrointestinal symptoms was observed in dehydrated runners who had lost more than 4% of body weight (Fig. 4). In controlled laboratory studies GE rate has been observed to be decreased with dehydration during exercise (Neufer et al, 1989; Rehrer et al, 1990) In the study we conducted, when a beverage was consumed during running exercise after dehydration (~3.5% body weight loss) six out of 16 subjects had GI symptoms and the GE rate was reduced.

Under euhydration conditions gastrointestinal symptoms were never observed during several gastric emptying studies in our laboratory. Whether the reduction in gastric emptying rate is a cause of or is a result of the symptoms, possibly being related to blood flow reduction to the gastrointestinal tract, can only be speculated upon at this time.

Practical considerations

When is carbohydrate supplementation warranted?

Recommendations for sportsmen and women should be based upon expected needs (CHO) and losses (fluid). Prediction can be made regarding CHO stores by taking into consideration the duration and intensity of exercise. Thus, in general, for maximal CHO utilisation during exercise which will last for >45 min at 70% VO$_2$max or above, supplementation with CHO is, in most cases, beneficial to delay fatigue and to enhance performance. There are a few studies which show a beneficial effect of CHO supplementation during intensive

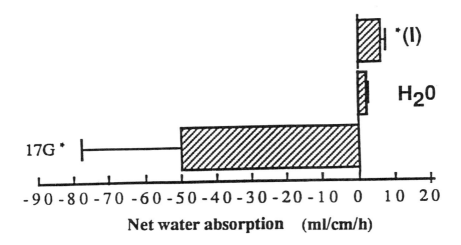

Fig. 5   Net fluid movement in the gut (negative figures = net absorption, positive figures = net secretion) after giving water, a 7% isotonic carbohydrate-electrolyte solution (ISO), (Isostar ®), or a 17 % hypertonic glucose solution (1223 mOsm) (17 G). ISO is significantly faster absorbed than water. The hypertonic glucose solution exerts a strong osmotic drive resulting in net water secretion into the gut.

interval type exercise of short duration (Murray et al, 1989; Neufer et al, 1987). One may speculate that the improvement observed with CHO supplementation, with an exercise regimen in which glycogen would not be expected to be exhausted, may be a result of preferential CHO oxidation, in place of fat, which would allow for exercise at a higher intensity. Thus, in conclusion, CHO supplementation during or shortly after warming-up or during exercise will, in most cases of endurance exercise, offer a potential delay in fatigue and thus improvement in performance.

When should consumption take place?

When a CHO containing beverage is ingested in rest, however, in the last hour preceding exercise, one may experience a rebound hypoglycaemia as a result of high insulin levels present in the blood when exercise begins, which may under some exercise conditions affect performance. This effect can be overcome by postponing ingestion until during or after warming-up (when performed immediately prior to competition), through which catecholamine release is sufficient to blunt the insulin response (Brouns et al, 1989).

Estimating fluid needs

Estimates of fluid losses can be made by measuring body weight changes as a result of exercise, since the majority of weight loss is a result of fluid loss due to sweating and evaporative losses from breathing. Because of additional substrate and metabolic water losses one will not have to maintain the exact same weight to maintain fluid balance. Thus, if an athlete can limit his weight loss to 1% during long-lasting (>1.5 h) exercise he may still be in fluid balance. Performance decrements have been observed with losses of 2% of body weight and greater (Saltin, 1964), thus the rehydration scheme should be such as to keep weight change below this level.

Confounding factors

The physiological situation an athlete finds himself in, in particular with reference to the endogenous reserves, plays a large role in determining exogenous needs. When glycogen reserves are large, the point at which CHO availability will become limiting to performance will be postponed. Similarly when one is fully hydrated at the onset of exercise one will less quickly become dehydrated to a level which will result in performance decrease.

How knowledge of gastrointestinal function can be put to use

Since normal gastrointestinal function results in a delay in the time between ingestion and when water and nutrients are available to tissues and the vascular compartment one should begin to drink in advance of losses. A pre-hydration regime, immediately prior to athletic endeavour, coupled with periodic supplementation during exercise, beginning early on, is the only way to maintain fluid balance and CHO supply when endogenous reserves of one or both will become limiting during the exercise session.

Furthermore, the knowledge concerning gastrointestinal symptoms and reduced gastric emptying rate observed with dehydration (>3% body weight) during exercise further underscore the necessity of maintaining fluid balance rather than attempting to reinstate it after dehydration has already occurred. Supplementation in anticipation of needs includes choosing a hydration regimen which is tailored to the situation. Based upon gastric emptying rates of fluids and CHO with solutions of varying CHO concentration one can deduce that for a situation in which fluid losses may become critical before CHO supply becomes limiting (eg. extremely warm and/or humid) one should select a moderately concentrated (2-8% CHO) solution, since this will provide the greatest rate of fluid delivery (Costill 1990; Rehrer 1991). Because of increased gastrointestinal secretions as a result of hypertonic beverage ingestion, one should also select a beverage which is hypo- or isotonic (<300 mosm.kg[-1]). This is, consequently, important with respect to net water absorption in the intestine. Ingestion of a carbohydrate containing beverage which is hypo- or isotonic will initially result in a greater rate of net water absorption than a similarly concentrated hypertonic solution.

A situation in which endogenous CHO supply becomes limiting before fluid losses are of such a magnitude as to impede performance, can also occur. This may be found particularly when endurance activity is conducted in a cold climate. In this situation a more concentrated solution may be more advantageous based upon the fact that the greater the concentration of CHO in a solution is the greater the rate of CHO delivery is. With more highly concentrated solutions it is of critical importance to be aware of the osmolality of a beverage.

As the concentration increases, greater use of di- and polysaccharides must be made in order to keep the osmolality low. This is important in order to minimise gastrointestinal secretions. At very high concentrations only long-chain polymers (maltodextrin) can allow the osmolality of a beverage to remain low. Carbohydrate concentration may be increased to 15% in cool/cold climatic conditions (Brouns 1991c). When considering whether a highly or less-concentrated beverage is in order for a particular situation, one must also consider the availability and possibility for intake as well as acceptability of a beverage during exercise. A situation of highly intensive, long-lasting bicycling, such as that conducted during the Tour de France induces large sweat losses. However, a continual supply and a high rate of beverage intake, which is possible during cycling, precludes fluid balance from becoming a limiting factor for performance before carbohydrate availability. Cyclists in this situation may therefore benefit from a more concentrated (up to 15%) carbohydrate containing beverage. When ingested frequently, this will increase carbohydrate availability while also supplying sufficient water.

When water provision is of sole concern, there is, based upon gastric emptying rates, no apparent advantage to a carbohydrate-electrolyte containing solution. However, the benefits of carbohydrate (glucose, or glucose containing di- or polysaccharides) and sodium in stimulating net intestinal absorption of water should be borne in mind. In support of data obtained by triple lumen perfusion experiments with respect to intestinal absorption are results from clinical trials. In disease states which result in large fluid losses from diarrhoea, rehydration with oral rehydration solutions (approximate composition: 100-300 mmol.l[-1] glucose, sucrose, glucose polymer or starch; 35-60 mmol.l[-1] sodium; hypo- or isotonic) results in better net fluid assimilation, evidenced by lower stool volume and reduced mortality, than with water. Extrapolating to the rehydration of a healthy individual during exercise is taking a large leap. Although blood flow to the splanchnic bed is reduced during exercise (Qamar and Read, 1987; Wade et al, 1956) and absorption may, in turn, be reduced, there is no evidence to suggest that this would alter the relative differences in absorption rates observed between various beverages at rest. Thus we may asssume that advantages in terms of absorption and fluid retention to a beverage with a particular composition, observed at rest may still be found during exercise.

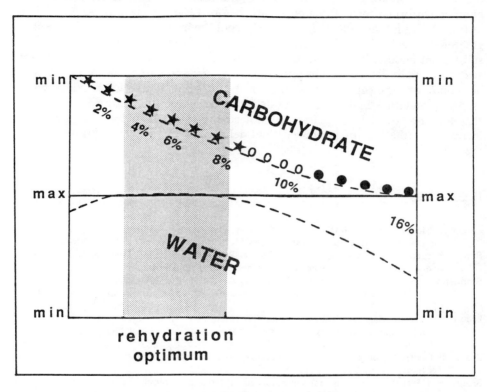

Fig. 6   Interaction of CHO and water on bioavailability of the 2 substances. A low carbohydrate content maximizes fluid absorption and thus availability. A high carbohydrate content maximizes CHO availability but reduces that of water. The symbols indicate CHO concentration which can be used under different climatological circumstances/sweat losses. * Hot, large sweatloss; *o warm, moderate sweat loss; *oo cool, small sweat loss

Summarizing advice

Depending on needs, dictated by CHO availability and fluid balance, one or the other may become limiting to performance. The exercise duration, intensity, climatic conditions and previous metabolic state (e.g. glycogen depleted versus loaded; hypo-versus euhydrated) will primarily determine whether CHO or water first becomes limiting. In general, in hot (and humid) conditions fluid deficit may hamper performance or threaten health before CHO deficit will occur. In long-lasting, fairly intense sports in relatively cool environments the possibility is far greater that lack of sufficient CHO will reduce performance before fluid losses are substantial enough to be detrimental. Thus climatic conditions and quantitative sweat loss both determine the priorities for water and carbohydrate ingestion. In hot conditions the carbohydrate content of drinks should allow a maximal gastric emptying and intestinal absorption rate for fluids. The carbohydrate content should therefore not exceed 80 g/liter. In cool conditions carbohydrate supply can be increased at the cost of a reduced fluid delivery to the intestine (Brouns, 1991c; Fig. 6).

References

Bonen A, McDermott JC, Hutber CA. (1989) Carbohydrate metabolism in skeletal muscle: an update of current concepts. Int J Sports Med, 10, 385-401.

Brandenberger G, Candas C, Follenius M, Libert JP, Kahn JM. (1986) Vascular fluid shifts and endocrine responses to exercise in the heat. Eur J Appl Physiol, 55, 123-229.

Brandenberger G, Candas V, Follenius M, Kahn JM. (1989) The influence of the initial state of hydration on endocrine responses to exercise in the heat. Eur J Appl Physiol, 58, 674-679.

Brouns F, Rehrer NJ, Saris WHM, Beckers E, Menheere P, ten Hoor F. (1989) Effect of carbohydrate intake during warming-up on the regulation of blood glucose during exercise. Int J Sports Med, 10, S68-S75.

Brouns F. (1991a) Etiology of gastrointestinal disturbances during endurance events. Scand J Med Sci Sports, 1, 66-77.

Brouns F. (1991b) Gastrointestinal symptoms in athletes: physiological and nutritional aspects. In: Brouns F, Saris WHM, Newsholme EA. (eds.) Advances in Nutrition and Top Sport; Medicine and Sport Science, 32, pp. 166-199 Karger, Basel.

Brouns F. (1991c) Dehydration-rehydration: a praxis oriented approach. J Sport Sci, 9 (special issue), 143-152.

Brouns F, Saris WHM, Beckers E, Adlercreutz H, van der Vusse GJ, Keizer HA, Kuipers H, Menheere P, Wagenmakers AJM, ten Hoor F. (1989) Metabolic changes induced by sustained exhaustive cycling and diet manipulation. Int J Sports Med, 10, Suppl 1, S49-S62.

Caballeria J, Frezza M, Hernandez-Munoz, R et al. (1989) Gastric origin of the first-pass metabolism of ethanol in humans: effect of gastrectomy. Gastroenterology, 97, 1205-1209.

Coggan AR, Coyle EF. (1991) Carbohydrate ingestion during prolonged exercise: effects on metabolism and performance. Ex Sport Sci Rev, 19, JO Holloszy (ed.), pp. 1-40.

Coggan AR, Coyle EF. (1989) Metabolism and performance following carbohydrate ingestion late in exercise. Med Sci Sports Exerc, **21**, 5965.

Costill DL. (1977) Sweating: its composition and effects on body fluids. In: The Marathon: Physiological, Medical, Epidemiological and Psychological Studies, pp. 161-174, P. Milvy (ed.), NY Academy of Sciences, New York.

Costill DL, Kammer WF, Fisher A. (1970) Fluid ingestion during distance running. Arch Environ Health, **21**, 520-525.

Costill DL, Saltin B. (1974) Factors limiting gastric emptying. J Appl Physiol, **37**, 679-683.

Costill DL. (1990) Gastric emptying of fluids during exercise. In: Gisolfi CV, Lamb DR (eds.); Fluid homeostasis during exercise. Benchmark Press, pp. 97-121.

Coyle EF. (1991) Timing and method of increased carbohydrate intake to cope with heavy training, competition and recovery. J Sport Sci, **9** (special issue), 53-70.

Coyle EF. (1991) Carbohydrate feedings: effects on metabolism, performance and recovery. In: Brouns F, Saris WH, Newsholme EA (eds.), Advances in Nutrition and Top Sport pp. 1-14, Med and Sport Sci, **32**, Karger, Basel.

Crane RK. (1962) Hypothesis for mechanism of intestinal active transport of sugars. Fed Proc, **21**, 891- 895.

Curran PF. (1960) Na, Cl and water transport by rat ileum in vitro. J Gen Physiol, **43**, 1137-1148.

Davis JM, Lamb DR, Pate RR, Slentz CA, Burgess WA, Bartoli WP. (1988) Carbohydrate electrolyte drinks: effects on endurance in the heat. Am J Clin Nutr, **48**, 1023-1030.

Davis JM, Burgess WA, Slentz CA, Bartoli WP, Pate RR. (1988) Effects of ingesting 6 % and 12 % glucose/electrolyte beverages during prolonged intermittent cycling in the heat. Eur J Appl Physiol, **57**, 563-569.

Farthing MJG. (1988) History and rationale for oral rehydration and recent developments in formulating an optimal solution. Drugs, **36** (supplement 4), 80-90.

Feldman M, Nixon JV. (1982) Effect of exercise on postprandial gastric secretion and emptying in humans. J Appl Physiol, **53**, 851-854.

Fink WJ, Costill DL, Stevens CF. (1983) Gastric-emptying characteristics of complete nutritional liquids. In: Nutrient Utilization During Exercise. Ross Symposium, Columbus, Ohio: Ross Laboratories, pp. 112-115.

Fordtran JS. (1975) Stimulation of active and passive sodium absorption by sugars in the human jejunum. J Clin Invest, **55**, 728-737.

Fordtran JS, Saltin B. (1967) Gastric emptying and intestinal absorption during prolonged severe exercise. J Appl Physiol, **23**, 331-335.

Foster C, Costill DL, Fink WJ. (1980) Gastric emptying characteristics of glucose and glucose polymer solutions. Res Q, **51**, 299-305.

Gisolfi CV, Summers RV, Schedl HP, Bleiler TL, Oppliger RA. (1990) Human intestinal absorption: direct vs. indirect measurements. Am J Physiol, **258**, G216-G222.

Gisolfi CV, Wilson NC, Claxton B. (1977) Work tolerance of distance runners. Ann NY Acad Sci, **301**, 139-150.

Greenhaff PL, Clough PJ. (1989) Predictors of sweat loss in man during prolonged exercise. Eur J Appl Physiol, **58**, 348-352.

Hargreaves M. (1991) Carbohydrates and exercise. J Sport Sci, **9** (special issue), 17-28.

Holdsworth CD, Dawson AM. (1964) The absorption of monosaccharides in man. Clin Sci, **27**, 371-379.

Houmard JA, Egan PC, Johns RA, Neufer PD, Chenier TC, Israel RG. (1991) Gastric emptying during 1 h of cycling and running at 75% VO$_2$max. Med Sci Sports Exerc, **23**, 320-325.

Hunt JN, MacDonald I. (1954) The influence of volume on gastric emptying. J Physiol, **126**, 459-474.

Hunt JN, Pathak JD. (1960) The osmotic effects of some simple molecules and ions on gastric emptying. J Physiol, **154**, 254-269.

Hunt, JN, Spurrell WR. (1951) The pattern of emptying of the human stomach. J Physiol, **113**, 157-168.

Leiper JB, Maughan RJ. (1986) Absorption of water and electrolytes from hypotonic, isotonic and hypertonic solutions. J Physiol, 373, 90P.

Leiper JB, Maughan RJ. (1988) Experimental models for the investigation of water and solute transport in man. Drugs, 36 (supplement 4), 65-79.

Marbaix O. (1898) Le passage pylorique. Cellule, 14, 249-330.

Maughan RJ. (1985) Thermoregulation and fluid balance in marathon competition at low ambient temperatures. Int J Sports Med, 6, 15-19.

Maughan RJ, Fenn CE, Leiper JB. (1989) Effects of fluid, electrolyte and substrate ingestion on endurance capacity. Eur J Appl Physiol, 58, 481-486.

Maughan RJ. (1991) Fluid and electrolyte loss and replacement in exercise. J Sports Sci, 9, 117-142.

McArthur KE, Feldman M. (1989) Gastric acid secretion, gastric release and gastric emptying in humans as affected by liquid meal temperature. Am J Clin Nutr, 49, 51-54.

Miller TG. (1949) Intestinal intubation. Cleveland Clin Q, 16, 68.

Mitchell JB, Costill DL, Houmard JA, Flynn MG, Fink WJ, Beltz JD. (1988) Effects of carbohydrate ingestion on gastric emptying and exercise performance. Med Sci Sports Exerc, 20, 110-115.

Mitchell JB, Costill DL, Houmard JA, Fink WJ, Robergs RA, Davis JA. (1989) Gastric emptying: influence of prolonged exercise and carbohydrate concentration. Med Sci Sports Exerc, 21, 269-274.

Mitchell JB, Voss KW. (1991) The influence of volume of fluid ingested on gastric emptying and fluid balance during prolonged exercise. Med Sci Sports Exerc, 23, 314-319.

Murray R, Paul GL, Seifert JG, Eddy DE, Halaby GA. (1989) The effects of glucose, fructose, and sucrose ingestion during exercise. Med Sci Sports Exerc, 21, 275-282.

Murray R, Eddy DE, Murray TW, Seifert JG, Paul GL, Halaby GA. (1987) The effect of fluid and carbohydrate feedings during intermittent cycling exercise. Med Sci Sports Exerc, 19, 597-604.

Murray R. (1987) The effects of consuming carbohydrate-electrolyte beverages on gastric emptying and fluid absorption during and following exercise. Sports Med, 4, 322-351.

Murray R, Seifert JG, Eddy OE, Paul GL, Halaby GA. (1989) Carbohydrate feeding and exercise: effect of beverage carbohydrate content. Eur J Appl Physiol, 59, 152-158.

Nadel ER, Wenger CB, Roberts MF, Stolwijk JAJ, Cafarelli E. (1977) Physiological defences against hyperthermia of exercise. Ann NY Acad Sci, 301, 98-109.

Nelson PB, Robinson AG, Kapoor W, Rinaldo J. (1988) Hyponatremia in a marathoner. Phys Sports Med, 16, 78-88.

Neufer PD, Costill DL, Fink WJ, Kirwan JP, Fielding RA, Flynn MG. (1986) Effects of exercise and carbohydrate composition on gastric emptying. Med Sci Sports Exerc, 18, 658-662.

Neufer PD, Costill DL, Flynn MG, Kirwan JP, Mitchell JB, Houmard J. (1987) Improvements in exercise performance : effects of carbohydrate feeding and diet. J Appl Physiol, 62, 983-988.

Neufer PD, Young AJ, Sawka MN. (1989) Gastric emptying during exercise: effects of heat stress and hypohydration. Eur J Appl Physiol, 58, 433-439.

Newsholme EA, Leech AR. (1983) Biochemistry for the Medical Sciences. John Wiley and Sons, Chichester, p. 337.

Noakes TD, Goodwin N, Rayner BL, Branken T, Taylor RKN. (1985) Water intoxication: a possible complication during endurance exercise. Med Sci Sports Exerc, 17, 370-375.

Noakes TD, Norman RJ, Buck RH, Godlonton J, Stevenson K, Pittaway D. (1990) The incidence of hyponatremia during prolonged ultraendurance exercise. Med Sci Sports Exerc, 22, 165-170.

Noakes TD, Rehrer NJ, Maughan RJ. (1991) The importance of volume in regulating gastric emptying. Med Sci Sports Exerc, 23, 307-313.

Nose H, Mack GW, Xiangrong S, Nadel ER. (1988) Role of osmolality and plasma volume during rehydration in humans. J Appl Physiol, **65**, 325-331. Qamar MI, Read AE. (1987) Effects of exercise on mesenteric blood flow in man. Gut **28**: 583-587.

Rehrer NJ, Beckers EJ, Brouns F, ten Hoor F, Saris WHM. (1989) Exercise and training effects on gastric emptying of carbohydrate beverages. Med Sci Sports Ex, **21**, 540-549.

Rehrer NJ, Brouns F, Beckers EJ, ten Hoor F, Saris WHM. (1990a) Gastric emptying with repeated drinking during running and bicycling. Int J Sports Med, **11**, 238-243.

Rehrer NJ, Beckers EJ, Brouns F, ten Hoor F, Saris WHM. (1990b) Effects of dehydration on gastric emptying and gastrointestinal distress while running. Med Sci Sports Ex, **22**, 790-795.

Rehrer NJ. (1991) Aspects of dehydration and rehydration during exercise. In: Brouns F, Saris WHM, Newsholme EA (eds.) Advances in Nutrition and Top Sport, Med and Sport Sci, **32**, pp. 128-146.

Rehrer NJ, van Kemenade MC, Meester TA, Brouns F, Saris WHM. (1991) Gastrointestinal complaints in relation to dietary intakes in triathletes. Int J Sports Nutr, (in the Press).

Rehrer NJ, Meijer GA. (1992) Biomechanical vibration of the abdominal region during running and bicycling. J Sports Med (in the Press).

Rehrer NJ, Wagenmakers AJM, Beckers EJ, Halliday D, Leiper JB, Brouns F, Maughan RJ, Westerterp K, Saris WHM. (1992) Gastric emptying, absorption, availability and oxidation of carbohydrate beverages and water during prolonged exercise. J Appl Physiol, (in press).

Riklis E, Quastel JH. (1958) Effects of cations on sugar absorption by isolated surviving guinea pig intestine. Can J Biochem Physiol, **36**, 347-363.

Saris WHM. (1991) Exercise, nutrition and weight control. In: Brouns F, Saris WHM, Newsholme EA (eds.) Advances in Nutrition and Top Sport; Medicine and Sport Science, Karger, Basel, **32**, pp. 200-215.

Saltin B. (1964) Aerobic work capacity and circulation at exercise in man. Acta Physiol Scand, **62** (suppl 238), 1-52.

Scholer JF, Code CF. (1954) Rate of absorption of water from stomach and small bowel of human beings. Gastroenterology, **27**, 565-577.

Schultz SG, Zalusky R. (1964) Ion transport in isolated rat ileum II. The interaction between active sodium and active sugar transport. J Gen Physiol, **47**, 1043-1059.

Sole CC, Noakes TD. (1989) Faster gastric emptying for glucose-polymer and fructose solutions than for glucose in humans. Eur J Appl Physiol, **58**, 605-612.

Sun WM, Houghton LA, Read NW, Grundy DG, Johnson AG. (1988) Effect of meal temperature on gastric emptying of liquids in man. Gut, **29**, 302-305.

Wade OL, Combes B, Childs AW, Wheeler HO, Cournand A, Bradley SE. (1956) The effect of exercise on the splanchnic blood flow and splanchnic blood volume in normal men. Cli Sci, **15**, 457-463.

Williams C, Nute MG, Broadbank L, Vinall S. (1990) Influence of fluid intake on endurance running performance. A comparison between water, glucose and fructose solutions. Eur J Appl Physiol, **60**, 112-119.

Dietary supplements, drugs and performance

M.H. Williams

Abstract. Experience suggests that athletes at various levels of competition, from the Olympian to the 45 minute 10-kilometer road racer, will always be in search of effective ergogenic aids. Although a variety of pharmaceutical ergogenics may effectively enhance performance, their use to enhance sports performance is not only illegal and unethical, but may also be unhealthy as well. Most nutrients are considered to be legal, but the use of several may contravene one aspect IOC antidoping rule which notes that athletes will not take any physiological substance in abnormal quantities with the sole intention of artificially enhancing performance. Nevertheless, all nutritional supplements are currently legal.
The first objective of the sports nutritionist should be the education of the athlete relative to planning and consuming a balanced, healthful diet that will meet specific individual calorific and nutrient requirements. Although genetic endowment and effective training are the determinants of sport success, proper nutrition may also be decisive under certain circumstances. Proper timing and composition of the pre-event meal, carbohydrate intake before and during prolonged exercise, rehydration during exercise in the heat, and maintenance of an optimal body weight and composition represent several nutritional practices which have been shown to influence sport performance. Research with several other nutritional practices, as noted in this review, show promise, but additional research is necessary for substantiation. Properly conducted research will provide sport nutritionists with the nutritional information essential to maximize sports performance in a safe, legal, and effective manner.

Keywords: Nutrition, anabolic streoids, blood doping, erythropoietin, alcohol, beta blockers, caffeine, amino acids, vitamins, minerals, phosphate, bicarbonate

Introduction

Success in sport at the highest levels of competition is determined primarily by two general factors. First, the athlete must be genetically endowed with the biomechanical, physiological, and psychological characteristics that appear to be critical for specific types of performance. Second, the athlete must receive appropriate training in order to optimize these characteristics during competition. At the international level of athletic competition, and even at lower levels of competition, these characteristics may be so evenly matched that the difference between first and second place is often determined in milliseconds. Thus, in order to get a competitive edge over their opponents, athletes over the years have attempted to enhance performance beyond the effects of training by resorting to various substances or techniques known as ergogenic aids, or ergogenics. (Lamb and Williams, 1991).

The primary purpose of an ergogenic is to enhance the <u>production</u>, <u>control</u>, or <u>efficiency</u> of human energy specific to a given sport. For example, anabolic steroids may stimulate muscle development and enhance energy <u>production</u> for power events; alcohol may reduce anxiety and hand tremor, enhancing energy <u>control</u> in marksmanship events such as pistol shooting and archery; diuretics may induce a rapid weight loss without impairing the ability to generate short-term power, enhancing the <u>efficiency</u> of the applied power generated by the high jumper to lift the center of gravity in competition.

Although Williams (1989a) has categorized ergogenics into five categories (mechanical; psychological; physiological; pharmacological; nutritional), he has noted that these categories are not rigidly defined, for a single ergogenic may elicit possible ergogenic effects related to each category. For example, caffeine is generally classified as a pharmacological ergogenic because it is a drug. However, it is also a component of certain beverages and foods, such as coffee and chocolate, and thus may be classified as a nutritional ergogenic. As a diuretic, caffeine may be classified as a mechanical ergogenic since it may enhance mechanical efficiency. It may also be classified as a physiological ergogenic because it enhances a variety of physiological processes deemed important to athletic performance, and as a psychological ergogenic because of its stimulating effect on mental processes.

It is important to note that ergogenics may elicit opposite effects if improperly applied. For example, beta blockers may enhance performance in marksmanship events by decreasing anxiety, but may impair performance in highly trained aerobic endurance athletes by mitigating appropriate cardiovascular and metabolic adjustments to high intensity aerobic exercise (Williams, 1991a). Agents that impair performance are referred to as ergolytics (Eichner, 1989).

Numerous ergogenics have been applied to sport for centuries, and the subject has been treated extensively in several texts (Lamb and Williams, 1991; Morgan, 1972; Wadler and Hainline, 1989; Williams, 1974; 1983A; 1989A). The purpose of this brief review is to highlight several of the pharmacological ergogenics that may have nutritional counterparts and a variety of nutritional ergogenics whose effectiveness has been studied in recent years and are not presented in other segments of this Congress meeting.

Pharmacological ergogenics

Literally hundreds of different drugs have been used by athletes in attempts to enhance performance, and the current list of banned drugs issued by the

International Olympic Committee (IOC) contains several hundred listed under the general categories of alcohol, anabolic steroids, human growth hormone, beta blockers, blood doping, corticosteroids, diuretics, local anesthetics, narcotic analgesics, and stimulants. This review will focus briefly on four general areas of pharmacological ergogenics that are related somewhat to nutritional ergogenics.

Anabolic steroids and human growth hormone (HGH)

Many athletes desire to increase muscle mass either for strength and power athletic events or for aesthetics in bodybuilding competition. Although nutritional supplements such as protein, amino acids, and chromium are popular, anabolic steroids have been used for years and human growth hormone (HGH) appears to becoming popular. Anabolic steroids represent a class of synthetic drugs designed to mimic the effects of the hormone testosterone. The structure of the testosterone molecule has been rearranged to maximize the anabolic effects and minimize the androgenic effects, although all anabolic steroids do produce some androgenic effects. Anabolic steroids may affect a variety of body cells that may impact upon athletic performance, such as the bone marrow to stimulate red blood cell production, and thus have some medical applications. However, the main target for most illegal users is the muscle cell. Although the mechanism is not totally understood, anabolic steroids are believed to enter the cell nucleus and bind to DNA, which then promotes the generation of RNA to direct the formation of muscle proteins. Other mechanisms also may be operative, and it is likely that the overall effect is generated by the interaction of several mechanisms (Lombardo et al, 1991)

Anabolic steroids have been used by strength and power athletes, as well as bodybuilders, for years because of their ability to increase muscle mass and the associated potential for power production. In the United States, they are also used by male nonathletes in attempts to enhance body image. Current estimates are that one million Americans use anabolic steroids, including approximately 5 percent of high school students. Most obtain steroids on the black market and a conservative estimate is over $100 million in yearly sales. To help stem the flow of these drugs, the United States Congress passed legislation leading to severe monetary and incarceration penalties to distributors.

The ergogenicity of anabolic steroids has been the subject of several major reviews (American College of Sports Medicine, 1987; Lombardo et al, 1991; Yesalis et al, 1989). Most reviewers agree that when combined with a proper resistance training program and adequate nutrient intake, anabolic steroids may increase lean body mass. Additionally, although the available data do not appear to be as consistent, most reviewers (American College of Sports Medicine, 1987; Lombardo et al, 1991; Williams, 1974) have suggested that anabolic steroids could increase muscular strength, a judgment based primarily on the fact that nearly

50 percent of the reported studies have shown statistically significant improvements in strength when anabolic steroids were used as an adjunct to the training program and no studies had shown an impairment. Other reviewers suggest that design flaws or vastly different methodologies in the available studies have led to such inconsistent results that a consensus is difficult to reach (Yesalis et al, 1989). One of the problems for researchers was the inability to duplicate the actual practices of the athlete in the laboratory because of the potential dangers of high dosages of steroids and techniques such as stacking and polydrug use; however, case studies with power-type athletes who would cycle on and off steroids have supported a potent ergogenic effect of such practices on muscular development and strength (Williams, 1989A).

Due to the increasing effectiveness of drug testing, there have been reports of increased interest among athletes relative to the efficacy of HGH as a possible substitute for anabolic steroids now that it is more readily available through biological engineering. One of the effects of HGH is to stimulate the production of another hormone, insulin-like growth factor-1, that spurs growth of muscle tissue, but other mechanisms may underlie its application as an ergogenic (Lombardo et al, 1991).

Very few data are available relative to the effect of HGH as an ergogenic. Crist and others (1988) and Yarasheski and colleagues (1990) noted increases in lean body mass when HGH was given to males during training, but Yarasheski and others suggested other tissues besides muscle must have accounted for the change since there were no significant increases in skeletal muscle protein synthesis and size, or in muscular strength, over the effects produced by weight training in the placebo group. Thus, at present, there are no data to support an ergogenic effect of HGH as a substitute for anabolic steroids. Because of the increased availability of HGH, its use as an ergogenic deserves increased research attention. The use of both these compounds is contraindicated for athletes since they are both proscribed by the IOC and both carry significant health risks (Lombardo et al, 1991; Williams, 1992).

Blood doping and erythropoietin (EPO)

Aerobic endurance athletes are interested in means to enhance oxygen delivery to the muscle, and they have supplemented with such nutrients as iron, folacin, and vitamins B_{12} and E in an attempt to maximize the oxygen transport capacity of the erythrocyte. Associated drug-related attempts include blood doping and erythropoietin (EPO).

The safest blood doping technique is the autologous procedure in which the athlete's blood is removed over a period of time and stored as frozen erythrocytes. The most effective results have been observed with dosages equivalent to approximately one liter of blood infused after normal hematological status is restored following the withdrawal. Within several days of competition, the stored blood is infused, leading to a significant increase in hemoglobin concentration and oxygen carrying capacity. When this protocol has been followed, laboratory studies have documented significant increases in maximal oxygen uptake and aerobic exercise tasks to exhaustion, and significant decreases in time to run eight kilometers (5 miles) (Spriet, 1991; Williams, 1983B).

In recent years, genetically engineered EPO has been used therapeutically to treat the anemia associated with certain forms of kidney disease that reduce the production of this natural hormone. As suggested at a recent American College of Sports Medicine symposium (Eichner, 1991), the use of EPO appears to be prevalent among certain athletic groups. Only limited data are available, but EPO appears to enhance aerobic endurance capacity similar to blood doping (Ekblom, 1989).

The use of blood doping and EPO is banned by the IOC; however, at the present time there is no test available that will successfully detect their use during athletic competition. Both techniques may possess serious side effects. Blood doping, particularly if homologous blood is used, increases the risk of disease transmission and incompatibility. EPO may be abused more readily, and large doses may increase the viscosity of the blood to dangerous levels, particularly during prolonged exercise under heat stress, and precipitate dangerous cardiovascular events.

Ethanol and beta blockers

In marksmanship sports such as pistol shooting and aesthetic endeavors involving precise timing such as diving, excessive anxiety may disrupt performance. Certain nutrients have been alleged to elicit a calming effect, but two of the most popular pharmaceuticals used over the years are ethanol and beta blockers. Ethanol is an anxiolytic and has been used for this purpose medicinally. Its use has been banned by the IOC, but only for certain sports involving marksmanship such as pistol shooting; it may actually be ergolytic in other events (Williams, 1991A). Unfortunately very few data are available relative to its effect on marksmanship performance. S'Jongers and others (1978) reported significant improvement in pistol shooting precision following one ounce of 80 proof ethanol, but the placebo group also improved performance. Reilly and Halliday (1985) studied the effects of ethanol on archery performance parameters, but the effects were inconsistent and no ergogenic effect on performance was documented.

Although developed primarily for the treatment of hypertension and cardiovascular disease, beta blockers are also anxiolytic and have been used in the treatment of benign essential tremor. Beta blockers have been applied to sports almost since their inception in the 1960s, and they appear to be effective. Several well-controlled studies have reported significant improvements in pistol shooting following beta blocker use by members of the British National Squad (Antal and Good, 1980) and amateur skilled pistol marksmen (Kruse et al, 1986). The dosage needs to be controlled, for excessive decreases in anxiety may also impair performance (Tesch, 1985).

The use of ethanol and beta blockers are both banned by the IOC for use in sports in which they may be ergogenic. Although their use is generally not banned for other athletes, both may be ergolytic, particularly the use of beta blockers by highly trained endurance athletes (Williams, 1991A)

Caffeine

Similar to alcohol, caffeine may be classified as a food drug, being readily available in many beverages and foods consumed on a daily basis. Caffeine has been used for ergogenic purposes since the turn of the century (Williams, 1974) and its effectiveness has been studied extensively, particularly in relation to aerobic endurance performance after research published in the late 1970s suggested that caffeine could enhance such performance (Costill et al, 1978; Ivy et al, 1979). Unfortunately, the available data still do not provide us with any definitive answers relative to the effect of caffeine on several physical performance parameters, possibly due to methodological differences between studies such as dosages and caffeine status of the subjects. The following discussion highlights the key points of several major reviews concerning the ergogenicity of caffeine (Conlee, 1991; Van Handel, 1983; Jacobson and Kulling, 1989; Wadler and Hainline, 1989; Williams, 1992).

Caffeine may increase alertness and improve reaction time, particularly so in individuals who are mentally fatigued. Large doses may induce anxiety, which could be ergolytic in events necessitating fine motor control. The vast majority of contemporary studies suggest that caffeine will not enhance performance in athletic events characterized by strength, speed, power,or muscular endurance. However, several studies have reported caffeine increased strength and power in subjects who abstained from caffeine use four days prior to the experiment, although it should be noted that the subjects took a variety of strength and power tests and only improved in several, not all (Williams, 1992).

The focus of much recent research has been the potential of caffeine to increase the serum level and muscle utilization of serum free fatty acids (FFA) during exercise which could provide a glycogen-sparing effect and enhanced performance in prolonged endurance tasks. Although it is well established that caffeine may raise serum FFA at rest, the data are equivocal as to whether or not this effect persists during exercise as the normal epinephrine response to exercise will elevate serum FFA and may abrogate the caffeine-induced effect. However, it appears that if subjects abstain from caffeine for 4-6 days and/or consume large doses (9-15 mg/kg), the FFA levels may be elevated beyond the independent effects of exercise. Using muscle biopsies, several studies have reported a glycogen sparing effect of caffeine, although the mechanism may be an increased utilization of muscle triglycerides.

The effect of caffeine on aerobic endurance performance is equivocal. As the duration of the endurance event increases to an hour or more the research data indicate, although not consistently, that caffeine may enhance performance. Although the sparing of glycogen may be involved, the mechanism of enhanced performance has not been elucidated, some investigators suggesting the stimulating psychological effect of caffeine. A recent presentation by Spriet and Graham (1991) noted significant elevations in epinephrine with caffeine ingestion of 9 mg/kg, a response which could enhance psychological stimulation. In this well-designed study, subjects experienced a phenomenal improvement in both running and cycling performance in tests to exhaustion at 85 percent VO_2max. Although not all data are supportive of an ergogenic effect, no study has reported a decrease in endurance performance with caffeine supplementation.

Although a potent stimulant, the IOC permits the use of some caffeine prior to competition; however, large doses may be grounds for disqualification. The permissible limit is a urine level of 12 $\mu g/ml$. Although body weight and composition may influence the results, 100 mg of caffeine will raise urine levels by about 1.5 $\mu g/ml$ in the average adult male; thus, 800 mg of caffeine, the equivalent of about 5-6 cups of brewed coffee, could exceed the legal limit.

Nutritional ergogenics

Because pharmacological ergogenics are illegal, and may pose a number of health risks, a variety of nutrients have been theorized to provide an effective, safe, and legal alternative. In this section we shall address some nutritional alternatives to pharmaceuticals, as well as other supplements marketed for athletes.

Amino acids

Various amino acid supplements have been advertised recently for athletes, suggestive of improved performance by diverse mechanisms. Although most amino acid supplements are targeted for strength athletes and bodybuilders, several are also designed for the endurance athlete. Research relative to the ergogenicity of such supplements is increasing, but the available data are somewhat limited. The following discussion is based upon several previous reviews (Bucci, 1989; Jacobson, 1990; Williams, 1991B; 1992) and several current investigations which appear only as abstracts because of only recent research interest concerning the ergogenicity of several amino acids.

Arginine and ornithine

The ingestion of arginine and ornithine may stimulate the release of HGH, although the dosages needed may cause gastric distress (Bucci et al, 1990). Five studies have been uncovered relative to the effect of arginine and/or ornithine supplementation on body composition or measures of muscular strength or power. Three of these studies indicated significant increases in lean body mass, but Williams (1992) indicated that the experimental methodology was so flawed in each study that the findings were invalid. Statistical significance was reported in two of the studies, but a recalculation using the appropriate statistical technique actually revealed no significant differences between the supplement and the placebo. The other two studies, presented at the 1991 meeting of the ACSM, appear only in abstract form; however, the methodological approach appears appropriate. Both studies reported no significant effect of arginine or a mixture of amino acids on measures of strength, power, or HGH in experienced weight lifters (Hawkins et al, 1991; Warren et al, 1991). Currently there are no sound research data to support an ergogenic effect of arginine and ornithine, which may be related to the general ineffectiveness of HGH noted previously. Additional research is merited to evaluate advertised claims of commercial products.

Tryptophan and branched chain amino acids (BCAA)

Tryptophan may also increase HGH, but its theoretical ergogenic effect is based upon another mechanism, the formation of 5-hydroxytryptamine and serotonin in the brain. Segura and Ventura (1988) postulate that these neurotransmitters might enhance performance by increasing the tolerance to pain during intense exercise. In support of their hypothesis, they found that 1,200 mg of tryptophan consumed in 300 mg doses over a 24 hour period increased time to exhaustion and a reduced rating of perceived exertion (RPE) on a treadmill run to exhaustion at 80 percent of VO_2max. Additional research is needed to confirm this finding. In contrast, Newsholme (1990) has hypothesized that serotonin may be involved in the etiology of fatigue because of its depressive activity; thus, entry of tryptophan into the brain may contribute to fatigue development. Based upon research with animals which suggests that low serum levels of branched chain amino acids (BCAA) may facilitate the entry of tryptophan into the brain, Newsholme theorizes that a decrease in serum levels of BCAA during the later stage of endurance exercise could be a contributing factor to fatigue. Theoretically, BCAA supplements could help delay the onset of fatigue. Unfortunately, few data are available to support this hypothesis. For example, some research has revealed no change in the tryptophan:BCAA ratio at the completion of a 42.2 km marathon. In a direct test of this hypothesis, Vandewalle and others (1991) depleted subjects of muscle glycogen and then subjected them to a cycle ergometer ride to exhaustion at 75 percent VO_2max; they reported no beneficial effect of BCAA supplementation. Nor did Galiano and others (1991), who supplemented BCAA during prolonged exercise to exhaustion at 70 percent VO$_2$max. Kreider and his associates (Kreider et al, 1991; Mitchell et al, 1991) provided BCAA supplements to five triathletes for 14 days prior to and during a half-Ironman triathlon (2 km swim; 90 km bike; 21 km run) under laboratory conditions. Although no significant differences were noted between the BCAA and placebo conditions, the authors suggested run performance in the last segment might be enhanced. Additional research with prolonged endurance tasks is necessary to test Newsholme's hypothesis.

Aspartates

Potassium and magnesium salts of aspartate, a nonessential amino acid, have been postulated to improve aerobic endurance performance by several mechanisms. The prevailing hypothesis is that aspartates will reduce the accumulation of ammonia during exercise; increases in serum ammonia have been correlated with muscular fatigue, although the mechanism has not been clarified. Research findings regarding the ergogenicity of aspartates are equivocal. A number of both earlier and contemporary studies have reported no ergogenic effect. As an example of a well designed study, Maughan and Sadler (1983) gave a placebo or 3 grams each of potassium and magnesium aspartate to eight subjects 24 hours prior to a cycle ergometer ride to exhaustion at 75-80 percent VO$_2$max, and reported no beneficial effects on serum ammonia levels or physiological and psychological variables important to aerobic endurance performance. Conversely, an equal number of both early and contemporary studies have documented an ergogenic effect of aspartates, some reporting greater than 20 percent improvement in aerobic endurance. As an example, Wesson and others (1988), also using an appropriate research design, gave a placebo or 10 grams of aspartates to subjects over a 24-hour period prior to exercise to exhaustion at 75 percent VO$_2$max, and reported a significant decrease in serum ammonia levels and an associated 15 percent increase in endurance capacity. It is clear that additional research is needed, particularly with dosages approximating 10 or more grams, for these dosages have often been associated with enhanced performance.

Vitamins, vitamin-like substances and minerals

Certain vitamins, vitamin-like substances, and minerals are theorized to have ergogenic potential because they are intimately involved in the regulation of a variety of physiological and metabolic processes critical to optimal exercise performance. Individual nutrients have been studied in relation to their specific potential benefit to the athlete, such as iron supplementation and oxygen transport, while broad-spectrum multivitamin\mineral supplements have been studied in relation to a wide variety of physical performance parameters. In general, the available research data suggest that physical performance will be impaired with a vitamin or mineral deficiency, but performance will be restored to normal if the vitamin or mineral deficiency is corrected by supplementation (Van der Beek, 1985; Van der Beek et al, 1988; Williams, 1989B). On the other hand, vitamin and mineral supplements are ineffective ergogenics when given to individuals who are well-nourished, although additional research is desirable with several nutrients or combinations of nutrients (Clarkson, 1991; Keith, 1989; Williams, 1989B).

Vitamin B complex

Thiamin (B_1), riboflavin (B_2), niacin, pantothenic acid, and pyridoxine (B_6) supplements have been studied, individually and in combination, for possible ergogenic effects because of their role in carbohydrate, fat, and protein metabolism. However, supplementation has not been associated with any ergogenic benefits. Cyanocobalamin (B_{12}) and folic acid supplements have been used in attempts to increase red blood cell production and hemoglobin concentration. Vitamin B_{12} is one of the most abused vitamins in the athletic arena, even though the available research indicates it is not an effective ergogenic to increase oxygen uptake or endurance performance. Folate supplementation has received little research relative to sports performance, but Matter and others (1987) reported that although folate supplementation to female runners who were diagnosed as being folate-deficient restored serum folate levels to normal, no improvements were observed in VO_2max, running speed at the lactate threshold, or maximal treadmill running time. It appears that neither vitamin B_{12} nor folic acid supplements are effective ergogenics for endurance capacity. Additionally, a coenzyme form of vitamin B_{12} known as Dibencobal has been marketed for bodybuilders to increase muscle and strength. However, no research appears to be available to support the advertised claims, which are based on fallacious data.

Although, in general, research does not support an ergogenic efficacy of the B complex vitamins to enhance energy production, some research suggests several B vitamins may enhance fine motor control, similar to the effect of beta blockers mentioned previously. Bonke (1986) reported that large doses of B_1, B_6, and B_{12} may increase fine motor control and pistol shooting accuracy. Bonke suggested these vitamins could promote the formation of neurotransmitters in the brain, possibly inducing an anxiolytic effect. Additional research is desirable to confirm this finding.

Vitamin E

Vitamin E is an effective antioxidant that is theorized to enhance aerobic endurance performance by mitigating the peroxidation of red blood cell or muscle cell membranes. However, an extensive review of over twenty studies (Williams, 1989B) has not supported any ergogenic effect of vitamin E megadoses on physiological processes or physical performance parameters when performed at sea level. Williams (1989B) cited several studies with vitamin E supplementation at altitude that have reported increased VO_2max or enhanced oxidative metabolism, presumably because red blood cells may be more prone to peroxidation at altitude. However, confirmation is desirable (Williams, 1992).

Vitamin E has also been coupled with other antioxidants, particularly beta-carotene, vitamin C, and selenium, in attempts to reduce exercise-induced muscle damage during eccentric exercise tasks. Although additional research is needed for confirmation, several investigators have reported supplementation with antioxidants may be beneficial, as several markers of muscle trauma or lipid peroxidation have been reduced (Goldfarb et al, 1989; Kanter et al, 1990; Viguie et al, 1989).

Carnitine

Carnitine is a vitamin-like compound that facilitates the transport of fatty acids into the mitochondria for oxidation and also facilitates the oxidation of several amino acids and pyruvate, functions that theoretically could lead to a sparing of muscle glycogen during exercise and a decreased production of lactate. Based on these theoretical considerations, Robert Haas (1986), in his book Eat to Succeed, suggested that carnitine would be an effective ergogenic for athletes, but the available data are not supportive of this viewpoint. Data from early studies were inconsistent due to inadequate research design or dosage utilized. For example, although several studies from Otto's research group (Otto et al, 1987; Shores et al, 1987) found no effect of 500 mg carnitine taken daily for four months on free fatty acid utilization, VO_2max, anaerobic threshold, exercise time to exhaustion, or work output on a cycle ergometer for 60 minutes, Bucci (1989) criticized these reports because of low dosage. However, three more recent studies, using doses up to 2 grams, also reported no effects of carnitine supplementation on fuel utilization at 50 percent VO_2max, maximal heart rate, anaerobic threshold, VO_2max, or exercise time to exhaustion (Greig et al, 1987; Oyono-Enguelle et al, 1988; Wyss et al, 1990).

Additional research is desirable, particularly regarding the potential for glycogen sparing in very prolonged endurance tasks. However, it should be noted that only L-carnitine should be used in research, for some forms of D- or DL-carnitine may be toxic (Wagenmakers, 1991).

CoQ10

CoQ10 is actually a lipid, but has characteristics comparable to a vitamin. It is found in the mitochondria, particularly in the heart, and has been used therapeutically for the treatment of cardiovascular disease because of its role in oxidative metabolism and as an antioxidant. Because CoQ10 has increased oxygen uptake and exercise performance in cardiac patients, it has been theorized to be ergogenic for endurance athletes. Unfortunately, only limited data are available, but several recent studies found that although CoQ10 supplementation may significantly increase serum CoQ10 levels, compared to a placebo there were no significant improvements in serum glucose or lactate at submaximal or maximal workloads, cardiovascular functions such as heart rate, VO_2max, or endurance performance (Braun et al, 1991; Roberts, 1990; Zuliani et al, 1989).

Additional research with CoQ10 is desirable because it is one of the compounds in a nutritional supplement marketed for endurance athletes. However, Demopoulos and others (1986) did suggest it may actually be ergolytic, for it may autooxidize and produce free radicals that could damage the mitochondria.

Inosine

Inosine is a nucleoside whose metabolic role in animals, studied primarily by infusion or perfusion techniques, appears to be variable and species specific. Some of these metabolic roles, such as facilitation of ATP replenishment, maintenance of glycogen breakdown, increased levels of 2,3-DPG, and vasodilation have been extrapolated by sports nutrition entrepreneurs to sports performance, suggesting both strength and endurance athletes could benefit from supplementation. Inosine is sold either separately or combined with other cofactors, such as CoQ10. One advertisement suggests that inosine supplementation may improve respiration, increase the ability to deliver oxygen to the muscles, metabolize blood sugars, reduce lactic acid buildup, and raise aerobic capacity.

These claims are based solely on theoretical considerations, not experimental research with humans. No research data are available relative to the effect of inosine on strength parameters, while only one study has investigated its effect on endurance parameters. Williams and others (1990) used a recommended supplementation protocol (6 grams of inosine for 2 days) and reported no significant effect on 2,3-DPG, glucose, or lactate during submaximal or maximal exercise tasks, nor did inosine supplementation improve performance in a treadmill run to exhaustion or a treadmill run designed to mimic a 3 mile (approximately

5 km) race.

Clearly additional research is needed to evaluate the advertised ergogenic claims, including research with strength performance as well as anaerobic and aerobic endurance performance.

Bee pollen

Chemical analysis of bee pollen reveals a mixture of vitamins, minerals, amino acids, and other nutrients. Although bee pollen does not appear to elicit any specific physiologic effects, its theoretical ergogenic effect may be based on the roles that vitamins and minerals may play in exercise metabolism. Advertising claims for bee pollen are based on one poorly controlled field study suggesting that supplementation may facilitate recovery between intense exercise bouts in an interval training workout. We tested this specific hypothesis with highly trained runners and reported no significant effect on the rate of recovery as measured by performance in repeated maximal treadmill runs to exhaustion with set recovery periods (Woodhouse et al, 1987). Additional well-controlled studies have reported no beneficial effects of bee pollen supplementation on VO_2max, other physiological responses to exercise, and endurance capacity (Chandler and Hawkins, 1984; Steben et al, 1976). Some individuals may also be allergic to bee pollen and experience an anaphylactic reaction (Dunnett and Crossen, 1980).

Vitamin B_{15}

Although advertised as an ergogenic for athletes, vitamin B_{15} is actually not a vitamin. As a matter of fact, compounds sold as vitamin B_{15} actually have no set chemical identity and are composed of different substances. The most common form has been marketed as calcium pangamate, a mixture of calcium gluconate and dimethylglycine (DMG), an amino acid. Soviet research with rats suggested that vitamin B_{15} could improve oxidative metabolism by stimulation of succinate dehydrogenase and cytochrome oxidase, but advertisements also claim it may increase muscular content of creatine phosphate and glycogen. The reputation of vitamin B_{15} as an ergogenic in the United States during the 1980s was magnified by anecdotal claims of several professional athletes.

However, the available data suggest that vitamin B_{15} will not enhance physical performance. Four well-designed studies have shown that B_{15} supplementation has no effect on cardiovascular and metabolic responses to exercise approximating 70 percent of VO_2max, anaerobic threshold, or exercise tasks to exhaustion (Gray and Titlow, 1982; Williams, 1985). Moreover, since vitamin B_{15} has no set chemical identity, marketed products may contain a variety of chemicals, some of them identified as mutagenic (Check, 1980).

Iron

As a constituent of hemoglobin, myoglobin, the cytochromes, and some respiratory enzymes, iron is essential for oxygen transport and utilization and thus is a critical nutrient for aerobic endurance athletes. Thus, iron supplementation was a forerunner of blood doping and EPO. Iron supplementation has been shown to correct iron deficiency anemia and restore physical performance to normal, but has no effect on performance in individuals who have normal iron and hemoglobin status prior to supplementation (Williams, 1985). However, the effect of iron supplementation on physical performance in individuals who are iron-deficient but nonanemic is uncertain, possibly because the effect on physical performance of iron deficiency without anemia is also uncertain (Williams, 1992). In support of iron supplementation to female runners who were iron deficient but nonanemic, Williams (1992) cited four studies indicating an enhanced iron status and significant improvements in treadmill running performance or competitive running performance. Conversely, he also cited several studies in which aerobic endurance performance was not improved with supplementation, even though iron status improved.

Many female endurance athletes, particularly runners, may be iron deficient because of diet and training, so this subject merits additional investigation.

Chromium

Chromium is an essential nutrient because it serves as an important constituent of the glucose-tolerance factor associated with insulin. Because insulin may also facilitate the transport of amino acids into the muscle cell, chromium has been advertised as an ergogenic aid for bodybuilders and weightlifters in order to enhance the development of lean body mass and strength. Limited research is available to support these claims. In a review article, Evans (1989) cited two of his unpublished studies involving the use of chromium picolinate supplementation as an adjunct to a weight training program with either college students or members of a university American football team. Supplementation was 200 μg daily for approximately forty days. Compared to the placebo groups, Evans noted that the chromium supplement significantly increased lean body mass and decreased body fat; no performance variables were measured. Unfortunately, these studies involved several defects, including no control over diet or other physical activity and the use of skinfolds to determine body composition. It is conceivable, however, that the subjects may have been chromium deficient, a distinct possibility in the United States (Anderson, 1988), and may have increased lean body mass through improved insulin activity with supplementation.

Additional research is merited along these lines, but also with endurance athletes who may possibly benefit from enhanced glucose utilization. It would appear to be important to evaluate chromium status of the individual prior to supplementation.

Phosphate salts

Phosphorus is an essential nutrient that functions in the body as several phosphate salts, being a cofactor or component for several B vitamins, ATP and phosphocreatine, 2,3-DPG, and an intracellular buffering system. Based on these metabolic roles, phosphate supplements have been theorized to possess ergogenic properties, and their use as an ergogenic has been studied for over sixty years. Early research suggested that phosphate salt supplementation was an effective ergogenic for several types of physical performance, and although Boje (1939) criticized these studies for design flaws, he indicated that phosphates probably could increase physical performance if consumed in quantities greater than normally found in the normal diet. Most of the current research has focused on the ability of phosphate salts to enhance oxygen uptake and endurance performance, and although a number of recent studies support the comment by Boje over 50 years ago, the data are still equivocal (Kreider, 1992; Williams, 1992).

Williams (1992) has cited four studies, all using appropriate experimental designs and dosages, reporting no beneficial effect of phosphate supplementation on such physical performance parameters as cardiovascular function and oxygen efficiency at 60 percent VO_2max, lactic acid production, VO_2max, or performance in an 8-kilometer (5 mile) bike race. In contrast, four other well designed studies reported significant increases in VO_2max approximating 10 percent, decreases in lactate production during submaximal exercise, enhancement of myocardial efficiency as evaluated by an echocardiogram, increases in treadmill running time and cycling endurance time, and decreases in the time to complete a 40 km race under laboratory conditions. The dosage in these studies approximated 4 grams daily of sodium phosphate consumed, usually consumed in one gram doses, for 3-6 days.

Additional research is needed to confirm these potential ergogenic effects and to determine the underlying mechanism. Although increases in 2,3-DPG were reported in two of the studies finding an ergogenic effect, the serum levels were not affected in the other two studies. Moreover, one of the studies that reported no improvement in performance did report significantly increased 2,3-DPG levels.

Sodium bicarbonate

Sodium bicarbonate is an alkaline salt found naturally in the body whose major function is to control acid-base balance. Its proposed role as an ergogenic is to buffer the lactic acid produced during high-intensity exercise generating ATP primarily via anaerobic glycolysis, theoretically delaying the onset of fatigue by facilitating the release of hydrogen ions from the active muscle tissue, although the exact mechanism has not been completely elucidated (Heigenhauser and Jones, 1991). Similar to phosphate salt supplementation, research relative to the ergogenic effect of sodium bicarbonate has been conducted for over 50 years, and yet its effectiveness is still debatable.

Several dozen studies have investigated the ergogenicity of sodium bicarbonate over the past fifteen years. The typical experimental design used 0.15-0.40 (most often 0.30) grams per kilogram body weight, administered 1-3 hours prior to executing an exercise task designed to maximize energy production via anaerobic glycolysis; laboratory tests usually involved tests to exhaustion at supramaximal workloads of approximately 125 percent of VO_2max, repeated bouts of high intensity exercise interspersed with rest periods and culminating with a supramaximal test to exhaustion; field tests such as 100-200 meter swims or 400-800 meter runs have also been used. The effects of sodium bicarbonate on other maximal exercise tasks involving shorter (less than 30 seconds) and longer (greater than 5 minutes) time periods have also been studied; however, these latter exercise tasks would not maximize the production of energy via anaerobic glycolysis.

Of all the published studies that used appropriate experimental designs, about 50 percent have shown a beneficial effect on actual physical performance and psychological perceptions of exertion; a similar ratio was evident for unpublished abstracts as well. Several major reviews regarding the effectiveness of sodium bicarbonate have been published (Gledhill, 1984; Heigenhauser and Jones, 1991; Maughan and Greenhaff, 1991). Based on their extensive review, Heigenhauser and Jones (1991) hypothesized that sodium bicarbonate supplementation with an appropriate dosage appears to have no effect on high-intensity performance of 30 seconds or less, nor on endurance performance that depends primarily upon oxidative metabolism, but will enhance performance in intense continuous exercise approximating 1-7.5 minutes in duration or repetitive bouts of intense exercise involving short rest intervals. Maughan and Greenhaff (1991) also concluded sodium bicarbonate may be an effective ergogenic.

At the present time, the IOC has not banned the use of sodium bicarbonate. Research is ongoing to confirm the potential ergogenicity of sodium bicarbonate and the underlying mechanisms.

This paper is based on previous reviews by the author in <u>Nutrition for Fitness and Sport</u> (3rd Edition), <u>Beyond Training: How Athletes Enhance Performance Legally and Illegally</u>, <u>Nutritional Aspects of Human Physical and Athletic Performance</u> (2nd Edition), and <u>Drugs and Athletic Performance</u>.

References

Anderson R. (1988) Selenium, chromium, and manganese. (b) Chromium, in Modern Nutrition in Health and Disease, (eds. M Shils and V Young), Lea & Febiger, Philadelphia, PA.

American College of Sports Medicine. (1987) Position stand on the use of anabolic-androgenic steroids in sports. Med Sci Sports Ex, **19**, 534-39.

Antal L, Good C. (1980) Effects of oxprenolol on pistol shooting under stress. Practitioner, **224**, 755-60.

Boje O. (1939) Doping: A study of the means employed to raise the level of performance in sport. League of Nations Bulletin of the Health Organization, **8**, 439-69.

Bonke D. (1986) Influence of vitamin B_1, B_6, and B_{12} on the control of fine motoric movements. Bibliotheca Nutritio et Dieta, **38**, 104-9.

Braun B, Clarkson P, Freedson P et al. (1991) The effect of coenzyme Q10 supplementation on exercise performance, VO_2max, and lipid peroxidation in trained cyclists. Int J Sport Nutr, **1**, 353-65.

Bucci L, Hickson J, Pivarnik J et al. (1990) Growth hormone release in bodybuilders after oral ornithine administration. FASEB J, **4**, A397, (abstract).

Bucci L. (1989) Nutritional ergogenic aids, in Nutrition in Exercise and Sport, (eds. J Hickson and I Wolinsky), CRD Press, Boca Raton, FL.

Chandler J, Hawkins J. (1984) The effect of bee pollen on physiological performance. Int J Biosoc Res, **6**, 107-14.

Check W. (1980) Vitamin B_{15} - Whatever it is, it won't help. JAMA, **243**, 2473-80.

Clarkson P. (1991) Vitamins, iron and trace minerals, in Enhancement of Performance in Exercise and Sport, (eds. D Lamb and M Williams), Brown & Benchmark, Dubuque, IA.

Conlee R. (1991) Amphetamine, caffeine, and cocaine, in Ergogenics: Enhancement of Performance in Exercise and Sports, (eds. D Lamb and M Williams), Brown & Benchmark, Dubuque, IA.

Costill D, Dalsky G, Fink W. (1978) Effects of caffeine ingestion on metabolism and exercise performance. Med Sci Sports. **10**, 155-58.

Crist D M, Peake G, Egan P et al. (1988) Body composition response to exogenous GH during training in highly conditioned adults. J Appl Physiol **65**, 579-584.

Demopoulous H, Santomier J, Seligman M et al. (1986) Free radical pathology: Rationale and toxicology of antioxidants and other supplements in sports medicine and exercise science, in Sport, Health and Nutrition, (ed.F Katch), Human Kinetics, Champaign, IL.

Dunnett W, and Crossen D. (1980) The bee pollen promise. Runners World, **15 (8)**, 53-54.

Eichner E. (1991) Dying to win: rEPO, blood doping, and athletics. American College of Sports Medicine Annual Meeting, Orlando, FL, May 29

Eichner E. (1989) Ergolytic drugs. Sports Science Exchange. **2 (15)**, 1-4.

Ekblom B. (1989) Effects of iron deficiency, variations in hemoglobin concentration, and erythropoietin injections on physical performance and relevant physiological parameters. Proceedings of the First IOC World Congress on Sport Sciences, United States Olympic Committee, Colorado Springs, CO.

Evans G. (1989) The effect of chromium picolinate on insulin controlled parameters in humans. Int J Biosoc Med Res, 11, 163-80.

Galiano F et al. (1991) Physiological, endocrine and performance effects of adding branched chain amino acids to a 6% carbohydrate-electrolyte beverage during prolonged cycling. Med Sci Sports Ex, 23, S14 (abstract).

Gledhill N. (1984) Bicarbonate ingestion and anaerobic performance. Sports Med, 1, 177-80.

Goldfarb A, Todd M, Boyer B et al. (1989) Effect of vitamin E on lipid peroxidation at 80% VO_2max. Med Sci Sports Ex, 21, S16 (abstract).

Gray M, Titlow L. (1982) B_{15}: Myth or miracle? Physician and Sportsmed, 10, 107-112.

Greig C, Finch K, Jones D et al. (1987) The effect of oral supplementation with L-carnitine on maximum and submaximum exercise capacity. Eur J Appl Physiol, 56, 457-60.

Haas R. (1986) Eat to Succeed, Rawson Associates, New York.

Hawkins C et al. (1991) Oral arginine does not affect body composition or muscle function in male weight lifters. Med Sci Sports Ex, 23, S15 (abstract).

Heigenhauser G, Jones N. (1991) Bicarbonate loading, in Ergogenics: Enhancement of Performance in Exercise and Sport, (eds. D Lamb and M Williams), Brown & Benchmark, Dubuque, IA.

Ivy J, Costill D, Fink W et al. (1979) Influence of caffeine and carbohydrate feedings on endurance performance. Med Sci Sports, 11, 6-11.

Jacobson B. (1990) Effect of amino acids on growth hormone release. Physician and Sportsmed, 18, 63-70.

Jacobson B, Kulling F. (1989) Health and ergogenic effects of caffeine. Br J Sports Med, 23, 34-40.

Kanter M, Nolte L, Holloszy J. (1990) Effects of antioxidant supplement on expired pentane production following low and high intensity exercise. Med Sci Sports Ex, 22, S86 (abstract).

Keith R. (1989) Vitamins in sport and exercise, in Nutrition in Exercise and Sport, (eds. J Hickson and I Wolinsky), CRD Press, Boca Raton, FL.

Kreider R. (1991) Phosphate loading and exercise performance. J Appl Nutr (In press)

Kreider R et al. (1991) Effects of amino acid supplementation on substrate usage during ultraendurance triathlon performance. Med Sci Sports Ex, 23, S16 (abstract).

Kruse P, Ladefoged J, Nielsen U et al. (1986) B-blockade used in precision sports: Effect on pistol shooting performance. J Appl Physiol, 61, 417-20.

Lamb D and Williams M (eds.). (1991) Ergogenics: Enhancement of Performance in Exercise and Sports, Brown & Benchmark, Dubuque, IA.

Lemon P. (1991) Protein and amino acid needs of the strength athlete. Int J Sport Nutr, 1, 127-45.

Lombardo J, Hickson R, Lamb D. (1991) Anabolic/androgenic steroids and growth hormone, in Enhancement of Performance in Exercise and Sports, (eds. D Lamb and M Williams), Brown & Benchmark, Dubuque, IA.

Matter M, Stittfall T, Graves J et al. (1987) The effect of iron and folate therapy on maximal exercise performance in female marathon runners with iron and folate deficiency. Clin Sci, 72, 415-22.

Maughan R, Greenhaff P. (1991) High intensity exercise performance and acid-base balance: The influence of diet and induced metabolic acidosis. In: Advances in Nutrition and Top Sport (ed. F Brouns). Medicine and Sport Science, 32, 147-165.

Maughan R, Sadler D. (1983) The effects of oral administration of salts of aspartic acid on the metabolic response to prolonged exhausting exercise in man. Int J Sports Med, 4, 119-123.

Mitchell M et al. (1991) Effects of amino acid supplementation on metabolic responses to ultraendurance triathlon performance. Med Sci Sports Ex, 23, S15 (abstract).

Morgan W. (1972) Ergogenic Aids and Muscular Performance, Academic Press, New York, NY.

Newsholme E. (1990) Effects of exercise on aspects of carbohydrate, fat, and amino acid metabolism, in Exercise, Fitness and Health, (eds. C Bouchard, R Shephard, T Stephens et al), Human Kinetics, Champaign, IL.

Otto R, Shores K, Wygard J et al. (1987) The effects of L-carnitine supplementation on endurance exercise. Med Sci Sports Ex, 19, S87 (abstract).

Oyono-Enguelle S, Freund H, Ott C et al. (1988) Prolonged submaximal exercise and L-carnitine in humans. Eur J Appl Physiol, 58, 53-61.

Reilly T, Halliday F. (1985) Influence of alcohol ingestion on tasks related to archery. J Hum Ergol, 14, 99-104.

Roberts J. (1990) The effect of coenzyme Q10 on exercise performance. Med Sci Sports Ex, 22. S87, (abstract).

Segura R, Ventura J. (1988) Effect of L-tryptophan supplementation on exercise performance. Int J Sports Med, 9, 301-5.

Shores K, Otto R, Wygard J et al. (1987) Effect of L-carnitine supplementation on maximal oxygen consumption and free fatty acid serum levels. Med Sci Sports Ex, 19, S60, (abstract).

S'Jongers J, Willain P, Sierakowski J et al. (1978) Effect d'un placebo et de faibles doses d'un betainhibiteur (oxprenolol) et d'alcohol etylique, sur la precision du tir sportif au pistolet. Bruxelles Medical, 58, 395-99.

Spriet L. (1991) Blood doping and oxygen transport, in Ergogenics: Enhancement of Performance in Exercise and Sport, (eds. D Lamb and M Williams), Brown & Benchmark, Dubuque, IA.

Spriet L, Graham T. (1991) Caffeine ingestion enhances running and cycling endurance performance in trained runners. Med Sci Sports Ex, 23, S116, (abstract).

Steben R, Wells J, Harless I. (1976) The effects of bee pollen tablets on the improvement of certain blood factors and performance of male collegiate swimmers. J Nat Ath Train Ass, 11, 124-26.

Tesch P. (1985) Exercise performance and B-blockade. Sports Med, 2, 389-412.

Van der Beek E, van Dokkum W, Schrijver J et al. (1988) Thiamin, riboflavin, and vitamins B_6 and C: Impact of combined restricted intake on functional performance in man. Am J Clin Nutr, 48, 1451-62.

Van der Beek E. (1985) Vitamins and endurance training. Food for running and faddish claims. Sports Med, 2, 175-197.

Vandewalle L et al. (1991) Effect of branched-chain amino acid supplements on exercise performance in glycogen depleted subjects. Med Sci Sports Ex, 23, S116 (abstract).

Van Handel P. (1983) Caffeine, in Ergogenic Aids in Sport (ed.M.Williams), Human Kinetics, Champaign, IL.

Viguie C, Packer L, Brooks G. (1989) Antioxidant supplementation affects indices of muscle trauma and oxidant stress in human blood during exercise. Med Sci Sports Ex 21, S16, (abstract).

Wadler G, Hainline B. (1989) Drugs and the Athlete, FA Davis, Philadelphia.

Wagenmakers A. (1991) L-carnitine supplementation and performance in man. In: Advances in Nutrition and Top Sport (ed. F Brouns). Medicine and Sport Science, 32, 110-127.

Warren B et al. (1991) The effect of amino acid supplementation on physiological responses of elite junior weightlifters. Med Sci Sports Ex, 23, S15 (abstract).

Wesson M, McNaughton L, Davies P et al. (1988) Effects of oral administration of aspartic acid salts on the endurance capacity of trained athletes. Res Q, 59, 234-239.

Williams M. (1992) Nutrition for Fitness and Sport, 3rd edn, Wm C Brown Publishers, Dubuque, IA.

Williams M. (1991A) Alcohol, marijuana, and beta blockers, in Ergogenics: Enhancement of Performance in Exercise and Sport, (eds. D Lamb and M Williams), Brown & Benchmark, Dubuque, IA.

Williams M. (1991B) Ergogenic aids, in Sports Nutrition for the 90s: The Health Professional's Handbook, (eds. J Berning and S Steen), Aspen Publishers, Gaithersburg, MD.

Williams M. (1989A) Beyond Training: How Athletes Enhance Performance Legally and Illegally, Leisure Press, Champaign, IL.

Williams M. (1989B) Vitamin supplementation and athletic performance. Int J Vit Nutr Res, Supplement 30, 161-91.

Williams M. (1985) Nutritional Aspects of Human Physical and Athletic Performance, 2nd edn, CC Thomas, Springfield, IL.

Williams M. (1983A) Ergogenic Aids in Sport, Human Kinetics, Champaign, IL.

Williams M. (1983B) Blood doping, in Ergogenic Aids in Sport (ed.M Williams), Human Kinetics, Champaign, IL.

Williams M. (1974) Drugs and Athletic Performance, CC Thomas, Springfield, IL.

Williams M, Kreider R, Hunter D et al. (1990) Effect of oral inosine supplementation on 3-mile treadmill run performance and VO$_2$peak. Med Sci Sports Ex, 22, 517-522.

Woodhouse M, Williams M, Jackson C. (1987) The effects of varying doses of orally ingested bee pollen extract upon selected performance variables. Athletic Training, 22, 26-28.

Wyss V et al. (1990) Effects of L-carnitine administration on VO$_2$max and the aerobic-anaerobic threshold in normoxia and acute hypoxia. Eur J Appl Physiol, 60, 1-6.

Yarasheski K et al (1990) Effect of strength training and growth hormone administration on whole body and skeletal muscle leucine metabolism. Med Sci Sports Ex, 22, S84 (abstract).

Yesalis C, Wright J, Lombardo J. (1989) Anabolic-androgenic steroids: A synthesis of existing data and recommendations for future research. Clin Sports Med, 1, 109-34.

Zuliani U, Bonetti A, Campana M et al. (1989) The influence of ubiquinone (CoQ10) on the metabolic response to work. J Sports Med Phys Fit, 29, 57-61.

Dietary habits of football players

L. Piearce

Abstract. The dietary habits of 17 male football players , aged 19-29 years, were analysed using a seven day weighed food intake method. Players trained for an average of 8.5 hours per week. Mean daily energy intake was 15.2±3.6 MJ (3626 kcal). Snacks contributed an average of 24% of total energy intake. Protein intake was 1.6 g/kg dody weight and fat intake was less than 33% of total energy intake, but alcohol intake was above the 5% maximum amount recommended for the general population. Average daily carbohydrate intake provided 49% of total energy intake, but 82% of the players had intakes of less than the 55% recommended for the general public as the basis of a healthy diet. Many players did not consume any carbohydrate in the first two hours following exercise. It appears that the carbohydrate intake of these players is insufficient, especially following exercise. Increased consumption of carbohydrate-rich snacks would help to overcome this shortfall.

Keywords: Football, dietary intake, protein, carbohydrate, energy, vitamins, alcohol.

Introduction

The nutritional status of a player is one of a number of factors which can have a profound effect, either beneficial or detrimental on physical performance. Other factors include genetics and training-induced physiological improvements. Indeed, nutrition has its greatest effects when it is supporting systematic and consistent training, because it is training that produces adaptation and subsequent improvements in performance.

The diets of seventeen football players were investigated, nine of these were rugby players and the remaining eight were soccer players. They were treated as a group as the physiological demands of both games are very similar, both involving periods of activity and rest which are unpredictable. Such intermittent exercise involves changes in intensity ranging from standing or walking to sprinting. The average exercise intensity during a football match has been estimated to be about 75% VO_2max for all players (Van Gool et al, 1988; Reilly, 1979). This is comparable with the average level of intensity measured during marathon running.

The importance of a high carbohydrate diet for the majority of athletes is well known, but many studies have also indicated that a large number of athletes do not eat sufficient carbohydrate (Short and Short, 1983). The present survey was carried out in order to investigate the adequacy of the diets of football players.

An important aspect of consuming a high carbohydrate diet is its role in maximizing recovery between frequent bouts of intense exercise, such as in football tournaments. It has been suggested that in order to achieve optimum refuelling of muscle glycogen stores in 24 hours following successive days of intense exercise, a carbohydrate intake of approximately 10g kg⁻¹ bw is required (Kirwan, 1988).

A comparison of the overall diets of the athletes with that of the general population was also made, using national dietary surveys (MAFF, 1989) of the general population. This was to identify (a) whether football players actually eat more carbohydrate than the general population, (b) if they have higher energy intakes than sedentary individuals, and (c) if they obtain sufficient vitamins and minerals from such high energy intakes to cover any increased requirements.

Only a limited number of dietary surveys have been carried out on games players. Nevertheless, such information is invaluable for dietitians and nutritionists involved in nutritional counselling. A good foundation of nutrition education should ideally be provided for athletes which can be used for the rest of their lives, providing long-term health benefits, rather than purely during their playing careers.

Methods

A seven day weighed food intake method was used to assess the dietary intakes of the seventeen players. Of the five methods of dietary assessment available, this method is believed to provide the most accurate and acceptable assessment of dietary intake (Stunkard and Waxman, 1981). Other methods available include unweighed dietary records, based on actual consumption, as with the weighed food intake method; 24 hour recall and diet history, both based on previous intake; and food frequency records, which can be based on either past or present intakes.

Each player was provided with a seven day food diary and a set of digital food scales accurate to the nearest gram. Detailed instructions on how to record all information on food, drinks and any supplements taken over a period of seven consecutive days were included in the front pages of the diary, together with pages of examples.

Players were asked to eat as normal and to be as accurate as possible in recording their food intakes, noting not only the quantity, but also the type of food, whether fresh, frozen or tinned for example, and how it was cooked. The food diaries contained a section for time when food was eaten, whether at home or away from home, brand name, method of cooking, food description, weight served and weight of leftovers. Athletes were also requested to record recipes for all home-made food, to allow coding of such recipes as separate ingredients. The accuracy of the nutrient analysis was improved by having a qualified dietitian code food items. Any necessary substitutions were made for food items not included in the database with the closest possible food item, or coded as its individual ingredients, as necessary for certain food items not included on the database or for home-made recipes.

The computer program used was developed within the Department, for use on an Apple Macintosh computer. It has a database of over 1160 foods and values for 38 nutrients for each food item. Values were based on McCance and Widdowson's "The Composition of Foods" (Paul and Southgate, 1978) and its most recent updates. Any supplements taken were noted but not included in the dietary assessments. Only one of the players took a supplement of any form, which did not provide any nutrients not supplied by the foods in his normal diet. The contribution made by these supplements to this player's nutrient intakes were therefore not included in the results.

The mean, standard deviation, minimum, and maximum intakes of each of the 38 macro- and micronutrients determined were calculated for all subjects. Results are shown in Tables 1 and 2. Reference Nutrient Intakes (RNIs) were used as comparisons for intake adequacy (DHSS, 1991). Such comparisons are not ideal, as RNIs are intended for whole populations, rather than individuals, however, they are useful in the identification of subgroups in which there is a risk of deficiency.

Results

Age range for the players was 19-26 years (mean 21 ± 2 years) and body weight of the players ranged from 65 - 103 kg (mean 78 ± 9 kg). Average time spent by the players in training was 8.5 hours (range 6 - 12.5 hours) per week. This corresponds to an energy expenditure of approximateiy 3.4 MJ (640kcal)/day. Assuming that the players have light occupations throughout the rest of the day, as can be assumed for the UK population in general (DHSS, 1991) then their Estimated Average Requirement (EAR) for energy would be approximately 14MJ (3350kcal)/day or 1.8 BMR units. The average daily energy intake of the male football players (see Table 1) was actually slightJy greater than this, namely 15.2 ± 3.6 MJ (3626 ± 847 kcal); range 10.2 - 23.3 MJ (2435 -5545 kcal). This is equivalent to 194.3 kJ (46.4 ± 9.8 kcal)/kg bw; range 127.3 - 263.6 kJ (30.4 - 63.0 kcal)/kg bw, similar to the energy intake of Dutch soccer players, namely 192 kJ/kg bw (range 118-287 kJ/kg bw reported by van Erp-Baart (1989). 65% of the players had energy intakes above the EAR.

Mean daily protein intake was 127 ± 37g (range 72 - 191g) which is equivalent to 1.6 ± 0.5g kg^{-1} bw (range 0.9-2.9g kg^{-1} bw), significantly greater than the RNI of 0.8g kg^{-1} bw (DHSS,1991). Mean percentage of the total energy intake which was provided by protein in the diets of the players was 16%, which was also well above the NACNE (1983) recommendation of 11%. This may be, in some part, a result of the belief that large amounts of protein are needed in the diet when attempting to increase muscle mass.

53% of the players had mean daily fat intakes which were below the Dietary Reference Value (DRV) (DHSS, 1991) recommendation of 33% of total energy intake for the population as a whole. Mean intake of fat for the players was 31 ± 7% (range 18 - 41%).

Table 1   Daily Dietary Intakes of Energy and Macronutrients for 17 Male Football Players

		Mean	SD	Range	*RNI
Energy	(MJ)	15.2	3.6	10.2-23.3	14
	(kcal)	3626	847	2435-5545	3350
Protein	(g)	127	37	72-91	56
Fat	(g)	128	35	61-200	
Carbohydrate	(g)	443	111		269-724
Alcohol	(g)	42	52	0-204	
Energy	(kJ/kg bw)	194	41	127-264	
	(kcal/kg bw)	46	10	30-63	
Protein	(g/kg bw)	1.6	0.5	0.9-2.9	0.8
Carbohydrate	(g/kg bw)	5.7	1.2	3.4-7.6	
Protein	(%E)	16	4	12-25	
Fat	(%E)	31	7	18-41	33
Carbohydrate	(%E)	49	7		40-6547
Alcohol	(%E)	5	4	0-14	

*   Reference Nutrient Intakes DHSS (1991)

Table 2 Daily Dietary Intakes of Micronutrients for 17 Male Football Players

		Mean	SD	Range	*RNI
Thiamin	(mg)	2.2	0.8	1.3-4.9	1.1
Riboflavin	(mg)	3.1	1.2	2.0-6.3	1.3
Niacin	(mg)	34.9	7.2	15.3-40.2	17
Vitamin B_6	(mg)	2.7	1.2	1.8-6.8	1.4
Vitamin B_{12}	(ug)	7.2	2.2	2.4-11.7	1.5
Folate	(ug)	367.8	175.3	148.1-955.5	200
Vitamin C	(mg)	122.8	82.3	41.7-352	40
Vitamin A	(ug)	582.2	270.7	215.4-1306	700
Calcium	(mg)	1427.0	480.2	757.2-2673.8	700
Phosphorus	(mg)	2273.1	727.1	1381.0-3825.6	550
Magnesium	(mg)	596.9	235.7	367.1-1286	300
Sodium	(mg)	4525.3	1243.1	2814.8-6988.0	1600
Potassium	(mg)	5765.0	1733.4	3468.1-9881.0	3500
Chloride	(mg)	7199.2	2081.2	4793.2-11464.4	2500
Iron	(mg)	23.3	9.1	14.4-45.8	8.7
Zinc	(mg)	16.8	5.5	8.7-26.3	9.5
Copper	(mg)	3.0	1.2	1.8-6.4	1.2

* Reference Nutrient Intakes DHSS (1991)

Only two of the players regularly used skimmed milk; the majority (12 players) used semi-skimmed milk most often and only three consumed full-cream milk on a regular basis. Eleven of the players used butter more often than margarine or low-fat spread, three of the players used polyunsaturated margarine, three used low-fat spread regularly.

Mean daily carbohydrate intake was 443 ± 111g (range 269 -724g) and equivalent to 5.7 ± 1.2g kg^{-1} bw (range 3.4 - 7.6g kg^{-1} bw), providing an average of 49 ± 7% (range 40-65%) of total energy. These intakes were far less than the 60-70% of total energy intake recommended for athletes, and were even below the 50-55% which should be supplied from carbohydrate, recommended by NACNE (1983) for the general population. The majority of the players (71%) had daily dietary intakes of carbohydrate which provided less than 55% of total daily energy intake, whereas only one of the players consumed a diet from which, on average, more than 60% of the total daily energy intake was provided by carbohydrate.

Mean daily dietary fibre intake for the group was 38 ± 22g (range 18 -109g), which is above the amount recommended for the general population of 30g per day (NACNE, 1983). It was interesting to note that only 3 of the players (18%) ate wholemeal bread regularly and 41% of the players ate mostly white bread and the same number ate mostly brown bread. Also, the average number of fruit eaten per week by the group as a whole was 5 per player. Four of the players ate no fruit at all over the seven days and one player ate twenty pieces of fruit per week, the majority of which were bananas, the most popular fruit eaten by the players.

Compared to the general population (MAFF, 1989) and University American football players (Short and Short, 1983), the diets of the players were only slightly better, as far as fat and carbohydrate intakes are concerned (NACNE, 1983). The players consumed, on average, 31% of their total energy intake in the form of fat, compared to 42% reported for both the general population and the American football players. They also consumed marginally more carbohydrate, 48% of total energy intake, as compared to 45% reported for the general population and 39-45% reported for American football players.

Sportspeople are usually discouraged from having high fat intakes as this can have a detrimental effect on carbohydrate intake. That is, if a high proportion of fatty foods are eaten, then less of the more bulky, high carbohydrate foods are likely to be eaten.

Figures 1 and 2 show the mean daily energy and carbohydrate intakes of the players. Figure 1 illustrates that snack foods make quite a considerable contribution to the overall energy intake, providing more than breakfast. Players obtained most energy from dinner, as would be expected. When the mean daily carbohydrate contents of breakfasts and snacks are compared in Figure 2, it can be seen that they are very similar. However, as can be seen in Figure 1, the average energy content of breakfast was lower than that of snacks, illustrating that breakfast was generally higher in carbohydrate. Figure 3 shows the average percentage of total daily energy intake supplied by carbohydrate in each meal, from which it can be seen that the mean percentage energy provided by carbohydrate in breakfast is 55% as compared to 45% for snacks. This difference, however, is probably a consequence of the high alcohol content of the players' snacks (providing 13% of the overall energy content of snacks). It is interesting to note that if the energy provided by alcohol were provided by carbohydrate instead, then the composition of snacks would then be improved, i.e. 58% carbohydrate, 24% fat and 18% protein. It can also be seen from Figure 3 that the fat content of both lunch and dinner, providing 36% and 34.5% of the total energy contents of these meals respectively, are above the ideal value of between 20-25% of overall energy content. Breakfast had by far the highest carbohydrate and one of the lowest fat content.

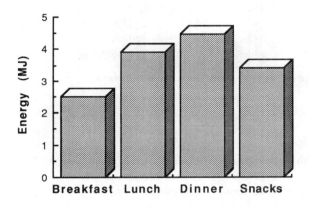

Fig. 1   Daily energy intake of male football players (n=17).

Higher alcohol intake has been reported amongst team sport athletes than amongst individual sport athletes. Two players (12%) recorded no alcohol intake over the seven day period. Mean daily intake of alcohol for the seven days was 42g, supplying 5% of total energy intake (range 0-204g; 0-14% of total energy). There was a high variation of alcohol intake over the seven days, with 76% of the players having their highest alcohol intake on a Saturday, as would be expected. Post-match binging appears to be an integral part of post-match relaxation for a large number of rugby or football players. Education on the detrimental effects of alcohol, both on performance and health in the short and long-term, appears to be ineffective in bringing about any favourable behaviour changes as far as alcohol consumption is concerned.

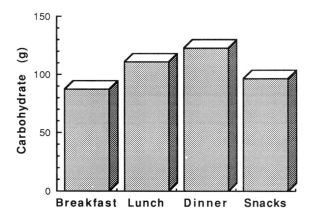

Fig. 2   Daily carbohydrate intake of male football players (n=17).

Three of the players had "poor" intakes (i.e. less than 66% of the RDA, as defined by Leverton, 1975) of vitamin A and the same number (but not the same players) had "poor" intakes of zinc.

Daily calcium intake for the group of players (300-700mg/1000kcal) was similar to that reported for University American football players (400-600 mg/1000kcal) (Short and Short, 1983). Daily intake of iron for the group (4.1-9.6 mg/1000kcal) was also similar to those reported by Short and Short (1983) (5.4-6.0 mg/1000kcal). Interestingly, the highest energy intakes did not correspond to the greatest intakes of these nutrients.

Only one of the players took a supplement of any form, which was a cod liver oil capsule, daily. The amount of vitamins and minerals supplied in his normal diet, were, however, above the recommended daily amounts, not taking into account the contribution made by such supplementation.

Discussion

It is well documented that the onset of fatigue can be delayed by maintenance of muscle and liver glycogen concentrations (Hermansen et al, 1967; Costill, 1988). The amount of glycogen used by the players during a game or training

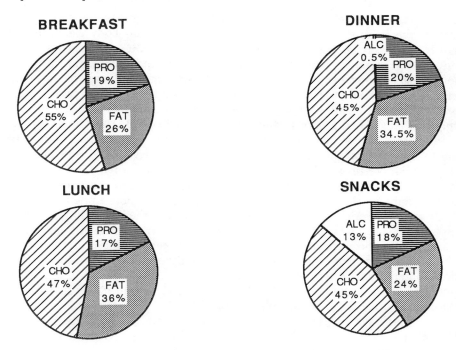

Fig. 3   Mean percentage energy intake from each meal.

session will depend not only on the relative intensity of exercise performed, how fit the players are and environmental conditions in which they are performing (Costill and Miller, 1980), but it will also depend on the players' diet (Bergstrom et al, 1967).

Mean daily energy intakes of the players were slightly above the recommended daily amount for energy for a very active man, namely 14MJ (3350 kcal). The percentage of overall energy intake supplied by fat in the diets of the players (31%; range 18-41 %) was lower than that observed for American University football players by Short and Short (1983) (38-42%) and for the general population (42%) (MAFF, 1989). The players' diets also provided an average of 49% (range 40-65% of energy) in the form of carbohydrate, slightly higher than that observed for the American University footballers (39-45%) and the general population (45%). Such an intake is well below that usually recommended for athletes, i.e. 60-70% energy intake (Devlin and Williams, 1991).

Average percentage of total daily energy intake provided by protein (16%) was well above the NACNE (1983) recommendation of 11%. This is equivalent to 1.6 (± 0.5)g kg^{-1} bw. A number of studies have been carried out in the area of protein requirements, but results have been contradictory. However, there is no evidence to support the claim that protein intakes in excess of 2g kg^{-1} body weight are of benefit to sportspeople. The National Research Council (NRC) published a report in 1989 which warned against protein intakes greater than twice the USA RDA value of 0.8g/kg body weight (NRCI 1989), as long term health may be adversely affected. This is based on evidence for a strong association between high protein intakes and certain forms of cancer and coronary heart disease.

Only one player had a poor intake (less than 66% of RDA) of vitamin A and zinc. Vitamin A is essential for normal function of the retina and it would be logical to assume that a deficiency in this vitamin may have an adverse effect in sports requiring keenness of vision. It is also essential for normal development of epithelial surfaces such as the skin and lining of the gut and bone growth. The fat-soluble vitamins can be stored in the body in quite considerable amounts. Indeed, the body stores of retinol are about 400mg, contained in the liver (Huque, 1979), which is sufficient to meet requirements for many months or years with no dietary intake. Clinical deficiencies are usually only seen in people whose diet has been deficient for a long time both in dairy produce and vegetables.

Zinc is important in enzyme function, it is a cofactor in RNA and DNA polymerases and is therefore essential for growth and protein synthesis (Krause, 1984). Zinc also has a significant role in wound healing. Effects of zinc intake on athletic injuries have not, however, been studied. Levels of zinc in the body are well regulated, thus increases in dietary intake of this trace element may have little effect on zinc nutritional status.

The low intakes of carbohydrate of these players indicates that they are not making full use of presently available knowledge on sports nutrition. The ultimate aim of surveys such as this is to improve sporting performance through ensuring that athletes consume a diet which optimises performance. This is more likely to happen if misbeliefs surrounding sports nutrition are dispelled and if athletes learn how to plan nutritious meals and obtain a sound nutritional education on which optimum food choices can be made.

A study conducted by Jacobs et al (1982) reported that a group of elite football players demonstrated relatively low muscle glycogen concentrations (46 mmol glucose units x kg^{-1} wet muscle weight) following a hard mid-season game of football. These concentrations slowly increased over the following 48 hours to a level still below that which would usually be observed for sedentary individuals (73 mmol kg^{-1} wet muscle weight) (Costill and Miller, 1980; Piehl, 1974). Thus, adequate recovery of glycogen levels between games was not achieved for these elite players. It was assumed that the muscle glycogen levels measured after 48 hours of rest and light physical exercise were approximately equal to pre-match levels. Based on this assumption, a decline in muscle glycogen levels to 63% of prematch values was observed. Such a decrease could have had significant effects on the performance of these players.

Sherman et al (1981), who observed that when a diet providing 50%

carbohydrate, 32% fat and 18% protein was consumed over six days, with a concurrent 5 day depletion-taper exercise sequence, muscle glycogen concentrations between days four and seven, only increased from 133.3 to 159.4 mmol kg^{-1} wet weight. Whereas, when a diet containing 70% carbohydrate, 20% fat and 12% protein was consumed, the increase in muscle glycogen levels was significantly greater (133.9 to 203.3 mmol kg^{-1} wet weight).

This supports the conclusion by Jacobs et al (1982) that the inability of these players to maintain normal glycogen levels between games was a consequence of their diets, providing only 47% of total energy as carbohydrate, 29% as fat and 14% as protein.

Such values are similar to those observed in the group of players in the present study, namely, 48% of total energy supplied by carbohydrate, 31% from fat and 16% as protein. Thus it appears that such an intake of carbohydrate for these players will be inadequate in maintaining optimum muscle glycogen levels and ensuring that performance remains unimpaired.

Considerable depletion of intramuscular glycogen levels has been reported in football players competing at high levels (Currie et al, 1981; Jacobs et al, 1982). Maintenance of muscle glycogen levels should be an important consideration for players. The performance of football players with low muscle glycogen stores does not compare favourably with that of players with adequate stores. It has been demonstrated during a football match that the former group of players actually covered less ground, at a slower average speed, than did the players with adequate stores (Saltin, 1973).

The physiological demands of a game of rugby or football vary between players, but a sufficient level of aerobic fitness is required by all in order to maintain high levels of activity throughout the game. Anaerobic capacity is also of importance, as brief bursts of intense action are an integral part of these games. During a game of rugby, frequent changes in pace and direction and angled runs, kicking, passing, carrying or travelling with the ball (usually at speed), catching or controlling the ball and tackling are involved. Players need the ability to maintain running at a high level of intensity, to recover quickly and move to a position to receive the ball.

During the 80 minutes of a game of rugby, the ball is actually in play for less than half an hour. Between play, time is spent preparing scrums and line-outs, preparing for kicks or re-forming after rucks or mauls. Williams (1976) calculated the average period of activity and rest during the game as 20s and 40s respectively.

Reilly and Thomas (1976) demonstrated that outfield players cover an average of 25% of total distance during the match walking, 37% jogging, 20% running at a submaximal speed, 11% sprinting and 7% of the distance is covered in moving backwards. During an international match, Williams (1976) estimated that approximately one-third of the total distance covered by forwards during the game was done at maximum speed. The fastest runs are, however, as would be expected, achieved by the wing three-quarters. Total distance covered during a game has been estimated as 5.5 km for forwards and 3.8 km for three-quarters, ranging from 4.8 km to 9.6 km (Reid and Williams, 1974).

Muscle glycogen stores can become depleted after only 15-30 minutes of exercise, performed at 90-130% VO_2 max in bouts of exercise lasting between 1-5 minutes, with rest between (Keizer et al, 1986). This is typical of a game of rugby, thus, it is possible that muscle glycogen stores can become depleted during the first half of a rugby match.

MacDougall et al (1977) suggested that following exercise of an intermittent nature, performed at a high level of intensity, as during a game of rugby, 24 hours should be adequate time to allow glycogen stores to be returned to levels similar to those usually observed for sedentary individuals. Piehl (1974) reported that up to 46 hours would normally be required if prolonged exercise has been performed. However, these suggestions rely on the provision of adequate carbohydrate to achieve such optimisation of muscle glycogen stores.

Kirwan et al (1988) suggested that a carbohydrate intake of 8g kg^{-1} bw following successive days of intense exercise aided glycogen repletion, but did not necessarily result in optimum muscle glycogen levels. Sherman et al (1981) observed that rate of muscle glycogen repletion over a three day period was significantly greater with a carbohydrate intake of 5g kg^{-1} bw compared to 7.7g kg^{-1} bw. Pascoe (1990) demonstrated that a carbohydrate intake of 5g kg^{-1} bw was insufficient to restore muscle glycogen stores following three days of exercise, each day consisting of a 60 min bout at 75% VO_2 max . Exercise of this type is comparable to that reported by Reilly (1979) for outfield soccer players - an average of 75% VO_2 max for the game. It therefore appears that during a tournament, when games are closely spaced and recovery time is limited, average carbohydrate intake should approximate 10g kg^{-1} bw per day (Hargreaves, 1991).

The mean carbohydrate intake of the players was 443g carbohydrate per day, equivalent to 5.7g carbohydrate kg^{-1} bw. In terms of food, this would mean that in order to achieve a daily intake of 10g carbohydrate kg^{-1} bw, the players would have to consume an additional intake of carbohydrate ranging from 32194% (average 85%) of their present intake. 76% of the players would require an additional intake of carbohydrate over 50% that of their present intake.

Simple and complex carbohydrates are equally effective in enhancing endurance performance (Brewer et al, 1988), implying that glycogen repletion from simple or complex carbohydrate sources is equal. However, rate of glycogen resynthesis is affected by the glycaemic index of a food. Foods with a moderate or high glycaemic index appear to produce similar rates of muscle glycogen resynthesis (Coyle, 1991). Whereas, the rate of muscle glycogen resynthesis produced by foods with a low glycaemic index may be significantly lower during the first 6 hours following exercise (Kiens et al, 1990).

As such a high carbohydrate intake is required here, muscle glycogen resynthesis may be compromised if chiefly complex carbohydrates or those with a low glycaemic index were consumed due to the sheer bulk of food involved, especially when appetite is suppressed. The more concentrated sources of carbohydrate, with moderate or high glycaemic indices would be required, such as boiled sweets, peppermints and other confectionery, raisins, bananas, jelly, jam, honey, sugar-coated breakfast cereals and biscuits, sugar-containing drinks such as fruit squashes and fizzy drinks. In addition to replacing fluid, drinks can also provide a useful way of replenishing glycogen stores, if appetite is suppressed following exercise, as is common.

During the first six hours post-exercise not only should foods with a low glycaemic index such as apples,grapefruit, baked beans, yoghurt and milk make up no more than one third of the total carbohydrate intake, for the reason mentioned above, but foods with a high fat or protein content should also be avoided if possible, as they hinder the recovery process, by slowing gastric emptying, suppressing hunger and consequently decreasing carbohydrate intake. Rate of recovery will be optimised by consuming foods or drinks with a high or moderate glycaemic index, a low-fat and low-protein content, such as bread, rice, boiled or baked potatoes, spaghetti, breakfast cereals, boiled sweets, raisins, bananas, grapes and oranges as soon after exercise as possible. Foods with a slightly higher protein content or lower glycaemic index could be included after six hours.

Summary

Players may be aware that they should eat high carbohydrate diets to optimise performance, but be unable to put these recommendations for nutrient intakes into practice through lack of practical knowledge. They may need advice in planning high complex carbohydrate meals, with slightly less fat. The emphasis must be on foods rather than nutrients, in order to provide the players with knowledge of which foods should be chosen to ensure that their diet is high in carbohydrate. Thus, when giving dietary advise to a sportsperson, this should be in terms of actual foods, rather than nutrients, preferably with consideration to how any suggested changes will fit in with the normal routine of each player.

Such high carbohydrate diets should ensure optimum carbohydrate reserves during the days leading up to an important game, maximize carbohydrate stores during the competition itself and enhance the rate of glycogen repletion following each game.

Acknowledgments

The author would like to thank Professor Clyde Williams for his invaluable help and support in the preparation of this paper. Both the author and the Sports Nutrition Service at Loughborough University are supported by the Sports Council.

References

Bergstrom J, Hermansen L, Hultman E et al. (1967) Diet, Muscle Glycogen and Physical Performance. Acta Physiol Scand, 71, 140-150.

Brewer J, Williams C and Patton H. (1988) The influence of high carbohydrate diets on endurance running performance. Eur J Appl Physiol, 57, 698-706.

Costill DL and Miller J. (1980) Nutrition for Endurance Sport: Carbohydrate and Fluid Balance. Int J Sports Med, 1, 2-14.

Costill, DL. (1988) Carbohydrates for exercise: dietary demands for optimal performance. Int J Sports Med, 9, 1-18.

Coyle E. (1991) Timing and method of increased carbohydrate intake to cope with heavy training, competition and recovery. J Sports Sci, 9, 29-52.

Currie D, Bonen A, Belcastro AN et al. (1981) Glycogen Utilization and Circulating Substrate Responses During Match Play Soccer and Soccer Training Sessions. Int J Sports Med, 2, 271 (Abstr.).

Devlin JT and Williams CW. (eds) (1991) Foods, Nutrition and Sports Performance: Final Consensus Statement. J Sports Sci, 9 (iii).

DHSS (1991) Dietary Reference Values for Food Energy and Nutrients for the United Kingdom. Report on Health and Social Subjects, 41, HMSO, London.

Erp-Baart AMJ van et al. (1989) Nationwide survey on nutritional habits in elite athletes, part 1: Energy, carbohydrate, protein, and fat intake. Int J Sports Med, 10, S3-S10.

Hargreaves M. (1991) Carbohydrates and exercise. J Sports Sci, 9, 17-28.

Hermansen L, Hultman E and Saltin B. (1967) Muscle Glycogen During Prolonged Severe Exercise. Acta Physiol Scand, 71, 129- 139.

Hickson JF and Wolinsky I. (eds.) (1990) Nutrition in Exercise and Sport, CRC Press, Florida.

Huque T and Truswell AS. (1979) Retinol content of human livers from autopsies in London. Prac Nutr Soc, 38, 41A.

Jacobs I, Westlin N, Karlsson J et al. (1982) Muscle Glycogen and Diet in Elite Soccer Players. Eur J Appl Physiol, 48, 297-302.

Karlsson J and Saltin B. (1971) Diet, Muscle Glycogen and Endurance Performance. J Appl Physiol 31, 203-206.

Kiens B et al. (1990) Benefit of dietary simple carbohydrates on the early postexercise muscle glycogen repletion in male athletes. Med Sci Sports Exerc, 22, 588.

Keizer H, Kuipers AH, van Kranenburg G and Geurten P. (1986) Influence of liquid and solid meals on muscle glycogen resynthesis, plasma fuel hormone response, and maximal physical working capacity. Int J Sports Med, 8, 99-104.

Kirwan JP, Costill DL, Mitchel JB et al. (1988) Carbohydrate Balance in Competitive Runners During Successive Days of Intense Training. J Appl Physiol, 65, 2601-2606.

Krause MV and Mahan LK. (1984) Food Nutrition and Diet Therapy, 7th edn, Saunders WB, Philadelphia.

Leverton RM. (1975)The RDAs are Not for Amateurs. J Am Diet Assoc, 66, 9.

MacDougall JD, Ward G, Sale D and Sutton J. (1977) Muscle Glycogen Repletion After High Intensity Intermittent Exercise. J Appl Physiol/Respirat Environ Exerc Physiol, 42, 120-132.

Ministry of Agriculture, Food and Fisheries (MAFF). (1989) Household Consumption and Expenditure: Annnual Report of the National Food Survey Committee, HMSO.

National Advisory Committee on Nutrition Education (NACNE). (1983) Proposals for Nutritional Guidelines for Health Education in Britain. Health Education Council, London.

National Research Council Committee on Diet and Health, Food and Nutrition Board. (1989) Diet and Health: Implications for Reducing Chronic Disease Risk. National Academy Press: Washington DC.

Pascoe (1990) Effects of exercise mode on muscle glycogen restorage during repeated days of exercise. Med Sci Sports Exerc, 22, 593-598.

Paul AA and Southgate DAT. (1978) McCance and Widdowson's: The Composition of Foods 4th edn, MRC Special Report Series No 297, London, HMSO.

Piehl K. (1974) Time Course For Refilling Of Glycogen Stores in Human Muscle Fibres Following Exercise-Induced Glycogen Depletion. Acta Physiol Scand, 90, 297-302.

Reid RM and Williams C. (1974) A Concept of Fitness and its Measurement in Relation to Rugby Football. British J Sports Med, 8, 96-99.

Reilly T. (1979) What Research Tells the Coach About Soccer. AAHPERD, Washington.

Reilly T and Thomas V. (1976) A motion analysis of work-rate in different positional roles in professional football match-play. J Human Movement Studies, 2, 87-97.

Saltin B. (1973) Metabolic Fundamentals in Exercise. Med Sci Sports, 5, 137-146.

Sherman WM et al. (1981) Effect of exercise-diet manipulation on muscle glycogen and its subsequent utilization during performance. Int J Sports Med, 2, 87-97.

Short SH and Short WR. (1983) Four-year Study of University Athlete's Dietary Intake. J Am Diet Assoc, 82, 632.

Spencer H, Kramer L, Osis D and Norris C. (1978) Effect of a High Protein (Meat) Intake on Calcium Metabolism in Man. Am J Clin Nutr, 31, 2167.

Stunkard AJ and Waxman M. (1981) Accuracy of Self Reports of Food Intake. J Am Diet Assoc, 79, 547-551.

Van Gool, D et al. (1988) The physiological load imposed on soccer players during real match-play. In Science and Football. E & FN Spon, London, pp. 51-59.

Williams R. (1976) Skilful Rugby. Souvenir Press, London.

Wilmore JH, Freund BJ. (1984) Nutritional Enhancement of Athletic Performance. Nutr Abstr and Rev, 54, 1-16.

Translating nutrition into diet: diet for training and competition

B. Kiens

Abstract

Dietary surveys often reveal that diet composition is not optimal to cover the needs of elite athletes in regular training. A diet rich in carbohydrate is important : an adequate carbohydrate intake is essential to support intense trainins and before competition. Total carbohydrate intake should be high (65-70% of total energy intake), but the types of carbohydrate also seem to be of significance for the resynthesis rate of muscle glycogen stores, especially early in the recovery period. moreover, eccentric exercise impairs glycogen resynthesis, and the exercise mode also has to be considered in the daily training schedule such that training sessions are planned according to fuel availability in the muscle. To achieve the high carbohydrate intake that is recommended a near-vegetarian diet is inevitable. However, there is no evidence that a lacto-ovo vegetarian diet is in any way less suitable than a mixed diet for the athlete, provided that the composition is such as to meet the athlete's needs.

Keywords: Diet, carbohydrate, muscle glycogen, exercise.

Introduction

The body continuously loses a certain amount of the different energy stores and structural proteins by metabolism. The main purpose of the diet is thus to supply the organism with nutrients necessary for cell resynthesis and with the energy necessary for cellular function and muscle contraction. If dietary intake does not cover the daily energy demand, the energy need is covered from energy stores within the body. The fat stores are large but the glycogen stores are limited. Carbohydrates are important for several metabolic functions, but primarily as a fuel for muscle during strenuous exercise. Some protein will be also be utilized, which, in the long run, results in a deterioration in muscle function. The diet must contain the essential nutrients to be adequate, and approximately 50 essential nutrients have to be supplied every day. Each of these has a special function and cannot be replaced. These include the essential amino acids, essential fatty acids, vitamins and minerals.

Questions arise whether nutrition can be a limiting factor in physical performance and whether nutritional requirements of athletes are quantitatively and qualitatively different from those of non-athletes. Today strong evidence indicates that, if the appropriate dietary considerations are not observed, performance both in training and competition will suffer.

The impact of diet on daily training performance

The training diet

The daily training of the athlete is frequently of long duration and high intensity. Thus the daily energy demand is large and must be covered by the diet. Unfortunately, most athletes spend a considerable amount of time and effort in perfecting skills and attaining top physical condition, but ignore proper nutrition and rest. It is not uncommon to trace the deterioration of an athlete's performance back to poor nutrition (Costill et al, 1988; Kirwan et al, 1988).

To gain some insight into the actual eating habits of athletes, diets of highly trained athletes from different sports were recorded during 3 days of training and one day of rest (Table 1). During these days all food was weighed and registered. Data on habitual energy and nutrient intake were calculated using computer data bases of foods from the national Food Agency of Denmark.

The findings revealed that there was little difference between the composition of the diets in athletes and the general population. The percentage of total energy intake in the form of carbohydrate was on the average of 50%. This is even lower than recommended for the general population. This means that for many of the athletes, the amount of carbohydrate in the daily diet was low in the light of the need of a carbohydrate-rich diet. The protein intake seems to be sufficient for the athletes. The fat intake, however, is high and should be replaced by more carbohydrates.

Due to the short duration of the dietary recording (4 days), it is difficult to get valid information on vitamin and mineral status of the athletes. However, the data on vitamins and minerals reveal that the variety in choice of food items is poor. Anyway, the findings from these four days reveal that 70-80% of the athletes questioned had a lower intake of vitamins B6 and E and of zinc compared to dietary recommendations. In regard to dietary iron, this also appears to be low, especially in the female athletes. These findings are frequently seen in athletes consuming relatively low energy diets. Intakes below 9 MJ are for example often associated with suboptimal dietary iron intake. Vegetarian diets are low in heme iron and have a poor iron bioavailability; athletes following such diets are also at risk of iron deficiency. Milk and dairy products have negligible amounts of iron while eggs, frequently reported to be iron-rich, are a poor source as the iron is not easily absorbed. The energy intake was rather low in some of the athletes, especially in the female athletes. It is, however, known that self-reported energy intake often is underestimated when compared with energy expenditure measured by the doubly labelled water method (Westerterp et al, 1988; Schoeller et al, 1989). This will, of course, also lead to an underestimation of the intake of all nutrients.

TABLE 1   Energy intake, dietary composition, vitamins and minerals in elite athletes in different sport activities (mean and range)

	SOCCER PLAYERS	SWIMMERS	FEMALE ATHLETES	Mixed aerobic endurance sports	NNA*
	Male (n=60)	Male (n=371)	Female (n=394)	(n=55)	
Energy (MJ)	14 (10-18)	8.7 (7.9-9.4)	12.4 (10.0-16.0)	9 (5-15)	
Carbohydrates (%)	47 (36-59)	51 (46-55)	53 (41-67)	52 (37-64)	55-60
(g)	379 (250-564)	263 (235-283)	376 (302-484)	280 (100-400)	
Proteins (%)	15 (10-19)	14 (13-16)	14 (11-18)	15 (14-16)	10-15
(g)	119 (93-193)	74 (67-80)	103 (84-132)	79 (22-135)	
Fat (%)	36 (27-47)	33 (30-35)	33 (26-41)	31 (21-48)	Max 30
(g)	128 (91-185)	79 (73-85)	111 (90-142)	77 (38-171)	
Dietary fibers (g)	29 (14-50)	22 (20-24)	31 (25-44)	26 (17-39)	3 g/MJ
B_6 Vitamin (mg)	2.0 (0.8-4.0)	1.2 (1.0-1.3)	1.5 (1.3-2.1)	1.3 (0.7-1.9)	1.5 (F);2.1 (M)
C-Vitamin (mg)	81 (24-94)	75 (58-106)	79 (69-107)	102 (27-159)	60
E-Vitamin (mg)	6.7 (5.0-16.0)	5.1 (4.7-5.5)	6.6 (6.0-9.0)	5.9 (0.7-8.3)	8 (F);10 (M)
Iron (mg)	20 (14-29)	12 (11-14)	17 (14-23)	13.8 (5-23)	12-18 (F);10 (M)
Zinc (mg)	16 (12-22)	8.6 (7.5-9.4)	12 (10-16)	10.2 (3-18)	12 (F); 12-15 (M)

* NNA: Nordic Dietary Recommendations (1989)
  (F) = Female   (M) = Male

177

The carbohydrate-rich diet

From early studies of muscle storage during repeated days of endurance running it was concluded that only a partial replenishment of glycogen stores occurred when the subjects were fed a mixed diet containing 250-300g of CHO per day (Costill et al, 1971). In that study, a consistent day-by-day decline in the glycogen content of m. vastus lateralis occurred despite the dietary carbohydrate intake. However, when the dietary carbohydrate intake was increased to 550-600g per day, the muscle glycogen stores were effectively restored in the 22 hours between the exercise sessions (Costill, 1985).

Thus it appears that dietary carbohydrates play a significant role in endurance exercise. Their inclusion in the daily diet of the athlete is essential for optimal training and competition. The question remains whether there is any benefit of different types of carbohydrates on the repletion of the muscle glycogen stores. Thus, as described by Coyle (this volume) some dietary carbohydrates exert a high glycemic response resulting in a high glycemic index (GI), whereas others exert a slow and low glycemic response, resulting in a low GI. In light of these differences in glycemic response exerted by the different types of carbohydrates, one might speculate whether a difference will appear in muscle glycogen resynthesis rate after ingestion of carbohydrate-rich meals consisting mainly of carbohydrates with a low GI in contrast to a diet containing carbohydrates with a high GI.

To address this question, we recently studied 7 well-trained athletes who were fed diets composed of 70 energy% carbohydrates for 2 days following an exercise bout on a cycle ergometer to deplete the glycogen stores in m. vastus lateralis (Kiens et al, 1989). In one trial the carbohydrate-rich diet comprised carbohydrate food items with high GI in contrast to the other trial, where the carbohydrate intake was mainly covered by carbohydrate food items of low GI. That study revealed a significantly faster glycogen storage in the muscles in the early recovery period after ingestion of carbohydrate food items with high GI compared with ingestion of the low GI carbohydrate food items. Thus, 6 hours after termination of exercise, muscle glycogen stores were restored to 70% of pre-exercise values as opposed to 34% on the low GI carbohydrate diet. In light of these findings, the type of carbohydrate in the diet of the athlete seems to be of significance for resynthesis rate of the muscle glycogen stores in the early recovery period. This is of particular importance when training is performed twice a day.

To arrive at such a large daily carbohydrate intake as recommended, the athlete must to a great extent make the dietary choice from vegetable food sources and will thus often approach a near-vegetarian diet with little meat and other animal food items. Increasing the intake of carbohydrates will increase the intake of dietary fibre, which may reduce the bioavailability of several nutrients, including minerals and vitamins (Helman et al, 1987) and amino acids (Acosta, 1988). Furthermore, vegetable non-heme iron is more poorly absorbed than the animal heme ion (Monsen et al, 1978). This may result in reduced iron stores and increased risk of sports anemia in the athlete who is training hard (Ehn et al, 1980).

In a recent study from our laboratory (Raben et al, in press) the effect of a vegetarian versus a mixed diet on physical performance was evaluated in heavily training male athletes (VO$_2$max :61-79 ml/kg^{-1}/min^{-1}). The experimental period consisted of six weeks on a lacto-ovo vegetarian diet and six weeks on a meat-rich mixed diet. The dietary composition in both diets was similar (57 E% carbohydrates, 13-15 E% proteins, 29 E% fat).The energy composition of the diet was not different from the athletes' habitual diet. The experimental and the habitual diet varied only in types of carbohydrates and the food sources of proteins. Thus, the lacto-ovo vegetarian diet was based primarily on food items with extensive use of protein rich vegetables and legumes. Some dairy products were included in order to reach the desired protein level. Most (83%) of the protein on the lacto-ovo vegetarian diet was supplied by vegetable sources and 17% by animal sources (dairy products). Soy protein amounted to 25% of the total protein content. The mixed diet was based primarily on food items typical of a Western diet including a daily amount of about 240 grams of meat or fish and with the carbohydrates supplied by vegetables and fruits which were low in protein. Animal protein thus amounted to 65% and vegetable protein to 35%.

Endurance performance to exhaustion measured on a Krogh ergometer cycle or a treadmill remained unchanged during both diet regimens (Fig. 1). Also no differences were obtained in maximum oxygen uptake or in isometric strength obtained from measurements of maximal voluntary contraction (MVC) and isometric endurance at 35% of MVC on quadriceps muscle and elbow flexors. Iron and transferrin concentrations in serum as well as blood haemoglobin concentration were unchanged during both dietary periods.

Thus, within the time frame of this study the data suggest that a lacto-ovo vegetarian diet has no detrimental effect on physical performance compared with a mixed diet. However, three important aspects need to be considered. First, the composition of the vegetarian diet was such that all known dietary needs for an athlete were covered, which might not always be the case for the diet consumed by the vegetarian athlete. Second, it may be that the dietary intervention period in this study was not long enough to detect an effect of the diets on physical performance. Finally, a third aspect of this study is that the large portion of dietary fibre and complex carbohydrates and consequently lower energy density and larger volume of the vegetarian compared with the mixed diet resulted in some gastrointestinal distress when on the vegetarian diet. Although some adaptation took place over the 6 weeks, it was still difficult for the athletes to consume the large quantities of food at the end of the vegetarian dietary period.

Protein does not play an essential role as an energy substrate during exercise. However,if the glycogen stores in the exercising muscles are low initially or depleted during exercise the contribution of proteins as an energy source is enhanced (Anderson and Sharp, 1990; Lemon and Mullin, 1980). For the general

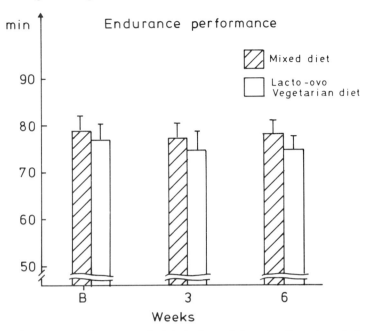

Fig 1. Endurance performance (min) before (B) and after 3 and 6 weeks on a mixed diet and a lacto-ovo vegetarian diet, respectively in well-trained male athletes.

population the recommended daily dietary protein intake is 0.8 g/kg body weight (WHO, 1985). However, today strong evidence exists indicating that the daily protein needs are increased as the result of regular strength or endurance training. Based on available data (Lemon, 1991) it appears that protein intakes should be about 1.2 - 1.4 g/kg body weight/day for most endurance training athletes, and slightly greater for those involved in strength/speed training.

Dietary protein can be derived from two sources: animal and vegetarian sources. Because the animal protein is of high biological value, which means that the amino acids are effectively utilized by the organism, it might be advantageous if the daily diet contained food items of animal origin. Moreover, animal food items usually have a high content of heme-iron and B vitamins. However, a vegetarian diet may also be of high biological value if food items which complement each other in their amino acid composition are chosen. In our recent study (Raben et al, in press) the 15 E% of proteins in the diet were either covered by proteins from vegetable food sources (83%) or from animal food sources (65 E%). Calculating the amino acid composition in these two dietary regimens revealed no significant differences between the two diets and all essential amino acids were supplied in amounts greatly exceeding the FAO/WHO recommendation (WHO,1985). Furthermore, fasting plasma amino acid concentrations were not different between the two diets after 6 weeks.

The mode of exercise seems to play an important role for the rate of muscle glycogen resynthesis. A study by O'Reilly et al (1987) may support this, as it was shown that muscle glycogen resynthesis was impaired for 10 days following an eccentric exercise bout. This is probably due to exercise induced muscle damage. Even with a high dietary carbohydrate intake the replenishment of the glycogen stores is delayed following eccentric exercise (Costill et al, 1990). Thus, in exercise training involving muscle damage an impaired restoration of muscle glycogen is expected, even though the dietary carbohydrate intake is high. This phenomenon should be taken into consideration in the daily training schedule such that training sessions are planned according to fuel availability in the muscles.

From principles to practice

For athletes who daily spend much of their time on training, it is difficult to follow the dietary advices as it is time consuming to prepare an adequate diet which covers the requirements of an athlete's diet. Therefore, there is a great need for diet plans and menus, based on readily available food, to assist athletes in the selection and preparation of food that meets their varied nutritional requirements.

There is no magic diet that in itself enhances performance. However, eating habits and food selection appropriate to the demands of training and competition are essential for optimum performance. An incorrect diet will negate much hard effort on the training field.

References

Acosta PB. (1988) Availability of essential amino acids and nitrogen in vegan diets. Am J Clin Nutr, **48**, 868-874.

Anderson DE, Sharp RL.(1990) Effects of muscle glycogen depletion on protein catabolism during exercise. Med Sci Sports Exerc **22**, S59.

Costill DL, Sparks KE, Gregor R, Turner C. (1971) Muscle glycogen utilization during exhaustive running. J Appl Physiol, **31**, 353-356.

Costill DL. (1985) Carbohydrate nutrition before, during, and after exercise. Fed Proc, **44**, 364-368.

Costill DL, Flynn MG, Kirwan JP, Houmard JA, Mitchell J, Thomas R, Park SH. (1988) Effects of repeated days of intensified training on muscle glycogen and swimming performance. Med Sci Sports Exerc, **20**, 249-254.

Costill DL, Pascoe DD, Fink WJ, Robergs RA, Barr SI, Pearson D. (1990) Impaired muscle glycogen resynthesis after eccentric exercise. J Appl Physiol, **69**, 46-50.

Ehn L, Carlman B, Hoglund S. (1980) Iron status in athletes involved in intense physical activity.

Med Sci Sports Exerc, **12**, 61-64.

Helman AD, Darnton-Hill I.(1987) Vitamin and iron status in new vegetarians. Am J Clin Nutr, **45**, 785-789.

Kiens B, Raben AB, Valeur AK, Richter EA. (1990) Benefit of dietary simple carbohydrates on the early postexercise muscle glycogen repletion in male athletes. Med Sci Sports Exerc, **22**, 588.

Kirwan JP, Costill DL, Mitchell JB, Houmard JA, Flynn MG, Fink WJ, Beltz JD. (1988) Carbohydrate balance in competitive runners during successive days of intense training. J Appl Physiol, **65**, 2601-2606.

Lemon PWR, Mullin JP.(1980) Effect of initial muscle glycogen levels on protein catabolism during exercise. J Appl Physiol, **48**, 624-629.

Lemon PWR. (1991) Effects of exercise on protein requirements. J.Sports Sci. (Foods, Nutrition and Sports Performance) **9**, 53-70.

Monsen ER, Hallberg L, Layrisse M, Hegsted M, Cook JD, Mertz W, Finch CA. (1978) Estimation of available dietary iron. Am J Clin Nutr, **31**, 134-141.

O'Reilly KP, Warhol MJ, Fielding RA, Frontera WA, Meredith CN, Evans WJ. (1987) Eccentric exercise-induced muscle damage impairs muscle glycogen repletion. J Appl Physiol, **63**, 252-256.

Raben AB, Kiens B, Richter EA, Rasmussen LB, Svenstrup B, Micic S, Bennett P. Serum sex hormones and endurance performance after a lacto-ovo vegetarian and a mixed diet. Med Sci Sports Exerc. (in the Press)

Schoeller DA, Bandini LG, Dietz W. (1990) Inaccuracies in self-reported intake identified by comparison with the doubly labelled water method. Can J Physiol Pharmacol, **68**, 941-949.

Westerterp KR, Brouns F, Saris WHM, ten Hoor F. (1988) Comparison of doubly labelled water with respirometry at low-and high-activity levels. J Appl Physiol, **65**, 53-56.

World Health Organisation (WHO) TECHNICAL REPORT SERIES 724, (1985). Energy and protein requirements. Reports of a joint FAO/WHO/UNU Expert Consultation.

PART TWO

Response to stress

Introduction   The immune system

The body relies on the immune system to protect it from assault from micro-organisms and this has been regarded as a generally efficient process. Nonetheless it can over-react or react in inappropriate ways (hypersensitivity) and its complexity is great. The extent to which its function is influenced by the state of training and fitness of the individual is now becoming recognized and this aspect is the subject of this section.

Training can potentiate the immune system, overtraining can undo this. Viruses can wreak havoc among the very fit and the unfit as anyone who has had genuine influenza, measles as an adult or glandular fever will testify. Moreover, the chronic fatigue syndrome has some of the features of the overtraining syndrome and may be linked to previous virus infections. Some viruses are known to infect muscle, both cardiac and skeletal, and the immune system may fail to eliminate them completely. Hence, there is the triad of viruses (with their intracellular habitat), the immune system (which should eliminate them) and fitness training (which can potentiate or sabotage the immune system). These factors act on each other and this section attempts to examine aspects of each, with chronic fatigue syndrome to confuse (or even clarify!) the picture.

C.R. Madeley

Viral myocarditis and myositis

J.E. Banatvala

Abstract. Although a number of viruses may induce an inflammatory response in the myocardium, studies on skeletal muscle implicate enteroviruses more than any other group of viruses in the pathogenesis of both acute and chronic inflammatory disease of skeletal muscle. This may reflect the fact that a systemic search for other causes has not been made, perhaps because, until recently, appropriate technology, notably molecular biological techniques, were not available for such studies. However, as enteroviruses are now implicated as the commonest cause of not only acute myocarditis but also of such chronic cardiac diseases as chronic relapsing pericarditis and dilated cardiomyopathy, this chapter is directed principally towards the role of enteroviruses in the pathogenesis of diseases of cardiac and skeletal muscle. However, in addition to their role in infecting and damaging cardiac and skeletal muscle, enteroviruses may also cause a number of different syndromes, disease being the result of an acute infection in various target organs (Table 1). Nevertheless, most persons infected by enteroviruses experience subclinical infection or a febrile illness wlth mild and non-specific features.

Keywords: Enteroviruses, Acute Myocarditis, Dilated Cardiomyopathy, Polymyositis, Chronic Fatigue Syndrome, Specific IgM Responses, Hybridisation Studies.

Enteroviruses

Enteroviruses are a family of small single-stranded RNA viruses, being approximately 27 nm in diameter and exhibitlng cubic symmetry. About 70 serotypes have been identified, including polioviruses (3 serotypes), coxsackie A viruses (23 serotypes), coxsackie B viruses (6 serotypes) and echoviruses (32 serotypes). More recently recognised viruses are no longer assigned to specific groups but listed numerically as enteroviruses 68-72.

Even among a particular enterovirus serotype, there is considerable genomic diversity; RNA viruses tend to undergo a high rate of mutation. Thus, there may be a number of variants even within a particular enterovirus isolate from a single patient and minor degrees of variation may alter such biological properties as affinity for specific
cell receptors (for example, cardiac muscle, CNS, etc). Employing a mouse model, there is evidence to suggest that the virulence of coxsackie B viruses may relate to a part of the viral genome coding for the capsid protein (Ramsigh et al, 1990).

This region may be recognised specifically by T-cells, which are involved partly in inducing cell-mediated immune responses, which result in damage to cardiac myocytes.

Table 1. Enterovirus induced acute infections

CNS (aseptic meningitis/encephalitis; poliomyelitis)
Skeletal muscle (Bornholm Disease)
Cardiac muscle (myocarditis)
Skin and mucous membranes (hand, foot and mouth; herpangina)
Respiratory tract
Generalised infection (newborn infants)

Enteroviruses are ubiquitous, person to person spread occurring by the faecal-oral route or by respiratory secretions after local replication in cells of the gastro-intestinal mucosa. In temperate climates, epidemics with one or more serotypes tend to occur in 3-5 year cycles and peak in summer and autumn months, although outbreaks of coxsackie B6 are rare; coxsackie B1 appears not to share this periodicity. The epidemiology of enterovirus infection has been reviewed by Banatvala (1983). Enterovirus infection is frequently subclinical and therefore only the more severely ill patients are investigated virologically. Infection is most frequently diagnosed in children, particularly in those less than 5 years of age, among whom CNS, muscular and respiratory symptoms predominate. Infection is much less commonly reported among adults, but they are more likely to develop cardiac complications following coxsackie B virus infection. Analysis of records of patients admitted to hospital with acute myocarditis showed that cases follow the seasonal pattern of coxsackie B virus infection in the community and that the disease is more common among males. Acute myocarditis is associated with a significant mortality, this being due to congestive heart failure or cardiac arrhythmias.

In developing countries, particularly in the tropics, where overcrowding and poor sanitation prevail, exposure to enteroviruses occurs in infancy and early childhood; up to 30% of infants under two may be found to be excreting enteroviruses. Although exposure to enteroviruses used also to be common in infancy in most western countries, improved standards of living during the last few decades have resulted in a shift in exposure from early childhood to older persons. This may result in an increase in the incidence of such clinically apparent infections as Bornholm disease, CNS infection
and acute myopericarditis.

Asymptomatic acute myocarditis followed by complete recovery is probably far commoner than is realised; indeed abnormalities in the electrocardiogram have frequently been observed during such viral infections as infectious mononucleosis, poliomyelitis and measles (reviewed by Woodruff, 1980). Some assessment of the incidence of asymptomatic acute myocarditis among previously healthy persons has been obtained from histological studies on the myocardium obtained at autopsy from those meeting a sudden and violent death. However, it must be appreciated that in many routine studies only a few sections of the myocardium are examined, and this may lead to considerable underestimates of the incidence of focal myocarditis. On the other hand, it is also important that undue significance should not be placed on the finding of a focus consisting merely of a few lymphocytes or neutrophils scattered between myocardial fibres. In a histological study of myocardial tissue obtained from British pilots killed in flying accidents in which an infiltrate of approximately 100 cells in a single focus. or about half this number with multiple foci were present, was accepted as significant evidence of myocarditis. Six of 263 (2.3%) pilots had a focal myocarditis, although these lesions were not thought to have contributed to the cause of the accidents. Myocardial tissue obtained at autopsy from 61 apparently healthy 18-50 year old civilian males dying from trauma was also examined and 3 of 61 (5%) also had evidence of focal myocarditis (Stevens and Underwood-Ground, 1970). A similar study carried out in the USA estimated that between 0.8-3.0% of pilots killed in flying accidents had focal myocarditis, although, as in the British study, pre-existing diseases were not considered to have played a role in causing the fatal accident (Sopher, 1974). Retrospective studies of unselected autopsy material suggests that acute focal myocarditis may also be detected in 3-4% of patients (Saphir, 1942; Gore and Saphir, 1947). Since a focal myocarditis might induce a fatal arrhythmia, it is not surprising that histological studies carried out on myocardial tissues on young persons dying suddenly have yielded an even higher proportion with myocarditis. Thus myocarditis was present in 10 of 47 (21%) Japanese schoolchildren (Okuni et al, 1973) and 15 of 90 (17%) US children who died suddenly (Noren et al, 1977).

Acute myocarditis

Acute myocarditis is defined as an inflammatory infiltration of the muscles of the heart with accompanying myocardial cell damage in a pattern not resembling ischaemic heart injury (Aretz, Billingham and Edwards, 1987). Both acute pericarditis and myocarditis will be considered together since, although the clinical features of one may predominate, histological studies show that in acute pericarditis there is invariably some myocardial involvement and usually vice versa. Indeed, since no electric potentials have been discovered in the pericardium, electrocardiographic changes in pericarditis are attributable to myocardial heart and pericardial fluid on a number of occasions (reviewed by Grist, 1977). Although such findings are obviously of considerable significance, providing aetiological evidence of the role of these viruses in acute myopericarditis, suitable specimens are only rarely available for isolation studies.

Until recently, most of the evidence linking enteroviruses with acute myocarditis has been serological. The presence of high neutralising antibodies to enteroviruses, particularly coxsackie B viruses, suggested that this group of viruses was involved in the pathogenesis of acute myopericarditis (Grist and Bell, 1964). However, tests to detect specific IgM responses were developed, which are indicative of a current or recent antigenic stimulus. They have shown that 45-50% of patients with acute myopericarditis had evidence of current or recent enterovirus infection (Banatvala, 1983). Most of the assays employed antigens containing shared enterovirus group determinants, which allow detection of many enterovirus infections without using antigens prepared from the homologous serotype.

Further evidence linking myocarditis with infection by enteroviruses was obtained more recently by techniques used to detect the presence of viral RNA in cardiac tissue, which can be detected in the absence of infectious virus or viral antigens. Thus, employing slot blot or in situ hybridisation, using labelled cDNA probes incorporating sequences which are highly conserved among enteroviruses, enterovirus RNA was detected in the myocardium of 20-40% of patients but not in controls (Archard et al, 1988b; Easton and Eglin, 1988; Kandolf et al, 1990). Since the distribution of pathological lesions and viral RNA is focal, variation in detection rates may merely reflect errors in sampling. The use of the more recently developed polymerase chain reaction (PCR), by which viral nucleic acid may theoretically be amplified a million fold or more, provides an assay which is likely to prove extremely versatile, much more sensitive and rapid when compared to other methods. Although, as yet, only a few patients with acute myopericarditis have been studied by this technique, enterovirus RNA has been detected in 20-50% of patients (Jin et al, 1990; Weiss et al, 1991).

Studies in experimental animals

Experimental studies have led to a greater understanding of the pathogenesis of acute myopericarditis, the mouse providing a model in which the histological features of infection closely resemble that found in humans. However, such factors as the breed of animal and the particular strain of virus employed are of importance. Most studies have been carried out comparing responses to cardiotropic strains of coxsackie B viruses (particularly B3) with non-cardiotropic strains.

Factors influencing susceptibility of coxsackie B virus induced myocarditis are listed in Table 2, from which it can be seen that among such factors is included exercise which enhances severity. Although there is little information relating to whether exercise also increases the severity of myocardial damage in humans, it is well-established that those who exercise whilst in the viraemic phase of poliovirus infection are likely to experience paralysis in the exercised limbs. Since the clinical features of infection by enteroviruses are essentially non specific, at least in the early phase of infection, it would be unwise to take exercise to "shake off a chill" lest athletes were experiencing an infection by an enterovirus.

Following experimental infection in the mouse with cardiotropic coxsackie B virus, virus appears in the myocardium within hours, peaks in 3-7 days and is then rapidly eliminated by the immune response. Thus, by days 5-7, neutralising antibodies develop and CD4 and CD8 T-cells infiltrate the myocardium. At first there are more CD4 cells but later CD8 T-cells predominate, these cells being involved in inducing cytotoxic damage to cardiac muscle fibres.

Thus, cardiac damage is a relatively late event following infection with enteroviruses and this may explain why it is unusual to be able to isolate enteroviruses from clinical specimens in patients who have developed the clinical features of myopericarditis.

Table 2.   Factors influencing susceptibility to coxsackie B virus induced myocarditis in the mouse model

Age.   Severe in weanling and post-pubertal mice.

Sex. M>F.   Androgens increase and oestrogens decrease severity.

Disease severity enhanced in third trimester and post-partum.

Exercise: Virus titres and severity increased.

Depletion of T-cells - is protective.

Persistent enterovirus infections and their role in chronic cardiac disease

It has long been established that enteroviruses induce acute lysis of the cells they infect. However, most medical virologists were reluctant to accept, until recently, that this group of viruses may persist and cause chronic disease although their veterinary colleagues have long recognised that similar viruses cause persistent infections in animals (Burrows, 1966).

Chronic relapsing pericarditis

Although many patients make an uninterrupted recovery after having experienced an episode of acute pericarditis, it has been estimated that about 20% of patients will subsequently experience one or more relapses over a period of months or years. We found that approximately 2/3rds of patients with chronic relapsing pericarditis of at least one year's duration had a persistent enterovirus specific IgM response (Muir et al, 1989), such responses persisting as long as symptoms were present - up to 10 years. Enterovirus specific IgM levels were significantly higher in such persons than among those with an acute self-limiting episode. Figure 1 shows that IgA and IgM responses among patients with non-relapsing pericarditis are of short duration compared with those who experience a relapsing course. In many patients monotypic IgM responses were observed throughout the follow-up period, which suggests that these patients had a specific enterovirus infection rather than repeated infections with different enteroviruses (Muir et al, 1989).

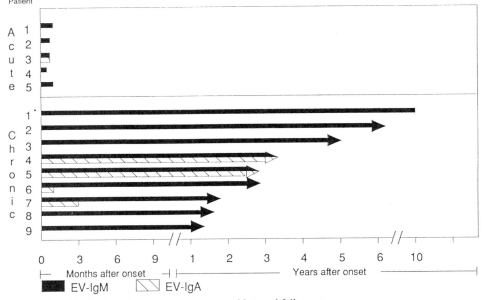

An arrowhead indicates that responses persisted beyond follow-up.
* Sera from this patient not available for EV-IgA testing.

Fig. 1 Enterovirus-specific IgM and IgA responses in acute and chronic relapsing pericarditis. Reproduced from Muir et al (1989) with permission from The Lancet.

Dilated cardiomyopathy

Dilated cardiomyopathy (DCM) is defined as a disease with intrinsic muscle dysfunction excluding such causes as valvular heart disease and ischaemic heart disease. The disease has an estimated annual incidence of about 1/100,000 persons in westernised industrial communities with end-stage disease being a significant cause of cardiac transplantation. Indeed, in Britain, next to ischaemic heart disease, DCM is the commonest reason for cardiac transplantation. Alcohol, amyloid, sarcoidosis, Chaga's disease, beri beri and other vitamin deficiencies may also induce DCM. However, until recently, no identifiable cause was found in most cases and disease was labelled as being of an idiopathic nature. However, the accumulated data from a number of studies, both serological and molecular biological, now implicate enteroviruses in the pathogenesis of DCM.

Enterovirus specific IgM responses have been detected in approximately 33% of patients with DCM, many of whom also have a persistent enterovirus specific IgA response. Figure 2 shows that, among patients undergoing transplantation, the enterovirus specific IgM response may be present for 18 months prior to transplantation and is likely to persist for periods extending to 4 years or more after transplantation (Muir et al, 1989).

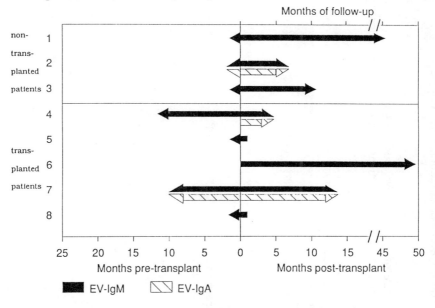

An arrowhead indicates that responses persisted prior to or beyond follow-up.

Fig. 2 Enterovirus-specific IgM and IgA responses in dilated cardiomyopathy. Reproduced from Muir et al (1989) with permission from The Lancet.

Supporting these observations are the findings that enteroviral RNA has been detected in explanted hearts from patients undergoing transplantation for end-stage disease. Table 3 summarises serological and molecular biological findings in patients with chronic cardiac disease. Serological evidence of infection is present in 1/3-2/3rds of cases of patients but among a significantly lower proportion of matched controls, presumably as a result of recent and often subclinical infection by this ubiquitous group of viruses. Enteroviral RNA has been detected in 15-41% of patients with DCM but only very rarely among controls.

Table 3 Evidence for enteroviral involvement in chronic heart disease

Patient diagnosis	Nature of evidence	No. positive (%) Patient group		Controlgroup		Reference
Dilated cardiomyopathy	High CBV-specific antibody titres	15/50	(30%)	1/50	(2%)	Cambridge et al (1979)
Dilated cardiomyopathy (chronic)	Enterovirus-specific IgM	28/86	(33%)	10/84	(12%)	Muir et al (1989)
Chronic relapsing pericarditis		9/14	(64%)	10/84	(12%)	Muir et al (1989)
Healed myocarditis/ dilated cardiomyopathy	Enterovirus RNA detection	17/44	(41%)	0/36	(0%)	Archard et al (1988b)
Dilated cardiomyopathy (recent onset)		10/33	(30%)	0/53	(0%)	Kandolf et al (1990)
Dilated cardiomyopathy (chronic)		6/21	(29%)	1/19	(5%)	Bowles et al (1989)
Dilated cardiomyopathy (chronic)		8/47	(17%)	0/53	(0%)	Kandolf et al (1990)
Dilated cardiomyopathy		3/20	(15%)*	0/9	(0%)	Jin et al (1990)

* Enterovirus RNA detected by PCR

Such findings may be of prognostic significance since recent evidence suggests that patients with enterovirus RNA in the myocardium have a poorer outcome than those without (Archard et al, 1991).

The mechanisms by which enteroviruses are involved in the pathogenesis of DCM have not been clearly established. However, there are two hypotheses: firstly, that defective replication of enteroviruses induces myocardial damage. Thus, patients with DCM have much higher relative amounts of viral negative template strand, which suggests that persisting virus fails to replicate normally (Archard et al, 1991). This may explain why infectious virus or viral antigens cannot be detected in the myocardium and also why immune responses in the myocardium are absent (Bowles et al, 1989). The second hypothesis proposes that autoimmune phenomena induce cardiac damage. It is possible that infection by enteroviruses alters major histocompatability complex antigen expression, which results in cardiac neoantigens being presented to the immune system. Alternatively, antiviral immune responses may react with host tissue; some enteroviral antigens have been shown to share epitopes with host tissue ("molecular mimicry") (Haspel et al, 1983). Although a number of autoantibodies have been detected, they may not be involved in inducing cardiac damage but merely represent epiphenomena.

Most patients with DCM will not have experienced an overt episode of acute myocarditis. It is more likely that patients may have experienced a subclinical infection with a cardiotropic enterovirus strain, which initially induces minimal damage but persists to eventually cause myocardial damage over an extended period.

Infections of skeletal muscle

Acute epidemic myalgia (Bornholm Disease)
This syndrome, which may occur sporadically or in epidemics, is characterised by fever and severe muscle pain, which may involve the limbs, chest and abdomen. Involvement of the pleura or pericardium may occasionally occur. The disease is self-limiting. Most cases are associated with infection by coxsackie B viruses. Virus may be recovered from the stools and nasal-pharyngeal secretions, and specific IgM responses may be detected within a few days of the onset of symptoms (McCartney, Banatvala and Bell, 1986; El Hagrassy, Banatvala and Coltart, 1980).

Polymyositis
Polymyositis is an inflammatory disease of skeletal muscles which may occur in children as well as adults. The disease is characterised by symmetrical weakness of the muscles of the hip girdle, shoulders and neck. The diaphragm, chest wall and pharynx may also be involved. In addition, a characteristic rash may also be present (dermatomyositis).

This disease has all the hallmarks of an autoimmune disease. Thus, there is a predominance of HLA-D8 and DR3 haplotypes, circulating antibodies to myosin and nuclear antigens may be present, and there can be a family history of other autoimmune diseases; 30% of patients have Sjogrens Syndrome and patients respond favourably to immunosuppressants. Histologically, patients in the acute phase have focal atrophy of striated muscles with perivascular mononuclear cell infiltration. These cells are mostly CD8 lymphocytes which are involved in damage to muscle by cytotoxic mechanisms.

Evidence that enteroviruses are involved in the pathogenesis of this disease comes from studies which reported the presence of enterovirus-like crystals in muscle biopsies (Chou and Gutmann, 1970; Benn-Bassat and Machtey, 1972) and the presence of enteroviral RNA in muscle biopsies of a small number of patients, but not controls (Bowles et al, 1987; Yousef, Isenberg and Mowbray, 1990). Serological studies to detect the presence of enterovirus specific IgM responses have not been reported and the mechanisms by which enteroviruses may induce autoimmune phenomena in genetically susceptible persons remains to be investigated.

Chronic Fatigue Syndrome

Chronic fatigue syndrome is characterised by severe fatigue of at least six months' duration, affecting physical and mental functioning, often accompanied by myalgia, mood and sleep disturbance. The diagnosis is by exclusion, and should not be made in patients with such known causes of chronic fatigue as anaemia, tuberculosis, schizophrenia, manic depressive illness, substance abuse, eating disorder or organic brain disease (Sharpe et al, 1991). The syndrome may follow an infectious illness, or may be associated with a current infection, in which case a sub-classification of post-infectious fatigue syndrome may be used. Research into this syndrome has often provided confusing or contradictory results, due mainly to lack of agreement over a case definition, poorly described sampling procedures and selection of control groups.

A number of different viruses have been implicated including Epstein Barr Virus, human herpes virus 6 and the human retroviruses. However, considerable research has been directed towards the role of enteroviruses, results of which are summarised in Table 4.

Although enteroviral RNA has been detected in muscle biopsies from patients with the chronic fatigue syndrome, the profound fatigue experienced by patients may not necessarily reflect enterovirus induced muscle damage. As is the case among patients with diluted cardiomyopathy, neither infectious virus nor viral antigens are present in skeletal muscle. Some psychiatric opinion favours the hypothesis that fatigue is central in origin although, as yet, there have been no published reports of enterovirus presence in the CNS among patients with chronic fatigue. Nevertheless, enteroviruses are potentially neurotropic and it is, therefore, quite possible that some of the psychiatric features, including disturbances in sleep as well as depression, may be the result of enteroviral involvement of the mid brain and limbic areas.

Table 4. Chronic Fatigue Syndrome:
Enteroviral Investigations

Virological Findings	CFS (%)	Controls (%)	References
Enterovirus (EV) VP1 antigen	30-65	0-12	Mowbray J (Pers Commun) Halpin & Wessely, 1989
EV-specific IgM	30	5-12	McCartney et al, 1986
	31	14	Muir et al, 1991
	24	24	Miller et al, 1991
Coxsackie B4 (IF)	90	65	Landay et al, 1991
EV in acid treated stools	22*	0	Yousef et al, 1988
Persistent EV excretion	7	0	Yousef et al, 1988
EV RNA in muscle biopsy (slot blot)	25+	0	Archard et al, 1988a
EV RNA in muscle biopsy (PCR)	53	15	Gow et al, 1991

* 22/22 had VP1 antigen in serum.
+ No VP1 antigen production and very little polymerase

There is a clear need to conduct further studies on patients, who fulfill the criteria for chronic fatigue syndrome, employing many of the virological investigations listed in Table 4. These patients should also be investigated for evidence of infection by Epstein Barr Virus (EBV) so that a more accurate assessment of the role of viruses in patients with the chronic fatigue syndrome may be obtained.

References

Archard LC, Bowles NE, Behan PO, Bell EJ and Doyle D. (1988a) Postviral fatigue syndrome: persistence of enterovirus RNA in muscle and elevated creatine kinase. J Royal Soc Med, **81**, 326-329.

Archard LC, Bowles NE, Cunningham L, Freeke CA, Olsen EGJ, Rose ML, Meany B, Why HJF and Richardson TJ. (1991) Molecular probes for detection of persisting enterovirus infection of human heart and their prognostic value. European Heart J, **12**, (Supp D), 56-59.

Archard LC. Freeke C, Richardson P, Meany B, Olsen EGJ, Morgan-Capner P, Rose M, Taylor P, Banner N, Yacoub M and Bowles N. (1988b) Persistence of enterovirus RNA in dilated cardiomyopathy: a progression from myocarditis in New Concepts in Viral Heart Disease (ed H-P Schultheiss), Springer-Verlag, Berlin, pp. 349-362.

Aretz HT, Billingham ME and Edwards D. (1987) Myocarditis - a histopathologic definition and classification. Am J Cardiovasc Pathol, **1**, 3-14.

Banatvala JE. (1983) Coxsackie B virus infections in cardiac disease in Recent Advances in Clinical Virology 3 (ed AP Waterson), Churchill Livingstone, London, pp. 99-115.

Benn-Bassat M and Machtey I (1972) Picornavirus-like structures in acute dermatomyositis. Am J Clin Path, **20**, 245-249.

Bowles NE, Rose ML, Taylor P, Banner NR, Morgan-Capner P, Cunningham L, Archard LC and Yacoub MH. (1989) End-stage dilated cardiomyopathy: persistence of enterovirus RNA in myocardium at transplantation and lack of immune response, Circulation, **80**, 1128-1136.

Bowles NE, Sewry CA, Dubowitz V and Archard LC. (1987) Dermatomyositis polymyositis and coxsackie-B virus infection. Lancet, **i**, 1120-1123.

Burrows R. (1966) Studies on the carrier state of cattle exposed to foot and mouth disease virus. J Hyg (Cambridge), **64**, 81-90.

Cambridge G, MacArthur CGC, Waterson AP, Goodwin JF and Oakley CM. (1979) Antibodies to coxsackie B viruses in primary congestive cardiomyopathy. Br Heart J, **41**, 692-696.

Chou SM and Gutmann L. (1970) Picornavirus-like crystals in subacute polymyositis. Neurology (Minneapolis), **20**, 205-213.

Easton AJ and Eglin RP. (1988) The detection of coxsackievirus RNA in cardiac tissue by in situ hybridization. J Gen Virol, **69**, 285-291.

El Hagrassy MMO, Banatvala JE and Coltart DJ. (1980) Coxsackie B virus specific IgM responses in patients with cardiac and other diseases. Lancet, **ii**, 1160-1162.

Gore I and Saphir O. (1947) Myocarditis: a classification of 1024 cases. Am Heart J, **38**, 827.

Gow JW, Behan WMH, Clements GB, Woodall C, Riding M and Behan PO. (1991) Enteroviral RNA sequences detected by polymerase chain reaction in muscle of patients with postviral fatigue syndrome. Br Med J, **302**, 692-696.

Grist NR. (1977) Coxsackie virus infections of the heart in Recent Advances in Clinical Virology 1 (ed AP Waterson). Churchill Livingstone, Edinburgh, pp. 141-150.

Grist NR and Bell EJ. (1964) A six-year study of coxsackie B infection in heart disease. J Hyg (Cambridge), **73**, 165-172.

Halpin D and Wessely S. (1989) VP-l antigen in chronic postviral fatigue syndrome. [Letter] Lancet, **i**, 1028-1029.

Haspel MV, Onodera T, Prabhakar BS, Horita MS and Notkins AL. (1983) Virus-induced autoimmunity: monoclonal antibodies that react with endocrine glands Science, **220**, 304-306.

Jin O, Sole MJ, Butany JW, Chia W-K, McLaughlin PR, Liu P and Liew C-C. (1990) Detection of enterovirus RNA in myocardial biopsies from patients with myocarditis and cardiomyopathy using gene amplification by polymerase chain reaction. Circulation, **82**, 8-16.

Kandolf R, Canu A, Klingel K, Kirschner P, Schonke H, Mertsching J, Zell R and Hofschneider PH. (1990) Molecular studies on enteroviral heart disease in New Aspects of Positive-Strand RNA Viruses (eds MA Brinton and FX Heinz), Am Soc Microbiol pp. 340-348.

Landay AL, Jessop C, Lennette ET and Levy JA. (1991) Chronic fatigue syndrome: clinical condition associated with immune activation. Lancet, ii, 707-712.

McCartney RA, Banatvala JE and Bell EJ. (1986) Routine use of u-antibody-capture ELISA for the serological diagnosis of coxsackie B virus infections. J Med Virol, 19, 205-212.

Miller NA, Carmichael HA, Calder BD, Behan PO, Bell EJ, McCartney RA and Hall FC. (1991) Antibody to coxsackie B virus in diagnosing postviral fatigue syndrome. Br Med J, 302, 140-143.

Muir P, Nicholson F, Tilzey AJ, Signy M, English TAH and Banatvala JE. (1989) Chronic relapsing pericarditis and dilated cardiomyopathy: serological evidence of persistent enterovirus infection, Lancet, i, 804-807.

Muir P, Nicholson F and Banatvala JE. (1991) Coxsackie B virus and postviral fatigue syndrome. [Letter] Br Med J, 302, 658.

Noren GR, Staley NA, Bandt CM and Kaplan EL. (1977) Occurrence of myocarditis in sudden death in children. J Forensic Science, 22, 188.

Okuni M, Mimaya J, Kabayashi H and Koshinaga H. (1973) Heart disease in childhood and sudden death syndrome. Pediatrics (Tokyo), 14, 1104 (in Japanese).

Ramsigh A, Hixon A, Duceman B and Slack J. (1990) Evidence suggesting that virulence maps to the P1 region of the coxsackievirus B4 genome. J Virol, 64, 3078-3081.

Saphir O. (1942) Myocarditis - general review with analysis of 240 cases. Arch Path, 33, 88.

Sharpe MC, Archard LC, Banatvala JE, Borysiewicz LK, Clare AW, David A, Edwards RHT, Hawton KEH, Lambert HP, Lane RJM, McDonald EM, Mowbray JF, Pearson DJ, Peto TEA, Preedy VR, Smith AP, Smith DG, Taylor DJ, Tyrrel DAJ, Wessely S, White PD, Behan PO, Clifford Rose F, Peters TJ, Wallace PG, Warrell DA and Wright DJM. (1991) A Report - chronic fatigue syndrome: guidelines for research. J Royal Soc Med, 84, 115-121.

Sopher IM. (1974) Myocarditis and the aircraft accident. Aerospace Medicine, 45, 963-967.

Stevens PJ and Underwood-Ground KE. (1970) Occurrence and significance of myocarditis in trauma. Aerospace Medicine, 47, 776-780.

Weiss LM, Movahed LA, Billingham ME and Cleary ML. (1991) Detection of coxsackievirus B3 RNA in myocardial tissues by the polymerase chain reaction. Am J Path, 138, 497-503.

Woodruff JR. (1980) Viral myocarditis. A review. Am J Path, 101, 427-479.

Yousef GE, Bell EJ, Mann GF, Murugesan V, Smith DG, McCartney RA and Mowbray JF. (1988) Chronic enterovirus infection in patients with postviral fatigue syndrome. Lancet, i, 146-150.

Yousef GE, Isenberg DA and Mowbray JF. (1990) Detection of enterovirus-specific RNA sequences in muscle biopsy specimens from patients with adult onset myositis. Ann Rheum Dis, 49, 310-315.

Immunological aspects of exercise, fitness and competition sport

N.C.C. Sharp

Abstract. Acute exercise of varying severity and corresponding levels of long term training have been found to affect various aspects of the immune system including lymphocyte subsets, immunoglobulins, the mononuclear phagocytic system, polymorphonuclear leukocytes and cytokines, especially IL-1, IL-2 IL-6 and TNF. Much work is contradictory and difficult to compare directly, but a tentative trend may be discerned whereby light to moderate exercise may increase immune responsiveness, but high-level competition sport, especially if it involves extensive endurance training, may lead to a degree of immunosuppression with a possible increase in susceptibility to infection.

Keywords: Competition Sport, Training, Immune Enhancement, Immune suppression.

Introduction

For nearly 15 years the author worked within the field of immunology (Sharp 1960; Jarrett and Sharp, 1963; Sharp and Garrett, 1968), however, since 1971 his work has been entirely in sports physiology. Originally there seemed little in common between the two disciplines, but now there is work linking muscle metabolism and the immune system (Parry-Billings et al, 1990), and there are extensive reviews on exercise and immunity (Asgeirsson and Bellanti, 1987; Fitzgerald, 1988; Calabrese 1990; Simon, 1990
and Shephard et al, 1991).

In reporting work involving sport, different authors interpret the word "elite" to represent collectively a broad range of standards. In the current review, "elite" refers to competitors of Olympic or National Team standard, while "moderate" refers to those of good club standard.

The immune system

A brief overview of the immune system may be useful. It probably originated early in evolution, on the formation of the metazoa from single-celled organisms, in order to keep cell clusters together as organisms became more complex. The original finding and recognition molecules were copied in an array of different forms within what is known as the Ig superfamily, and which now serves three main functions: antigen recognition, e.g. IgM; cell function regulation, e.g. CD4 and CD8 molecules as markers for helper and suppressor T-lymphocytes respectively; and brain cell organisation, e.g. the neurone organiser contactin.

Cells of the immune system originate from a multipotential stem cell which develops either through the thymus to form T-lymphocytes, or through bone marrow as B-lymphocytes. In human peripheral blood, T-cells account for some 75% and B-cells approximately 10% of mononuclear leukocytes. The former provide a cell-mediated response to micro-organisms and parasites, together with delayed hypersensitivity reactions. T-cells also form subsets designated Th (helper), Tc (cytotoxic) and Ts (suppressor), they are important in immunological surveillance (for which they undergo T-cell-eduction in the thymus for "non-self" recognition), and they secrete a number of regulatory proteins within the class of cytokines.

B-lymphocytes can be triggered to differentiate into plasma cells which produce the five immunoglobulin (Ig) subclasses. Ig provides defence against micro-organisms and may assist the 15% of "null" or "non-T non-B" mononuclear leukocytes, almost all of which are lymphocytes. If appropriate antibody is present, null cells may serve a direct cytotoxic function, inducing cell membrane lysis via their perforins, or pore-forming proteins.

Antibody may also activate the complement sytem, a 20-protein cascade which may augment the effects of antibody-antigen combination, and produce cellular lysis through the membrane-attack-pathway, as well as attracting and activating neutrophils, and mediating mast cell degranulation. The non-phagocytic null cells, together with the non-T natural killer (NK) cells and large-granule lymphocytes (LGL) are all part of a cell killing population. Much of this killing may be activated by cytokines, and may be of particular importance against neoplasia (Rosenberg at al, 1985).

The mononuclear phagocytic system, including tissue macrophages, monocytes, Kupffer cells and osteoclasts (and which was formerly known as the reticulo-endothelial system), in addition to its scavenging function also presents antigen to T-cells, thus triggering immune responses, as well as secreting, and reacting to, cytokines, and producing prostaglandins. A good recent summary of the whole immune system is that of Reeves and Todd (1991).

Responses to exercise and training

Lymphocytes

A mild lymphocytosis occurs during and after bouts of acute exercise (Robertson et al, 1981; Soppi et al, 1982 and Niemen et al, 1989). Kendall et al, (1990) found that the T-suppressor population was very resistant to change on exercise of either high intensity (75% of VO_2 max) or long duration (120 minutes), and that the T's response was not related to levels of aerobic fitness, whether these were low (i.e. a mean VO_2 max of 44.9ml O_2/kg/min), moderate (mean VO_2 max of 55.2ml O_2/kg/min) or reasonably high (mean VO_2 max of 63.3ml O_2/kg/min) in male subjects. They also found that the percentages of T-4 helper lymphocytes were reduced immediately after the exercise, with the highest intensity of exercise (i.e. at 75% of VO_2 max for 60 min producing the largest Th drop, followed closely by the group who worked longer at lower intensity (at 65% of VO_2 max for 75 min). The lowest intensity of exercise (30% of VO_2 max for 60 min.) resulted in some reduction in Th lymphocytes, but not as dramatically or as consistently as the higher work sessions. These results were independent of the fitness levels of the subjects. Finally, Kendall et al noted marked rises in the percentage of NK cells, with the greatest increases occurring at the highest work intensity. No clinical histories of the three fitness groups were taken, so disease incidences could not be matched.

Green et al (1981) found that the resting lymphocyte counts were low (<1500/mm³) in marathon runners, especially in those who could run the distance in under 2h 25 min.

So much for numbers, but a vital attribute of lymphocytes is their responsiveness. Kendall's group (MacNeil et al, 1991), utilising subjects of the same three fitness levels, exercised by the same four randomly ordered cycle ergometer tests (30 min at 65% of VO_2 max; 60 min at 30%; 60 min at 75% and 120 min at 65%),studied lymphocyte responses to the mitogen concanavalin A by the incorporation of radiolabeled thymidine. They found that a consistent depression in mitogenesis was present at two hours post exercise in all groups, with a trend towards greater reduction when the exercise intensity was increased in their highest fit group. Exercise duration did not affect the degree of reduction in mitogenesis, and all values had returned to pre-exercise baselines by 24 hours. Interestingly, the group with the lowest fitness showed the lowest pre-exercise lymphocyte proliferation rate, but their T-cell response was not as severely depressed by the high-intensity exercise as the other two fitter groups.

It is interesting in the above studies that, although lymphocyte subset numbers have returned to normal by two hours after exercise, lymphocyte function, as assessed by mitogenesis, may then be at its lowest level. Eskola et al (1978) also found that in-vitro lymphocyte function was markedly reduced in elite runners after a fast marathon, whereas lymphocytes from moderate but not elite runners in the same study showed no reduction in responsiveness after a training run.

Similarly, Gmunder et al (1988) found depressions of from 30% to 70% in lymphocyte responsiveness to concanavalin A in seven moderate marathon runners sampled from four to six minutes after the finish, and found their results to be similar to those of Skylab and Space-shuttle astronauts, who showed similar depressions of responsiveness. Gmunder and colleagues believed that cortisol was responsible for such lymphocyte functional depression in the runners, as six of them had immediate post-race plasma cortisol levels of 1000 to 1250 nmol/l, compared to their pre-race levels of 276 to 690 nmol/l. However, the effect of cortisol on lymphocyte function may depend on its particular local concentration, as small increases in which may act as an immune stimulant, rather than a depressant (Jeffries, 1991).

Nearly 50 years ago Rusch and Kline (1944) demonstrated a reduction in the growth of transplanted tumours in vigorously exercised rats, compared to controls, and there is a growing body of data (Calabrese, 1990; Simon, 1990) which suggests that exercise may lessen the risk of some neoplasms, especially mammary and colon carcinomata, mainly for reasons unconnected with immunity. Nevertheless, it is quite possible that exercise-associated increases in NK cells may contribute to this resistance, as they are part of the effector series against neoplastic cells. Calabrese (1990) concluded that, apart from numerous other factors; "The potential for physical activity to influence the immune response and possibly enhance tumour surveillance is a hypothesis that deserves serious consideration" .

Complement and immunoglobin

Niemen et al (1989) compared levels of IgG, IgA and IgM and the complement factors C3 and C4 in 11 marathon runners and sedentary controls before, during and after a maximal treadmill test. The antibody levels rose by between 8.3% and 18.5% from pre-exercise to 5-minutes post-exercise in both groups, and C3 and C4 rose by 11.3% and 17.1% respectively. The authors attributed most of this rise to haemoconcentration as they considered that there was a 12% to 16% reduction in plasma volume following such exercise. However, the C3 and C4 levels, but not the immunoglobulins, were significantly lower throughout in the marathon runners, during rest, exercise and post-exercise (from 11 blood samples from indwelling catheters), suggesting complement depression may also follow long term endurance exercise. However, within the running group, no significant correlations were found between the weekly training mileage, the body fat percentage or the level of competition performance, and resting C3 and C4 levels. The runners were of moderate standard, as indicated by a group mean VO_2 max of 54.2ml O_2/kg/min and a mean body fat percentage of 12.5% (utilising the skinfold regression formula of Jackson and Pollock (1979).

Poortmans (1970) reported that IgA and IgG significantly increased by 11.8% and 14.4% respectively, following maximal exercise in 28 Olympic competitors, and that this was more than could be accounted for by a decreasing plasma volume. Nieman et al (1989) quote Poortmans and Haralambie as finding a significant 7% increase in IgG following a 100 km run, despite no change in plasma volume. Tomasi et al (1982) found resting levels of salivary IgA to be depressed in elite cross-country skiers, with further depressions after racing. They found IgG to be unaffected, although Fitzgerald (1998) found low resting levels of serum IgG in elite distance runners. She considered that because these were end-of-season findings a possible cumulative effect of repeated training and racing may have occurred.

Cytokines

A number of regulatory proteins, synthesised and secreted by lymphocytes and other cells have a role in orchestrating immune activity, under the generic name of cytokines. They form four main groups: at least eight interleukins (IL1-8); tumour necrosis factors (TNF); three interferons; and colony stimulating factors. Probably all cytokines have multiple biological activities. Collectively, they stimulate T and B lymphocytes, e.g. IL-1 enhances T-cell activation; IL-2 stimulates cytotoxic T-cells and NK cells; and IL-6 contributes to the differentiation of B-cells into plasma cells. Cytokines also promote haemopoiesis and contribute to the inflammatory process including the stimulation of fibroblasts, while more specifically interferons and TNF may inhibit cellular replication. Cytokines tend to function in networks and cascades and although they may show only a modest rise in blood levels, this may indicate much higher local concentrations in the cellular milieu.

Lewicki et al (1988) studied 11 elite road cyclists (mean VO_2max 76ml O_2/kg/min) after a bout of maximum exercise, and found that in vitro IL-1 production rose from 27.4 units/ml before exercise to 48.7 during, and to 57.2 after two hours recovery. IL-2 production, however, fell from a resting 68.9 units to 49.6 during the exercise and down to 41.4 two hours after. On the other hand, NK activity increased by 100% in the same subjects. By contrast, Esperson et al (1990), working with 11 runners (mean VO_2max 72ml O_2/kg/min) after a moderate 5000m run, found that the IL-2 levels were significantly decreased immediately after the run, compared to resting values, that they were back to rest levels two hours later and that they were significantly increased 24 hours after. TNF values in plasma were significantly elevated at two hours after, but nearly normal at 24 hours. Like Lewicki and colleagues they found that the T-helper/T-suppressor ratio had dropped immediately post-exercise, but increased above rest values at two hours and was back to rest levels at 24 hours. Interestingly, the Th/Ts resting ratio was higher in the competitors than their matched controls, at 1.7 compared to 1.4, which is a ratio at which susceptibility to infection may increase due to a decrease of appropriate lymphocyte response (Keast, Cameron and Morton, 1988)

Esperson and colleagues explained the increase in IL-2 by the increased numbers of HLA-DR- or "activated" lymphocytes, which are known to express an increased number of IL-2 receptors. Possible muscle micro-trauma, with resulting micro-foci of inflammation and cytokine release, may explain the higher IL-2 levels found at 24 hours post-exercise. Similarly, Dufaux and Order (1989) found that IL-2 receptor concentration was significantly raised 24 and 48 hours after a 2.5-hour race in moderate runners. They also found an increase in plasma elastase-alpha-1-antitrypsin complex to twice resting values after one hour of the run, with a threefold increase at the end. This rise in elastase is indicative of lysosomal enzyme release from polymorphonuclear leucocytes, suggesting an exercise-induced proteolysis in muscle.

Northoff (1991), working with 16 marathon runners, observed that the systemic levels of IL-6 were significantly increased two hours after their race, and had fallen to resting levels by 24 hours.

Most authors working on cytokines and exercise remark on the striking similarities between the response to strenuous acute exercise and the acute inflammatory response to infection, including marked leukocytosis, moderate fever and an increase in cytokines, influencing leucocyte function.

Polymorphonuclear leukocytes

Although not strictly part of the immune system, this cell type is included because of close links with it, especially the acute inflammatory response and the defence against pyogenic and other bacterial infections. Smith et al (1990) have shown that regular moderate exercise (e.g. one hour at 60% of VO_2max) may increase non-specific resistance to infection by priming the "killing capacity" of neutrophils to produce hydrogen peroxide, for example. Such priming may last for up to six hours after exercise. However, they also found that prolonged periods of intensive training may curtail this activity by up to 50%. Fehr, Lotzerich and Michna (1988) and Michna (1988) have shown similarly that macrophage chemotactic and phagocytic activity increased after a bout of strenuous exercise, but were diminished by long-term endurance training, however Macha, Shlafer and Kluger (1990) found that one hour of moderate exercise (at 50% of VO_2max) may indeed elevate the neutrophil count, but it reduced the cell's ability to generate hydrogen peroxide. Moreover, by adding post-exercise plasma to pre-exercise neutrophils, Macha and colleagues could diminish the production of hydrogen peroxide, suggesting the presence of an exercise-induced inhibitory factor. Finally, Ferry et al (1990) studied cyclists on a longitudinal basis and found that the absolute number of blood neutrophils at rest was significantly lower after five months of intensive training, than before.

Effects of training and sport on clinical aspects of immunity

There is little doubt that frequent moderately strenuous aerobic exercise is beneficial to health, especially on the functional and disease aspects of the cardiovascular system, as shown by the major studies of Paffenbarger et al (1986) and Morris et al (1990). However, there is a general feeling among coaches, ccmpetitors and team doctors that more severe competition and training schedules render athletes more liable to illness and infection, on a spectrum of severity whose upper end may encompass the "overtraining syndrome". There is also a tendency, indeed an increasing necessity, for the elite competitor to become virtually full-time in his or her sport. For example, in gymnastics about 35 hours of training per week are required to seriously challenge for a place in an individual apparatus Olympic or World Championship final. Swimmers spend two to four hours daily in the water, and cyclists, distance runners and cross-country skiers more than that on the road, track or trail. Squash players may play and practise for five hours each day, most days per week, and triathletes, pentathletes, heptathletes and decathletes may spend even longer. Yet there exist very few clinical data charting the disease prevalence of such competitors.

Clinical data

Several reports of outbreaks of mainly viral diseases have been reported in sporting groups, usually of moderate ability levels. Some workers suggest an increased susceptibility to infection among competitors, others indicate that training or competing within the incubation period may exacerbate the condition.

Weinstein (1973) reported an outbreak of poliomyelitis in a school at which, because of religious convictions no-one had been vaccinated. All nine boys who contracted the disease suffered paraplegia, attributed to the fact that they were active sportsmen. Exercise during incubation is known to worsen polio, and paresis tends to affect those muscles specific to the sport. Morse et al (1972) reported an outbreak of infectious hepatitis which affected 90 out of 97 college footballers, during which no other students or staff became ill. Baron et al (1982) reported an outbreak of echovirus meningitis in which 43 of 51 footballers were affected, while non-team members suffered half the morbidity and less severe symptoms.

Gastro-intestinal infections, respiratory diseases and skin conditions seem more frequent in sports competitors (Asgeirsson and Bellanti, 1987), and Hanley (1976) reported the common occurrence of tracheitis and tracheobronchitis in American Olympic distance runners, rowers and speed skaters, and speculated that a combination of cold air with their high ventilation rates might have been a more important cause than alterations in immune status. More recently, Halvorsen (1989) has reported an increased incidence of disease in elite competitors which "may have to do with an impairment of the body immune response caused by clinical exercise". Part of the clinical response to possible effects of severe training on the immune system may relate to what has been termed the "overtraining syndrome", biochemical aspects of which are comprehensively reported elsewhere in Section 4 of this Congress by Parry-Billings, and physiological aspects of which have been studied in the author's laboratory (Koutedakis, Budgett and Faulmann, 1989), while there is an excellent review by Budgett (1990), also from the British Olympic Medical Centre, who deals more with the clinical details.

At the highest levels of competition, especially associated with high expectations of success, the contribution of psychological stress may be added to any effects of exercise stress on the immune system. In the forthcoming Rugby World Cup,very high expectations will rest heavily on players in key positions, thus imparting a major psychological burden on the players concerned. Many studies have shown that various types of stress, including life-stress, bereavement and examination stress affect immune function (Asgeirsson and Bellanti, 1987). High competition stress would seem likely to produce similar effects, although the modern elite competitor receives ever-increasing help from good sports psychologists. Roberts (1986) in a comprehensive review on viral illness and sports performance specifically indicates that "recent evidence has shown that people undergoing severe mental or physical stress may have reduced immunity to viral infections".

HIV disease and sport

There are numerous publications on HIV disease and sport (e.g. Calabrese and Kelley, 1989; Loveday, 1990) but these mainly concentrate on appropriate precautions against sporting risks, especially in body contact sports. Nevertheless, Calabrese and Kelley (1989) state, "A growing body of scientific data supports the contention that most individuals infected with human immunodeficiency virus can and should remain physically active". Given that moderate physical activity may benefit immmune function, such advice seems sound; but if, as the trend of this review implies, and as Parry-Billings will also suggest at this Congress, very high levels of exercise may lead to a degree of immunodeficiency in its own right, then one should perhaps counsel HIV-poitive competitors not to over-do their training, a piece of advice which is always very unwelcome to high-training performers. Conversely, there are conditions associated with an overactive immune system, e.g. some forms of chronic arthritis, where strenuous exercise (if possible) might be positively indicated, while immune deficiency ccnditions, such as in the aged, might benefit from moderate exercise.

Finally, although sports allergies are commonly reported (e.g. Blumenthal, 1990), it is hard to find evidence whether these are immunologically potentiated through moderate training or diminished through overtraining.

Mechanisms of alteration in immune function

These are complex, as would be expected, and fall into at least three areas; hormonal, metabolic and, possibly, psychoneural.

On the endocrine side, Maki (1989) found that a significant increase in lymphocyte beta-adrenoceptor density from 45 to 81 fmol/mg protein occurred during the first hour of a three-hour run by moderate subjects. Receptor densities did not change further, but remained elevated. Similarly, isoproterenol-stimulated cyclicAMP increased during the first hour from 190 to 269 pmol/mg protein, returning to resting levels at the end of the run, while mean levels of catecholamines increased sixfold during the first hour and remained high throughout the three hours. Thus the exercise activated state of the lymphocytes became attenuated two to three hours into the run as indicated by the diminishing ability of the beta-adrenoceptors to mediate catecholamine-induced cyclicAMP production. Similarly, Graafsma et al (1990) studied the effect of cycle exercise (up to 75% of VO_2 max) on beta-2-adrenoceptors and cyclicAMP in lymphocytes and found that the receptor density increased from 1207 to 1776 sites per cell, and isoprenaline-induced cyclicAMP synthesis increased by 68% compared to pre-test resting values, indicating that the new receptors were functional.

Budgett et al (1989) found no significant difference in plasma cortisol and testosterone levels between nine Olympic endurance competitors suffering "overtraining", and matched controls, while Adlercreutz et al (1986) noted also that moderate exercise did not cause changes in plasma cortisol or testosterone. However, Vervoorn et al (1991) showed that the plasma free-testosteronetcortisol ratio had decreased by 5% to 50% in Olympic rowers at rest following a heavy two-week training period, but the ratio rose again following less intensive periods of training.

Interestingly, Calabrese and Kelley (1989), noting that gonadal steroids help regulate immunological function, showed that prolonged strength training combined with high anabolic steroid usage was immunosuppressive, with IgG, IgM and IgA serum levels reduced by 16%, 33% and 35% respectively, compared to controls, possibly through the steroid's enhancement of suppressor cell activity, (NK activity was also increased). However, the steroid users showed no clinical evidence of reduced incidence to infections.

In the current session, Parry-Billings will discuss metabolic influences on the immune function of elite competitors, including lowered levels of plasma glutamine, an amino acid which may provide over 30% of the energy substrate for lymphocytes, as well as being vital in their regulation of nucleotide synthesis. Other work is in progress (Fitzgerald (1991) personal communication) to determine the effect of elite level training on the lymphocyte glucose transporter protein, which may be activated by stress to transfer from intracellular inactive sites to the plasma membrane where it becomes fully functional (Warren and Pasternak, 1989).

Various forms of psychological stress have been shown to affect immune status, via mechanisms which are often considered to be hormonal, e.g. cortisol and other "stress hormones". However, within the context of psychoneuro-immunology Felton (1991, personal communication) appears to have shown direct neural contact with immune cells through lymph node innervation. It seems not unreasonable to suggest that the CNS and the immune system may communicate by means of specific proteins of the Ig superfamily. Also, on a rather different line, Newsholme's group are producing increasing evidence linking muscle, brain and the immune system (Parry-Billings et al, 1990).

Recommendation

If the basic tenet is correct, that high levels of training stress combined with high psychological stress from competition and the compulsion to win may adversely affect immune function, and predispose to disease, then coach and competitor need to know how to break the cycle. The general principle should be to reduce the multiple stressors. At the BOMC we have found that two to five weeks rest from training and competition may help to alleviate the "overtraining syndrome", and such rest might help to restore immune function. Lowering training volume does not necessarily lower performance, and may even increase it. Costill et al (1990) have shown that reducing swimming training from two 90-minute session per day down to one such session did not lessen performance, but increased both swimming speed and the ability to generate muscle force, partly through beneficial effects on muscle glycogen.

Conclusion

The effects of exercise, fitness and competition on the immune system are very complex to review, partly because there are so many variables regarding exercise and fitness, viz. aerobic, anaerobic, strength, speed, power, body fat level, upper body, lower body, whole body, short or long duration, continuous or intermittent (or both, as in multiple sprint sports such as rugby), level of exertion as a percentage of individual maxima, and level at which the sport is performed, from recreational through club class to Olympic medallist. These exercise, fitness and sport variables have to be matched to an equal complexity of immune system variables, some of which are indicated in this review. Hence it is difficult to compare much of the reported work.

What is needed is a database of resting immunological values of the superfit, to see if they do differ from norms. Also, many more good clinical data are needed on whether the superfit have higher incidences of infection. Thirdly, it is also important to know whether different sporting categories of the superfit are differently affected immunologically. For example, at the BOMC we believe that the overtraining syndrome occurs primarily in continuous endurance sports such as rowing, distance running and cross-country skiing, rather than in the sprints or power sports. Depressive alterations in the immune system may be similarly distributed.

In the literature, a discernible trend seems to be that if a sedentary life - other factors being equal - is associated with a given level of immune function, then moderate exercise may increase it, but that somewhere up the scale towards world class sporting performance the training required may decrease immune function. Thus training quality and quantity, diet and psychological status all need to be individually optimised. This could be achieved for our sports teams, but at considerable cost.

Acknowledgements

For their willing and excellent help in the preparation of this review, I am extremely grateful to Steve Hewitt and Heather Medcalf of the Sports Documentation Centre, University of Birmingham Library; to Kathryn Walter, librarian of the London Sports Medicine Institute; to Dr Lynn Fitzgerald of St George's Hospital Medical School; to Drs Richard Budgett and Yiannis Koutedakis of the British Olympic Medical Centre; and to Duncan Sharp for his illustration used in the slide presentation.

References

Adlercreutz H, Harkonen M, Kuoppasalmi K, Naneri H, Huhtaniemi I, Tikkanen K, Remes K, Dessypris A and Karvonen J. (1986) Effect of training on plasma anabolic and catabolic steroid hormones and their response during physical exercise. Int J Sports Med, **7**, S27-S28.

Asgeirsson G and Bellanti JA. (1987) Exercise, immunology and infections. Seminars in Adolesc Med, **3**, 199-204.

Baron RC, Hatch MH, Kleeman K and MacCormack JN. (1982) Aseptic meningitis among members of a high school football team. JAMA, **248**, 1724-1727.

Blumental MN. (1990) Sports aggravated allergies. Phys Sportsmed, **18**, 2-66.

Budgett R, Koutedakis Y, Walker R, Parry-Billings M and Newsholme EA. (1989) The overtraining syndrome/staleness. Proc IOC 1st World Congress on Sports Sciences, US Olympic Committee, Colorado Springs, USA, pp. 140-142.

Budgett R. (1990) Overtraining syndrome. Br J Sport Med, **24**, 231-236.

Calabrese LH and Kelley D. (1989) AIDS and athletes. Phys Sportsmed, **17**, 127-13 .

Calabrese LH. (1990) Exercise, immunity, cancer and infection. In: Exercise Fitness and Health (ed. C Bouchard) Human Kinetics, Champaign, Ill, USA, pp. 567-579.

Costill DL, Thomas R, Robergs RA, Pascoe D, Lambert C, Barr S and Fink WJ. (1990) Adaptations to swimming training: influence of training volume. Med Sci Sports Ex, **23**, 231-236.

Dufaux B and Order U. (1989) Plasma elastase-alpha-1-antitrypsin, neopterin, tumor necrosing factor and soluble interleukin-2 receptor after prolonged exercise. Int J Sport Med, **10**, 434-438.

Eskola J, Ruuskanen O, Soppi E, Viljaner MK, Jarvinen M, Toivoren H and Kouvalainen K. (1978) Effect of sports stress on lymphocyte transformation and antibody formation. Clin Exp Immunol, **32**, 339-345.

Esperson GT, Elbaek A, Ernst E, Toft E, Kaalund S, Jersild C and Grunnet N. (1990) Effect of physical exercise on cytokines and lymphocyte subpopulations in human peripheral blood. APMIS, **98**, 395-400.

Fehr HG, Lotzerich H and Michna H. (1988) The influence of exercise on peritoneal macrophage functions: histochemical and phagocytic studies. Int J Sport Med, **9**, 77-81.

Felten D. (1991) Professor of Neurobiology, Rochester University, New York State, USA. Personal communication.

Ferry A, Picard F, Weill Bb, Duvallet A and Rieu M. (1990) Changes in leucocyte populations induced by acute maximal and chronic submaximal exercise. Eur J Appl Physiol, **59**, 435-442.

Fitzgerald L. (1988) Exercise and the immune system. Immunol Today **9**, 337-339.

Fitzgerald L. (1991) Senior Reserch Fellow, Division of Immunology, St George's Hospital Medical

School, London. Personal communication.

Gmunder FK,. Lorenzie G, Bechler B, Joller P, Muller J, Ziegler WH and Cogoli A. (1988) Effect of long-term exercise on lymphocyte reactivity: similarity to spaceflight reactions. Aviation Space Environ Med, **62**, 146-151.

Graafsma SJ, van Tits LJH, Willems PHGM, Hectors MPC, Rodrigues de Miranda, JF, De Pont JJHHM and Thien Th. (1990) Beta-2-adrenoceptor up-regulation in relation to cAMP production in human lymphocytes after exercise. Br J Clin Pharmac, **30**, 142S-144S.

Green RJ, Kaplan SS, Rabin BS, Stanistki CL and Zdziarski U. (1981) Immune function in the marathon runner. Ann Allergy, **47**, 73-75.

Halvorsen R. (1989) The effect of exercise and elite athletics on the immune system. Tidsskrift for den Norske Laegeforening, **109**, 2859-2862.

Hanley DF. (1976) Medical care of the US Olympic team. JAMA, **236**, 147-148.

Jackson AS and Pollock ML. (1979) Generalised equations for predicting body density of men. Br J Nutr, **40**, 497-503.

Jarrett WFH and Sharp NCC. (1963) Vaccinations against parasitic disease: reactions in vaccinated and immune hosts in Dictyocaulus viviparus infections. J Parasitol, **49**, 177-189.

Jeffries WM. (1991) Cortisol and immunity. Med Hypoth, **34**, 198-208.

Keast D, Cameron K and Morton AR. (1988) Exercise and immune response. Sport Med, **5**, 248-267.

Kendall A, Hoffman-Goetz L, Houston M, MacNeil B and Arumugam Y. (1990) Exercise and blood lymphocyte subset responses: intensity, duration and subject fitness effects. J Appl Physiol, **69**, 251-260.

Koutedakis Y, Budgett R and Faulmann L. (1989) The role of physical rest for underperforming elite competitors. Proc IOC 1st World Congress on Sports Sciences, US Olympic Committee, Colorado Springs, USA, pp. 140-142.

Lewicki R, Tchorzewski,H, Majewska E, Nowak Z and Baj Z. (1988) Effect of maximal physical exercise on T-lymphocyte subpopulations and on interleukin 1 (IL 1) and interleukin 2 (IL 2) production in vitro. Int J Sport Med, **9**, 114-117.

Loveday C. (1990) HIV disease and sport. In Medicine, Sport and the Law (ed SDW Payne). Blackwell Scientific Publications, Oxford, England, pp. 81-86.

Macha M, Shlafer M and Kluger MJ. (1990) Human neutrophil hydrogen peroxide generation following physical exercise. J Sport Med, Physical Fitness, **30**, 412-419.

MacNeil B, Hoffman-Goetz L, Kendall A, Houston M and Arumugam Y. (1991) Lymphocyte proliferation responses after exercise in men: fitness, intensity and duration effects. J Appl Physiol, **70**, 179-185.

Maki T. (1989) Density and functioning of human lymphocyte beta-adrenergic receptors during exercise. Acta Physiol Scand, **136**, 569-574.

Michna H. (1988) The human macrophage system: activity and functional morphology. Bibliotheca Anat, **31**, 1-84.

Morris JN, Clayton DG, Everitt MG, Semmence AM and Burgess EH. (1990) Exercise in leisure time: coronary attacks and death rates. Br Heart J, **63**, 325-334.

Morse LJ, Bryan JA, Murle JP. (1972) Infectious hepatitis, an outbreak in college footballers. JAMA, **219**, 706-708.

Nieman DC, Tan SA, Lee JW and Berk LS. (1989) Complement and immunoglobulin levels in athletes and sedentary controls. Int J Sport Med, **10**, 124-128.

Northoff H. (1991) The systemic cytokine reaction after strenuous exercise. Immunol Today, 12, in press.

Paffenbarger RS, Hyde RT, Wing AL and Hsieh CC. (1986) Physical activity; all-cause mortality of college alumni. N Engl J Med, **314**, 605-613.

Parry-Billings M, Blomstrand E, McAndrew N and Newsholme EA. (1990) A communication link between skeletal muscle, brain and cells of the immune system. Int J Sport Med, **11**, S122-S128.

The immune system

Poortmans JR. (1970) Serum protein determination during short exhaustive physical activity. J Appl Physiol, 30, 190-192.

Reeves G and Todd I. (1991) Lecture Notes on Immunology, 2nd edition. Blackwell Scientific Publications, Oxford, UK.

Robertson AJ, Ramesar KCRB, Potts RC, Gibbs JH, Browning MCK, Brown RA, Hayes PC and Beck JS. (1981) The effect of strenuous physical exercise on circulating blood lymphocytes and serum cortisol levels. J Clin Lab Immunol, 5, 53-57.

Rosenberg SA, Lotze MT, Muul LM, Leitman S, Chang AE, Ettinghausen SE, Matory YL, Skibber JM, Shiloni E, Vetto JT, Seipp C, Simpson C and Reichart CM. (1985) Observation of the systemic administrtion of autologous lymphokine-activated killer cells and recombinant interleukin-2 to patients with metastatic cancer. N Engl J Med, 313, 1485-1492.

Roberts JA. 1986 Viral illnesses and sports performance. Sports Med, 3, 296-3 .

Rusch HP and Kline BE. (1944) The effect of exercise on the growth of mouse tumor. Cancer Res, 4, 116-118.

Sharp NCC. (1960) The world's first parasitic vaccine. Manuf Chemist, 31, 469-473.

Sharp NCC and Jarrett WFH. (1968) Inhibition of immunological expulsion of helminths by reserpine. Nature, 218, 1161-1162.

Shephard RJ, Verde TJ, Thomas SG and Shek P. (1991) Physical activity and the immune system. Can J Sport Sci, 16, 163-185.

Simon HB. (1990) Exercise, immunity, cancer and infection. In Exercise, Fitness and Health (ed C Bouchard), Human Kinetics, Champaign, Ill, USA, pp 581-588.

Smith JA, Telford RD, Mason IB and Weidemann MJ. (1990) Exercise, training and neutrophil microbicidial activity. Int J Sport Med, 11, 179-184.

Soppi EP, Varjo P, Eskola J and Latinen LA. (1982) Effect of strenuous physical exercise on circulating lymphocyte number and function before and after training. J Clin Lab Immunol, 8, 43-46.

Tomasi TB, Trudeau FB, Czerwinski D and Erredge S. (1982) Immune parameters in athletes before and after strenuous exercise. J Clin Immunol, 2, 173-178.

Vervoorn C, Quist AM, Vermulst LJM, Erich WBM, de Vries WR and Thijssen JHH. (1991) The behaviour of plasma free-testosterone/cortisol ratio during a season of elite rowing training. Int J Sport Med, 12, 257-263.

Warren AP and Pasternak CA. (1989) Common pathway for the induction of hexose transport by insulin and stress. J Cell Physiol, 138, 323-328.

Weinstein L. (1973) Poliomyelitis: a persistent problem. N Engl J Med, 288, 370-372.

The overtraining syndrome: some biochemical aspects

M. Parry-Billings, V.J. Matthews, E.A. Newsholme, R. Budgett and J. Koutedakis

Abstract. The overtraining syndrome is a complex clinical condition with a range of signs and symptoms, including immunosuppression, central fatigue and depression. Little evidence exists to explain the biochemical aetiology of the condition. This paper presents the hypothesis that the metabolism of certain key amino acids may be altered following prolonged exercise and in overtrained athletes and may contribute to the development of the overtrained state.

Keywords: Overtraining, Exercise, Amino Acids, Glutamine, Tryptophan.

The overtraining syndrome

When exercise is performed on a regular basis, "adaptation" occurs and the athlete's performance improves. This is the **training** effect. All exercise elicits a "stress" response and results in a degree of short term fatigue, from which the athlete recovers. However, if exercise periods are too frequent, too intense and/or too prolonged, possibly combined with inadequate nutrition and psychological stress, recovery after each exercise bout is not complete, less adaptation and hence less improvement in performance occurs. If continued, this can lead to **overtraining** (Noakes, 1986). The overtrained athlete may be said to be suffering from **the overtraining syndrome.**

The overtraining syndrome is a complex of clinical conditions, which has been described by a number of authors (see Noakes, 1986). Athletes suffering from this syndrome present with a large number of signs and symptoms (see Table 1). Thus, it is unlikely that a single biochemical defect is responsible and it is concluded that the biochemical explanation for overtraining is multifactorial. A number of studies have proposed metabolic changes thought to be associated with overtraining, including negative nitrogen balance and decreased muscle glycogen content (see Fry et al, 1991). However, it must be emphasized that many of these studies were performed on a small number of subjects, did not demonstrate good case definition and included subjects who may not have been truly overtrained. Thus, a biochemical basis for any of the signs and symptoms of overtraining is missing.

Table 1. Some signs and symptoms of the overtraining syndrome

Impaired exercise performance
Chronic fatigue
Depression
Increased incidence of infections
Slower wound healing
Increased early morning heart rate
Retarded recovery of heart rate after exercise
Increased resting blood pressure
Postural hypotension
Disturbed sleep
Loss of appetite
Loss of drive and enthusiasm
Amenorrhoea
Loss of libido

The effects of exercise on the immune system

Exercise, particularly low-intensity exercise, appears to be beneficial for the immune system. Thus, there is evidence that low-intensity exercise enhances the lymphocyte response to mitogenic stimulation in vitro, increases the number of natural killer cells and increases the number of circulating lymphocytes ("leukocytosis") (Keast et al, 1988, Oshida et al, 1988). These effects would be expected to enhance immune function.

In contrast, there is considerable evidence which suggests that exercise of high intensity or long duration is associated with adverse effects on immune function (Keast et al, 1988). A period of training may prevent or reduce the magnitude of the postexercise leukocytosis. Although the total number of lymphocytes may increase following exercise, changes in the numbers of lymphocytes in specific subpopulations may not enhance the overall potential immunological activity; thus, the ratio of CD4[T4](helper) cells: CD8[T8](suppressor) cells is decreased post-exercise (Keast et al, 1988; Lewicki et al, 1988). In addition to the effect of exercise on the **number** of circulating leukocytes, a decrease in immune **function** following exercise has also been reported. In general, high intensity exercise and training appear to cause a marked decline in the functioning of cells of the immune system. The response of T lymphocytes to mitogenic stimulation in vitro may therefore be decreased and antibody syntheisis may be impaired: immunoglobulin levels in blood and saliva are decreased post-exercise in trained subjects; training decreases neutrophil and monocyte adherance, monocyte bacteriocidal activity, levels of the complement components C3 and C4 and total thrombocytic clotting capacity (Keast et al, 1988; van Wersch et al, 1989, Nieman and Nehlsen-Cannarella, 1991).

No systematic studies of the immunological status of overtrained athletes have been performed. However, it is well established that these individuals show an increased incidence of viral infections, which may be associated with decreased lymphocyte number and function (Noakes, 1986; Fry et al, 1991).

Until now, a biochemical mechanism to explain this immunosupppression has not been put forward. We suggest that intense and long duration exercise, particularly if it is regular, can cause a marked decrease in the plasma glutamine level and this can result in immunosuppression. In order to understand the evidence for this hypothesis, it is necessary to consider the nutrition of the immune system.

Nutrition of the immune system

Until recently, it had been generally considered that both lymphocytes and macrophages obtained most of their energy from glucose and, furthermore, that cells which had not been subjected to an immune stimulus (resting or quiescent) were metabolically inactive. However, the rates of both glucose and glutamine utilisation by these cells are very high. Indeed, the rates of utilisation of glucose plus glutamine by resting lymphocytes is about 25% of the rate of glucose utilised by a maximally, physically working heart (Table 2). In addition, both substrates are only partially oxidized by these cells, suggesting that ATP generation is not the major role of these "fuels".

This work has led to a new hypothesis to explain these high rates of fuel utilisation in lymphocytes and macrophages. It proposes that the high rates provide optimal conditions for the precise regulation of the rates of purine and pyrimidine nucleotide synthesis, which utilise intermediates of both glycolysis and glutaminolysis when needed during proliferation of cells: the high rates provide a dynamic buffer for the use of intermediates of these pathways for biosynthesis. The mechanism for providing precision in regulation is known as **branched point sensitivity** in metabolic control (Newsholme et al, 1985). Understanding the metabolic control theory that underlies this hypothesis is less important than appreciating the prediction to which it gives rise. It predicts that, if the plasma glutamine level is decreased below the physiological level, the rate of proliferation of lymphocytes and the function of the macrophage will be decreased: this would be expected to impair the immune system. This prediction has been tested and shown to be true. Thus, a decrease in the concentration of glutamine decreases the maximum rate of proliferation of human or rat lymphocytes in culture, despite the presence of all other amino acids and fuels (Parry-Billings et al, 1990a). Similarly, a decrease in the glutamine concentration has been shown to decrease the rate of antibody synthesis by lymphocytes and the rate of phagocytosis by macrophages (Schneider & Lavoix, 1990, ParryBillings et al, 1990a). Furthermore, a decrease in the plasma glutamine level **in vivo,** following administration of the enzyme glutaminase, has been shown to result in immunosuppression (Brambilla et al, 1970).

The important point to emerge from this discussion is that glutamine is used at a high rate by cells of the immune system even when they are quiescent. The immune response to invasion by a micro-organism must be rapid: hence, the rate of glutamine utilisation must always be high and the plasma glutamine level must always be maintained to provide optimal conditions for response to an immune challenge. Therefore a decrease in the plasma concentration of glutamine could be an explanation for the immunosuppression experienced in the overtraining syndrome.

Table 2.   Rates of utilisation of glucose and glutamine by lymphocytes and macrophages and other tissues in mouse, rat and man

Animal	Tissue	Rates of utilisation (nmoles/h/mg) protein)	
		Glucose	Glutamine
mouse	macrophage	355	186
rat	mesenteric lymphocyte	42	223
	maximally-working heart	1000	-
man	peripheral lymphocyte	65	190
	brain	200	-

Effects of exercise on the plasma concentration of glutamine

In human subjects the response of plasma glutamine to exercise varies according to the duration and intensity. Short-term exercise (sprinting) increases the plasma level of glutamine, whereas endurance exercise (marathon race) decreases the level (Decombaz et al, 1979, Babij et al, 1983, Parry-Billings et al, 1990b, see Table 3). To some extent, similar results were observed in rats: plasma glutamine levels decreased after exercise to exhaustion in trained rats, but was unchanged following exercise in sedentary rats, who ran for a markedly shorter time than the trained rats (Parry-Billings et al, 1988).

Table 3. Effects of different exercise regimens on plasma glutamine concentrations in man. The significance of the differences between pre- and post-exercise means is indicated by **(p<0.001) and *(p<0.05)

Condition	Plasma glutamine concentration (uM)			
	marathon	30km run race	70%VO$_2$max	sprints cycle(10x6s)
Pre-exercise	592	641	558	556
Post-exercise	495**	694	581	616*

A study of athletes with the overtraining syndrome

The concentrations of glutamine, glutamate, alanine and branched chain amino acids (BCAA) have been measured in a large sample of trained and overtrained athletes. The concentrations of alanine and BCAA were similar in the plasma of trained and overtrained athletes, whereas the concentration of glutamate was increased in overtrained athletes. However, of importance for the present discussion, the plasma concentration of glutamine was **lower** in overtrained compared to that in trained athletes (Parry-Billings et al, unpublished data, Table 4). Since samples were taken from **resting** subjects sometime after performance had been impaired, these results suggest that overtraining may have a long-term effect, specifically on plasma glutamine levels. Furthermore, although this is a small change, it is possible that in overtrained athletes **following** prolonged exercise the decrease in plasma glutamine levels may be considerably greater.

It is hypothesized that such a decrease in plasma glutamine concentration in overtraining or following prolonged exercise may contribute to the impairment of the immune function observed in these conditions in vivo. This hypothesis is supported by the observation that the overtraining syndrome is rarely seen in sprinters or power athletes, but affects endurance athletes, suggesting that repeated **prolonged** exercise is a predisposing factor. Thus, the present study provides evidence that glutamine may play a key role in the pathophysiology of this condition. The important question arises as to the source of glutamine in the bloodstream.

Skeletal muscle as part of the immune system

A number of tissues can synthesize and release glutamine into the bloodstream,

Table 4.   The effect of overtraining syndrome on plasma amino acid concentrations in man. The significance of the differences between control and overtrained means are indicated by *(p<0.02) and **(p<0.01)

| | Plasma amino acid concentration(uM) | | | |
	Glutamine	Glutamate	Alanine	BCAA
Control	550	125	392	398
	n=36	n=35	n=37	n=37
Overtrained	503*	161**	379	408
	n=40	n=35	n=40	n=40

including skeletal muscle, liver and lung. Since the cells of the intestine have a large capacity to utilize glutamine, most of the glutamine that enters the body via the diet is utilized by the intestine. Muscle may be quantitatively the most important tissue. Thus, glutamine production and release by muscle becomes of considerable physiological and immunological importance. Furthermore, analysis of the process of glutamine release from muscle and glutamine metabolism by the immune system by metabolic-control-logic indicates that glutamine release from muscle is the flux generating step in the pathway of glutamine utilisation by cells of the immune system (Newsholme & Parry-Billings, 1990). Thus, the release process is considered to be non-equilibrium and to approach saturation with its substrate. The pathway of glutamine utilisation by cells of the immune system is not saturated with this substrate, so that changes in the rate of glutamine release by muscle, via changes in the concentration of glutamine in plasma, will change the rate of glutamine utilisation by immune cells. This emphasizes the important nutritional link between the two tissues. And, it is also of importance that any insult to muscle may lead to an impairment of the rate of glutamine release by muscle. Could this be the explanation for the decrease in plasma glutamine concentration following prolonged exercise or in overtraining ?

The effect of exercise and overtraining on the rate of glutamine release from muscle

The rate of glutamine release is decreased from incubated soleus and epitrochlearis muscles of the rat following prolonged exercise and is decreased from the perfused rat hindlimb following sciatic nerve stimulation (Goodmann & Lowenstein, 1977; Nie et al, 1987; Parry-Billings et al, 1988). These findings support the view that the decrease in the plasma glutamine level after prolonged exercise is caused, at least in part, by a decreased rate of release from muscle. However, measurements of arteriovenous differences across skeletal muscle of rats and man after exercise are essential to provide further support. Furthermore, these measurements have never been performed in overtrained athletes and represent an area for future research.

In conclusion, the decrease in the plasma glutamine concentration in overtrained athletes and following prolonged exercise may cause, at least in part, the observed immunosuppression. We can not, of course, rule out the possibility that changes in other metabolites, hormones or cytokines may also play a role in this immunosuppression. Indeed it is likely that the cause of this immunosuppression is multifactorial. For example, the plasma concentration of cortisol is elevated in overtrained athletes (Barron et al, 1985) and glucocorticoids are generally considered to be immunosuppressive. However, this effect of glucocorticoids on the immune system may only be evident at supraphysiological concentrations and a small increase in circulating cortisol levels may in fact stimulate the immune system (Jefferies, 1991).

The role of changes in amino acids in other symptoms of overtraining

Athletes suffering from the overtraining syndrome may experience, not only a state of immunosupppression, but a number of psychological/central changes including central fatigue, depression, loss of appetite and insomnia, they may also experience cardiovascular changes and females may present with amenorrhoea (Table 1). It is proposed that excessive exercise may affect the metabolism of other key amino acids and which may in turn explain some of these symptoms.

One important role of some amino acids is that they act as precursors for certain neurotransmitters in the brain. One of these amino acids is tryptophan which is converted in the brain to the neurotransmitter known as 5-hydroxytryptamine (5-HT). There are two important additional facts, tryptophan competes for entry into the brain with the BCAA and BCAA are taken up primarily by muscle where they may be oxidized.

A decrease in the level of BCAA in the blood, due to an increase in the rate of utilisation by muscle, will increase the ratio of tryptophan:BCAA in the bloodstream and favour the entry of tryptophan into the brain. This will increase the formation of 5HT and hence increase the level of this neurotransmitter in the brain. A further important point is that the blood level of free fatty acids may play an additional role: an increase in the free fatty acid level above approximately 1mM increases the concentration of free tryptophan - and it is the free concentration, rather than the total concentration, that influences the rate of entry of tryptophan into the brain. Hence, an increase in the plasma free fatty acid level plus a decrease in that of BCAA could markedly influence the plasma concentration ratio of free tryptophan:BCAA. This has been shown to be the case in endurance activity in man (Blomstrand et al, 1988). Furthermore, endurance exercise in rats produced similar changes in the free tryptophan:BCAA concentration ratio in the plasma. However, more complete experiments are possible with animals and it has been shown that when the plasma concentration ratio increases, the concentration of 5-HT in the hypothalamus and the brain stem increases (Blomstrand et al, 1989). Such changes, especially if chronic, in the level of 5-HT in both the brain and the peripheral nerves could cause a number of symptoms of overtraining.

5-HT and the overtraining syndrome

Neurones containing 5-HT are widely distributed in the brain. However, the physiological functions of 5-HT in the brain can be grouped into at least three areas: wakefulness and mood; motor neurone excitability; autonomic and endocrine function.

Wakefulness: Lesions in the raphe nuclei or the administratioon of p-chlorophenylalanine (an inhibitor of 5-HT synthesis), abolish sleep. Could this neurotransmitter, therefore, also be involved in the central fatigue and disturbed sleep pattern experienced in overtraining?

Motor neurone excitability: Descending 5-HT neurones increase motor neurone excitability and in doing so increase monosynaptic reflexes and decrease polysynaptic reflexes. Inhibition of polysynaptic reflexes may include those involved in exercise, such as running, and may contribute to the decreased maximal work capacity in the overtrained state.

Autonomic and endocrine: 5-HT neurones project into the hypothalamus, which is considered to be the major centre for autonomic, endocrine and neuronal integration. 5-HT inhibits the release of factors from the hypothalamus that act to control the rate of release of pituitary hormones. A low rate of gonadotrophin-releasing hormone (GnRH) secretion by the hypothalamus would be expected to decrease the rate of release of luteinizing hormone and follicle-stimulating hormone from the pituitary and hence lower the plasma level of these hormones. A decrease in the luteinizing hormone pulse frequency and in the amplitude of luteinizing hormone secretion has been reported in overtrained men. This would be expected to lower the rate of testosterone synthesis and release, with a subsequent decline in the plasma levels of testosterone. In the female, such a decrease would be expected to interfere in the complex endocrine system that controls the menstrual cycle and could thus lead to irregular menses or amenorrhoea.

Peripheral 5-HT and the overtraining syndrome

Similar considerations regarding the entry of tryptophan and its conversion to 5-HT apply to peripheral nerves as to central nerves. Hence peripheral 5-HT levels could be altered in the overtrained state. An increase in 5-HT is known to stimulate sympathetic afferent nerves in the heart which cause an increase in heart rate and an increase in resting heart rate is a well established sign of overtraining. In contrast, it causes an inhibition of the rate of noradrenaline release from sympathetic nerve endings on blood vessels; this would be expected to have a general vasodilatory effect and could explain changes in blood pressure in the overtrained athlete.

The question therefore arises as to whether the plasma concentration ratio of free tryptophan:BCAA is altered in overtrained athletes. A preliminary cross-sectional study of trained and overtrained athletes at rest showed that the plasma concentrations of total tryptophan, free tryptophan and BCAA were unaffected by overtraining (VJ Matthews, unpublished data). However, a longitudinal study which examined the effect of an intensive period of training in elite female rowers (some of whom developed symptoms of overtraining) showed that following a period of very intense training the plasma concentration of free tryptophan and the ratio of free tryptophan:BCAA were significantly decreased (Table 5, VJ Matthews, unpublished data)

Table 5. The effect of training load on the plasma concentrations of branched chain amino acids (BCAA), total tryptophan and free tryptophan in a squad of elite female rowers. Periods 1-4 represent consecutive samples taken during the same season, as training loads were progressively increased. The significance of the differences between period 1 and other periods are indicated by * ($p < 0.02$) and ** ($p < 0.001$).

	total tryptophan	Plasma amino Acid concentration (uM) free tryptophan	BCAA	free tryptophan BCAA ratio
Period 1	47	8.0	344	2.15
Period 2	56*	5.8	384	1.46
Period 3	50	3.6	398	0.91**
Period 4	52	3.6*	397	0.92**

Thus, some preliminary evidence supports the hypothesis that tryptophan and 5-HT may play a role in the aetiology of the overtraining syndrome. However, future work is required to examine the possibility that overtraining alters the function of the 5-HT pathway or the inherent **sensitivity** to this neurotransmitter. Indeed, the overtraining syndrome is a clinical condition which requires future detailed and systematic studies of its biochemistry, physiology and immunology . This may allow nutritional or pharmacological treatment strategies to be developed.

Acknowledgement

We acknowledge the financial support of the Medical Research Council and are indebited to Professor C Williams and Dr S Brooks, Department of PE and Sports Science, Loughborough University, for their help in the experiments presented in Table 3.

References

Barron JL, Noakes TD, Levy W, Smith C and Millar RP. (1985) Hypothalamic dysfunction in overtrained athletes. J Clin Endocrinol Metab, **60**, 803-806.

Babij P, Matthews SM and Rennie MJ. (1983) Changes in blood ammonia, lactate and amino acids in relation to workload during bicycle ergometer exercise in man. Eur J Appl Physiol, **50**, 405-411.

Blomstrand E, Cesling F and Newsholme EA. (1988) Changes in the concentration of aromatic and branched chain amino acids during sustained exercise in man. Acta Physiol Scand, **133**, 115-121.

Blomstrand E, Perret D, Parry-Billings M and Newsholme EA. (1989) Effect of sustained exercise on plasma amino acid concentrations and on 5-HT metabolism in six different brain regions in the rat. Acta Physiol Scand, **136**, 473-481.

Brambilla G, Pardodi S, Cavanna M, Caraceni CE and Baldini L.(1970) The immunodepressive activity of E coli L-asparaginase in some transplant systems. Cancer Res, **30**, 2665-2670.

Decombaz J, Reinhardt P, Anantharaman K, von Glutz G and Poortmans JR. (1979) Biochemical changes in a 100km run: free amino acids, urea and creatinine. Eur J Appl Physiol, **41**, 61-72.

The immune system

Fry RD, Morton AR and Keast D. (1991) Overtraining in athletes. Sport Med, 12, 32-65.

Goodmann MN and Lowenstein JM. (1977) The purine nucleotide cycle: studies of ammonia production by skeletal muscle in situ and in perfused preparations. J Biol Chem, 252, 5054-5060.

Jefferies WM. (1991) Cortisol and immunity. Med Hypoth, 34, 198-208.

Keast D, Cameron K and Morton AR. (1988) Exercise and the immune response. Sports Med, 5, 248-267.

Lewicki R, Tchorzewski H, Majewska E, Nowak Z and Baj Z. (1988) Effect of maximal physical exercise on T-lymphocyte sub-populations and on interleukin- 1 and -2 production in vitro. Int J Sport Med, 9, 114-117.

Newsholme EA, Crabtree B and Ardawi MSM. (1985) Glutamine metabolism in lymphocytes: its biochemical, physiological and clinical importance. Q J Exp Physiol, 70, 473-489.

Newsholme EA and Parry-Billings M. (1990) Properties of glutamine release from muscle and its importance for the immune system. J Parent Enter Nutr, 14, 63S-67S.

Nie ZT, Wallberg-Henriksson H, Johansson S, Henriksson J. (1989) Effects of adrenaline and prior exercise on the release of alanine, glutamine and glutamate from incubated rat skeletal muscle. Acta Physiologica Scandinavica, 136, 395-401.

Nieman DC and Nehlsen-Cannarella SL. (1991) The effects of acute and chronic exercise on immunoglobins. Sport Med, 11, 183-201.

Noakes TD. (1986) The Lore of Running. Oxford University Press, Cape Town.

Oshida Y, Yamanouchi K, Hayamizu S and Sato Y. (1988) Effect of acute physical exercise on lymphocyte sub-populations in trained and untrained subjects. Int J Sport Med, 9, 137-140.

Parry-Billings M, Blomstrand E, Leighton B, Dimitriadis GD and Newsholme EA. (1988) Does endurance exercise impair glutamine metabolism? Can J Sport Sci, 13, 27P.

Parry-Billings M, Evans J, Calder PC and Newsholme EA. (1990a) Does glutamine contribute to immunosuppressio after major burns? Lancet, 336, 523-525.

Parry-Billings M, Blomstrand E, McAndrew N and Newsholme EA. (1990b) A communicational link between skeletal muscle, brain and cells of the immune system. Int J Sport Med, 11, S122-S128.

Schneider YJ and Lavoix A. (1990) Monoclonal antibody production in semi-continuous serum and protein-free culture. J Immunol Method, 129, 251-268.

van Wersch JWJ, Kaiser V and Janssen GME. (1989) Platelet system changes associated with a training period of 18-20 months: a transverse and longitudinal approach. Int J Sport Med, 10, S181-S185

Chronic fatigue syndrome, what is it?

P.O. Behan and W.M.H. Behan

Abstract. The postviral fatigue syndrome is defined and a brief outline of its history and epidemiology given. The clinical features are discussed. Recent findings, metabolic, electro-physiological, pathological, neuroendocrinological and immunological are reported. The evidence for an aetiological role of enteroviruses, as opposed to other viruses, including retroviruses, is presented. It is suggested that this disorder may be due to a persistent viral infection in which there is no cell necrosis but cellular function is severely disturbed.

Keywords: Postviral Fatigue Syndrome, Chronic Fatigue Syndrome, Myalgia, Persistent Virus, Enteroviruses, Neuroendocrine Function, Fatty Acids.

Introduction

The causes of chronic fatigue are legion so that the case definition of chronic fatigue syndrome, a predominantly American or psychiatric term, is one based largely on a process of exclusion (Holmes, Kaplan, Gantz et al, 1988; Sharpe, Archard, Banatvala et al, 1991). Postviral fatigue syndrome (PFS), however, in which incapacitating fatigue follows a definite viral infection is a specific entity and it is this which we discuss here.

PFS has received enormous attention from both the medical and lay press in which it has been viewed as a modern illness. Sir Richard Manningham, however, described its salient features in the 18th century (Manningham, 1750). He drew attention to the fever which initiated the illness and described "listlessness with great lassitude, weariness all over the body: little flying pains sometimes the patient is a little delirious and forgetful". He also drew attention to the occurrence of the illness following infections. The neurologist George Beard introduced the term "neurasthenia" in a discussion of the illness (Beard, 1869). Beard stated that "the diagnosis is obtained partly by positive symptoms and partly by exclusion". About the same time Da Costa (1871) published a classic study on "Irritable heart: a clinical study of a form of functional cardiac disorder and its consequence". This astute physician noted that his patients often developed their illness after an acute febrile infection, especially one including the gastrointestinal tract. During World War I there were 60,000 cases of Soldier" (Irritable) Heart in the British Army, of which 44,000 received a medical pension (Lewis, 1940). It would be interesting to see the results of modern, physiological studies on the patients observed by the 19th century physicians.

In the first half of this century, the great Paul Wood had formed the opinion that "they should be treated as psychoneurotics" (Wood, 1941). Investigators reported however, that there were significant physiological differences between the patients and the controls, ie a greater amount of lactic acid was produced on exercise and their oxygen consumption was different (Cohen, White and Johnson, 1948). These studies are very similar to later, modern work (Riley, O'Brien, McCluskey et al, 1990; Montague, Marrie, Klassen et al, 1989; Stevenson R, Bakheit AMO and Behan PO, in preparation).

The confusion surrounding the diagnosis of PFS is exemplified by the many names it has been given in different epidemics, including "a disease resembling or simulating poliomyelitis", "atypical poliomyelitis", "abortive poliomyelitis", "encephalitis simulating poliomyelitis", "encephalitis resembling poliomyelitis", "Akureyri disease", "Iceland disease", "Demadien's ache", "epidemic malaise", "persistent myalgia following sore throat", "virus epidemic in recurrent waves", "Royal Free disease", "epidemic vegetative neuritis", "lymphoreticular encephalomyelopathy", "encephalomyelitis", "benign encephalomyelitis", "myalgic encephalomyelitis", "benign myalgic encephalomyelitis", benign subacute encephalomyelitis", "epidemic myalgic encephalomyelitis or encephalomyelopathy", "acute infective encephalomyelitis", epidemic diencephalomyelitis", "epidemic pseudoneurasthenia", "epidemic neuromyesthenia", and "encephalo-neuro-myasthenia (Acheson, 1959; Henderson and Shelekov, 1959; Behan and Behan, 1988).

The first well-described epidemics occurred in Los Angeles in 1934; the many outbreaks occurring since then have been reviewed in great detail by Acheson and others (Acheson, 1959; Henderson and Shelekov, 1959). More recently, Behan and Behan (1988) have drawn attention to the fact that the illness occurs in sporadic cases, as well as in epidemics. It is worth stressing that PFS is indeed an endemic disease with periodic epidemic outbreaks. In both the epidemic and sporadic form, however, there is a central core of clinical symptoms which is virtually identical, irrespective of the time or place in which it is described. It was stated in an editorial in the British Medical Journal in 1957, that "the pattern is so similar that it seems justifiable at the present to consider them as a clinical entity" (BMJ, 1957a).

The symptoms may vary somewhat so that, for instance, in some epidemics the myalgia has attracted most attention, whilst in others it is the abnormal psychiatric state which causes the most concern. Sometimes the illness begins with an acute stiff neck or generalized myalgia, sometimes with symptoms of myocarditis, occasionally as epidemic vertigo (Pedersen, 1959). These latter patients clearly have the same syndrome since "intense asthenia which develops in 5 - 10% of the cases often becomes the predominant symptom in the late course" (Pedersen, 1959). The author continues, "In many of our patients, the asthenia was complicated by depression and anxiety so that it was difficult to differentiate the condition from depressive neurosis; several of our cases were, in fact interpreted as such at some phase of the disease".

In the early epidemics, the investigators were convinced that the disorder was infectious but no pathogenetic agent was ever found. Several physicians therefore raised the possibility of hysteria or a relationghip to neurosis (McEvedy and Beard, 1970). It is clear, however, on analysing the world literature, that some patients have not had any psychiatric illness before the infection, while others never complain of any psychiatric symptoms. In contrast there are cases with a history of neurosis which is accentuated by the illness.

Studies by Pedersen were important in that they drew attention to how often the brain stem is involved in this disorder; he placed the lesion in and around the second vestibular nucleus, suggesting that the illness was similar to vestibular neuronitis (Pedersen, 1959). He states: "In recapitulation it may be said that an infection of the brain stem seems to be the most plausible cause, but as the disease is undoubtedly infectious in nature, it cannot be excluded that the localization may vary from patient to patient both in the central and peripheral vestibular system".

The close temporal relationship of the illness to outbreaks of poliomyelitis and a peculiar form of jerking on voluntary movement was mentioned by several investigators (Behan and Behan, 1988). Others have commented on the night sweats. Few investigators noted any endocrine effects, but in some instances "the jerking of spasmodic involuntary contractions of the limbs and back increased and the tremors became more noticeable" during the menstrual period. Indeed, "the association of exacerbation of both physical and mental symptoms with the menstrual phase was striking, especially in the latter stages of the disease" (Deisher, 1957).

It is plain from descriptions of the epidemics that, when the patients were observed over a long period, their fatigue and mental symptoms did not remit and often became chronic. This feature was stressed in many of the classical descriptions of the disease, including that of the famous outbreak at the Royal Free Hospital in 1955 (BMJ, 1957b).

Importance - modern controversy

PFS is an important disease in many respects. It has severe economic consequences for the general population and the individual and it can have a devastating result on the individual's life style. It may also give us an insight into how a chronic viral infection can affect the body and produce the varied effects on the nervous, neuroendocrine (and possibly gastrointestinal) systems. Its analysis may help us to understand the pathogenesis of some common psychiatric and neurological syndromes. It may be that PFS is the human counterpart of the curious animal syndromes described by Oldstone, in which viruses cause disease purely by interfering with cellular function and not by causing cell death (de la Torre, Borrow and Oldstone, 1991). We already know that simple viral infections such as colds can have an important effect on performance (Cohen, Tyrrell and Smith, 1991). In highly trained athletes, in the industrial workforce, or indeed among any workers, the relevance of such an effect is readily apparent.

Clinical findings

The clinical spectrum of postviral fatigue syndrome has been described in detail in other publications, (Behan and Behan, 1988; Behan and Bakheit, 1991), so that only a brief account is given here. The illness can occur at any age, but is most common in young and middle-aged adults, with perhaps a greater frequency in females. In many epidemics attention has been drawn to the increased susceptibility of hospital personnel, perhaps denoting greater exposure to the infective agent. In the majority of cases the mode of presentation is acute, following, or concurrent with, an acute viral infection such as a sore throat, gastroenteritis, labyrinthitis or myocarditis. Occasionally, the illness begins with a type of chest pain similar to that in Bornholm's disease. Symptoms invariably include headache, nausea, dizziness and generalized myalgia, the latter tending to affect the neck and trapezius muscles.

The characteristic fatigue may be present from the start, so conspicuous that the patients are unable to comb their hair or rise from a lying position or it may first be noticed when they attempt to resume work. By mid-day or even earlier, they are incapacitated. This symptom, which appears to be identical to that in patients with certain forms of multiple sclerosis, is not cured by bed rest, qood food or relaxation although it may be ameliorated. It does, however, fluctuate with relapses and remissions occurring, the former sometimes related to exercise or infection.

The myalgia can at times be very severe, resembling an acute myocardial infarction when it involves the chest muscles. At other times there is a deep, generalized ache, and the muscles are tender to touch. Those involved are usually the muscles of the neck and shoulder, but virtually any muscles, including those of the chest wall and abdomen can be affected. Tightening the muscle or palpating it, causes an exacerbation of pain. Occasionally the myalgia is flitting, affecting part of one muscle on one day and a different muscle some days later.

The mental symptoms are varied but one of the commonest we observe is emotional lability: under stress there is a tendency for the patient to exhibit great irritability, anxiety and often crying. Patients have difficulty in carrying out tasks, although strangely enough, on formal testing, there are no differences in memory tests between patients and controls (Smith A, Behan PO and Bell W, in preparation). They complain of forgetfulness and poor concentration. They never complain of hallucinations, nor do they experience anhedonia, (an inability to experience pleasure) or guilt. Anomic aphasia of the chronic type is particularly common. In the majority of patients sleep is increased. Some children and younger adults tend to sleep in the day and stay awake at night. Often patients exhibit a curious sensitivity to light and noise with " a tendency to startle, have frightening hypnagogic hallucinations, lack of concentration and listlessness" (Slater and Roth, 1970). Hypochondriasis may be present, with the patient taking enormous care to document each feature of his illness.

Patients often describe attacks of severe sweating, occurring during the night or day. In more than two-thirds of patients, early satiety, bloating and diarrhoea, alternating with constipation, suggest gastrointestinal involvement as does the abdominal pain and increased gut mobility which also occur. Some women patients find that they put on weight, sometimes amounting to ten or twelve pounds, between periods: a feature characteristic of the idiopathic fluid retention syndrome.

In summary to make a firm diagnogis of PFS, we require a history of a viral infection followed by severe fatigue, together with at least two of the following symptoms: generalized myalgia, depression, persistent labyrinthine symptoms, symptoms suggestive of irritable bowel syndrome, and or severe night sweats.

Differential diagnoses

The differential diagnoses in postviral fatigue syndrome are many because of the numerous clinical conditions that may mimic this syndrome. In all our patients a search for these other causes is carried out before a firm diagnosis of postviral fatigue syndrome is made. A working case definition drawn up by American physicians indicates the large list of disorders to be excluded (Holmes, Kaplan, Gantz et al, 1988). An example of this is given by the fact that, of the last ten patients referred to one of us (POB) with a possible diagnosis of PFS, in all of whom the illness began insidiously, and was not related to an acute viral infection, we identified one case each of haemachromatosis, ulcerative colitis and occult multiple sclerosis, and two cases of disseminated carcinoma.

Recent findings in the syndrome

Metabolic

Patients have been found to have a reduced aerobic work capacity when compared with healthy control subjectsg (Riley, O'Brien, McCluskey et al,

1990). The patient's heart rate shows a different pattern of response to graded exercise, when compared with controls. "The reduction in peak oxygen consumption indicates that this is due to decreased work capacity". We have confirmed those findings in a detailed study of patients with PFS (Stevenson R, Bakheit AMO and Behan PO, in preparation). These findings clearly rule out hyperventilation, an explanation first put forward by psychiatrists (McEvedy and Beard, 1970). Other invegtigators have shown that these patients have a limited exercise capacity with an inability on their part to achieve the target heart rate (Montague, Marrie, Klassen et al, 1989). Excessive intracellular acidosis on exercise, suggesting increased glycolytic activity, has been found by using nuclear magnetic resonance spectroscopy (Arnold, Radda, Bore et al, 1984).

Electrophysiological

A reduced recruitment pattern of voluntary motor units, particularly during recovery, was described but regarded as non-specific by some workers. Other investigators have used single fibre electromyographic (EMG) techniques: - we found that, of 40 patients with PFS, 75% had abnormal single fibre EMG (Behan, Behan and Bell, 1985; Jamal and Hansen, 1985). This can be regarded as evidence of an abnormality in the peripheral part of the motor unit, with the muscle fibre as the likely site of involvement. Patients have shown no abnormality in fibre density but they all have high jitter values, not associated with impulse or concomitant blocking. The above findings were considered to confirm the organic nature of the disease (Jamal and Hansen, 1989). It is known that patients with myalgia secondary to acute viral infection may have similar findings (Friman, 1977).

Pathology

An analysis of muscle biopsies in a very large series of patients studied by us showed mild to severe atrophy of type 2 fibres (Behan and Behan, 1988). Sometimes a mild to moderate excess of lipid was demonstrated. These are non-specific features. On ultrastructural examination there is evidence of muscle damage with secondary lysosomes and occasional myelin figures (Behan, More and Behan, 1991). In addition, the mitochondria show both reactive (hyperplastic) and degenerative changes with proliferation of cristae and focal or complete vacuolation. These latter again are non-specific features but they do indicate that PFS is associated with mitochondrial damage. The abnormalities we describe are in obvious contrast to control biopsies, where such changes, if ever found, are extremely mild (Friman, 1977). The best example of severe mitochondrial abnormalities following viral infection are those which occur in Reye's syndrome, which follows influenza or varicella virus infections. Mitochondrial changes identical to what we have seen occur in acute viral infections of muscle (Astrom, Friman and Pilstrom, 1976; Patten,

Shalbot, Alperin et al, 1977). Similar, nonspecific, findings have been observed in chronic fatigue syndrome by other workers (Warner, Cookfair, Heffner et al, 1989).

Neuroendocrine

Since 5-hydroxytryptamine (5-HT) pathways have been implicated in the control of a variety of hypothalamic functions, including temperature regulation, sleep, mood, appetite and memory, we decided to study 5-hydroxytryptamine in patients with PFS, comparing the results to age and sex-matched controls. We used the Buspirone Challenge Test to determine the functional activity of hypothalamic 5-HT receptors (Behan and Bakheit, 1991), since it is known that this substance, an anxiolytic with 5-HT1A receptor agonist properties, stimulates prolactin release by acting on hypothalamic 5-HT receptors. We found that there was a greater prolactin response to buspirone in patients with PFS, than in the two control groups. The first control group was of healthy subjects while the second was of those with primary depression. The buspirone test is known to be flattened or blunted with patients with depression. These results add further weight to the idea that PFS is different to primary depression (Bakheit, Behan, Dinan et al, in press).

Immunological findings

A variety of immunological abnormalities have been claimed to occur in patients with PFS and chronic fatigue syndrome, eg an increase in auto-antibodies and abnormalities in various immunoglobulin concentrations (reviewed by Morrison, Behan and Behan, 1991). Low levels of circulating immune complexes and abnormalities of complement metabolism have been recorded (Behan, Behan and Bell, 1985; Borysiewicz, Haworth, Cohen et al, 1986) and the presence or absence of increased levels of circulating peripheral blood cytokines reported (Landay, Jessop, Lennette et al, 1991). T-cell function has been reported to be depresced with abnormalities in the phenotypic expression of circulating T-cells (Buchwald and Kamaroff, 1991). In one group of patients with PFS compared with healthy controls, significantly increased percentageg of CD56+ cells (a natural killer cell subset) were found (Morrison, Behan and Behan, 1991). It was suggested that these changes provided evidence for disturbed immunological mechanisms, consistent with persistent viral infection. An increase in total natural killer cells has also been reported, as has a change in their phenotypic expression and function. These changes have usually been put forward as evidence of infection (Morrison, Behan and Behan, 1991; Landay, Jessop, Lennette et al, 1991).

Virological studies

The early epidemiological studies of PFS, its incubation period, the myalgia and fever, the upper respiratory or gastrointestinal symptoms, all suggested an infective aetiology. The failure to identify an infectious agent and the similarity to other viral infections suggested, as a vector, a virus with an incubation period of about six to seven days. Exhaustive virological testing, however, did not reveal an aetiological agent in any of the epidemics although viruses have been found in rare cases. For example, enteroviruses have been isolated from the faeces or throat of some patients, echovirus 9 from the stool of four others, and coxsackie B2 and echovirus type 3 from two further cases (Behan and Behan, 1988).

It is curious that the illness appears to follow a wide variety of viral infections such as rubella, influenza, hepatitis and infectious mononucleosis. The association with Epstein-Barr virus has been reported so frequently that in America this virus was considered the prime suspect (Straus, Tosato, Armstrong et al, 1985). Serological and immunological studies, however, have not supported an aetiological role for this agent (Straus, Tosato, Armstrong et al, 1985).

The role of enteroviruses and particularly coxsackie viruses has assumed much greater importance. Serological tests of neutralising and specific IgM antibodies to coxsackie B viruses are unhelpful, since virtually equal results are found in both patients and (age and sex-matched) controls (Miller, Carmichael, Calder et al, 1991). Other studies, however, have suggested that enteroviral antigen is present in circulating immune complexes (Al Khadiry, Gold, Behan et al, 1983). Using dot-blot hybridization techniques, genomic enteroviral RNA has been identified in skeletal muscle biopsies from cases of PFS (Bowles, Archard, Behan et al, 1987).

The best evidence to date for the role of coxsackie virus in PFS is provided by the finding of enteroviral RNA sequences in muscle biopsies of well-studied cases, using the polymerase chain reaction (Gow, Behan, Clements et al, 1991).

Claims by De Freitas that there is a novel retrovirus in this syndrome (De Freitas, Hilliard, Cheney et al, 1991) have been ruled out by comprehensive studies, demonstrating beyond doubt that the retroviral sequence found is of an endogenous type, present equally in patients and controls (Gow JG, Rethwilm A, Cavanagh H et al, in preparation). It is still an unanswered question as to whether the illness is due to one virus or a variety. Further work in this area is clearly indicated.

Treatment

It has long been recognized that viral infections lower plasma levels of essential fatty acids (EFAs) and inhibit 6-desaturation of dietary EFAs (Williams, Doody and Horrocks, 1988). EFAs themselves have definite antiviral effects. For these reasons, we carried out a double-blind, placebo controlled study to test the efficacy of EFAs in patients with PFS. We showed conclusively that a significant number of patients reported benefit although not cure (Behan, Behan and Horrobin, 1990). EFAs therefore provided a rational, safe and sometimes effective treatment for patients. Fatty acids are known to reduce serum levels of cytokines, which might be one reason for the improvement in symptoms.

In carrying out studies of 5-HT metabolism and the effect of 5-HT1 agonists on hypothalamic function, we noted that patients taking 5-HT1 agonists rapidly had their symptoms exacerbated. This led us to suggest that there might be a reduced level of intrasynaptic 5-HT. Preliminary studies with a 5-HT1 re-uptake inhibitor (Sertraline), have demonstrated encouraging results.

Conclusion

The cumulative data point to an organic aetiology for the postviral fatigue syndrome and modern biological techniques indicate that this may be a persistent virus. How such a persistent virus could cause symptoms is not known but an analogy may be made with certain animal diseases where the chronic infection produces severe disturbance of cellular function in the absence of any cytopathic effect (de la Torre, Borrow, and Oldstone, 1991).

References

Acheson ED. (1959) The clinical syndrome variously called benign myalgic encephalomyelitis, Iceland disease and epidemic neuromyasthenia. Am J Med, 26, 569-595.

Al Khadiry W, Gold RG, Behan PO and Mowbray JF. (1983) Analysis of antigens in the circulating immune complexes of patients with Coxsackie infections, in Immunology of Nervous System Infections. Progress in Brain Research, (eds PO Behan, V ter Meulen and FC Rose), Elsevier, Amsterdam, Vol 59, pp. 61.

Arnold DL, Radda GK, Bore PJ, Styles P and Taylor DJ. (1984) Excessive intracellular acidosis of skeletal muscle on exercise in a patient with postviral exhaustion/fatigue syndrome. Lancet, 1, 1367.

Astrom E, Friman G and Pilstrom L. (1976) Effects of viral and mycoplasma infections on ultrastructure and enzyme activities in human skeletal muscle. Acta Path Microbiol Scand, 84, 113-122.

Bakheit AMO, Behan PO, Dinan TG, Gray C and Kane, V. (1991) Possible upregulation of hypothalamic 5-HT receptors in patients with the postviral fatigue syndrome. Brit Med J (in press).

Beard G. (1869) Neurasthenia, or nervous exhaustion. Boston Medical and Surgical Journal, 3(new series), 217-220.

Behan PO and Bakheit AMO. (1991) Clinical spectrum of postviral fatigue syndrome, in Postviral Fatigue Syndrome, British Medical Bulletin, Churchill Livingstone, London, pp. 793-808.

Behan PO, Behan WMH and Bell EJ. (1985) The postviral fatigue syndrome - an analysis of the findings in 50 cases. J Infect, 10, 211-222.

Behan PO and Behan WMH. (1988) Postviral fatigue syndrome. Crit Rev Neurobiol, 4, 157-178.

Behan PO, Behan WMH and Horrobin D. (1990) Essential fatty acids in the treatment of the postviral fatigue syndrome. Acta Neurol Scand, 82, 209-216.

Behan PO, Goldberg DR and Mowbray JF. (eds) (1991) Postviral Fatigue Syndrome British Medical Bulletin, Churchill Livingstone, London, 47, No. 4.

Behan WMH, More IAR and Behan PO. (1991) Mitochondrial abnormalities in the postviral fatigue syndrome. Acta Neuropathol, (in press).

Borysiewicz LK, Haworth SJ, Cohen J, Mundin J, Rickinson A and Sigsons JCP. (1986) Epstein-Barr virus-specific immune defects in patients with persistent symptoms following infectious mononucleosis. Quart J Med, 58, 111-121.

Bowles NE, Archard LC, Behan WMH, Bell EJ and Behan PO. (1987) Detection of Coxsackie B virus-specific RNA in skeletal muscle biopsies of patients with the postviral fatigue syndrome. Ann Neurol, 22, 126.

British Medical Journal. (1957a) Epidemic myalgic encephalomyelitis. Brit Med J, II, 927-928.

British Medical Journal. (1957b) An outbreak of encephalomyelitis in the Royal Free Hospital Group, London, in 1955. Brit Med J, II, 895-904.

Buchwald D and Kamaroff AL. (1991) Review of labortory findings for patients with chronic fatigue syndrome. Rev Infect Dis, 13(Suppl 1), S12-18.

Cohen ME, White PD and Johnson RE. (1948) Neurocircualatory asthenia, anxiety neurosis or the effort syndrome. Arch Intern Med, 81, 260-281.

Cohen S, Tyrrell DAJ and Smith AP. (1991) Psychological stress and susceptibility to the common cold. New Engl J Med, 325, 606-612.

Da Costa JM. (1871) On irritable heart: a clinical study of a form of functional cardiac disorder and its consequence. Am J Med Sci, 121, 17-52.

De Freitas E, Hilliard B, Cheney PR, Bell DS, Kiggundu E, Sankey D, Wroblewska Z, Palladino M, Woodward JP and Koprowski H. (1991) Retroviral sequences related to human T-lymphotrophic virus type II in patients with chronic fatigue immune dysfunction syndrome. Proc Natl Acad Sci, USA, 88, 2922-2926.

Deisher JB. (1957) Benign myalgic encephalomyelitis (Iceland disease) in Alaska. Northwest Medicine, 56, 1451-1456.

de la Torre JC, Borrow P and Oldstone MBA. (1991) Cytopathology in the absence of cytolysis, in Postviral Fatigue Syndrome, British Medical Bulletin, Churchill Livingstone, London, pp. 838-851.

Friman G. (1977) Effect of acute infectious disease on isometric muscle strength. Scand J Clin Invest, 37, 303.

Gow JW, Behan WMH, Clements GB, Woodall C and Behan PO. (1991) Enteroviral RNA sequences detected by polymerase chain reaction in muscle of patients with postviral fatigue syndrome. Brit Med J, 302, 692-696.

Gow JW, Rethwilm A, Cavanagh H, Behan WM, Simpson K, Morrison L, ter Meulen V and Behan PO. Analysis of retroviral sequences in the chronic fatigue syndrome (in preparation).

Henderson DA and Shelokov A. (1959) Epidemic neuromyasthenia: clinical syndrome? N Engl J Med, 260, 757-764.

Holmes GP, Kaplan JE, Gantz NM, Komaroff AL, Schonberger LB, Straus SE, Jones JF, Dubois RE, Cunningham-Rundles C, Pahwa S, Tosato G, Zegans L, Purtilo DT, Brown N, Schooley RT and Brus I. (1988) Chronic fatigue syndrome: a working case definition. Ann Intern Med, 108, 387-389.

Jamal GA and Hansen S. (1985) Electrophysiological studies in the post-viral fatigue syndrome. JNNP, 48, 691-694.

Jamal GA and Hansen S. (1989) Post-viral fatigue syndrome: evidence for underlying organic disturbance in the muscle fibre. European Neurology, 29, 273-276.

Landay AL, Jessop C, Lennette ET and Levy JA. (1991) Chronic fatigue syndrome: clinical condition associated with immune activation. Lancet, 338, 707-712.

Lewis T. (1940) Soldiers Heart and the Effort Syndrome. 2nd ed. Shaw Publishing Co, London.

McEvedy CP and Beard AW. (1970) Concept of benign myalgic encephalomyelitis. Brit Med J, 1, 7-11.

Manningham R. (1750) The symptoms, nature, causes and cure of the febricula or little fever: commonly called the nervous or hysteric fever, the fever on the spirits; vapours, hypo, or spleen. 2nd ed. J Robinson, London, pp. 52-53.

Miller NA, Carmichael HA, Calder BD, Behan PO, Bell EJ, McCartney RA and Hall FC. (1991) Antibody to coxsackie B virus in diagnosing postviral fatigue syndrome. Brit Med J, 302, 140-143.

Montague TJ, Marrie TJ, Klassen GA, Berwick DJ & Horacek BM et al. (1989) Cardiac function at rest and with exercise in the chronic fatigue syndrome. Chest, 95, 779-784.

Morrison LJA, Behan WMH and Behan PO. (1991) Changes in natural killer cell phenotype in patients with post-viral fatigue syndrome. Clin Exp Immunol, 83, 441-446.

Patten BM, Shalbot JM, Alperin J and Dodson RF. (1977) Hepatitis-associated lipid storage myopathy. Annals of Int Med, 87, 417-421.

Pedersen E. (1959) Clinical picture, epidemiology and relation to encephalitis. Brain, 82, 566-580.

Riley MS, O'Brien CJ, McCluskey DR, Bell NP & Nichols DP. (1990) Aerobic work capacity in patients with chronic fatigue syndrome. Brit Med J, 301, 953-956.

Sharpe MC, Archard LC, Banatvala JE, Borysiewicz LK, Clare AW, David A, Edwards RHT, Hawton KEH, Lambert HP, Lane RJM, McDonald EM, Mowbray JF, Pearson DJ, Peto TEA, Preedy VR, Smith AP, Smith DG, Taylor DJ, Tyrrell DAJ, Wessely S, White PD, Behan PO, Rose FC, Peters TJ, Wallace PG, Warrell DA, and Wright DJM. (1991) Chronic fatigue syndrome; Guidelines for research. J Roy Soc Med, 84, 118-121.

Slater E and Roth M. (eds) (1970) Clinical Psychiatry. Balliere, Tindall & Cassell, London p.350.

Smith AP, Behan PO and Bell WP. Behaviour problems associated with the chronic fatigue syndrome (in preparation).

Stevenson R, Bakheit AMO and Behan PO. A physiological study of patients with postviral fatigue syndrome (in preparation).

Straus SE, Tosato G, Armstrong G, Lawley T, Preble OT, Henle W, Davey R, Pearson G, Epstein J, Brus I and Blaese RM. (1985) Persisting illness and fatigue in adults with evidence of Epstein-Barr virus infection. Ann Intern Med, 102, 7-16.

Warner CL, Cookfair D, Heffner R, Bell D, Ley D and Jacobs L. (1989) Neurologic abnormalities in the chronic fatigue syndrome (abstract). Neurology, 39, (Suppl 1), 420.

Williams LL, Doody DM and Horrocks, LA. (1988) Serum fatty acid proportions are altered during the year following acute Epstein-Barr virus infection. Lipids, 23, 981-988.

Wood P. (1941) Da Costa's syndrome (or effort syndrome). The mechanism of the somatic manifestations. Brit Med J, 1, 805-811.

Chronic fatigue syndrome and its effect on exercise capacity

D.R. McCluskey

Abstract. Chronic Fatigue Syndrome (CFS) is a disorder which is characterised by fatigue both during and after exercise. Patients complain that minimal exertion often results in exhaustion and a variety of other subjective symptoms. In an effort to determine which of the many suggested pathophysiological mechanism operate in this condition our department has performed objective measurement of aerobic work capacity using a symptom limited exercise treadmill test. Patients with CFS show a significantly reduced exercise capacity compared to normal subjects or a patient control population. The CFS patients also display an alteration in their subjective perception of the severity of the exercise which they undertake. These findings would indicate that while deconditioning plays a role in this disorder, patients with CFS also have a central disorder of sensory perception, the exact nature of which remains uncertain but may occur as a result of a primary sleep disorder.

Keywords: Chronic fatigue syndrome, exercise, aerobic work capacity, perceived exertion, infection

Introduction

Although Chronic Fatigue Syndrome (CFS) has become very topical within the past few years, with much appearing in both the popular press and medical journals, it is by no means a new condition. The first well documented epidemic of this disorder occurred in Iceland in the 1930s at which time it became known as Icelandic Disease. In the mid-1950s a large number cf health care workers employed in The Royal Free Hospital developed an acute 'flu-like illness which was followed by a prolonged period of ill-health; the condition was then referred to as Royal Free Disease. Since then it has been called a variety of names and most recently the name Myalgic Encephalomyelitis (ME) (Anon, 1978) has become associated in the popular press with this condition. This term is a misnomer however, since examination of muscle biopsies from patients or brain tissue obtained from individuals who have committed suicide while suffering from the disorder fail to show any evidence of inflammation. Because the vast majority of patients develop their chronic symptoms after an acute pyrexial illness it has been called Post-Viral Fatigue Syndrome, (Behan et al, 1985) however, in some patients there ls no history of preceding pyrexial illness and it may be that other stimuli can precipitate this condition. Since all patients, whatever the precipitating event or the assumed pathophysiological mechanism, suffer from chronic fatigue, the name Chronic Fatigue Syndrome (CFS) should be used.

Fibromyalgia

The condition fibromyalgia shares many of the clinical manifestations of CFS. Patients with this painful musculoskeletal disorder of unknown aetiology also usually fail to show any abnormality on laboratory investigation. It has been suggested that the two conditions may be closely related and common pathophysiological mechanisms may be involved in both disorders.

Over the past four years we have seen more than 800 patients with symptoms consistent with CFS and this chapter outlines our understanding of the condition at present and describes some objective research which has been performed in our department on patients who fulfil the diagnostic criteria for CFS.

Table 1. Diagnostic criteria for the CFS

Major criteria	Minor Criteria Symptom	Physical
1 New onset of fatigue, that does not resolve with bedrest, and is severe enough to impair daily activity to below 50% of premorbid levels. 2 Careful exclusion of physical conditions that may cause similar symptoms (eg hypothyroidism)	1 Feverishness/chills. 2 Sore throat. 3 Painful cervical or axillary lymph nodes. 4 Unexplained muscle weakness. 5 Muscle discomfort. 6 Prolonged post-exercise fatigue. 7 New generalised headaches. 8 Arthralgia, without swelling or redness. 9 Neuropsychologic complaints, eg memory loss, poor concentration. 10 Sleep disturbance. 11 Onset of condition over a few hours to a few days.	1 Low grade fever (oral temperature 37.6-38.6 C). 2 Non-exudative pharyngitis. 3 Palpable or tender anterior or posterior cervical or axillary lymph-adenopathy < 2cm.

Definition

Chronic Fatigue Syndrome is a disorder which lasts for more than six months and is characterised by profound fatigue and disorders of higher cerebral function. The Centers for Disease Control (Holmes et al, 1988) have suggested the fulfilment of major and minor criteria in a fashion analogous to the diagnosis of rheumatic fever. The criteria are summarized in Table 1. Symptoms must be present either continuously or intermittently over a period of at least six months from the onset of fatigue and physical criteria must be noted by a physician on at least two separate occasions one month or more apart. In order to sustain a diagnosis, both major criteria must be present in addition to either at least 6 symptom and 2 physical criteria or 8 or more symptom criteria.

Aetiology

Although the exact aetiology is unknown there are clear aetiological factors which appear constant throughout various parts of the world. This disease affects mainly young and middle-aged adults. The most common age of onset is between 20 and 40 years. It can occur in children although this is not common and onset is also unusual in older age groups. The female to male ratio is 3:1, this may possibly be explained by the fact that the condition occurs more commonly in certain occupational groups, particularly school teachers and nurses.

The role of virus infection in CFS

The vast majority of patients who develop CFS describe an acute pyrexial illness. This is usually an upper respiratory infection, a glandular fever type illness, or an episode of gastro-enteritis. Patients describe influenza-like symptoms with fever, general malaise and myalgia and having developed this acute 'flu-like illness the patients feel they never make a full recovery. A small proportion (less than 10%) however, do not describe an acute onset and simply develop symptoms of fatigue and weakness.

Because of the association with acute pyrexial illness, the role of a virus has been suspected. By far the most likely candidate would be one of the enteroviruses and much effort has been directed at trying to identify chronic enterovirus infection in patients suffering from this condition. Enteroviruses, which include coxsackie and herpes, seem the likely putative agents, since these viruses are capable of causing chronic infection in humans; for example, herpes zoster is known to cause chronic latent infection which can persist for many years. Coxsackle viruses which are known to cause Bornholm Disease are capable of causing myositis as a result of chronic infection, the virus becoming incorporated into the muscle cell. Some workers have suggested that the majority of patients with CFS show evidence of chronic enterovirus infection (Yousef et al, 1988). However, there remains considerable controversy with regard to the role of viruses in this condition.

It may be that the symptoms of CFS can be triggered by any one of a number

Table 2.   Possible aetiological factors in the development of the chronic fatigue syndrome

Chronic virus infection	Post-viral syndrome
Immunological reaction	Hyperventilation syndrome
Deconditioning	Primary sleep disorder
Psychiatric illness	Psychosomatic disorder

of initiating events. Indeed, CFS is likely to be a spectrum of disorders which comprises a number of sub-groups differing according to either the initiating event or the pathophysiological mechanism. A number of mechanisms have been suggested (Table 2) and it would seem likely that one or more of these is responsible for the clinical manifestations of the condition in a given patient.

Clinical features

The initial pyrexial illness may be severe and the patient often describes in dramatic detail a severe and often prolonged 'flu-like disorder. Following this, most patients complain that they never seem to fully regain normal health and can then develop a wide variety of symptoms, the most common of which are tiredness, weakness and post-exercise fatigue. Patients describe marked fatigue during and, for a variable period, after exertion. The other cardinal feature is some defect in higher cerebral function, with loss of short-term memory, difficulty with mental concentration, or alteration in mood especially depression. Virtually all patients describe some disorder in sleep with the majority complaining of difficulty in getting to sleep while others experience early morning wakening. Nearly all patients state that even if they can get a reasonable night's sleep they do not feel rested.

Despite the wide variety of symptoms, clinical examination usually fails to show any demonstrable abnormality, ie the clinical features of this condition are mainly subjective. Despite the complaints of muscle weakness, on clinical testing or indeed on objective measurement, muscular weakness is usually not demonstrable (Stokes et al, 1988).

In keeping with these clinical features, laboratory investigation is usually unhelpful. If patients are studied over a prolonged period of time with serial measurements taken, some may show either a transient relative lymphocytosis or elevation in serum immunoglobulins. However, there is no reproducible laboratory test, and even those which are non-specific, such as the erythrocyte sedimentation rate or C-reactive protein level, remain normal.

Exercise testing

Since fatigue, particularly that induced by exercise, is such a prominent symptom, we thought it would be of interest to study the exercise capacity and associated symptoms of these patients objectively. Using treadmill exercise and concurrent measurement of respiratory gas exchange, we examined a group of patients with CFS and compared them with a normal sedentary control group and group of patients with the irritable bowel syndrome (Riley et al, 1990). The latter group was included as this condition, like CFS, is essentially a symptom complex without positive investigations. After prior familiarisation, exercise was performed to an incremental modified Bruce protocol with 3 minute stages until exhaustion. In order to reduce observer bias, the investigator conducting the tests was blinded to the subjects' diagnosis. Heart rate, respiratory gas exchange and end-tidal CO_2 were monitored throughout exercise and for three minutes into the recovery phase. In addition venous lactate, glucose and free fatty acids were sampled intermittently during the same period. Subjects were asked to indicate their subjective impression of the severity of the exercise at the end of the test by means of a perceived exertion score (Borg, 1982). Perhaps not surprisingly, we found that the CFS patients had a somewhat lower exercise capacity than the other two groups, both in terms of their treadmill time (Fig. 1) and their peak oxygen consumption (Fig. 2). The latter measurement indicates that the maximal aerobic capacity of the body was impaired and that the lower treadmill time could not simply be explained on the basis of inefficiency of gait. In contrast, the CFS group indicated significantly greater subjective scores of **perceived** exertion, suggesting that they found the exercise very severe (Fig. 3). The impairment of exercise capacity did not appear to be due to poor motivation as peak heart rate, peak lactate and peak respiratory exchange ratio (quotient of CO_2 production and O_2 consumption) were similar in the 3 groups. No fall occurred in the circulating levels of glucose or free fatty acids, suggesting that lack of substrates did not play a part, and no differences were seen in the end-tidal CO_2 values, tending to discount hyperventilation. When compared at equal treadmill exercise stages, i.e. at similar submaximal absolute workloads, the CFS group displayed higher heart rates and lactate levels than the other two groups (Fig 4 & 5). This pattern is similar to that found in unfit or deconditioned individuals (Saltin et al, 1968 & Holloszy et al, 1976) and suggests that physical deconditioning may partially account for the excess fatigue so characteristic of this condition. The greater scores of perceived exertion might suggest a disorder in the perception of fatigue whether occurring at a central or peripheral level, and this finding may hold an important clue to the symptoms experienced by these patients.

If deconditioning was the only mechanism operating then one would expect the exercise capacity of patients to remain relatively constant or display a gradual deterioration. One of the characteristic features of this disorder is the fluctuation in exercise capacity and fatigue which can occur over periods of days or weeks.

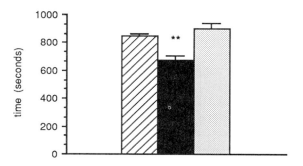

Fig 1   Treadmill time achieved in the controls (hatched bars), chronic fatigue
syndrome patients (filled bars) and the irritable bowel syndrome patients
(dotted bars). Bars represent standard errors . ** p<O.OOO1; * p<O.O5
compared to other groups.

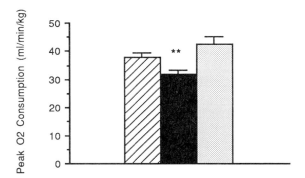

Fig. 2   Peak O$_2$ consumption achieved in the controls, chronic fatigue syndrome
patients and the irritable bowel syndrome patients. Key as Fig. 1.

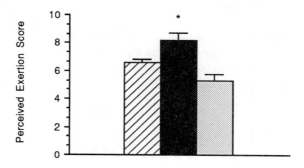

Fig. 3   Perceived exertion score at peak exercise in the controls, chronic fatigue syndrome patients and the irritable bowel syndrome patients. Key as Fig. 1.

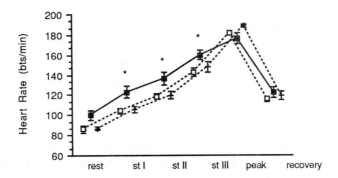

Fig. 4   Heart rates at rest, stages 1-3 of the exercise protocol, peak exercise and after 3 minutes recovery in the controls (open squares), chronic fatigue syndrome patients (filled squares) and the irritable bowel syndrome patients (crosses) Points are mean ± SEM. * $p < 0.05$

Patients can have profound weakness and lethargy and after a few days their exercise capacity improves dramatically only to relapse at a later date. Clearly some central mechanism such as a disorder of perception of fatigue must also operate. This could occur as a result of a primary sleep pattern disturbance which may alter the sensory threshold for pain afferents coming from muscles and joints. When the sleep pattern is grossly disturbed then more symptoms are experienced and at times when the sleep pattern is relatively normal, then fewer and less severe fatigue is experienced.

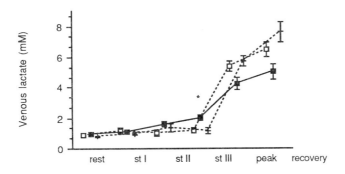

Fig. 5   Venous lactate levels at rest, stages 1-3 of the exercise protocol, peak exercise and after 3 min recovery in the controls, chronic fatigue syndrome patients and irritable bowel syndrome patients. Key as Fig. 4.

Diagnosis and differential diagnosis

The diagnosis of this condition is one of exclusion. It is based on the clinical history and the criteria which have been outlined above. There is no definitive laboratory test which can be performed at present for diagnosis, but, since many of the symptoms are shared by other organic and psychiatric disease, it is important first to rule out a number of other conditions (Table 3).

Table 3. Differential Diagnosis

1	Thyroid disease	5	Immuno-deficiency
2	Malignancy	6	Sarcoidosis
3	Infection	7	Psychosomatic
4	Auto-immunity	8	Psychiatric disorder

Treatment

At present there is no specific therapy. The mainstay of treatment is to re-assure the patient that there is no evidence of any other serious underlying organic disease or psychiatric illness. The patient should be advised to rest during the acute phase of their illness and then attempt to increase their level of physical exertion in a graded way to reverse the deconditioning which occurs as part of the disorder. Until more is known about the precise pathogenesis of the condition it will remain difficult to plan rational therapeutic strategies. The symptoms described by many patients usually follow a cyclic relapsing and remitting pattern and many reports of useful therapies are either anecdotal or based on small numbers of patients. Assessment of response is often purely on subjective parameters and therefore assessing effectiveness of therapy is difficult. The types of treatments currently used for CFS can be classified broadly into:

1. Those directed against a presumed underlying pathophysiological mechanism.
2. Those which provide symptomatic relief.

A variety of treatments used have been aimed at trying to eradicate a presumed chronic virus infection. These include anti-viral drugs, such as, acyclovir (Straus et al, 1988) and amantadine. However, the small number of clinical trials which have been performed fail to show any benefit using these forms of therapy. Although no control trials of interferon have been performed for this condition we have treated a small number of patients with subcutaneous alpha interferon with no evidence of improvement in their symptoms.

Many patients resort to a variety of alternative therapies. Since these are scientifically implausible, usually expensive and may even be potentially harmful, patients should be discouraged from complying with such exploitation. The vogue for such treatments is a reflection of the patients' dissatisfaction with current medical management and of their desperation to find a cure. Table 4 lists some of the many alternative therapies used by CFS patients.

The best approach to treatment therefore is reassurance and explanation of the natural history of the condition. Patients should be told that although they may have severe and chronic symptoms, there is no evidence of any serious or life threatening disorder and that the vast majority of patients (over 85%) will make a full and complete recovery. The specific management plan adopted for any individual patient should be directed to the relief of symptoms which they find most troublesome. Unfortunately the majority of patients will experience symptoms over a prolonged period of time. The mean time to recovery is 2.5 years. Patients usually experience relapses and remissions in their symptoms and the remissions begin to last for longer periods of time and occur more frequently until the patient eventually recovers completely. It has been of some interest to us to try and identify factors which are associated with remissions and it would appear reasonably clear that when a patient's sleep pattern improves and they start to have normal restful sleep they usually enter a remission. Conversely a disordered sleep pattern often heralds a relapse in the condition. It has been our experience that normally prescribed hypnotic drugs are of no real benefit to this group of patients. Since some of the tricyclic group of antidepressants are known to alter patterns of rapid eye movement (REM) sleep and non REM sleep we have used these drugs with limited success in a number of patients.

Table 4. Alternative Therapies

Candida eradication	Colonic irrigation
Herbal remedies	Alexander technique
Homeopathy	Yoga
Acupuncture	Spiritual healing
Aromatherpy	Hypnosis
Bach flower remedies	Transcendental meditation
Royal jelly	Visualisation
Reflexology	Hydrotherapy
Autogenic training	

Summary

Chronic Fatigue Syndrome appears to represent a spectrum of disorders in which a variety of pathophysiological mechanisms may operate. While the initiating event in the majority of patients is a pyrexial illness, possibly due to enterovirus infection, evidence of persisting infection or inflammatory changes in muscle and/or brain remain unconvincing. CFS patients display a definite reduced aerobic work capacity compared to normal control subjects but this may reflect a state of deconditioning resulting from prolonged physical inactivity. They also have an altered perception of their level of exertion and premorbid fitness.

The characteristic fluctuation in symptoms, with periods of relapses and partial remissions, may indicate that some central disorder of sensory perception is operational. It may be that a primary sleep disorder results in a reduced sensory threshold for afferent stimuli from muscle. This could well account for many of the subjective symptoms which patients experience.

We are currently assessing the effects of altered sleep patterns and sleep deprivation on aerobic exercise capacity and sensory pain thresholds in normal subjects.

Clearly much more objective research of this type is necessary to achieve a better understanding of the pathophysiologic mechanisms which operate in this distressing and at present enigmatic disorder.

References

Anonymous. (1978) Epidemic myalgic encephalomyelitis. Br Med J, i, 1436-1437.

Behan PO, Behan WHM, Bell EJ. (1985) The post-viral fatigue syndrome - an analysis of findings in 50 cases. J Infect, 10, 211-222.

Borg GAV. (1982) Psychophysical basis of exertion. Med Sci Sports Exerc, 14, 377-381.

Holloszy JO, Booth FW. (1976) Biochemical adaptations to endurance exercise in muscle. Ann Rev Physiol, 38, 263-291.

Holmes GP, Kaplan JE, Gantz NM, Komaroff AL, Schonberger LB, Straus SE, Jones JF, Dubois RE, Cunningham-Rundles C, Pahwa S, Tosato G, Zegans LS, Purtilo DT, Brown N, Schooley RT. (1988) Chronic fatigue syndrome: a working case definition. Ann Intern Med, 108, 387-389.

Medical Staff of the Royal Free Hospital. (1955) An outbreak of encephalomyelitis in the Royal Free Hospital Group, London. Br Med J, ii, 895-904.

Riley MS, O'Brien CJ, McCluskey DR, Bell NP, Nicholls DP. (1990) Aerobic work capacity in the chronic fatigue syndrome. Br Med J, 301, 953-956.

Saltin B, Blomqvist B, Mitchell JH, Johnston RL, Wildenthal K, Chapman CB. (1968) Response to submaximal and maximal exercise after bedrest and training. Circulation, 38 (suppl 7), 1-78.

Stokes MJ, Cooper RG, Edwards RHT. (1988) Normal muscle strength and fatigability in patients with effort syndromes. Br Med J, 297, 1014-1017.

Straus SE, Dale JK, Tobi M, Lawley T, Preble O, Blaese M, Hallahan C, Henle W. (1988) Acyclovir treatment of the chronic fatigue syndrome. N Eng J Med, 319, 1692-1698.

Yousef GE, Bell EJ, Mann GF, Murugesan V, Smith DG, McCartney RA, Mowbray JF. (1988) Chronic enterovirus infection in patients with post-viral fatigue syndrome. Lancet, i, 146-150.

Discussion: the immune system, the hyperfit athlete and chronic fatigue

R. Budgett

Budgett Your Royal Highness, ladies and gentlemen, I have been asked to lead this discussion on this important subject of the immune system, the hyperfit athlete and chronic fatigue.

Since the British Olympic Medical Centre was opened in 1987 by Her Royal Highness The Princess Royal, I have seen a large number of chronically fatigued athletes and, as was mentioned earlier, they have all been endurance athletes except for one decathlete. That is the nearest we have actually got to a sprinter! We have investigated these individuals with the help of a physiologist working with Dr Craig Sharp and in cooperation with the Department of Biochemistry at Oxford University.

One of the main problems is the definition and diagnosis of the chronically fatigued athletes. We have heard that there is disagreement on the terms, disagreement on the definition and, if you look at the literature, people talk about different things when they talk about chronic fatigue in athletes. I use the large number of subjective symptoms which have been described today so I will not go through them again. It is very important to exclude treatable or serious disease, such as viral myocarditis. I think that the message is at last getting through that athletes should not exercise when they have got a viremia.

We have also got to look at glycogen depletion, which was discussed yesterday, and depression which no doubt some of these athletes suffer from. There is one symptom which the athletes cannot ignore and it is objective, as opposed to all the others which are subjective, and is uniquely important to athletes. When present they have to take notice of it. It is under-performance. Athletes are used to being fatigued, as any of you who have been serious athletes will know. You feel tired most of the time when you are training hard and you probably feel low a lot of the time as well. Your sleep may be disturbed but, when you start to underperform, then you really notice it. It is probably why these athletes present earlier than the other individuals which I may see in general practice for chronic fatigue. The athletes are actually functioning normally in everyday life; they are able to continue with their jobs but their athletic performance declines. They have to perform at such a high level that they notice the deterioration far earlier and then, on direct questioning, all the other symptoms become apparent.

A common picture that we see is a cycle of hard training and competition, leading to under-performance and chronic fatigue. Other stresses and infection may be important and we have talked about these today. These eventually lead to a period of enforced rest. Athletes hate resting but eventually they have to. They literally break down. They do recover to some extent, but then go back into training too soon. They are driven back to training by a determination to win and their own conscientiousness. They feel guilty when they are not training hard and it is ironic that these are the very qualities which lead them to success in the first place. To us, one of the most interesting aspects is this story of immunosuppression and infection. We are all aware of the fascinating changes in the immune system described by Dr Craig Sharp and it is very likely that, in athletes who are training very hard, there are bodily changes which lead to immunosuppression and, in turn, to infection accompanied by the changes in amino acid and hormone levels which Dr Mark Parry-Billings described. These are all relevant in leading to an increased vulnerability to infection and even more importantly, maybe, to an increased vulnerability to chronic fatigue. Both athletes and coaches, however, are most interested in the bottom line. To them, prevention and management, the practicalities, are very important and we are still very limited here. Prevention would be fine but there is a conflict between maximal training, supposedly leading to maximal physical adaptation, and overtraining. In my opinion, and it has also been mentioned by various speakers, the majority of athletes, the very top athletes, do overtrain. They train harder than is actually necessary to reach full physiological adaptation. Even more importantly, they leave inadequate time for muscle recovery and consequently do not even benefit from the training they do do. It was fascinating to hear yesterday how long it takes muscle to regenerate glycogen stores. Top class athletes train twice a day; I am sure that the majority of them do not replace their glycogen stores fully thus making them more vulnerable to the stresses of training, and maybe to the overtraining syndrome or chronic fatigue.

We have heard Dr Coyle talk about the World back-stroke record holder, a swimmer from Texas, who trains far less than her competitors. But her training is intense and specific and of high quality, giving herself time to recover. I tell the athletes who come to the Olympic Centre that it is far better to undertrain than overtrain but this concept is anathema, even heresy, to most of them and their coaches. How about the management of overtraining? Here we are still very limited. Some exciting ideas have come up today but the basis still has to be rest and it is very difficult to persuade a top-class athlete to do this. I try to be more positive and encourage them to use various regeneration strategies. These have been used in Eastern Europe and include anything to make the athlete feel better; everything from counselling and relaxation therapy to sauna, massage and hydrotherapy, with careful attention to diet and general mollycoddling of the athlete. They will eventually get better, in my experience, probably because they are not as severely affected as some of these chronically fatigued non-athletes we have heard about. Because they are aiming at the highest possible standards they have to take notice earlier. Other treatment strategies may also be important.

Branched-chain amino acids are going to be important both in treatment and in prevention and I know there are various studies in progress around the world to see if giving branched-chain amino acids throughout the training season has any effect on the immune system. Maybe we should also be helping these athletes to sleep. On occasion I have used anti-depressants and one wonders if these drugs have an additional role in promoting sleep as well as helping the depression and other symptoms. In a previous study, we have shown that 3-6 weeks of physical rest will lead to a significant improvement in both mood state and performance. The majority of athletes however need to keep their training at a very low level for a lot longer than that and we have seen athletes break down again after about three months so that it is essential that they are careful over how quickly they get back into full training. All the athletes we have seen have eventually recovered.

After this brief outline of my views on the overtraining syndrome, or chronic fatigue in athletes, I would like to open the discussion to the floor and invite further question to any of the speakers.

Prof C R Madeley (Chairman)   Well what do we think? We would not be here if we did not have muscles. I guess that if most of us ran down to Waverley Station from here, we would discover a few muscles we either never knew we had or had forgotten about but we would not necessarily develop chronic fatigue. How important are coaches in tackling prevention and treatment? It seems to me that the individual athletes can drive themselves more or less into the ground but does the coach ever restrain them?

Budgett   We do see athletes from the same squad, I am afraid to say, so one wonders whether the particular programmes, or the attitude within the squad in some cases, does predispose to an overtraining syndrome. But more and more coaches are becoming aware. They are prepared to pull an athlete back when they start to underperform, but other coaches still do not believe there is such a thing as the overtraining syndrome.

HRH The Princess Royal   It is a very good point that it is very difficult to get athletes to rest properly. Not only that, and I think this may apply to everyone, does the quality of rest, the type of break, matter in helping to break the cycle? Sending someone home and saying "do not train" is not in itself enough.

Budgett   I quite agree. What I get these overtrained athletes to do is to rest completely for a week. I do not think you can really ask them to rest any more than that because they begin to become more ill from not training. Psychologically they are used to training and you have to try to be more positive about it. For instance, if you are training a runner, he knows the area over which he normally trains and there is always a temptation for him to look at his watch to see how fast he is going, to see if he can go a bit better and push himself a little bit harder. During the period when they are supposed to be exercising at a very low level (I do not call it training because otherwise they are looking for a training response even at a very low level), I will get them to do different types of exercise. I may send them for a gentle cycle ride or a gentle swim, something completely different to keep them active, keep them ticking over, but they are not looking for a training response and are not pushing themselves hard.

HRH The Princess Royal   So the old adage "a change is as good as a rest" would apply.

Budgett   I think it would help.

Madeley   Is there an argument for some other forms of positive distraction? Not just doing some other form of exercise but going to look at an Art Gallery - something like that? There are all sorts of possibilities in the way of distractions - could one take this further?

Budgett   I think the athletes who have interests outside sport are at an advantage. The pressure of Olympic competition is so specific and so professional that some athletes give up all their outside interests to concentrate on their sport but for those who have outside interests this helps in their recovery.

Prof P O Behan (Glasgow)   There are two kinds of stress. There is stress that is pleasurable and there is stress that is unpleasurable and, I believe, a study was done on the girls at Radcliffe College in Ireland. Those who trained extremely hard found that their periods stopped very quickly whereas those who had other interests regarded the training as less stressful and progressed in a more physiological way. But there are other aspects which are more controversial. It has been suggested that patients who receive an injury may be more likely to develop multiple sclerosis, motor neurone disease or other unpleasant complications. It has been shown that if you damage a nerve, the neurones subserving that nerve metabolically are turned on to produce all sorts of glyco-protein receptors and ornithine decarboxylase. You can test this very quickly by giving an injection of viruses to a mouse and the infection in the mouse goes quiescent. Stick the mouse into ice cold water and let him swim around for a few hours and the virus becomes apparent again, affects his heart and he gets a myocarditis. Similarly, if you section the nerve and then leave the mouse for three days and then inject him with a virus, the virus will go straight to the muscle which has been damaged when its nerve supply was cut and will damage the muscle further. But there are all sorts of factors including the endocrine system and so forth as well as infection which are all inter-related. I think that is important.

<u>Budgett</u> I think stress is in the eye of the beholder, in the athlete. We do see some athletes who have been getting good results in training, say at College, and decide to take it more seriously. They give up their studies to take the game professionally, taking a year off to do so, and then things start to go wrong.

<u>Mr P Edmond</u> (Vice-President, Royal College of Surgeons of Edinburgh) Patients in general, and athletes in particular, love to have a measurement, a time or a value. We were nearly driven crazy during the Commonwealth Games by athletes wanting to know their serum ferritin levels. Without having a level they thought appropriate, they did not want to compete and we consulted every known biochemist. None of them could tell us what levels were significant but nevertheless, to the athletes, this was terribly important. I have an indirect question then to Craig Sharp. I would like to be reassured that athletes will not want to know in the future how their lymphocytes perform.

<u>Dr N C C Sharp</u> (British Olympic Centre)   I am afraid I cannot answer the question of how they would know how their lymphocytes function. Nevertheless, one might be able to know this one day. However, if one brings athletes into the laboratory and puts them on a treadmill or a rowing machine or other device then measures their lactic acid levels, they learn to remember pretty quickly how much exertion produced that level. If, at a much later date on the river or on the track you can ask them what you think their lactic acid level is and they can tell you pretty accurately. They might say that they feel 10.5 millimoles or 14 millimoles today. Now if one had a similar marker in terms of immune response, one might be able to answer the query.

<u>Madeley</u> These thoughts raise some important questions of who is in charge? If you tell the athletes what levels of this, that or the next parameter they have reached, it encourages a degree of what you might call navel gazing. On the other hand, if the coach is the only person who monitors these levels then it makes the athlete into a clockwork mouse. How we get a balance is, I suppose, a matter for individual athletes.

<u>Sharp</u> It is and I think Richard should have learnt this very well having performed at the top level.

<u>Budgett</u> Yes, I did not realise it at the time but my coach said "I think you are overtrained", took me out for two weeks and then we started low level training again and I felt a lot better.

<u>Sharp</u> Your own coach took you out. At the highest level the coach does not really tell the athlete what to do. It is more of a partnership, though here I am not talking about gymnastics or swimming where the athlete is very young. John

Anderson worked with David Moorcroft but did not tell him what to do. They would debate between them and Moorcroft would say "I feel like working to this level today". This was partnership at the highest level and both contributed.

Budgett   Morgan in the States has used profile of mood state questionnaires and there have been other questionnaires which have been used to follow, particularly swimmers, through a period of training. They have shown those swimmers who do break down have very dramatic changes in various psychological profiles such as fatigue, depression and vigour. If you monitor their progression you may hope that they will be able to prevent the overtraining syndrome from developing.

Mr G McLatchie (Hartlepool)   Sleep disturbance seems to be a feature of chronic fatigue syndrome in overtraining. Is there any evidence that using hypnotics improves performance in athletes who are overtraining?

Budgett   No, it is the first time today that I have thought of actually using hypnotics because of course coaches and other advisers are all extremely prejudiced against using them.

McLatchie   It would seem to be a reasonable thing to do as sleep disturbance is part of the problem.

Budgett   I think if you talk to many athletes before a major competition a large proportion of them hardly sleep at all because of the tension and anxiety. I am certainly happy to give them hypnotics then, but during long term heavy winter training I do not think it is justifiable.

McLatchie   I was certainly aware when I was involved in the British Karate team for many years that, before major competitions, they would be requested not to take hypnotic drugs because they then found it difficult to cope. They would wake up the next day for the fight feeling stiff and it was obviously vital that they relaxed. I think in other major international sports hypnotics are occasionally used before major competitions.

Dr D R McCluskey (Belfast)   In patients with chronic fatigue syndrome, and I am not talking about athletes now, hypnotics do not work. If you gave them a large dose of some hypnotic drug they still do not sleep and there is some disturbance of their sleep centre which hypnotics do not act on. Alternatively, one might use 5-HT agonists, or anti-depressants might work but athletes are probably different. We are going to study this shortly.

Madeley   In these cases perhaps a little of the national beverage might help?

McCluskey   Well, they cannot take that either because they feel worse when they drink.

Prof J E Banatvala (London)   You talked about infection and immunity particularly in top athletes training for something like the Olympics. When you go to the Olympics as an athlete, you are stuck in the Olympic village, aren't you? Now, is that the right environment to avoid infection. From the outside it seems like going back to Preparatory School. Numbers of young adults living together, eating together and bedding close to one another. It is a super place to get infected!

Budgett   It is a real problem and has occurred in various situations, particularly in the Training Camps, because the trend now is to spend 2 or 3 weeks before the competition in a Training Camp before you go to the Olympic Village. So you may have, say, the whole rowing squad, 50-plus individuals, all living close together. Infections, particularly gastro-enteritis, can run rife as well as upper respiratory tract infections. Apart from educating them, I think it is very difficult to prevent this.

Banatvala   You do not have the choice. Could one say "Look I am going to win this event. I do not want to be near any of these people. I want to stay by myself and arrive on the day". Is that not important?

Budgett   Yes, it is, I suppose, so long as you are in the right time zone but some of the top athletes can do that because they have the resources and the discipline to go and prepare on their own.

HRH The Princess Royal   Ben Johnson did just that, lived entirely by himself in the hotel and kept himself to himself. As it happens, it did not make a lot of difference but there is no question that it is one of the problems. It is one of the unique aspects of the Olympics that this mix of athletes from all over the world come to one place, sharing similar ambitions. This does pose a problem of infection in such living conditions but that, in a way is inevitably part of going to the Olympics. If you feel really strongly about the risk, and without doubt, some will use this as an excuse. They can become very neurotic during the last stages of their training and any excuse will be better than none. Gastro-enteritis is a good one - it is easily come by and can be due just as much to nerves as to bacteria. It is difficult to judge how important these various influences are on individuals at a particular moment in their career. I find it interesting that the chronic fatigue syndrome involves people who are not at that level of fitness and it may be difficult to know how to treat them.

Behan   We have begun treating people with a substance that acts on depleted levels of hormones. So far all the data are not in but I can say categorically that we have patients such as school teachers who have not been able to do any work for the last five years, have no signs of depression whatsoever and are unable to walk up hills. If you put them on this drug they do not feel too well in the first three weeks but at the end of the month their sleep and everything comes back to normal. Within three months they are back to square one. These data will be published shortly but there is no doubt that you can treat them when they do respond. On the other hand there are other individuals who do not respond to the same treatment but when you look carefully at them, some of them have Parkinson's disease in which there is idio-pathic fluid retention which has not been mentioned in athletes but which can occur particularly in women. There are other transmitters probably and it is not simple hypothalamic dysfunction.

Budgett   I think that every symptom you can think of has been described in over-training. The list is a very long one when you look at all the literature.

Mr D A D Macleod (SRU, Edinburgh)   I work with the Scottish Rugby Team and one of the things we have noticed that our coaches have become much more amenable to rest and allowing players to relax during training sessions. During the build-up to a major competition like the World Cup, you have to prescribe it positively. You have to specify a work-rest ratio of, for example, one to one, one to two or one to three depending on the stage of the build-up. In addition, it is very unusual for rugby players to get into a situation like the World Cup unless they go on tour. Here the players' own curiosity may help. During the first week they are all out and about, seeing what is happening in the rest of the world away from home but, by the second week, they have all gone back to the routine of going to bed in the afternoon for two hours, particularly if they have a two-training session day. As a result, rest is being recognised as an integral part of a training programme, even in Rugby Football now. The message is beginning to get across.

Budgett   No-one talked about that in 1984 but now the message is being recognised.

Madeley   I wonder how widely this applies through the world? However, I think we must now bring this to a close.

Your Royal Highness, it has been a pleasure to have you with us and to have your contributions to the discussion. As an Olympic athlete yourself, I am sure you are aware of some of these problems, particularly I guess from time to time that of dozy horses, but may I invite you to bring this particular session to a close with some words of your own. Thank you.

<u>Her Royal Highness, The Princess Royal</u> Thank you very much. I must admit that on these occasions it is much more fun sitting in the audience, being allowed to listen in and take part in the discussion. Obviously, from the point of view of sport, I feel I have some knowledge of the problems, but horses are seldom mentioned at this type of conference. It must be the Irish influence which we have today. Both speakers from Ireland have referred to examples of problems in horses, particularly with chronic fatigue.

I mention this because, certainly in terms of viral infections in horses, controls have got much better, but have left a problem of recognising symptoms which used to be pretty obvious, particularly with breathing difficulties. Horses have been running while infected with viruses that otherwise would have been noticed but, because they have had vaccinations and treatment, the infection was not recognised. What was noticed was that they took far longer to recover their form. The effect of having run with a virus left them with a difficulty of getting back to fitness. And this was so despite the fact that they appeared and trained as if they were perfectly all right. Nevertheless, as far as actually running in competition, they were definitely <u>not</u> fit. This is one kind of observation and another also briefly touched on was the trend towards testing for every conceivable thing. I have to admit that I got to the point when I was forced to say to a trainer that I was not surprised that the horse did not run well. He must have been so full of holes from the number of times he was blood tested that he did not actually feel like running. There has to be a balance, obviously, between what you can achieve and what fashion indicates you ought to be looking for in blood levels.

As for this sort of conference, perhaps people think sports medicine is an unnecessary addition to medical sciences, but what has been highlighted today for me, both during this session and the first session I went to, is what it brings in increased knowledge of a variety of different conditions in overall terms. Everybody encounters much the same problems of fluctuations in physical fitness and, under sporting conditions, these obviously occur more often and possibly in greater depth. Sporting activities provide an opportunity to look at severe fatigue that may develop under a variety of conditions. The information that you gain as specialists in the particular fields of sports medicine can be transferred into, for instance, general practice and be used to help people who are not involved in sport at the highest level. Their fitness in general terms can be better understood and even the diseases that everybody suffers from day by day.

The reference, for instance, to teachers and the amount of viruses carried around by children is a particularly interesting one; certainly I think I have noticed at the end of the summer holidays, within a week of the schools going back (be it my children's schools or anybody else's), the incidence of people having cold, feeling ill and generally being under the weather is extraordinary. Now I must admit that I had put it down to "just one of those things that children suffer from" and not noticed it particularly until I realised that there was a couple that I knew with no children who for years never suffered from any of these problems. With teachers I suspect that it is very common and maybe it is that regularity of assault on their immune systems that makes it so difficult for them to withstand. This kind of information is often difficult to analyse in medical science because it is so anecdotal and, as I have noticed in dealing with doctors in the past, if you cannot prove it with figures, it does not exist. I have noticed this particularly over Riding for the Disabled as a therapy. Because we cannot prove scientifically the improvements we see in individuals, they are dismissed as trivial, not real or valid.

This is patently nonsense, but the kind of information transfer, discussion amongst people dealing with specialist problems, seen in this conference has tremendous potential for everybody. For that reason alone, I am delighted that so many have come to this conference and hope that, apart from satisfying your own curiosity and improving your own lines of work, links between you can be made and made much more broadly as a result. As we have heard, some of you are general practitioners. Therefore it has provided a very good opportunity for some of the specialist expertise that has been on offer here to be transferred into the general community. For that alone, thank you for taking part in the conference. Enjoy the rest of it - I very much enjoyed my opportunity to join you, albeit briefly. Thank you.

Introduction   Cartilage and the soft tissues

The continuing improvement in performance in all fields of high quality sporting activity is exhilarating for participants and exciting for the spectating public. However such improvements inevitably lead to increasing mechanical stress on body tissues with the potential consequence of damage, even to the extent of failure, of that tissue. In addition, even at a lower level of achievement, the active participation in sport of all kinds by an increasing number of the population has produced an expanding crop of similar stress-induced injuries or conditions.

In both groups these injuries arise either from a sudden acute load applied to the tissue which usually results in failure (rupture) or repetitive stressing, which leads to the 'over-use' condition. The only means by which we will be able to prevent such injuries is to understand better the mechanisms by which they arise. In addition it is incumbent upon us to know and understand their potential for spontaneous repair. Sports people expect and demand this of us.

In this section, authors of differing backgrounds present some facets of their work which offer some understanding of a few of the effects of stressing the musculo-skeletal system. In the opening paper Professor Paul presents work illustrating the surprising magnitude of forces which act across joints during even normal use, far less sporting activities. Such forces will have an effect not only on bone but also ligaments, tendons and muscle and perhaps of more importance, the articular cartilage. Following this Professor Bentley describes the repair process which can occur following injury to articular cartilage in both experimental animals and in humans. He also describes methods by which this may be enhanced or assisted. Dr Armstrong then discusses the cellular changes which occur in contracting skeletal muscle in experimental animals, which may extend to a form of cellular injury and could explain in some part muscle stiffness and soreness after a bout of exercise. Finally Professor Whitehouse and Dr Williams describe their work with ultrasound, computerized tomography and magnetic resonance imaging which have so greatly advanced the diagnosis of injuries of the soft tissues in the past five years. They illustrate this with particular reference to musculo-tendinous injuries and injuries of the ligaments and menisci of the knee.

J. Graham

Biomechanics related to sport

J.P. Paul

Abstract. This application of methods of mechanics to study the loads imposed on the structures of human joints is a complicated process. Force actions from the environment will produce tendencies to rotate particular joints in three dimensions and will require sophisticated muscle control for balance or equilibrium. Biomechanical analyses have been performed for level walking which can produce joint forces of several times body weight. For higher speeds and for turning and jumping activities these forces are multiplied several times and the injury potential is significant.

Keywords: Biomechanics, Joint Forces, Equilibrium, Muscle Forces, Gait.

The study of mechanics usually relates to inanimate objects such as automobiles, bridges, power plants, etc where the basic analysis depends on Newton's laws of motion. It is a surprise to many that these same laws of motion can be applied to the movements of the human body. However, one is accustomed to measuring the weight of the human body and its dimensions and, consequently, the study of biomechanics has been established since the time of Leonardo da Vinci. A complicating factor in biomechanics is generally that only external measurements can be made on the human body and the interpretation of their effects in respect of tension in muscles, ligaments or stresses in bone can only be calculated with some difficulty. One of the major difficulties is exemplified by the fact that, conceptually, since muscles can develop tension only, one could consider the need for six muscles at the hip joint, one to control flexion, one for extension, one for abduction, one for adduction and one each for internal and external rotation. If this were the case one could calculate the tensions in them from measurements of the loads transmitted between the leg and the trunk. However, there are 21 muscles which act between the trunk and the leg, and the mechanics' equations are not sufficient to solve this problem. Some cases are dealt with using EMG, the electrical signals picked up by electrodes placed on the skin over selected muscles, in association with the equations corresponding to the physiological characteristics of muscle. These analyses frequently use the concept that the body will so organise the use of muscles as to minimise the rate of energy consumption at any instant. This, however, is obviously not a relevant rule in situations where there may be a risk of a fall, or there is a requirement for very precise control of movement as in writing. An alternative method of approach is to work with a simplified anatomical system where muscles situated anatomically close to each other in respect of areas of origin or insertion or of lines of action are taken to correspond to a single effective muscle force. In this way, simplifications can be made to determine the relevant loads.

Before the analysis of loads of the body structure is undertaken, however, it is necessary to determine in any activity what the external loads are. A major load is the body's own weight due to gravity and the forces due to acceleration which in whiplash injuries can be of high magnitude. The second and probably more important load is that exerted by the environment on the body. It is a curious fact that there is effectively no resistance to the body in walking on a level surface provided that the wind velocity is not high. If a ball or a javelin is thrown, then the force necessary to accelerate either of these has its reaction on the hand and is an external force. In walking and running the ground exerts forces on each foot in turn and these forces correspond to body weight together with the acceleration being undertaken. It is not possible to calculate these ground to foot forces throughout the cycle of walking since the definition of walking is locomotion during which the body is supported continuously by one or two feet. During the period of support by two feet, the ground to foot force cannot be calculated. This may be appreciated by a simple exercise as follows. Stand with legs apart and tense the muscles on the inside of each leg tending to pull the feet together. Because of friction at the ground, this is very difficult to do and because there is no movement, one cannot analyse velocities or accelerations to obtain the forces. The same holds true during the double support phase of walking. During running, it is theoretically possible to calculate the ground to foot force during each support phase, but this requires detailed measurement of the positions and accelerations in space for each body segment and for accuracy one should take account of the fact that the trunk is not rigid but has deformation of the shoulders relative to pelvis, etc. One needs also accurate values for the mass properties of the body segments and although there are publications quoting average data for these, the applications in particular cases are not precise.

Sophisticated instruments have been designed to measure the ground to foot forces and these usually give signals corresponding to six quantities; the upward, forward and medio/lateral components of force, together with the moments about the reference axes of the force platform. From two of these moments, one can infer the position of the line of resultant force between ground and foot on the force platform, together with the twisting moment about the vertical axis through the centre of the force platform. The curves of variation of these components of force during the walking cycle are well known. The values of the forces are expressed as a percentage of body weight and time is expressed as a fraction of the time for one complete walking cycle. The greatest force is obviously the vertical component which for each foot has two peaks with comparable magnitude each being greater than body weight for most styles of walking. Each peak occurs approximately at the time when the other foot is leaving the ground or making ground contact again. Between them there is a trough of about 80% of body weight and this occurs when the body is supported solely on one leg or the other. The difference between this value and body weight corresponds to the vertical acceleration being undertaken at that time. The magnitude of the maximum is frequently taken as being approximately 1.2 times body weight. Since it corresponds to the vertical accelerations, it will respond to the style of walking, for instance, a long stride length involves a larger range of vertical movement from the trunk and therefore a higher ground to foot force. If one walks with bent knees as in carrying a liquid filled vessel, then the variations of the value of this component of force from body weight will be small.

The forward or backward force on the foot has a maximum value of approximately 25% of body weight, and from heel contact in walking until mid-stance, the force is directed backwards on the foot corresponding to deceleration of the forward velocity of the body from the maximum which it may reach at the time of changeover from left foot to right. The maximum and minimum forward speeds may be ±10% of the mean walking speed. Consequently, in the late stages of the stance phase of walking, the ground to foot force is accelerating the body forwards again so that it is moving faster than the mean speed, then the ground force on the other foot decelerates, and so the cycle goes on. It is interesting to note that while both feet are on the ground, the body has received a backwards force from the foot which is in front, and at the same time there is a forwards force from the foot which is behind. This may seem a waste in terms of energy consumption, but in fact the presence of this component of force reduces the loading on the muscles round the hip and therefore the loading on the hip joints, and is beneficial in the walking cycle. If one tries to walk on a very slippery surface, this force cannot be developed and walking becomes very tiring. In the same way if this force is enhanced as in walking through sand, the tiring effect is noticed again. In situations where someone is walking at uniform forwards speed the faster periods must balance the slower periods, and thus the forward accelerations balance the backward accelerations and there is no resultant work done on the body during walking on a level surface. In engineering terms the efficiency is defined as the work obtained from a machine divided by the work put into it. According to this definition, walking has an efficiency of zero since energy is involved in the development of force in the muscles producing the movement without any work being done against the environment.

The side to side force on each foot is smaller in magnitude than the other two components, being approximately 8% of body weight at maximum. Throughout most of the walking cycle, it is acting inwards on the foot and corresponds to the necessity to move the trunk over from the right leg on to the left leg when it is next supporting, and so on. It might be thought that the smaller value of this force makes it less important, and in straight line walking it does. Although it must be remembered it acts at the knee and hip with a very considerable lever arm and its effect at these joints may be almost as great as the moments or turning actions due to the vertical component of force.

In running the body is airborne between the periods when there is contact between one foot or the other on the ground. Since on average the body does not rise from the ground or sink towards it, the effective vertical forces transmitted at the foot must be considerably higher than body weight. For a running style with long airborne periods, the ground to foot force may easily exceed three times body weight. In fast running there is the resistance of the air to be taken into account and therefore the forces by the ground on the feet forwards are much greater than in level walking. Just after foot contact however there is a backwards component of force by the ground on the foot, initially turning rapidly to a forwards direction.

If we think of the structures of the knee which are involved in the activities of walking or running, the straightening of the leg or its prevention from bending at the knee is due to the quadriceps muscle mainly, although the knee can be kept straight by action of the muscles at the hip tending to extend the thigh. This occurs late in the stance phase when the ground to foot force is on the ball of the foot tending to dorsiflex the ankle. This is resisted by the muscles inserted into the Achilles tendon, namely, soleus and gastrocnemius. Soleus is attached to the structure of the calf, but gastrocnemius is attached to the back of the femur above the knee joint and therefore tends to flex the knee and the knee is prevented from collapsing in this situation by action of the gluteal muscle.

The hip joint is situated deep within soft tissues and controlled by powerful muscles for all its movements. The knee bends or extends under the action of strong muscles in the thigh and the calf. However the knee is "held together" largely by ligaments at each side and internally so any tendency for external forces to make the leg knock-kneed or bowed outwards are generally resisted by the ligaments joining the femur to the tibia. The tibia is prevented from moving forwards or backwards relative to the femur by the cruciate ligaments. The anterior cruciate ligament prevents the tibia from moving forward as it might under the action of a strong push-off in running and also as it might due to the load in the quadriceps muscle translated into a force with a forwards component by the patella. Side to side movement is not a problem because the areas of the joint surface on the tibia are shallow and saucer shaped in form to engage with the curved ends of the femur. However, none of these ligaments is well positioned to resist twisting on the lower leg relative to the upper. The ideal form of such a ligament would be from an origin on the femur to wrap around the joint for about half of the circumference and then join up with the tibia matched by others in helical form round the joint. This would not be altogether effective because as the knee bent the ligaments at the back would go slack and be unable to resist twisted load. In fact, with the knee slightly bent, twisting is resisted by tension in one or other of the cruciate ligaments in association with tension in the appropriate collateral ligament at the side. Since neither of these ligaments is laid out in the most effective form, it is not surprising that many injuries of the knee joint occur due to twisting movements. However, the situation is not so bad as it might be in that the saucer shape of the tibia joint surface and the curved shape of the end of the femur, even that when the leg is carrying load, the femur is kept to the bottom of the saucer shape on the tibia and is therefore resistant to sliding out either by twisting or other movement.

In level walking at normal speeds the force transmitted at the knee joint is mainly in the medial compartment at the inside of the leg and may be of value three to four times body weight. This high value compared to the ground to foot force is due to the tension in the muscles controlling the knee joint pulling it together and augmenting the external force. The same phenomenon occurs at the hip joint, standing on one leg requires a force of nearly 2.5 times body weight at the hip joint, since the muscles of the rump have to stop the trunk bending over sideways since the centre of gravity of the trunk is several centimetres away from the centre of the hip joint. This muscle force of about 1.5 times body weight combines with the ground force to give the high value mentioned. The forces are even higher in straight line walking because there is then the additional effect of the muscles used to control the leg as it transmits load while bent forward from the hip and backwards from the hip. In very rapid walking, these hip joint forces may be seven to eight times body weight, or easily half a ton! If the calculations are done for people of different weights, walking at different speeds, it is found that the joint force in different people corresponds closely to a constant multiplied by the product of their body weight and stride length. So the advice to people with painful joints is to lose weight and walk with a short stride!

The discussion so far is related to straight line walking or running. The real trouble arises when sharp turns are made when walking, or more so when running. To run round a tight corner and change direction by 90° means that the force on the feet has to stop the body's forward movement and start its sideways movement in a very short time and very short distance. Thus ground to foot forces sideways on the foot can rise to a half of body weight, if not more, and since much of the time these are acting sideways on the foot, the bending effect on the knee may be very large and calculations have shown that the knee joint force in right angle turns from moderate speed running may be as high as twelve times body weight.

Most of the studies on the loading of joints in the leg have been undertaken with a view to obtaining information relating to the design of joint replacements for patients with degenerative disease. Thus there are few studies of joint loading for contact sports or for rapid moving indoor activities such as squash. There are two reasons for this. Firstly, it is presumed that the patient with a joint replacement will have been strongly advised not to undertake any such active sports. The second reason is that the instrumentation available for the measurement of such recreations would be too imprecise to give realistic values to the end results.

Stress injury and repair of articular cartilage

G. Bentley

Abstract. Stress injury to articular cartilage of joints is extremely important to athletes and all young active individuals because it is frequently missed and, even if diagnosed, is difficult to treat. This is because articular cartilage has no nerve endings, therefore not indicating its damage by pain and also the cartilage has little capacity for repair. Recent work has shown that early diagnosis by arthroscopy and MRI scanning can be valuable and that methods of repairing articular cartilage by stimulating the cartilage itself to repair by growth factors and drugs may be possible. Later repair of cartilage may be stimulated by a combination of articular grafts and cartilage cell grafts for the use of composite grafts composed of synthetic fabrics together with living cartilage cells. Thus disability produced by stress injury of cartilage will be considerably reduced in future.

Keywords: Injury, Repair, Articular Cartilage, Allografts, Chondrocytes, Matrix Support.

Introduction

Stress injury is extremely important to athletes and to all young active individuals because it is frequently missed and, even if diagnosed is difficult to treat. This is because articular cartilage is a unique structure which after skeletal maturity, shows little or no tendency to repair spontaneously. Therefore concentrated efforts to investigate the causes for breakdown of cartilage and possible mechanisms to repair it after injury have been pursued in this unit.

Articular cartilage is characterised by its unique structure which can be likened in a simplistic way to a sponge inflated with water. The cell-to-matrix ratio in cartilage is low and the essential strength of the cartilage lies in its fibrill meshwork which is composed uniquely of type II collagen. The arrangement of the collagen fibres is complex but essentially the meshwork is held in a state of turgor by the osmotic pressure of the large long-chain proteoglycan aggregates which lie interposed between the collagen fibres. The negative charge of the proteoglycans draws in water by osmosis so that the total water composition of cartilage is 75%. Thus the resilience of the cartilage is maintained by the water. It follows that loss of water or loss of proteoglycans which maintains the water within the substance of the cartilage will lead to loss of turgor and to early failure of the cartilage due to the mechanical stresses of compression and shear occurring during normal movement. This situation is particularly so if the joints are highly stressed.

The surface of articular cartilage is not smooth and the irregularity of the surface is necessary for the complex lubrication mechanism of cartilage which depends on the presence of hyaluronic acid and other proteins within the synovial fluid. The consequent effect of this highly efficient lubrication system is to produce a coefficient of friction which is at least eight times better than the best artificial joint presently available.

The earliest changes observed in cartilage undergoing degenerative change secondary to stress are loss of matrix from the superficial zones of the cartilage which is accompanied by death of superficial cells and fibrillation of the surface of the cartilage. However, since the cartilage has no nerve endings within it, this change produces no pain or symptoms in the patient. It is not until destruction of cartilage is sufficient to expose the bone beneath the cartilage which does contain nerve endings that pain is felt. The cartilage receives its nutrition entirely from the synovial fluid and has a very low metaboic turnover rate. This, combined with the low number of cells in the cartilage, produces a situation where repair does not occur.

It is thus of paramount importance to develop methods of identifiying early cartilage damage in the hope of preventing further damage and possibly of inducing repair at an early stage before disruption of the cartilage matrix has occurred. In the case of the knee joint, the advent of arthroscopy has allowed this to happen and the development of more refined imaging with MRI may very well allow early identification of cartilage damage in a non-invasive manner.

So at present the situation is that damage to joints is frequently not recognised until the articular cartilage is badly eroded and the changes are irreversible.

We have developed a simple categorisation of cartilage damage which is useful in assessing patients and also in assessing the appropriate method of treatment for them.

In the first stage there is damage to the articular cartilage alone.

In stage two there is damage to the articular cartilage exposing the subchondral bone but with no involvement of the bone.

In stage three there is extensive destruction of the subchondral bone.

Stage 1: Articular cartilage damage and repair

In stage one damage, caused for instance by lacerations or shearing of small amounts of articular cartilage during sporting activity, or following other types of trauma, the potential for repair may be greater than previously thought. In the clinical situation stage one injuries may present as small cartilaginous loose bodies or more commonly as manifestations of early cartilage damage in the condition of chondromalacia patellae. This condition may occur in non-active young females, but also is a great problem in athletic males and females who transmit excessive loads through the patello-femoral joint. Thus in sporting activity involving squatting and jumping, loads through the joint of three to four times body weight may occur. This condition therefore is clinically important and also offers an opportunity to study the early damage in human cartilage and the repair capacity.

In a study of 21 patients with chondromalacia patellae, full thickness specimens of cartilage were removed from the damaged area of the patella as part of the treatment. These were examined by hisotology, histochemistry, auto-radiography and electron microscopy. The findings were of great interest since it was observed that definite evidence of cellular division in the chondromalacia patellae cartilage was occurring. This was confirmed by auto-radiography and electron microscopy. In addition it appeared that metaplasia of the superficial damaged area of the cartilage could occur producing a smoothing of the surface. It is thus possible that with conservative methods of treatment such as physiotherapy and also following operative methods to alter loading on the patella such as quadriceps realignment, that healing of cartilage can occur. This would also explain the resolution of symptoms which occurs in approximately 50% of patients with conservative treatment.

The question of inducing cartilage repair is hotly debated. A number of agents such as non-steroidal anti-inflammatory drugs and growth hormone have been claimed to produce healing, but evidence on this is scant. In an animal experiment in which lacerations were made into the articular cartilage of mature femoral heads, healing of simple cuts within the cartilage was observed in between 25% and 75% of cases when Aspirin was administered for a three month period in therapeutic dosages. However, a clinical study of 30 patients with chondromalacia patellae treated for three months with Aspirin showed no evidence of improvement in the cartilage changes whatsoever. It is thus concluded that early damage of human cartilage is much more refractory to treatment than the simple lacerations of the experimental model. However, further research in this area is obviously urgently required.

Stage 2: Articular cartilage damage and repair

When the articular cartilage is completely lost from the surface and the subchondral bone is exposed, then any repair that would occur would be by fibro-cartilage formed from tufts of granulation tissue which arises from the marrow of the subchondral bone. This can be facilitated by drilling the surface or even by an osteotomy close to the joint which will alter the circulation and stimulate the growth of such tufts. Our experiments have shown that although such tufts may appear by histology and histo-chemistry to be formed of good quality cartilage, antibody studies reveal that the matrix of this cartilage is made up of type I collagen principally and does not contain type II collagen of normal hyaline cartilage. In addition there is evidence that the proteoglycans of this repair tissue are not normal. This fits in with the clinical experience that fibrocartilage formed following drilling of a surface is soft and gradually breaks down over the course of one or two years.

One solution to this type of problem has been to employ allografts of cartilage. The original allografts were made up of articular cartilage with an attached piece of subchondral bone to give stability to the graft and enable it to be attached to the bone of the recipient. Initial experience with these was unsatisfactory because of the intense immunological response generated by the subchondral bone component of the graft. This led us to develop the concept of isolating articular cartilage cells alone and growing them in culture to form a cartilage bank. This method together with transplantation of whole pieces of cartilage has been tested in experimental animals. Results show that cultures of cartilage and also intact plugs of cartilage transplanted as allografts into the knees of experimental animals do survive without rejection for a period of one year.

Recent work with osteochondral allografts in humans has shown that the results can be much better than those originally reported. Based on the work of Langer and Gross in Toronto, we have carried out a small osteochondral allograft programme in patients with osteochondritis dissecans, traumatic injuries to the articular cartilage, and also depressed fractures of the articular surface. Provided the graft completely replaces the damaged area of the joint and provided the loading of the joint is normal, then good incorporation of the grafts and good function can be achieved. However there is the small but definite risk of transmission of infections, in particular, HIV and hepatitis and thus we are carrying out experiments on storage of living cartilage for 90 days to exclude the possibility of transmission of such infections.

Meanwhile, we have been studying the alternative method of using a matrix of carbon fibre or other fibrous mateial to reinforce the repair fibrocartilage formed on the surface of joints after drilling. This technique, developed by Muckle and Minns, has been reviewed in 96 patients and has been shown to give approximately 70% of satisfactory results in lesions secondary to trauma and in stage one and two cartilage damage.

We are now conducting a prospective study on this method to assess its validity with annual arthroscopic assessment of the joints.

A completely new approach to the concept of replacement of early cartilage damage uses not only a fibrous matrix (a matrix support prosthesis, but also the incorporation of living chondrocytes within such a meshwork. Our early experiments in animals have shown that chondrocytes will grow within such a meshwork for a three week period and produce normal matrix, collagen and proteoglycans. The transplantation of such composite grafts of carbon fibre and chondrocytes shows incorporation of these grafts and maintenance of the phenotype, i.e. the collagen and proteoglycans over a three month period after implantation in experimental animals. This method offers great promise for the future.

In summary the aim and object of the research programme has been to achieve early identification of articular cartilage damage and treatment of early defects in order to prevent detioration of the joints and osteoarthritis. It appears that there is great promise in detecting early damage by MRI and applying methods for promoting healing in the most early stages by drugs and by growth hormones and also by the use of matrix support prostheses. The osteochondral allograft remains an option in some cases where articular cartilage damage is more extensive, but where the joint is otherwise normal. It is thus anticipated that the disability produced by early articular cartilage damage will be minimised and osteoarthritis prevented in a substantial proportion of such patients.

References

Langer F, Gross AE, West M. Urowitz EP. (1978) The Immunogenicity of Allograft Knee Joint Transplants. Clin Orthop, **132**, 155-162.

Muckle DS, Minns RJ. (1979) The Use of Filamentous Carbon Fibre for the Repair of Osteoarthritic Articular Cartilage. J Bone Joint Surg (Br), **61b**, 381.

Strain-induced skeletal muscle fiber injury

R.B. Armstrong and G.L. Warren III

Abstract. Type I strain injury is associated with delayed-onset muscular soreness, elevated plasma enzyme activities, elevated muscle [Ca^{2+}], reduced muscular performance, and disruptions of muscle fiber and basal laminar ultrastructure. The injury appears to have a mechanical etiology; initiation of the pathology is most closely related to the stress developed during eccentric contractions, and, secondarily, to the velocities of lengthening during the contractions. Data are consistent with the interpretation that these mechanical factors induce localized injury to the sarcolemma of active fibers, permitting influx of Ca^{2+}. If this influx surpasses the Ca^{2+} buffering and translocation capacity of the fiber, free [Ca^{2+}] rises, activating various Ca^{2+}-dependent phospholipolytic (e.g., phospholipase A_2) and proteolytic mechanisms in the local regions. These activated pathways degrade contractile and membrane components of the fibers, with consequent appearance of ultrastructural abnormalities and loss of soluble enzymes, respectively. By 2-6 h following initiation of the injury, phagolytic cells are in evidence proximal to the damaged fibers; the time course of this phagocytic phase corresponds to that of the delayed soreness. By 4-5 d following the injury, regenerative processes are in evidence, and the localized damage may completely heal within 2 wk. Training the muscle with high stress eccentric contractions prevents the injury; it is unclear whether acute preventative measures (e.g. warm up and stretching) attenuate Type I muscle strain injuries.

Keywords: Muscle Injury, Concentric Contraction, Muscle Cell Changes, Calcium Irons, Muscle Cell Repair

Introduction

Safran et al (1989) recommend classifying sports-related muscle injuries into 3 categories. Type I injury results from unaccustomed muscular exertion and is associated with reductions in muscle performance and delayed onset muscle soreness. The underlying pathology appears to be "micro-lesions" in both the muscle fibers and supporting connective tissue elements (for reviews see Armstrong, 1984; Stauber, 1989), and is precipitated by eccentric (lengthening) contractions.

Type II injury is identified as frank tears of the muscle-tendon unit resulting in acute disabling pain. Type II injuries are graded according to the amount of tissue involvement: Grade 1, tearing of a few fibers with the fascia intact; Grade 2, tearing of a moderate number of fibers with the fascia intact; Grade 3, tearing of

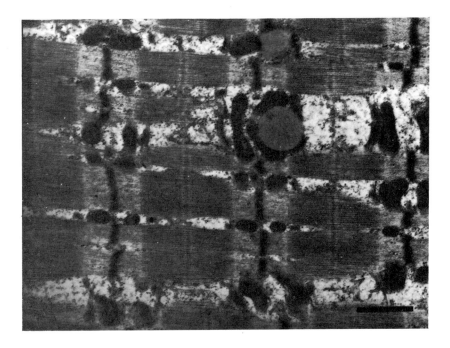

Fig. 1 Transmission electron micrograph illustrating dissolution of a sarcomere in a rat soleus muscle that performed 5 brief (200 ms) eccentric contractions (150% P_o). Note the enlarged fat droplet and the altered appearance of the adjacent mitochondria. The scale bar represents 1 micron.

many fibers and of fascia with ecchymosis; and Grade 4, complete tearing of the fibers and fascia. Like Type I injuries, these usually result from high stress lengthening contractions. Type II injuries most commonly occur in muscles with high fast-twitch fiber populations that cross more than one joint, e.g. the hamstrings (for review see Safran et al, 1989).

Type III injury occurs during or immediately after muscular exertion in the form of pain or cramp. Less is known about the etiology of Type III injury, but it may result from accumulation of metabolic products or ionic imbalances.

The focus of this brief review is on Type I muscular injury. Although this pathology is usually subclinical, it has important practical consequences and clearly has a higher incidence in athletes than the other classes of soft tissue injury.

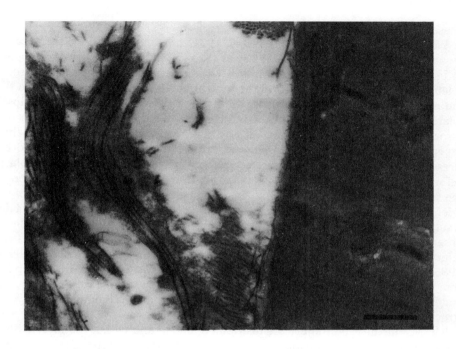

Fig. 2 Transmission electron micrograph demonstrating basement membrane disruption in a rat soleus muscle that performed 5 brief (200 ms) eccentric contractions (150% P_o). Bar represents 1 micron.

Description of Type I muscle injury

The strain-induced lesions in the muscles in Type I injury are subcellular (Armstrong et al, 1983; Friden et al, 1983; Newham et al, 1983; Kuipers et al, 1983; Ogilvie et al, 1988), so the pathology may be referred to as "microinjury" in contrast to Type II injuries. The extent of the injury is related to the stresses produced during the eccentric contractions and the duration of the exercise (McCully and Faulkner, 1985). Clinical symptoms associated with the pathology include muscular pain, elevated plasma levels of intramuscular enzymes (e.g, creatine kinase, CK), myoglobin, and protein metabolites from the injured muscles (e.g. 3-methylhistidine), and structural damage to subcellular components as indicated by light and electron microscopic examination (for reviews see Armstrong, 1984; Stauber, 1989; Ebbeling and Clarkson, 1989). Figure 1 depicts

277

the ultrastructural damage to a muscle fiber following high stress eccentric contractions.

Phases of Type I muscle injury

We (Armstrong, 1990; Armstrong et al, 1991) previously described the apparent sequence of strain-induced Type I injury as follows. An initial event, which appears to be mechanical in nature, inaugurates the injury process. Using an in vitro rat soleus muscle preparation, we (Warren et al, unpublished observations) found that the magnitude of the injury resulting from eccentric contractions is most closely related to the stress produced in the muscle (Fig. 2); the degree of injury is also associated with the strain rate during the contractions. Data from these experiments indicate that strain-induced muscle injury occurs by both normal stress theory and materials fatigue mechanisms. According to the former, plastic deformation of a structural component can occur during only one contraction if the stress exceeds the yield strength of the component. In fact, performance of one brief (167 ms) high stress (175% maximal isometric force) lengthening contraction results in significant reduction in force during a second contraction (unpublished observations). Regarding the materials fatigue hypothesis, the magnitude of strain injury is related to the number of eccentric contractions (McCully and Faulkner, 1985). These observations support the concept that ruptures in susceptible components from plastic deformations grow with successive contractions, i.e. materials fatigue. Interpretation of these observations is complicated by the structural complexity of skeletal muscle.

The lesions in Type I injury are distributed among and within the muscle fibers in seemingly random fashion (Armstrong et al, 1983; Kuipers et al, 1983), although they occur in greater numbers in the distal and proximal thirds of the injured muscle (Ogilvie et al, 1988). This distribution supports the hypothesis of injury suggested by Morgan (1990). Inhomogeneities in the length of sarcomeres in series occur during eccentric contractions (Julian and Morgan, 1979). If individual sarcomeres are stretched beyond the length where maximal interaction of thick and thin filaments can occur (L_o) their ability to produce active tension is reduced, and the tension must be borne by parallel passive elements (e.g. sarcolemma). Thus, the seemingly random distribution of the lesions in sarcomeres or small groups of sarcomeres may reflect which sarcomeres in series in the active fibers were "weakest" and were stretched to the greatest extent during the eccentric exercise.

The initial event appears to lead to a focal loss of Ca^{2+} homeostasis at the site of injury in the muscle fiber, referred to as the Ca^{2+} overload phase. This condition may result from damage to the sarcolemma, which normally serves to prevent Ca^{2+} from entering the cell down its steep concentration gradient. Much of the energy lost during stretch-shortening cycles of muscle fibers is in the sarcolemma (Tidball, 1986; Tidball and Daniel, 1986) and passive tension at relatively long muscle lengths (>140-150% of resting length) is primarily contributed by the sarcolemma

(Rapoport, 1972; Higuchi and Umazume, 1986). Stauber and colleagues (1988) have presented evidence that eccentric contractions damage the interfiber matrix, which is composed of the sarcolemma of adjacent fibers, and we have observed disruption of the basal lamina of injured fibers (Fig. 3). Also, it is known that following exercise with eccentric contractions there is an elevation in muscle $[Ca^{2+}]$ (Duan et al; 1990, Warren et al, 1991) as in diseased muscles with sarcolemmal abnormalities (e.g. Jackson et al, 1985), that elevation of muscle $[Ca^{2+}]$ with Ca^{2+} ionophores can induce muscle damage (Duncan and Jackson, 1987) qualitatively similar to that caused by eccentric exercise, and that prevention of Ca^{2+} influx in ionophore-induced muscle injury attenuates the damage (Duncan and Jackson, 1987). Thus, it is reasonable to hypothesize that loss of Ca^{2+} homeostasis follows the initial disruption of cell structural elements, and plays a role in subsequent events.

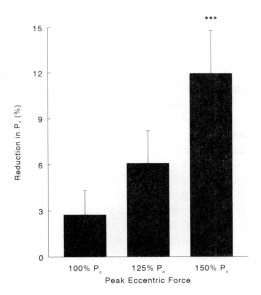

Fig. 3 Reduction in strength in a rat soleus muscles immediately following performance of 5 brief eccentric contractions at different peak stresses. *** The reduction in P_o was greater in the muscles performing eccentric contractions at 150%P_o than in the other two groups (P < 0.05).

The <u>autogenetic phase,</u> which commences within minutes of the <u>initial event</u> at the local injury sites, presumably involves disruption of normal mitochondrial function from excessive uptake of Ca^{2+} and activation of Ca^{2+}-dependent phospholipolytic and proteolytic pathways. Mitochondria serve to buffer cytosolic $[Ca^{2+}]$, and during periods of Ca^{2+} overload in the cell, these organelles can accumulate large quantities ($\sim$3 ,umol/mg mitochondrial protein) of the ion (Gillis, 1985), which depresses mitochondrial oxidation (Wrogemann and Pena, 1976). Elevations in free cytosolic $[Ca^{2+}]$ also activate various proteases (Murachi et al, 1981; Baracos et al, 1984; Mellgren, 1987) that degrade specific protein structures in the fiber, e.g. Z-discs (Busch et al, 1972; Cullen and Fulthorpe, 1982) and contractile filament components (Cullen and Fulthorpe, 1982; Dayton et al, 1976). Phospholipase A2 (PLA2) may also be activated by Ca^{2+} (Chang et al, 1987; Scheuer, 1989); this enzyme, which is located in sarcolemma and organelle membranes (van der Vusse et al, 1989), produces arachidonic acid using membrane phospholipids as substrates. Arachidonic acid in turn serves as substrate for production of prostaglandins, leukotrienes, and thromboxanes. There is good evidence that activation of PLA_2 plays an important role in muscle damage resulting from electrical stimulation of isolated mouse muscles in the presence of dinitrophenol (Jackson et al, 1984) and in damage caused by Ca^{2+} ionophore (Duncan and Jackson, 1987). Indomethacin blockade of prostaglandin (specifically, prostaglandin E_2) production attenuates injury induced by stretching of cultured chick skeletal muscle cells (Vandenburgh et al, 1990). Thus, the muscle fibers contain intrinsic degradative enzyme systems that can be activated as part of the injury sequence to begin the breakdown of the damaged structures. Products resulting from these pathways probably play a role in attracting phagocytic cells to the local injury sites in the muscles to complete the degradation of the focal injury sites.

Several hours following the induction of the injury, mononuclear cells begin to appear at the sites of injury (Armstrong et al, 1983). During this time period there is also an activation of complement and increase in circulating cytokines (Evans and Cannon, 1991). It is reasonable to assume that the delayed muscle soreness resulting from Type I injury is associated with this local "inflammatory" response. This phagocytic phase lasts up to about 4 days, at which time there is evidence of regeneration of myofibrils in the localized sites of injury (Armstrong et al, 1983). In the conscious rat model we (Armstrong et al, 1983) have used to study Type I muscle injury, healing of the fibers is complete in about 2 weeks, at which time there is no evidence of the sites of injury. However, the time required for the regeneration is related to the extent of the injury (McCully and Faulkner, 1985).

Effect of Type I muscle injury on athletic performance

Type I injury occurs when muscles perform eccentric contractions of an intensity or duration for which they are not accustomed. Professor A.V. Hill referred to this fact when he related that "once, I remember, when in excellent training for running I climbed a rope in gymnasium; I had not done this for years, though [I was] accomplished at it as a boy. I became abominably stiff afterwards" (1951).

In practical terms, any time an athlete performs eccentric contractions employing stresses that the muscles have not been trained for, the injury occurs. Thus, the extra effort expended in competition normally results in sore muscles and reduced performance for several days, even though the athlete may be at a relatively high state of training.

The practical consequences of Type I injury are two-fold. Most obvious is the discomfort during the several days following the effort. Perhaps of greater importance for the athlete is the attenuation in muscle performance following induction of the injury. Muscle force production, whether elicited voluntarily or through electrical stimulation, is significantly reduced for varying periods of time during and following the exercise (Hough, 1902; Davies and White, 1981; Newham et al, 1983). This reduction in strength is immediate. For example, performance of just two brief (167 ms) high stress eccentric contractions (175% of maximal isometric force) results in an immediate 6% reduction in maximal isometric strength; performance of 10 such contractions results in a 35% loss in force (unpublished data from isolated rat soleus muscle studies). Thus, performance of high stress lengthening contractions during a match competition could immediately and dramatically affect muscular performance during the match.

Prevention of Type I skeletal muscle injury

Acute preventative interventions

Whether or not Type I muscle injury can be prevented through acute interventions remains an enigma. Although stretching and warming up prior to muscular exertion are widely recommended for prevention of muscle injury by clinical practitioners (see Safran et al, 1989) and fitness and training experts (see Beaulieu, 1981), there is no compelling scientific evidence supporting the contention. Theoretically, both warm up and stretching could attenuate strain-induced Type I muscle injury by increasing the compliance of a susceptible component of the series elastic element in the muscle, warming by increasing the elasticity of the component (Williford et al, 1986; Strickler et al, 1990), and stretching through stress-relaxation mechanisms (Taylor et al, 1990). Evidence that these mechanisms may be invoked to protect the muscles from strain injury comes from the recent work of Garrett and colleagues at Duke University (see review by Safran et al, 1989). Their model for muscle injury involves stretching passive rabbit muscles to failure, i.e. the point on the stress-strain curve at which the muscle tendon unit tears (Type II injury). It is not clear how applicable their findings are to Type I injury, because failure in their model occurs at lengths in excess of normal anatomical excursion for the muscles, and at passive stresses that would not normally occur. Nonetheless, these investigators have reported that preconditioning rabbit extensor digitorum longus (EDL) muscles with isometric contractions prior to stretching them to failure increases the force to failure (8%)

and the length at failure (11%) (Safran et al, 1988). Strickler and colleagues (1990) reported that rabbit EDL muscle passively warmed at 39°C increased length at failure by 9% compared to muscles at 35°C. During cyclic passive stretching of rabbit EDL muscle to 10% beyond normal resting length, peak passive tensions decreased significantly during the first 4 stretches (Taylor et al, 1990). By the tenth cycle, peak passive tension had decreased by about 17%; subsequently, a greater length could be attained without tearing the muscle tendon unit (Safran et al, 1989). Thus, these studies on in situ rabbit muscle suggest that stretching and warm up prior to high stress eccentric contractions may attenuate strain injury. As discussed above, a significant amount of the energy absorbed by the muscle during stretching occurs in the sarcolemma, so it is reasonable to hypothesize that these preventative measures may in part affect this component.

A number of studies on human subjects have been done to estimate the influence of stretching and warm up on attenuation of muscle soreness (see reviews by Franks, 1983; Armstrong, 1984; Safran et al, 1989). The results from these studies are mixed, with some authors reporting benefits, and others, no benefit. In most cases, the ambiguity could result from the design of the studies and/or the criteria for injury (e.g. subjective ratings of soreness).

Effects of training on Type I muscle injury

Repeated performance of a particular exercise with eccentric contractions results in adaptation that attenuates or alleviates the injury (Armstrong, 1984; Ebbeling and Clarkson, 1989). Three points regarding this adaptation may be noted. First, it is relatively rapid. Using a conscious rat downhill walking model, we (Schwane and Armstrong, 1983) found that one relatively short conditioning session of downhill walking protected muscles against injury during a prolonged bout of downhill walking the following week. Similarly, Clarkson et al (1985) reported that one bout of exercise with eccentric contractions in human subjects resulted in a reduction of plasma CK activity and soreness after a second bout performed the following week. Secondly, the training or conditioning exercise must be specific for the injury-inducing eccentric exercise. For example, a conditioning session of uphill walking in rats did not protect the muscles against injury during prolonged downhill walking the following week (Schwane and Armstrong, 1983). Thirdly, the protective effect of the conditioning is finite. For example, if a second bout of eccentric exercise is performed by human subjects three or six weeks following the initial conditioning bout, CK release and soreness are attenuated, but by nine weeks, the injury markers are similar to those after the first bout (Byrnes et al, 1985).

Two contrasting hypotheses for this training adaptation can be suggested. The protection against further injury may result from structural or biochemical adaptations within the muscles per se; alternatively, adaptation in motor unit recruitment patterns may be initiated to distribute the stresses produced in the muscles during the eccentric contractions over larger cross-sectional areas of active motor units, thus decreasing the specific stresses on susceptible components in the muscles. There is no conclusive proof for either of these hypotheses. However, in a recent abstract, Stassen and colleagues (1991) reported that a bout of stretching of tibialis anterior muscle in an anesthetized rat during electrical stimulation protected the muscle from injury during repetition of the same protocol three weeks later. The electrical stimulation presumably maximally activated the muscle in both bouts, so the attenuation of injury in the second bout could not be attributed to central nervous system adaptation (i.e. altered recruitment patterns). These findings support the contention that adaptation of some structural entities within the muscle accounted for the training effect. If in fact the adaptation is in some component(s) in the muscle, further research is required to identify the component and elucidate the mechanisms underlying the response.

References

Armstrong RB. (1984) Mechanisms of exercise-induced delayed onset muscular soreness: a brief review. Med Sci Sports Exerc, 16, 529-538.

Armstrong RB. (1990) Initial events in exercise-induced muscular injury. Med Sci Sporys Exerc, 22, 429-435.

Armstrong RB, Ogilvie RW and Schwane J. (1983) Eccentric exercise-induced injury to rat skeletal muscle. J Appl Physiol, 54, 80-93.

Armstrong RB, Warren GL and Warren JA. (1991) Mechanisms of exercise-induced muscle fiber injury. Sports Med, 12, 184-207.

Baracos VE, Greenberg RE and Goldberg AL. (1984) Calcium ions and the regulation of intracellular protein breakdown in muscle, in Calcium Regulation in Biological Systems (eds S Ebashi, M Endo, K Imahori, S Kakiuchi and Y Nishizuka), Academic Press, Tokyo, pp. 227-242.

Beaulieu JE. (1981) Developing a stretching program. Physician and Sports Med, 9, 5960.

Busch WA, Stromer MH, Goll DE and Suzuki A. (1972) Ca^{2+}-specific removal of Z lines from rabbit skeletal muscle. J Cell Biol, 52, 367-381.

Byrnes WC, Clarkson PM, White, JS, Hsieh SS, Frykman PN and Maughan RJ. (1985) Delayed onset muscle soreness following repeated bouts of downhill running. J Appl Physiol, 59, 710-715.

Chang J, Musser JH and McGregor H. (1987) Phospholipase A2: function and pharmacological regulation. Biochem Pharmacol, 36, 2429-2436.

Clarkson PM, Litchfield P, Graves J, Kirwan J, and Byrnes WC. (1985) Serum creatine kinase activity following forearm flexion isometric exercise. Eur J Appl Physiol Occupat Physiol, 53, 368-371.

Cullen MJ, and Fulthorpe JJ. (1982) Phagocytosis of the A band following Z line and I band loss. Pathology, 138, 129-143.

Davies CTM and White MJ. (1981) Muscle weakness following eccentric work in man. Pflugers Arch, 392, 168-171.

Dayton WR, Reville WJ, Goll DE and Stromer MH. (1976) A Ca^{2+}-activated protease possibly involved in myofibrillar protein turnover. Biochemistry, 15, 2159-2167.

Duan C, Delp MD, Hayes DA, Delp PD and Armstrong RB. (1990) Rat skeletal muscle mitochondrial [Ca^{2+}] and injury from downhill walking. J Appl Physiol, 68, 1241-1251.

Duncan CJ and Jackson MJ. (1987) Different mechanisms mediate structural changes and intracellular enzyme efflux following damage to skeletal muscle. J Cell Sci, **87**, 183-188.

Ebbeling CB and Clarkson PM. (1989) Exercise-induced muscle damage and adaptation. Sports Med, **7**, 207-234.

Evans WJ and Cannon JG. (1991) The metabolic effects of exercise-induced muscle damage. Exerc Sports Sci Rev, **19**, 99-125.

Franks BD. (1983) Warm-up in Ergogenic Aids in Sport (ed M Williams), Human Kinetics, Champaign, IL, pp. 340-375.

Friden J, Sjostrom M, and Ekblom B. (1983) Myofibrillar damage following intense eccentric exercise in man. Int J Sports Med, **37**, 506-507.

Gillis JM. (1985) Relaxation of vertebrate skeletal muscle. A synthesis of the biochemical and physiological approaches. Biochim Biophys Acta, **811**, 97-145.

Higuchi H, and Umazume Y. (1986) Lattice shrinkage with increasing resting tension in stretched, single skinned fibers of frog muscle. Biophys J, **50**, 385-389.

Hill AV. (1951) The mechanics of voluntary muscle. Lancet, **261**, 947-954.

Hough T. (1902) Ergographic studies in muscular soreness. Am J Physiol, **7**, 76-92.

Jackson MJ, Jones DA and Edwards RHT. (1984) Experimental skeletal muscle damage: the nature of the calcium-activated degenerative processes. Eur J Clin Invest, **14**, 369-374.

Jackson MJ, Jones DA and Edwards RHT. (1985) Measurements of calcium and other elements in muscle biopsy samples from patients with Duchenne muscular dystrophy. Clin Chim Acta, **147**, 215-221.

Julian FJ and Morgan DL. (1979) The effect on tension of non-uniform distribution of length changes applied to frog muscle fibres. J Physiol **293**, 379-392.

Kuipers J, Drukker J, Frederiks P, Geurten P and van Kranenburg G. (1983) Transient degenerative changes in muscle of untrained rats after non-exhaustive exercise. Int J Sports Med, **4**, 45-51.

McCully KK and Faulkner JA. (1985) Injury to skeletal muscle fibers of mice following lengthening contractions. J Appl Physiol, **59**, 119-126.

McCully KK and Faulkner JA. (1986) Characteristics of lengthening contractions associated with injury to skeletal muscle fibers. J Appl Physiol, **61**, 293-299.

Mellgren RL. (1987) Calcium-dependent proteases: an enzyme system active at cellular membranes? FASEB J, **1**, 110-115.

Morgan DL. (1990) New insights into the behavior of muscle during active lengthening. Biophys J, **57**, 209-221.

Muriachi T, Tanaka K, Hatanaka M and Murakami T. (1981) Intracellular Ca^{2+}-dependent protease (calpain) and its high-molecular weight endogenous inhibitor (calpastatin). Adv Enzyme Regul, **19**, 407-424.

Newham DJ, Mills KR, Quigley BM and Edwards RHT. (1983) Pain and fatigue after concentric and eccentric muscle contractions. Clin Sci, **64**, 55-62.

Ogilvie RW, Armstrong RB, Baird KE and Bottoms CL. (1988) Lesions in the rat soleus muscle following eccentrically-biased exercise. Am J Anat, **182**, 335-346.

Rapoport SI. (1972) Mechanical properties of the sarcolemma and myoplasm in frog muscle as a function of sarcomere length. J Gen Physiol, **59**, 559-585.

Safran MR, Seaber AV and Garrett WE Jr. (1989) Warm-up and muscular injury prevention. Sports Med, **8**, 239-249.

Scheuer W. (1989) Phospholipase A2 - regulation and inhibition. Klin Wochenschr, **67**, 153-159.

Schwane JA and Armstrong RB. (1983) Effect of training on skeletal muscle injury from downhill running in rats. J Appl Physiol, **55**, 969-975.

Stassen F, Kuipers H and van der Meulen J. (1991) Peripheral adjustment after one bout of forced lengthening contractions. Med Sci Sports Exerc, **23**, S110.

Stauber WT. (1989) Eccentric action of muscles: physiology, injury, and adaptation. Exerc Sports Sci Rev, **17**, 157-185.

Stauber WT, Fritz VK, Vogelbach, DW and Dahlmann B. (1988) Characterization of muscles injured by forced lengthening. I. Cellular infiltrates. Med Sci Sports Exerc, **20**, 345-353.

Strickler T, Malone T and Garrett WE. (1990) The effects of passive warming on muscle injury. Am J Sports Med, **18**, 141-145.

Taylor DC, Dalton JD, Seaber AV and Garrett WE. (1990) Viscoelastic properties of muscle-tendon units. Am J Sports Med, **18**, 300-309.

Tidball JG. (1986) Energy stored and dissipated in skeletal muscle basement membranes during sinusoidal oscillations. Biophys J, **50**, 1127-1138.

Tidball JG and Daniel TL. (1986) Elastic energy storage in rigored skeletal muscle cells under physiological loading conditions. Am J Physiol, **250**, R54-R64.

Vandenburgh HH, Hatfaludy IS and Shansky J. (1990) Stretch-induced prostaglandins and protein turnover in cultured skeletal muscle. Am J Physiol, **259**, C232-C240.

van der Vusse GJ, van Bilsen M and Reneman RS. (1989) Is phospholipid degradation a critical event in ischemia- and reperfusion-induced damage? New Physiol Sci, **4**, 49-5.

Warren G, Hayes D, Lowe D, Guo W and Armstrong R. (1991) Mechanical factors in exercise-induced muscle injury. FASEB J, **5**, A1036.

Williford HN, East JB, Smith FH and Burry LA (1986) Evaluation of warm-up for improvement in flexibility. Am J Sports Med, **14**, 316-319.

Wrogemann K and Pena SDJ. (1976) Mitochondrial calcium overload: a general mechanism for cell-necrosis in muscle diseases. Lancet, **1**, 672-674.

Imaging of soft tissue and joint injuries

L.A. Williams and G.H. Whitehouse

Abstract. Imaging of injuries to the soft tissues and joints involves the use of plain radiographs, nuclear medicine studies and arthrography, the latter being occasionally combined with computed tomography (CT). Although these techniques are still valuable and extensively used, they are gradually being replaced by ultrasound and magnetic resonance imaging (MRI) which are non-invasive and do not use ionising radiation. Some of the current applications of these newer - imaging techniques are described, with particular emphasis on magnetic resonance imaging which is probably the imaging method of choice in most cases. The main restriction of the use of MRI is its limited availability.

Keywords: Tendon Injuries, Knee Injuries, Muscles, Magnetic Resonance Imaging.

Introduction

Many injuries sustained by sports people are straight forward fractures and dislocations requiring no special expertise in diagnosis. However, there are specific problems seen in the sports person which have been recognised over the last few years, particularly stress fractures. These may occur in almost any bone and are often invisible on plain radiography, but isotope bone scanning techniques have enabled us to solve this particular group of problems.

The diagnosis of joint abnormalities induced by trauma has been partially solved by the use of arthrography, sometimes combined with CT, and also by the use of diagnostic arthroscopy. A combination of arthrography and arthroscopy leads to almost 100% accuracy in the diagnosis of complex knee problems. Imaging of the soft tissues has been, until recently, very inadequate. The use of conventional X-rays, even when augmented by CT scanning, has not contributed a great deal. Although the ever-improving modality of ultrasound has given us a readily available and safe technique to look at muscles and tendons, the most exciting development has been Magnetic Resonance Imaging (MRI).

Magnetic resonance imaging

The principle of nuclear magnetic resonance (NMR) was described independently by Bloch and Purcell in 1946. Until recently, the use of NMR has been in chemical analysis, where nuclear magnetic resonance data are presented as a spectrum indicating the relative quantities of the atomic nucleus of interest within various molecules. Lauterbur (1973) invented a method of localising the information from NMR, thus giving the data a spatial orientation. This principle was applied by pioneer units in Nottingham and Aberdeen who developed magnetic resonance images (Mansfield, 1977; Edelstein et al, 1980).

The physical principles underlying MRI are based on the fact that hydrogen nuclei within the body, under the influence of a strong magnetic field, absorb short bursts of radiofrequency pulses. This results in the hydrogen nuclei gaining energy, which is then emitted as signals. The spatial relationships of these signals is then built up by a computer into images which reflect the distribution and concentration of hydrogen nuclei, as well as their physico-chemical environment. Hydrogen is the most suitable element for imaging, not only because of its abundance in the body but also the susceptibility of hydrogen nuclei to the external influences of a magnetic field and radiofrequency transmission. Depending on variations in the applied radiofrequency pulsation, the emitted signals result in different information on the resultant images. The factors responsible for these differences are proton density, which is the number of hydrogen nuclei per unit volume and two time constants termed T1 and T2.

MRI is expensive in terms of both capital cost and recurrent expenditure. However, MRI gives exquisite anatomical detail and, despite limited tissue specificity, demonstrates a wide range of pathological conditions. The comparatively narrow and elongated bore of the magnet, in which the patient lies, results in claustrophobia in some subjects and restricts access to the patient. The magnetic field will cause dysfunction of standard patient monitoring devices, cardiac pacemakers and other electrical equipment. Under the influence of the magnetic field, paramagnetic metallic implants and foreign bodies may move within the body. This is clearly a danger, especially in the case of ferrous surgical clips. Large metallic implants cause artefacts which can severely degrade image quality.

The value of MRI in the investigation of the central nervous system quickly becomes apparent during the development of the technique.

Gradually, MRI has established an important role in the investigation of musculoskeletal abnormalities.

Although bone does not emit magnetic resonance signals, the bone marrow gives out strong signals which, when contrasted with the signal void of osseous tissue, provides a considerable amount of information concerning a wide range of bone pathology. Flowing blood also gives a signal void, thus providing contrasting delineation of the vascular compartment.

The advantages of MRI in imaging the musculoskeletal system, including soft tissue injuries, are: the excellent soft tissue contrast, the ability to image in any plane, the good spatial resolution, the reproducibility of the method and the relatively short scanning time. The local application of surface coils, which have the ability to both transmit and receive the radiofrequency pulsations, improves the signal to noise ratio and enhances the spatial resolution, has particular application in injuries and other localised pathology within the limbs. By varying the applied RF pulsation, it is possible to demonstrate and discriminate between differemt pathological conditions.

Knee injuries

The knee is probably the commonest joint to be injured in sport and the standard investigation for the last 20 years has been double contrast knee arthrography (Stoker et al, 1981). This is an inexpensive out-patient investigation with-a high degree of accuracy in demonstrating meniscal tears, although it has limitations in the assessment of ligaments and other intra-articular tissues. The demand for arthrography has generally decreased since the introduction of arthroscopy, although it is still a useful adjunct to arthroscopy. The combination of both procedures increases the overall diagnostic accuracy to almost 100%. It can certainly prevent the arthroscopist missing the peripheral detachment of the posterior horn of the medial meniscus, which can be a difficult region to assess with the arthroscope.

If the arthrogram is combined with CT, other structures, such as the ligaments and articular surfaces, can be more clearly demonstrated (Pavlov et al, 1979). These techniques have gradually disappeared in establishments where magnetic resonance imaging has become available.

MRI clearly demonstrates the internal normal anatomy of the knee, menisci being shown in the sagittal and coronal planes. The combination of both planes helps in resolving difficult cases and increases the overall accuracy (Fig. 1). The cruciate ligaments are also readily demonstrated. The anterior cruciate is straight and gives a grey signal, while the posterior cruciate is curved and quite black (Fig. 2). The collateral ligaments and patellar tendon, together with the surrounding muscles and soft tissues are easily and clearly shown. It should be stressed that plain films are essential in all cases as it is easy to miss intra-articular loose bone fragments on MRI. Articular cartilage can be demonstrated, appearing white on T2 weighted scans. Defects due to osteochondritis dissecans are clearly visible. As already mentioned, the underlying bone marrow can be imaged; so that incidental tumours, infection and avascular necrosis are occasionally discovered. An entity that has not previously been recognised but which is now being diagnosed is the "bone bruise" (Lynch et al, 1989) (Fig. 3). While complete tears of the cruciate and collateral ligaments are often diagnosed by the apparent absence of the normal structure, partial tears are shown by deformity and alteration in the usual signal.

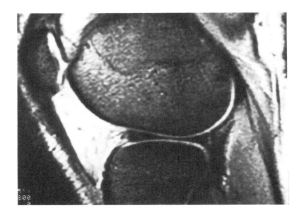

Fig. 1a   MRI of normal menisci. T2 weighted sagittal slice through the periphery of the lateral meniscus.

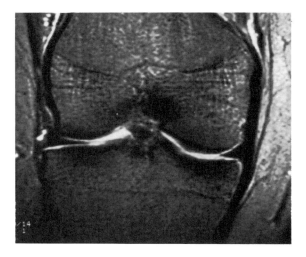

Fig. 1b   MRI of normal menisci. T2 weighted coronal slice through the menisci.

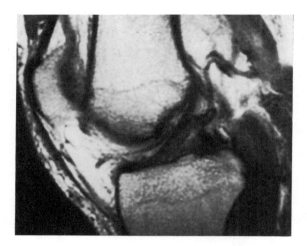

Fig. 2a   MRI of normal cruciate ligaments. T1 5mm slice showing the anterior cruciate ligament.

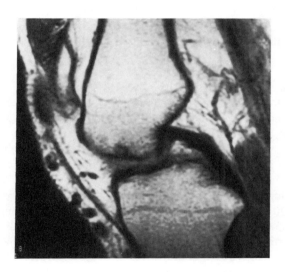

Fig. 2b   MRI of normal cruciate ligaments. T1 weighted sagittal scan of the posterior cruciate. Note the area of osteochondritis dissecans in the femoral condyle.

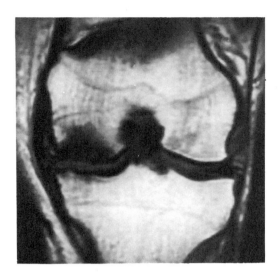

Fig. 3 Coronal MRI of the knee demonstrating a large "bone bruise" in the medial femoral condyle. Note the absence of the medial meniscus due to its complete disintegration of the meniscus.

Although tears of the minisci are usually easily demonstrated by a focus of high signal extending to the meniscal surface (Fig. 4), false positive diagnoses may be made if one is not aware that a quite marked increase of signal within the meniscus may be associated with a macroscopically normal meniscus. However, histology of the internal structure of the meniscus shows degeneration in these cases of increased signal. These patients often go on to develop cleavage tears and should therefore be counselled accordingly.

In the detection of meniscal tears there is concordance between MRI and arthroscopy in 90-98%, with a specificity of 84-100% and negative predictive values of 95-100% (Jackson et al, 1988; Mink et al, 1988; Polly et al, 1988) for MRI. Although arthroscopy is the gold standard against which MRI is set, it may well be that false positive examinations on MRI are arthroscopic false negatives - perhaps occurring in a posterior horn of the medial meniscus which has been difficult to see on arthroscopy. High signal may persist for some time in healed meniscal tears . There are several normal variants which may be misinterpreted as tears (Bassett et al, 1990).

The overall accuracy of MRI in the diagnosis of ACL tears is 95-97% (Mink et

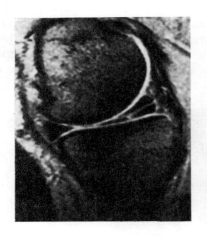 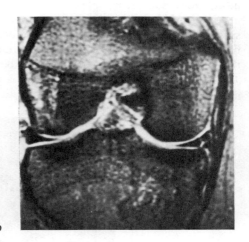

a   b

Fig. 4 MRI of torn menisci. T2 weighted sagittal scan (a) showing a complex tear
of the posterior horn of the medial meniscus. T2 weighted coronalscan (b)
showing a full thickness peripheral tear of the medial meniscus.

al, 1988; Polly et al, 1988). Associated fractures and other bone lesions such as
marrow haematoma may be visible on MRI in the presence of soft tissue knee
injuries (Lynch et al, 1989).

The sensitivity of MRI may lead to the detection of asymptomatic abnormalities
in the knee. Brunner et al (1989), reviewing MRI scans of the knee in
asymptomatic professional basketball and collegiate football players, found that
50% had significant abnormalities on the scans but there was no history of knee
surgery or significant injury in half of the players with abnormal scans. Clinical
judgement must always be applied in the light of MRI findings.

Other joints

Any joint in the body can be demonstrated by MRI with varying degrees of
success, depending on the experience of the radiographer and the radiologist. The
internal and surrounding anatomy of the shoulder can be demonstrated without
the necessity of injecting contrast medium. Whilst the ability to demonstrate the
rotator cuff and glenoid is extremely useful (Kneeland et al, 1987; Kieft et al,
1988a) the best technique for demonstrating instability of the shoulder is still
undecided. CT arthrography combined with screening still has a major role to play
(Braunstein and O'Connor, 1982; Danzig et al, 1982; Cove et al, 1984; Kleinman

et al, 1984; Raffi et al, 1987).

Wrist problems are becoming of increasing interest with the ability of the surgeon to repair defects using the operating microscope. Damage to the triangular fibrocartilage can be the cause of persistent wrist pain. Traditionally we investigate this by arthrography but again MRI is beginning to replace arthrography (Pierre-Jerome and Shahabpour, 1991). MRI is also able to make an early diagnosis of avascular necrosis of the carpal bones, in particular the scaphoid (Fig. 5).

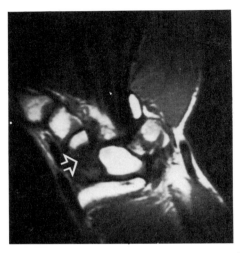

Fig. 5 MRI of the wrist. Coronal weighted scan. Note complete loss of signal in the proximal half of the scaphoid due to a fracture of the waist of the scaphoid (arrow) with resultant avascular necrosis of the proximal pole.

Soft tissue injuries

Although conventional X-rays and CT have a role in the demonstration of soft tissue abnormalities, the two major imaging modalities at the present time are ultrasound and MRI. Ultrasound is readily obtainable in most X-ray departments. The availability of small portable machines makes it possible to investigate injured players in the dressing room of tne stadium immediately following injury. The larger machines combining Doppler techniques enable very subtle diagnoses to be made. It is possible to demonstrate complete muscle tears (Fig. 6) or partial tears. Acute and chronic haematomas are also easily visualised (Fig. 7).

Tendon problems can be assessed using suitable probes. Complete rupture of large tendons, such as the Achilles tendon, is not usually a difficult diagnosis to make on clinical grounds, but partial tears and chronic inflammation are much more difficult. However, it is possible to demonstrate these abnormalities on

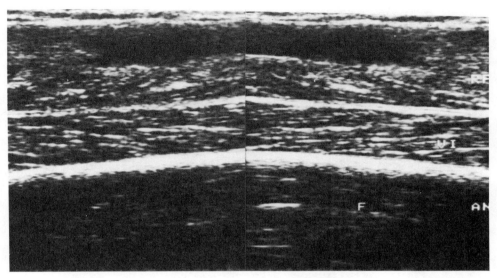

Fig. 6 Ultrasound scan through the length of the rectus femoris muscle. The muscle is completely disrupted with a large hypoechoic gap between the torn muscle ends.

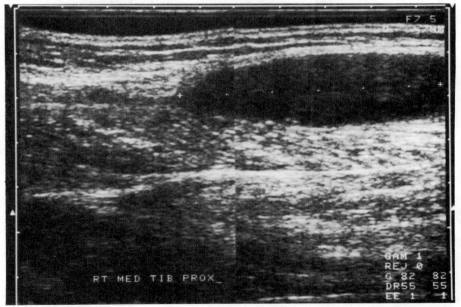

Fig. 7 Ultrasound scan of the calf. The large hypoechoic area is an acute haematoma in the gastrocnemius muscle.

ultrasound. Ligament tears around the knee, ankle and shoulder can be demonstrated by experienced ultrasonographers. The main drawback to ultrasound is that the images are difficult to interpret and to obtain accurate results it requires an experienced and expert ultrasonographer. The alternative to ultrasound is MRI which will demonstrate the anatomy with great clarity.

On MRI, muscle tears result in increased signal intensity, especially on T2 weighted sequences. Proton density and T1 weighting gives less of an increase in signal, but provide better anatomical detail than T2 weighted images. The high signal may persist for several months after the injury, although the development of low signal may be a result of fibrosis (De Smet et al, 1990) or chronic haemosiderin deposition. Muscle tears may give rise to atrophy or a focal mass effect on MR scans. The point of pain and even tenderness may occur some distance away from the site of injury as seen on the scan, for instance in hamstring injuries (Fig. 8).

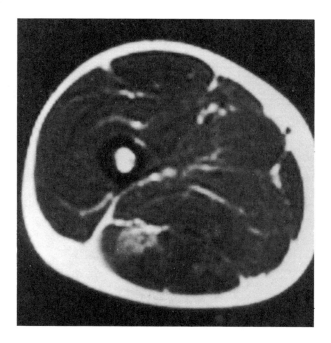

Fig. 8 Hamstring injury. High signal area in semitendonosus muscle on T2 weighted axial section.

Tears within the adductor longus muscle are particularly frequent in footballers (Fig. 9). Other causes of groin pain, such as hip abnormalities and iliopsoas bursitis, can also be seen on MRI.

Areas of high signal have been noted at the periphery of muscles which were painful after exercise (Fleckenstein et al, 1989).

Compartment syndromes, where increased pressure due to muscle oedema develops within a fascial space and results in diminished capillary perfusion and hence ischaemia, is associated with a diffuse, reticular increase in signal intensity on T2 weighted images (Fig. 10).

Bruises to muscles are seen in the superficial portions or muscles in contact sports, often as incidental findings (Fig. 11).

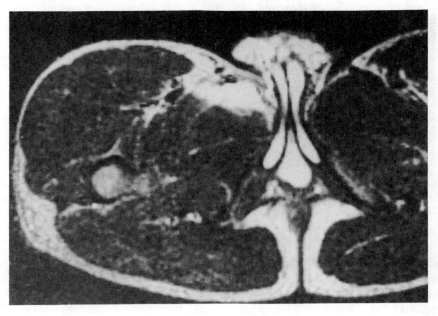

Fig. 9 Adductor longus tear. Large area of high signal within muscle on T2 weighted axial image.

Normal tendons have an absence of signal and are often silhouetted against the high signal intensity of surrounding fat. MRI is helpful in the diagnosis of traumatic disruptions, both partial and complete, as well as inflammatory conditions within and around tendons. For instance, complete tears of the Achilles tendon are seen as discontinuity of the tendon, retraction of the upper part of the tendon and increased signal intensity on T2 weighting at the site of injury (Daffner et al, 1986; Quinn et al, 1987). Incomplete ruptures can result in

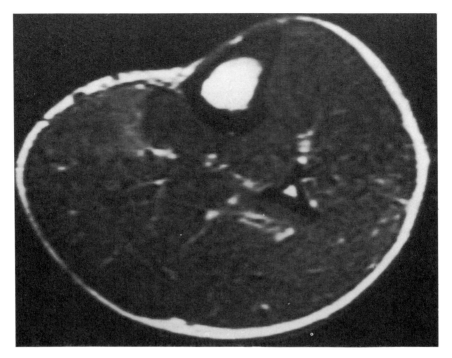

Fig.10   Compartment syndrome. Reticular area of high signal intensity in medial
          head and gastrocnemius and soleus muscles on T2 weighted axial image.

localised thickening of the Achilles tendon, with or without areas of high signal
intensity within the substance of the tendon, but with continuity of the outline.
Chronic Achilles tendinitis gives similar changes to partial rupture and the two
conditions may require differentiation on the clinical history (Fig. 12).
Peritendinitis and bursitis are other causes of pain in the region of the Achilles
tendon which can be diagnosed by MRI (Fig. 13).

Patellar tendinitis, or "jumper's knee", occurs in basketball players and other
athletes who have repeated stressful extension of the knee joint. MRI shows focal
enlargement and high signal intensity within the proximal part of the tendon (Fig.
14) (Davies et al, 1991).

Tears in other tendons, for example around the ankle, may be seen on MR
imaging (Fig. 15). Tenosynovitis is shown on axial images by a high signal
intensity fluid layer surrounding the low signal intensity tendons.

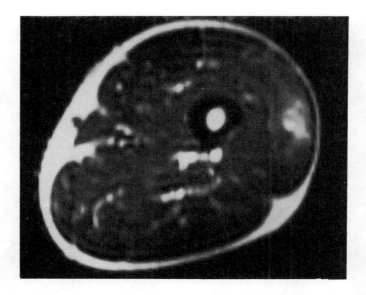

Fig. 11 Haematoma in vastus lateralis muscle seen as an incidental finding in a footballer. T2 weighted axial image.

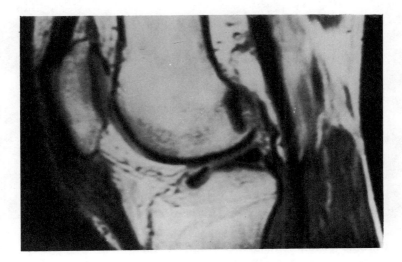

Fig. 14 Jumper's knee. High signal within thickened proximal portion of patella tendon on T2 weighted sagittal scan.

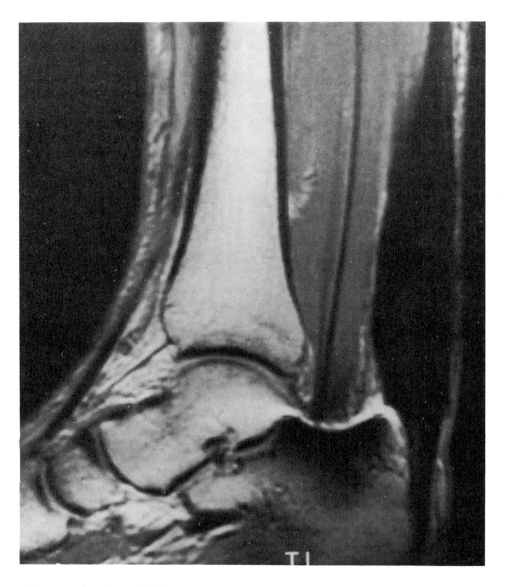

Fig. 12 Chronic Achilles tendinitis. Marked thickening of Achilles tendon, containing some patchy increase in signal intensity on T2 weighted sagittal scan.

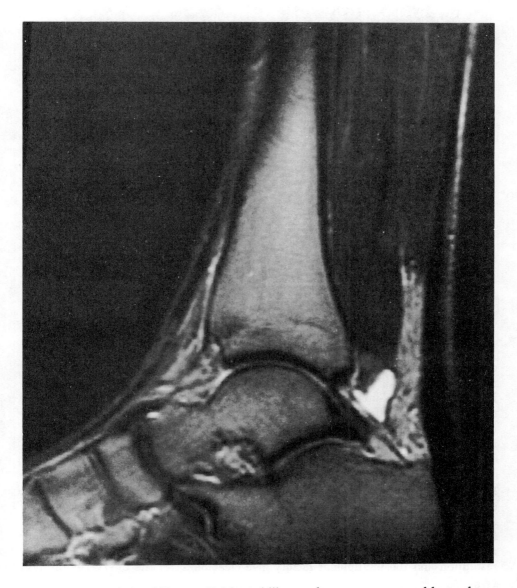

Fig. 13 Suspected Achilles tendinitis. Achilles tendon appears normal but enlarge bursa is seen anterior to the tendon on T2 weighted sagittal scan.

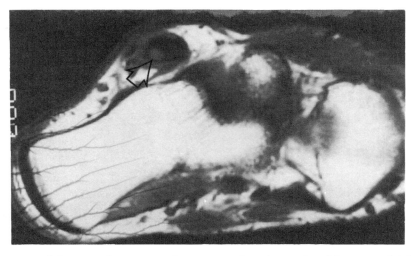

Fig. 15   Partial tear of peroneus longus tendon (arrow) with some thickening
around the tendon (arrow). Axial scan through tarsus with T1 weighting.

Spinal injuries

In neck injuries, plain radiograghs and CT remain the first line investigation for
demonstrating fractures and subluxation. However, sagittal MRI allows an easy and
rapid evaluation of possible spinal cord compression, ligamentous injury and
intervertebral disc damage in the cervical region. Spinal cord damage which is not
associated with significant osseous abnormality can be due to contusion or possibly
ischaemia resulting from impairment of the anterior spinal artery. T2 weighted
images may then show a focal area of high signal intensity at the site of cord
contusion.

In the lumbar spine, spondylolysis is usually diagnosed on plain radiography.
Radionuclides bone scans may be useful for detecting early and unilateral
spondylolysis, especially in young athletes. CT is useful for demonstrating fractures
and for evaluating spondylolisthesis. MRI is now regarded as the most appropriate
first line investigation in cases of suspected intervertebral disc prolapse, having
replaced myelography and giving more information than CT. The excellent
resolution and the multiplanar facility give clear detail of the intervertebral disc
(Fig. 16).

There is often discrepancy between abnormalities shown on MRI and clinical
symptoms (Fig. 17).   Approximately a third of asymptomatic adult males have
abnormal MR scans of their lumbar spine while almost half of all subjects who
have experienced low back pain have normal scans (Savage, 1991).

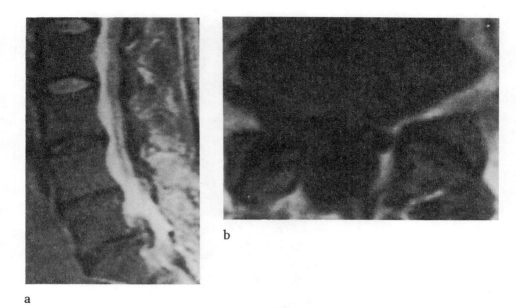

b

a

Fig. 16 Large posterior protusion of L5/S1 disc, encroaching upon right lateral recess and neural foramen, impinging upon nerve root. Note reduced signal from L3/4 to L5/S1 discs, indicating disc degeneration shown on T2 weighted sagittal (a) and proton density weighted axial scans (b).

Summary

There is no doubt that magnetic resonance imaging is now the investigation of choice in sports injuries of joints and soft tissues. The only limitation to the application of this technique is the availability of magnetic resonance machines. However, a rapid expansion of their numbers is occurring in the UK and, with changing financial structures within the NHS, it is now quite acceptable for sporting organisations to enter into contracts with MRI departments to provide a service for their individual athletes and players. The use of MRI should be encouraged as it saves young people having invasive tests and exposure to ionising radiation. However, where MRI is still unavailable, radiologists with suitable ultrasound experience in soft tissue problems can provide a fast, safe and accurate diagnosis in cases of sports injury.

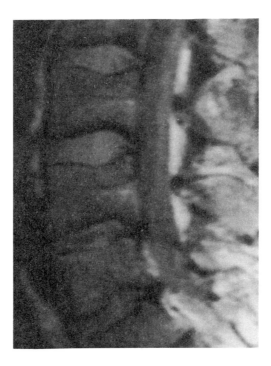

Fig. 17 International footballer with only occasional moderate backache. Disc degeneration at L4/5 and L5/S1. Some posterior protrusion of L5/S1 disc. Proton density saggital scan.

References

Bassett LW, Grover JS and Seegar LC. (1990) Magnetic resonance imaging of knee trauma. Skel Radiol, **19**, 401-405.

Bloch F, Hanson W and Packard ME (1946) Nuclear Induction Physical Review, **69**, 127.

Braunstein EM and O'Connor G. (1982) Double contrast arthrotomography of the shoulder. J Bone Joint Surg, **64(A)**, 192.

Brunner MC, Flower SP, Evancho AM et al. (1989) MRI of the athletic knee. Invest Radiol, **24**, 72-75.

Cone RO III, Resnick D and Danzig L. (1984) Shoulder impingement syndrome: radiographic evaluation. Radiology, **150**, 29.

Daffner RH, Riemer BL, Lupetin AR et al. (1987) Magnetic Resonance Imaging in acute tendon ruptures. Skel Radiol, **15**, 619-621.

Danzig LA, Resnick D and Greenway G. (1982) Evaluation of unstable shoulders by CT. Am J Sports Med, **10**, 138.

Cartilage & soft tissue

De Smet AA, Fisher DR, Heiner JP and Keene JS. (1990) Magnetic resonance imaging of muscle tears. Skel Radiol, 19, 283-286.

Edelstein WA, Hutchison JMS, Johnson G and Redpath TW. (980) Spin-warp NMR imaging applications to human whole body imaging. Phys Med Biol, 25, 751-756.

Fleckenstein JL, Weatherall PT, Parkey RW et al. (1989) Sports-related muscle injuries: evaluation with MR imaging. Radiology, 172, 793-798.

Jackson DW, Jennings LD, Maywood RM et al. (1988) Magnetic resonance imaging of the knee. Am J Sports Med, 16, 29-37.

Kieft GJ, Bloem JL and Roging PM (1988a) Rotator cuff impingement syndrome: MR Imaging. Radiology, 166, 211-214.

Kleinman PK, Kanzarai PK, Goss TP and Pappas AM. (1984) Axillary arthrotomography of the glenoid labrum. Am J Roentgenol, 141, 993.

Kneeland JB, Middleton WD, Carrera GF et al. (1987) MR imaging of the shoulder: diagnosis of rotator cuff tears. Am J Roentgenol, 149, 333-347.

Lauterbur PC. (1973) Image formation by induced local interreactions: examples emphasising nuclear magnetic resonance. Nature, 242, 190-191.

Lynch TCP, Crues JV, Morgan FW et al. (1989) Bone abnormalities of the knee: prevalence and significance at MR imaging. Radiology, 171, 761-766.

Mansfield P. (1977) Multi-planar image formation using NMR spin echoes. J Phys Chem, 10, 55-58.

Mink JH, Levy T and Crues JV. (1988) Tears of the anterior cruciate ligament and menisci of the knee: MR imaging evaluation. Radiology, 167, 769-774.

Pavlov H, Hirschy JC and Torg JS. (1979) Computer tomography of the cruciate ligaments. Radiology, 132, 389.

Pierre-Jerome C and Shahabpour M. (1991) The Wrist Joint in Magnetic Resonance Imaging and Spectroscopy in Sports Medicine (eds M Osteaux, K DeMeirleir and M Shahabpour). Springer-Verlag, Berlin, pp.139-149.

Polly DW, Callaghan JJ, Sikes RA et al. (1988) The accuracy of selective magnetic resonance imaging compared to the findings of arthroscopy of the knee. J Bone Joint Surg, 70A, 192-198.

Purcell EM, Torrey HC and Pound RV (1946) Resonance absorption by nuclear magnetic moments in a solid. Physical Review, 63, 37-38.

Savage RA. (1991) A critical review of the potential role of magnetic resonance imaging in the evaluation of low back pain. PhD thesis, University of Liverpool.

Stoker DJ, Enton B and Fulton A. (1981) The value of arthrography in the management of internal derangement of the knee. Clin Radiol, 32, 557.

Turner DA, Prodromos CC, Petasnick JP and Clark JW. (1985) Acute injury of the ligaments of the knee: magnetic resonance evaluation Radiology, 166, 865-871.

PART THREE

Damage limitation

Introduction   Damage limitation

Preparation for performance at the top level of sport subjects the body to significant biomechanical, physiological and immunological stress. These stresses are particularly apparent in a highly competitive, contact, intermittent high intensity sport such as soccer or rugby, and have been highlighted in earlier papers in this publication.

Appropriate preparation can minimize stress by balancing training programmes, diet, the use of suitable equipment and adopting a realistic expectation of what can be achieved. The importance of work/rest ratios in training cycles are increasingly well understood. Injuries will happen and the physical disruption of tissue must be minimized, accurately assessed and both treatment and rehabilitation programmes instituted in conjunction with maintaining overall fitness if recovery is to be rapid and effective.

A series of papers are included in this section of the Proceedings which look at 'damage limitation' by identifying the principles of care of sports injuries in conjunction with critical reviews of the value of ultrasound and laser therapy, hyperbaric oxygen, non-steroidal anti-inflammatory drugs and movement against rest.

As already indicated much can be done to enhance performance and minimize injuries by appropriate preparation. This concept can be extended to include the playing surface, the choice and style of footwear and the use of orthoses.

In these days of international travel, politicians, conference speakers and delegates, and top class athletes can be seen jet-setting all over the world and they are expected to perform on arrival. The physical and pyschological consequences of jet lag and heat are reviewed, identifying strategies which will help achieve early acclimatization.

D.A.D. Macleod

The principles of care for soft tissue injuries

M.A. Hutson

Abstract. The majority of sports injuries involve the soft tissues of the musculoskeletal system, of which muscles, tendons and ligaments are pre-eminent. Although the anatomical, physiological, and biomechanical characteristics of these tissues vary widely, their response to injury is very similar. The essential features of the healing process - pathophysiological and pathomechanical - are examined in this paper and related to the clinical presentation and the principles of management. Injury to the musculotendinous unit is used as a model.

Keywords: Soft Tissues, Healing Process, Pathophysiological, Pathomechanical, Musculotendinous Unit, Management.

Characteristics of soft tissues

All soft tissues have cellular and non-cellular components, and a high water content (70% on average). The musculotendinous unit is composed of a highly cellular contractile component (muscle) and a relatively hypocellular component offering tensile strength (collagen).

Muscle
Each muscle fibre contains hundreds or thousands of myofibrils in which the polymerised myosin filaments slide past the actin filaments to produce contraction. The myofibrils are contained within a matrix of sarcoplasm and connective tissue, principally collagen. The many branches of this tree-shaped arrangement of connective tissue within a muscle coalesce to form large fascial sheaths and connections with tendons. This intramuscular connective tissue has considerable importance: it contributes to the viscoelastic properties of the musculotendinous unit. If a muscle is preloaded (stretched by eccentric contraction) prior to concentric contraction, elastic storage energy may be utilised to increase efficiency and to reduce potential for injury by shock absorption.

Tendon
Tendon has entirely different characteristics. It is composed of two proteins, collagen and elastin, embedded in a proteoglycan matrix. The distribution of the two proteins is usually considered to be: elastin 2%, collagen 30%. Collagen accounts for 70% of the dry weight of tendon and is the most important structure to impart tensile strength to all soft tissues.

Collagen synthesis is under the control of fibroblasts which secrete tropocollagen, the most fundamental molecular unit, which is a helical structure and bonds in a staggered fashion to form a microfibril. Aggregation of units allows the development of fibrils which are crossed-striated under EM because of the staggering of tropocollagen molecules. Collagen fibres are wavy when relaxed and are arranged in parallel; they straighten longitudinally when stretched. When the tensile load is relaxed the elastin fibres reorient the collagen in its wavy, or crimped configuration.

During physiological loading elastic deformation occurs up to 2-5% strain (defined as the percentage increase in length over the original length). Microscopic collagen failure begins at the yield point, approximetely 7-8% strain, beyond which plastic deformation occurs (during which there is failure to resume resting length). Ultimately rupture results.

Ligaments
Ligaments are very similar in composition to tendons. They have a slightly higher elastin content (2-5%) and are arranged in fascicles along the axis of a limb, connecting bone to bone. They have a more exaggerated weave of collagen fibres than tendons, bestowing on them a greater capacity for elongation - at the expense of stiffness.

Joint capsules
Joint capsules are also predominantly collagen by dry weight, with collagen fibres orientated along different lines of stress, producing a criss-cross effect. Some fibres are then available to resist tensile loads, whatever the direction of the applied stress.

Effects of immobilisation
Of considerable clinical importance are the grave consequences to the musculotendinous units and other connective tissues as a result off disuse, and particularly of immobilisation. Following injury fibril deposition in ligaments and joint capsules, for instance, becomes haphazard, and their parallel lines disorganised. Yield strengths are compromised. Noyes et al (1987) have identified a 39% decrease in maximum failure load and decreased stiffness in the anterior cruciate ligaments of monkeys after cast immobilisation for eight weeks. Following twenty weeks of reconditioning there was a partial recovery only. (In surgically treated medial collateral ligament tears at the knee, wound strength is about 50% of normal at twelve months, confirming that a long period of time is required for maturation of collagen by restoration of cross-linkages and increase in cross-sectional area.)

It is estimated that there is a 20% loss of muscle strength after one week of muscle immobilisation. A further 20% loss of residual strength is experienced with every subsequent week. Atrophy is more rapid if muscle is immobilised in a shortened position; type I fibres are particularly affected (47% loss by the fifth week of immobilisation).

The biomechanical changes in collagen are also profound: reduced collagen mass, increased degradation (and synthesis) rate, increased turnover overall. Proteoglycan changes, in the form of reduced total glycosaminoglycans, are also observed. Morphological, biomechanical, and biochemical changes in other tissues, notably articular cartilage, as a result of stress deprivation are well documented and are not described further here. Clearly the advantages of early mobilisation for soft tissue injuries are considerable.

Muscle Injury

Soft tissue injuries, in general, may be classified into direct (contact trauma) and indirect (overload - acute or chronic). As far as the musculotendinous unit is concerned, tendon is resistant to the compressive effect of direct trauma, but muscle may be contused.

Contusion
During contusion muscle fibres are ruptured with the development of a haematoma, and healing takes place in the same way as is described subsequently for a muscle tear; however, there is an additional propensity for the development of myositis ossificans if the degree of contusion has been considerable.

Indirect strain
Indirect strain results from excessive tensile force causing tearing of both muscle fibres and the intricate collagen lattice with which it is intimately associated. In common with other connective tissue injuries, it may be graded as:

grade 1 = muscle "pull" (less than 5% disruption)
grade 2 = partial tear
grade 3 = complete tear

Eccentric loading
Muscle injury is more likely to arise during an <u>eccentric</u> <u>contraction:</u> greater force development is possible, and more force is produced by the connective tissue in muscle during stretching. It arises principally in athletes engaged in sprint running, and in team sports in which bursts of speed or rapid acceleration are demanded such as rugby football, soccer, American football, field hockey, and squash rackets. The muscles commonly affected are those which span two or more joints, such as the hamstrings, quadriceps, and gastrocnemii. Associated features of these muscles are:

a. they often limit joint mobility (e.g. tightness in the hamstrings limits knee extension when the hip is flexed).
b. they act eccentrically in sport (e.g. the hamstrings decelerate the joints over which they act in sprinting)
c. they have a relatively high percentage of type 2 (fast twitch) fibres and fast contractions

The common site for muscle strain is close to the musculotendinous junction. Tears may occur at any point of the musculotendinous unit, however, and sometimes muscle or tendon is avulsed from its attachment to bone.

Risk factors
Factors which increase the predisposition to injury are:

a. inadequate training (conditioning)
b. imbalance (e.g. between quadriceps and hamstrings)
c. inadequate flexibility (loss of storage energy potential) d. insufficient warm up
e. localised muscle fatigue
f. generalised fatigue
g. excessive scarring

Unaccustomed activity
To complete the picture of muscle injury in sport, in addition to contusion and strain, muscle damage may also arise as a result of unaccustomed eccentric muscle activity (e.g. arising during the first day of preseason training for rugby and soccer, or after exhausting activity such as marathon running. Pathological changes include disruption of the sarcolemma, contractile apparatus and mitochondria in the gastrocnemii of marathon runners. After eccentric exercise myofibrillar disorganisation is observed with particular damage to the Z-lines. Other features of excessive or unaccustomed eccentric exercise are elevation of muscle enzymes (principally creatine kinase) in the blood, delayed-onset muscle pain and tenderness, and reduction in performance.

Pathophysiology

Soft tissue healing is characterised by a number of phases which merge with overlap into each other. The histological characteristics are related to the clinical appearances of a muscle tear in Table 1.

Injury
Tensile failure of collagen is a primary characteristic of soft tissue injuries involving muscle, tendon, or ligament. Clearly myofibrillar disruption and

retraction of the torn ends occur in muscles strain. The connective tissue elements, composed primarily of collagen within the muscle and encapsulating the muscle, are also disrupted and bleeding occurs into the gap with the formation, over several hours, of a haematoma. Careful examination of a patient immediately after a grade 3 soft tissue tear, prior to the onset of swelling in the inflammatory phase, will reveal a palpable gap or loss of muscle definition.

Inflammatory (proliferative) phase

The essential features of this stage are the release of chemotactic agents from platelets and mast cells, and the subsequent invasion of inflammatory cells, such as mononuclear cells (macrophages and T lymphocytes) and polymorphs. Vasodilatation and increased capillary permeability occur with the development of interstitial oedema. Degranulation of mast cells releases serotonin and histamine. Degradative enzymes are released from assorted inflammatory cells. Localised coagulation within the haematoma gives rise to a fibrin clot. Infiltration of this clot by primitive blood vessels, resulting from endothelial budding, and by proliferating immature connective tissue cells (fibroblasts) results in granulation tissue.

Prostaglandins are formed from the metabolism of arachidonic acid which is released from tissue membranes consequent upon the activity of digestive enzymes from polymorphs, and probably from other cells. Among their many actions prostaglandins contribute vasodilatation and chemotaxis, and lower the pain threshold of nerve endings to histamine and other substances (i.e. they potentiate the inflammatory response). Since excessive bleeding and formation of tissue oedema at this stage are counter-productive, the use of non-steroidal anti-inflammatory drugs which inhibit prostaglandin synthesis is seen to be anti-inflammatory. Similarly, cryotherapy, rest and elevation have an anti-inflammatory effect. The inflammatory phase; nevertheless, is essential for healing; in some respects therapeutic modalities such as the use of ultrasound may be considered to accelerate this phase of healing (in other words are "pro-inflammatory").

Clinically this phase is characterised by the cardinal signs of inflammation: swelling, warmth, pain and redness. (To these features, which were recorded by Celsus in the first few years A.D., Galen added a fifth sign: loss of function). Tissue oedema may be seen some distance away from the injury site. Early bruising may be observed, tracking down the limb, if the initial haematoma was intermuscular (or was released to become intermuscular) rather than intramuscular. The clinician welcomes the sight of extensive bruising and/or ecchymoses as the likelihood of the development of a tense haematoma is reduced. Should tissue oedema around a muscle contusion, for instance in a charley-horse injury to the quadriceps, be profound there is a substantial risk of myositis ossificans, and the initial phase of immobilisation (see under "Treatment") should be extended.

The inflammatory phase lasts for at least several days, often peaking at seventy

Table 1   Characteristics of muscle tear

	Clinical	Pathophysiological
Injury	Sudden pain during overload Dysfunction Pain - worse after few hours Palpable gap Painful stretch Muscle weakness	Disruption of fibres Contraction of torn ends Haemorrhage into defect Intramuscular collagen disruption

Inflammation	Pain (on use)
	Swelling
	Warmth
	Redness
	Discolouration:
	  bruising
	  ecchymoses
	Oedema:
	  localised (boggy)
	  distal
	Granulation tissue
		Release of vasoactive and chemotactic factors
		Invasion of cells:
		  macrophages
		  polymorphs
		Fibrin clot
		Prostaglandin release
		Degranulation of mast cells
		Fibroblastic activity
		Endothelial budding

Repair	Palpable (scar) thickening
	Intramuscular haematoma palpable
	Myositis ossificans palpable
	Oedema:
	  localised = improving
	  distal = may persist
	Bruising gradually disappears
		Fibroblastic proliferation
		Collagen deposition - disorganised lattice
		Increased vascularisation
		Persistent macrophage and polymorph activity
		Maturation of satellite cells

Remodelling	Moderate restoration of function: flexibility improves, power improves Palpable scar (in superficial injuries) Muscle bulge on contraction Maturation of myosotis Haematoma may persist Effective result = replacement of torn muscle fibres by relatively inelastic scar	Maturation of collagen (orientation of fibres along lines of wound stress) High % immature collagen still Increasing tensile strength Mucopolysaccharide content decreases Reduced vasculature ?Hypertrophy of remaining muscle fibres

two hours. It may be prolonged, regrettably, by overeager mobilisation which provokes further bleeding. It is suppressed by cortisone which has an adverse effect on the invasion of macrophages and on the proliferation of fibroblasts. Occasionally a very irritable lesion is found with shiny, tender skin overlying and tethering a fluctuant haematoma.

Repair phase

This phase lasts from days to several weeks and commences towards the end of the inflammatory phase. A proliferation of fibroblasts is seen, and tropocollagen is produced within the cell membrane. Maturation of the primitive collagen by bonding, then aggregation into fibrils and fibres, takes place. There is increased vascularisation as a result of the formation of larger blood vessels, and continued phagocytic activity to remove cellular debris. There is evidence for regeneration of muscle by the maturation of primitive satellite cells into myoblasts, then myotubes, then into muscle fibres following relatively minor muscle trauma (for instance secondary to unaccustomed eccentric exercise.

The principle feature of this phase is the synthesis and deposition of collagen which is arranged in a disorganised lattice. Proteoglycan ground substance, also secreted by fibroblasts, probably plays an important role in determining fibre size and direction and cross-linkages. Both type I and type III collagen are produced. Clinically, this highly collagenised area may be palpated, in superficial injuries, as a cord-like, nodular or band-like structure. Soft tissue swelling due to oedema resolves steadily over a two week period if healing progresses satisfactorily. A large haematoma, either intramuscular or at the site of muscle/tendon avulsion from bone, may become cystic with a granulomatous/fibrotic lining, and its fluctuant nature detectable.

Remodelling phase

During this phase, which lasts from several weeks after injury to several months or years, remodelling of the anatomical configuration of collagen occurs in response to mechanical stress. This maturation of collagen is associated with increasing tensile strength. Further intermolecular bonding between collagen fibrils occurs, and there is a high turnover overall of collagen which probably lasts for up to two years.

In ligament injuries there is a high proportion of immature type III collagen during the early weeks of healing. Maturation, with the establishment of cross-linkages, takes many months/years. Gradually the mucopolysaccharide content of ground substance and the degree of vascularisation decrease. Hypertrophy of remaining muscle fibres may occur. Some degree of penetration of muscle fibres through the developing connective tissue is possible, though penetration through dense scar tissue is unlikely. Since too early mobilisation after soft tissue trauma may delay the development of tensile strength in granulation tissue (yet often leads subsequently to dense scar formation) it is desirable for a short period (of

3-5 days) of relative immobilisation to be allowed after muscle injury. (This period should be extended to 10-14 days in the case of severe direct contusion.) Following this, however, early mobilisation is desirable on both clinical and histochemical grounds. Experimental studies have shown that when mobilisation follows a short period of immobilisation, there is more rapid return of tensile properties to muscle, better penetration and orientation of muscle fibres through the connective tissue scar, and more rapid development of the essential features of the repair and remodelling stages.

The clinical features of this phase relate to the moderate restoration of function. Flexibility is restored to normal (unless complicated by surgery and/or prolonged immobilisation) and improvement of muscle power is seen. In superficial injuries a scar may be palpated and in the case of grade III muscle rupture, a muscle bulge proximal to a cicatrised scar may be seen on muscle contraction. In respect of muscle tears, the effective result is the replacement of muscle fibres by relatively inelastic scar following which residual dysfunction may persist.

In respect of intramuscular collagen, Lehto and Jarvinen (1991) suggest that normalisation of the usual collagen cross-link structure does not take place before six weeks from injury, indicating that at least this length of time should be allowed for the development of tensile strength in the collagenised tissue which replaces the wound granulation tissue.

Graduated resistive exercises aimed at strengthening injured or disused muscle are an essential requirement prior to the imposition of large impact forces, for instance in running, which provide the tensile stresses necessary for collagen maturation and compression stresses necessary for increasing bone strength.

Treatment

The time honoured modalities of ICE - ice, compression, and elevation - continue to be promoted as a valuable first-aid measure which should be started as soon as possible after injury and continued for 1-3 days. These treatments are mainly designed to minimise the degree of tissue disruption due to haemmorhage and oedema. Ice packs or commercial cold preparations, when used for 15-20 minutes every 1-2 hours, may reduce intramuscular temperature substantially, thereby restricting further bleeding. Prolonged cold immersion should be avoided as this gives rise to secondary vasodilatation and increased bleeding. Adequate elevation of the affected limb and the use of appropriate non-adhesive compression bandaging or intermittent pressure compression and non-steroidal anti-inflammatory drugs help reduce the likelihood of prolonged bleeding and tissue oedema further. Rest should be added for the first few days for reasons already given: in particular it is important to allow sufficient time for
a.   the development of a basic level of tensile strength within granulation tissue.
b.   the restriction of the size of granulation tissue.

In certain cases of a severe muscle tear the early application of a Plaster of Paris cast may also be of value to ease pain and reduce the risk of myositis ossificans. After three days, that is during the repair phase, gentle active and passive movements are encouraged and isometric contractions begun. A graded stretching programme is instituted and combined with a gradually increasing regime of resistive exercises in conjunction with hydrotherapy and effleurage. Friction massage is helpful once the developing collagen is palpable as a recognised bundle of tissue fibres, thought should be gentle at first: this improves the alignment of fibres and reduced unwanted fibrous adhesions within and around the developing scar. Local heat, ultrasound or laser therapy may be used to accelerate and improve the effectiveness of the repair phase. Strength training should include attention to the antagonist muscles; appropriate rehabilitation exercises should be included for co-ordination, and balancing of agonist/antagonist muscle groups in affected and non-affected limbs.

The presence of a substantial amount of bleeding into a muscle such as quadriceps femoris after a charley-horse (contusion) injury, associated with extensive tissue oedema and gross restriction in passive flexion of the knee joint, calls for utmost caution for the first two weeks. It is one of the few occasions when a cast (groin to ankle) may be used for two weeks to minimise muscle activity and avoid the chance of overeager stretching of the developing granulation tissue. By this means the possibility of myositis ossificans in which heterotopic calcification, then ossification, occurs in the haematoma is reduced.

Should the clinical condition, after a muscle tear, not improve steadily over two to three weeks, the possibility of an encysted intramuscular haematoma should be suspected. Despite the fluctuant nature of the injury, however, aspiration is usually unrewarding. Should it be attempted, a needle with a minimum diameter of 20g should be used. Incision and evacuation of the haematoma may be necessary after diagnostic ultrasound assessment of the lesion.

Conclusions

Disruption of muscle and/or connective tissue, whether by direct or indirect trauma, gives rise to bleeding and the formation of a haematoma. In the presence of tissue necrosis and a fibrin clot, the essential features of the inflammatory and repair phases of healing are the invasion of polymorphs and macrophages, intense vascularisation, and subsequent collagen synthesis following fibroblastic activity, resulting in the formation of granulation tissue. Maturation of collagen takes place over several months during the remodelling phase.

Early mobilisation (following a short period of relative immobilisation) with graduated resistive exercises is required to accelerate the healing phases, and in particular to allow realignment of collagen fibres and restoration of tensile strength. Furthermore the value of early mobilisation in respect of reduction in muscle atrophy, maintenance of proprioceptive reflexes, and maintenance of nutrition of articular cartilage is well documented.

References

Akeson WH et al. (1987) Effects of immobilisatlon on joints. Clin Orthop, **219**, 28-37.

Garrett WE. (1987) Muscle injuries and inflammation. Ann Sports Med, **3**, 71-2.

Garrett WE. (1990) Muscle strain injuries: clinical and basic aspects. Med Sci Sports Exerc, **2**, 436-43.

Lehto M, Duance VC, Restall D. (1985) Collagen and fibronectin in a healing skeletal muscle injury. J Bone Joint Surg, **67-B**,820-8.

Lehto MUK and Jarvinen MJ. (1991) Muscle injuries, their healing process and treatment. Ann Chir Gynaecol, **80**, 102-8.

Medoff RJ. (1987) Soft tissue healing. Ann Sports Med, **3**, 67-70.

Muir's Textbook of Pathology. llth Ed. (1980) (ed. JR Anderson), Edward Arnold, pp. 43-87.

Noyes FR. (1987) Functional properties of knee ligaments and alterations induced by immobilisation: a correlative biomechanical and histological study in primates. Clin Orthop, **123**, 210-42.

Renstrom P. (1991) Sports traumatology today: a review of common current sports injury problems. Ann Chir Gynaecol, **80**, 81-93.

Zarins B, Cuillo JV. (1983) Acute muscle and tendon athletes. Clin Sports Med, **2**, 167-82.

The effect of ultrasound and light therapy on tissue repair

S.R. Young and M. Dyson

Abstract. Electrotherapeutic modalities are widely used by physiotherapists to accelerate repair and reduce pain. It is important that the underlying mechanisms and effects that they produce are fully understood, together with any underlying adverse effects which may arise from their use. Ultrasound has been used therapeutically for over 50 years and a recent survey on the use of ultrasound in physiotherapy showed that 20% of all physiotherapy treatments in the public sector and 54% in the private sector involved the use of ultrasound. Ultrasound has been shown to be effective on both acute and chronic conditions, in particular with injuries to soft tissue. The laboratory evidence that ultrasound at therapeutic levels can cause biological effects, which would be expected to stimulate tissue repair, is described. Light therapy is a relatively new addition to the physiotherapy arsenal and the mechanisms of action have not yet been fully identified. There is clinical evidence suggesting that it is effective in promoting tissue repair and pain relief. This, together with some recent laboratory evidence showing light to be effective in stimulating cells, involved in the repair process, to produce wound mediators, is described. The weight of evidence suggests that, if used correctly, both ultrasound and light therapy can induce bioeffects which are beneficial to the patient.

Keywords: Ultrasound, Laser, Light, Wound Healing, Macrophage, Fibroblast, Pain Relief.

Introduction

Most of the injuries treated by physiotherapists involve soft tissue, for example, that located in the dermis, joint capsules, ligaments and tendons. The repair of such tissue consists of three overlapping stages: acute inflammation, proliferation and remodelling. Inflammation is an essential precursor of the proliferative stage of repair, and is generally short in duration, but in some pathological conditions it may persist, delaying healing. Healing, the repair of injured tissue, is a result of the movement, division, and death of specific cells, and the synthesis of intracellular and extracellular materials. The principal cellular responses immediately after injury of the dermis involve the interaction of platelets with thrombin and collagen. This results in local blood coagulation, accompanied by mast cell degranulation, which results in the liberation of an array of chemical mediators many of which are involved in the inflammatory phase of tissue repair

(Yurt, 1980). On completion of the coagulation process there begins a chronological sequence of events characterised by the appearance of various cellular infiltrates in the wound. Part of this sequence was recognized by Metchnikoff (1891), and it was elaborated upon and quantified by Ross and Benditt (1961). The rate at which this sequence changes is a measure of the rate of dermal repair (Dyson et al, 1988).

Leucocytes are the first cells to appear at the site of injury; within a few hours, the edge of the injured area is infiltrated with granulocytes and macrophages. Within a few days the proliferative phase of repair begins; fibroblasts arrive at the wound bed, attracted and stimulated to proliferate by mediators released from macrophages (Wahl, 1981). These fibroblasts gradually replace the majority of the leucocytes, and, as they do, the rate of collagen synthesis increases. Neovascularisation of the wound bed is essential for successful repair, and by the third or fourth day after injury the presence of endothelial cells marks its commencement. As with fibroblasts, this process is apparently influenced by macrophage-derived mediators (Banda et al, 1982; Polverini and Leibovich, 1984; Knighton et al, 1986).

In mammalian skin the end product of the healing process is scar tissue, covered on its superficial aspect by epidermal cells. Scar tissue generally forms rapidly, but is a poor substitute for natural dermis, and can cause immense physical and psychological problems, some life threatening. Control of the development of scar tissue and its replacement by tissue more closely resembling the dermis is thus of considerable importance.

Various modes of electrotherapy are now used widely as therapeutic agents in medicine and dentistry to accelerate repair, modify scar tissue production, and to reduce pain. The aim of this paper is to talk about the effect of two modes of electrotherapy, ultrasound and light, on tissue repair.

Ultrasound

Ultrasound can produce a wide range of effects depending on the parameters of the ultrasonic field and also the cell and tissue type irradiated.

Ultrasound is one of the most widely used forms of treatment in physiotherapy. A survey in 1985 revealed that in the UK 54% of all physiotherapy treatments in the private sector, and 20% in the NHS, involved the use of ultrasound (ter Haar, Dyson and Oakley, 1988). It is clearly important that any form of treatment as widely used as ultrasound should be used correctly. To do this we need to know what changes ultrasound can produce in tissues and by what mechanisms these changes are achieved.

There is clinical evidence that ultrasound affects the inflammatory phase of repair, for example, it reduces oedema (ElHag et al, 1985). In this study the effect of dexamethasone was compared with that of ultrasound in the reduction of oedema after wisdom tooth extraction. It was shown that very low levels of ultrasound (O.1W/cm², spatial average temporal average [SATA]) produced a reduction of post operative oedema. Although ultrasound did not reduce oedema to the same extent as the dexamethasone, ultrasound does not have the undesirable side-effects of anti-inflammatory steroids, e.g. suppression of the hypothalamopituitary-adrenal axis. Even though ultrasound and an anti-inflammatory drug both reduce oedema after injury, it does not necessarily follow that ultrasound is truly anti-inflammatory in its action. A paper published by Goddard et al (1983), looked at the effect of ultrasound irradiation on sites where bacteria-laden sponges had been implanted subcutaneously. It was found that ultrasound had no effect upon the production of fluid exudate or the infiltration of inflammatory cells.

The weight of the evidence in the literature suggests that ultrasound is not anti-inflammatory. It should be remembered that anti-inflammatory agents may inhibit repair, while the acceleration of the inflammatory phase can accelerate the whole process of healing. There is no evidence that ultrasound inhibits repair, on the contrary, it can speed it up. It is likely that ultrasound causes oedema reduction in trauma-induced inflammation by reducing the length of the inflammatory phase, so accelerating repair. Therefore early treatment may speed up the release of wound factors and so stimulate repair.

Work by Young and Dyson (1990a and b) showed that ultrasound at an intensity of O.1W/cm² SATA, and a frequency of either 0.75 or 3.0 MHz can accelerate the repair process when applied during the early inflammatory phase. In the experiment wounds treated with ultrasound, by 5 days after injury, contained more extensive granulation tissue, fewer inflammatory cells, and more fibroblasts (aligned in a manner conducive to efficient wound contraction) than the control wounds that received only sham-irradiations.

Many investigations have been carried out to find out what the underlying mechanisms of action of ultrasound are. Because ultrasound appears to be most effective when used during the early phase of repair many studies have looked at the interaction of ultrasound with cells known to be prevalent during this phase, e.g. mast cells and macrophages.

Mast cells are stationary sentinels found at sites prone to injury. Their degranulation initiates the response of the body to injury. Their granules are packed with pharmaco-logically active agents, some of which are of great significance in the repair process:

> Histamine, which stimulates exudation
> Heparil, which stimulates angiogenesis
> Chemotactic mediators, which stimulate leucocyte invasion

Fyfe and Chahl (1982) showed that a single treatment of ultrasound at an intensity O.1W/cm² SATA and at frequency of 3MHz induced mast cell degranulation in injured tissue. Even in intact skin, mast cell degranulation can be induced (Dyson and Luke, 1986), but the cells are less sensitive and, therefore, require higher ultrasound intensities (over 1.5W/cm² SATA).

Young and Dyson (1990c) examined the effect of ultrasound on another major inflammatory phase cell, the macrophage. They found that the treatment of macrophages in vitro with ultrasound, at an intensity of 0.5W/cm² SATA and at a frequency of either 0.75 or 3.0 MHz, stimulated the production of chemical mediators which were stimulatory in their effect on fibroblast proliferation. This observation explains, in part, why physiotherapists find ultrasound particularly effective when used during the inflammatory phase of repair, as this is when the macrophage is the predominant cell type.

There are a number of possible ways in which ultrasound could be stimulating cell activity. There is a lot of evidence to suggest that ultrasound alters cell membrane permeability to various ions, in particular calcium (Mummery, 1978; Mortimer, 1981; Mortimer and Dyson, 1988). Changes in cell permeability to calcium ions may have a dramatic effect on cell behaviour. Calcium ion fluxes, in response to membrane permeability changes, act as chemical signals (second messengers) which control the enzymatic activity of the cell and stimulate, for example, the increase in synthesis of specific proteins and their secretion (Katz, 1966; Douglas, 1968; Webster et al, 1978; Fyfe and Chahl, 1982).

Because the evidence suggests that therapeutic ultrasound affects the inflammatory phase of dermal repair, it is recommended that it be applied during this phase. Also, relatively low intensity levels (0.1W/cm² SATA) have been shown to be effective in producing the desired biological effects, therefore, there is no need to use the higher, potentially damaging, levels of ultrasound.

Light

There has been much interest in the biological effects of low level laser radiation since the pioneering work of Mester in the early 70s (Mester et al, 1985). However, despite the rapid expansion in the number of investigations into this modality, doubts still exist with regards to its efficacy. There are a number of reasons for this (Basford JK, 1986; King PR, 1989). The main reasons appear to be the anecdotal nature of the many reports on the clinical use of laser where trials have been carried out without adequate control groups and also with very low numbers of patients. The reports often do not give adequate information with regard to the physical parameters of the laser used which precludes attempts by other research groups to repeat the work.

One of the characteristics of laser radiation is that it is coherent; however, it has been shown that significant biological effects can be achieved by exposure to noncoherent light (Young et al, 1989; Karu, 1988). Even with a question mark hanging over the efficacy of light therapy, laser and light therapy machines can now be found in many physiotherapy departments and are being used routinely for pain relief and to accelerate tissue repair. This section of the paper looks at some of the clinical and laboratory evidence showing areas where light therapy may be effective.

Light therapy has been used to produce relief from chronic pain. Walker (1983) looked at the effect of laser treatment on 26 patients suffering from either trigeminal neuralgia, post-herpatic neuralgia, sciatica or osteoarthritis. The laser used was a He-Ne operating at a wavelength of 632nm. The laser was pulsed at a frequency of 20Hz. The treatment was found to be successful in 19 out of the 26 patients. Successful treatment was associated with a temporary elevation in serotonin metabolism, i.e. an increase in 5 hydroxy indole acetic acid excretion. It was claimed that since there were no placebo responders in the group, the effect was not a placebo effect. Although it was suggested by Walker that the results obtained could be explained by an increase in serotonin production by a pain relief centre such as the raphe magnus nucleus, there are other possible sites that the serotonin could have come from, e.g. platelets.

Moore (1988) published results of a double blind cross over trial of low level laser therapy in the treatment of post herpatic neuralgia. The laser used was a galliumaluminium-arsenide model with a wavelength of 820nm. The power output was 60 mW (continuous wave) and the treatments 20 minutes in length, twice weekly. The patients were divided into 2 groups, one given 4 laser treatments followed by 4 sham-irradiations, and the other given the 4 sham-irradiations first. Pain was assessed on a linear analogue scale before each treatment. All patients experienced a reduction in pain and in a limited follow up it was shown that pain relief was maintained in the majority of patients.

Work on the effect of light on tissue repair was initiated by Mester 1971 (Mester, 1985) who showed that exposure of partial thickness skin wounds to a ruby laser increased the rate of epithelial growth. More recently Dyson and Young (1986) showed that full-thickness excised lesions could be stimulated to repair more rapidly when exposed to a combined pulsed infrared and continuous He-Ne laser. Laser irradiated wounds were shown to contract more than the control wounds when the infrared radiation was delivered at a frequency of 700Hz, however, wound contraction was inhibited when the infrared was pulsed at a frequency of 1200Hz. Differential cell counts carried out on histological sections of the wound bed showed that there were significantly more fibroblasts in the granulation tissue of the 700Hz treated wounds and they were aligned in a specific orientation, parallel to each other, at right-angles to the direction of blood vessel growth. This orientation is indicative of a wound undergoing active contraction. The lack of this parallel orientation of the fibroblasts seen in the control wounds and those treated with 1200Hz infrared indicates that they were not yet fully cooperating with each other in inducing contraction, and this is probably why there was less contraction seen in these wounds.

As with ultrasound, it appears that light therapy is particularly effective when used during the inflammatory phase of repair, therefore, it is possible that its mode of action on the wound healing process is similar, i.e. the light interacts with the macrophages, encouraging them to release wound mediators which in turn stimulate the onset of the later stages of repair. Work was carried out by Young and Dyson (1989) to test this hypothesis. U-937 cells (Sundstrom and Nilsson, 1976) were either sham-irradiated (control group) or exposed in vitro to one of a range of wavelengths of light. Some of the light sources were coherent, others noncoherent. The average power output of all the probes was 15mW, the power density 2.4J/cm^2, and the wavelengths were 660, 820, 870 and 880nm. After irradiation the macrophages were placed in an incubator for 12 hours to allow the synthesis and secretion of wound mediators into the surrounding medium. The medium was then removed and placed on fibroblast cultures and their proliferation assessed over 132 hours. It was found that the following wavelengths, 660, 820 and 870nm encouraged the release of wound mediators which stimulated fibroblast proliferation, whereas 880nm had the opposite effect. It was also noticed, that as far as the response is concerned, the light need not be coherent.

El Sayed and Dyson (1990) showed that another important inflammatory cell, the mast cell, can also be stimulated by light therapy. Wavelengths which appeared to be the most effective in causing an increase in mast cell number and degranulation were 660, 820, 940 and 950 nm.

Many investigators have tried to produce hypotheses which explain how light can stimulate cells. First of all, to cause an effect, light as with any form of energy has to be absorbed. It has been proposed (Karu, 1988) that the photoabsorbers in mammalian cells are the respiratory pigments or cytochromes which are found in the mitochondria of all cells. The hypothesis is that light is absorbed by these photoacceptors causing short-term respiratory chain activation and oxidation of the electron acceptor NAD (nicotinamide adenine dinucleotide). This leads to changes in the redox status of both the mitochondria and the cytoplasm. As a result there is an increase in the ATP pool and cytoplasmic H+ concentration. The change in cytoplasmic pH can lead to cell membrane permeability changes to a variety of ions such as calcium which in turn can modify cell activity.

Work by Young et al (1990d) has shown that light therapy can modify calcium uptake in macrophages. The effect was shown to be wavelength, energy density and frequency dependent.

Summary

Evidence suggests that both ultrasound and light may be useful therapeutic modalities. Although, physically, they are very different in their nature (ultrasound being a form of mechanical, vibrational energy, and light an electromagnetic energy) the effects they can produce in injured tissues are very similar. They can both interact with cells such as macrophages and mast cells, stimulating the production of wound mediators. The mechanism of action on cells, however, appears to be different for the two modalities. With ultrasound the energy appears to exert its effect directly upon the membrane causing permeability changes, whereas with light the energy appears to be absorbed initially within the cell (by the mitochondria) triggering a series of intracellular events which lead eventually to a membrane permeability change.

There is a need for more carefully controlled clinical trials (in particular in the field of light therapy) to assess the clinical value of electrotherapy. Also, more work is needed to investigate the mechanisms of action to discover how best to achieve the desired biological effects. As yet, no conclusive experimental or clinical evidence exists to compare the effectiveness of ultrasound to light therapy.

References

Banda MJ, Knighton DR, Hunt TK and Werb Z. (1982) Isolation of a nonmitogenic angiogenesis factor from wound fluid. Proc Natl Acad Sci, USA, **79**, 7773-7777.

Basford JK. (1986) Low-energy treatment of pain and wounds: Hype, hope or hokum? Mayo Clinic Proceedings, **61**, 671-675.

Douglas WW. (1968) Stimulus-secretion coupling. The concept and clues from chromaffin and other cells. Br J Pharmacol, **34**, 453-474.

Dyson M and Luke DA. (1986). Induction of mast cell degranulation in skin by ultrasound. IEEE Transactions Ultrasound, Ferroelectrics, and Frequency Control, UFFC-33(2), 194-201.

Dyson M and Young SR. (1986) Effect of laser therapy on wound contraction and cellularity in mice. Lasers in Medical Science, **1**, 125-130.

Dyson M, Young SR, Pendle CL, Webster DF and Lang SM. (1988) Comparison of the effects of moist and dry conditions on dermal repair. J Invest Dermatol, **91**, 434-439.

ElHag M, Coghlan K, Christmas P, Harvey W and Harris M. (1985) The anti-inflammatory effects of dexamethasone and therapeutic ultrasound in oral surgery. British Journal of Oral and Maxillofacial Surgery, **23**, 17-23.

Fyfe MC and Chahl LA. (1982) Mast cell degranulation. possible mechanism of action of therapeutic ultrasound. Ultrasound Med Biol, **8**, 62.

Goddard DH, Revell PA, Cason J, Gallagher S and Currey HLF. (1983) Ultrasound has no anti - inflammatory effect. Ann Rheum Dis, **42**, 582-584.

ter Haar G, Dyson M and Oakley S. (1988) Ultrasound in physiotherapy in the United Kingdom; results of a questionnaire. Physiotherapy Practice, **4**, 69-72.

Karu TI. (1988) Molecular mechanisms of the therapeutic effect of low-intensity laser irradiation. Lasers in Life Sciences, **2**, 53-74.

Katz B. (1966) Nerve, muscle and synapse. New York, McGraw-Hill pp. 63-85.

King PR. (1989) Low level laser therapy: a review. Lasers in Medical Science, **4**, 141-150.

Knighton DR, Ciresi KF, Fiegel VD, Austen LL and Butler CL. (1986) Classification and treatment of chronic nonhealing wounds. Successful treatment with autologous platelet-derived wound healing factors (PDWHF) Am Surg. **204**, 323-330.

Mester, E, Mester AF and Mester A. (1985) The biomedical effects of laser application. Lasers in Surgery and Medicine. **5**, 31-39.

Metchnikof E. (1891) Lectures on the comparative Pathology of Inflammation. Dover, New York.

Moore KC, Hira N, Kumar PS et al. (1988) A double blind crossover trial of low level laser therapy in the treatment of post herpatic neuralgia. Laser Therapy. Pilot Issue, pp. 7-9.

Mortimer AJ. (1981) Effects of ultrasound on membrane electrophysiology. In: Mortimer AJ and Lee N. (eds) Proc Intnl Symp on Therapeutic Ultrasound. Canadian Physiotherapy Association, pp. 67-92.

Mortimer AJ and Dyson M. (1988) The effect of therapeutic ultrasound on calcium uptake in fibroblasts. Ultrasound Med Biol, 14, 499-506.

Mummery CL. (1978). The effect of ultrasound on fibroblasts in vitro. University of London. PhD Thesis.

Polverini PJ and Leibovich JS. (1984) Induction of neovascularisation in vivo by tumor associated macrophages. Lab Invest, 51, 635-342.

Ross R and Benditt EP. (1961) Wound healing and collagen formation 1. sequential changes in components of guinea pig skin wounds observed in the electron microscope. J Biophys Biochem Cytol, 11, 677-700.

El Sayed SO and Dyson M. (1990) Comparison of the effect of multiwavelength light produced by a cluster of semiconductor diodes and of each individual diode on mast cell number and degranulation in intact and injured skin. Lasers in Surgery and Medicine, 10, 559 -568.

Sundstrom C and Nilsson K. (1976) Establishment and characterisation of a human histiocytic lymphoma cell line (U-937). Int J Cancer, 17, 565-577.

Wahl SM. (1981) The role of mononuclear cells in the wound repair process in: The Surgical Wound, (P Dineen and G Hildick-Smith, eds), Lea and Febiger, Philadelphia, pp. 63-74.

Walker JB. (1983) Relief from chronic pain by low power laser irradiation. Neuroscience Letters, 43, 339-344.

Webster,DF, Pond JB, Dyson M and Harvey W. The role of cavitation in the in vitro stimulation of proteinsynthesis in human fibroblasts by ultrasound. Ultrasound Med Biol, 4, 343-351.

Young SR, Bolton PA, Dyson M, Harvey W and Diamantopoulos C. (1988) Macrophage responsiveness to light therapy. Lasers in Surgery and Medicine, 9, 497 -505.

Young SR and Dyson M. (1990a) Effect of therapeutic ultrasound excised skin lesions on the healing of full-thickness Ultrasonics, 28, 175-180.

Young SR and Dyson M. (1990b) The effect of therapeutic ultrasound on angiogenesis. Ultrasound Med Biol, 16, 261-269.

Young SR and Dyson M. (1990c) Macrophage responsiveness to therapeutic ultrasound. Ultrasound Med Biol, 16, 809-816.

Young SR, Dyson M. and Bolton PA. (1990d) Effect of light on calcium uptake by macrophages. Laser Therapy, 2, 53-57

Yurt RW. (1981) Role of the mast cell in trauma. cited in: The Surgical Wound, (P Dineen and G Hildick-Smith, eds) Lea and Ferbiger, Philadelphia pp. 37-62.

Rehabilitation following anterior cruciate ligament reconstruction - considerations related to immobility

J.P. Long

Abstract. The effects of immobility have been observed related to post-traumatic and postoperative cases of the knee. Changes can be observed in articular cartilage and subchondral bone, the ligament-bone complex and peri-articular musculature. Recent surgical and rehabilitative modifications have been developed to allow acceleration of rehabilitation following anterior cruciate ligament reconstruction prior to final maturation of the substitute graft. It is the responsibility of the clinician to individualize each rehabilitation program to coordinate biological healing with functional return.

Keywords: Anterior cruciate ligament, ligament reconstruction, repair, immobilisation

Introduction

Rehabilitation following anterior cruciate ligament (ACL) reconstruction continues to move in accelerated fashion in an effort to overcome complications such as prolonged knee stiffness, limitation of complete extension, delay in strength recovery, and anterior knee pain. At the same time, knee stability must be preserved.

Effects of immobilization upon the knee

Immobilization has been shown to affect the joint capsule with histochemical changes at 6 weeks including a decrease in the water content, increased collagen cross-linking, and a decrease in glycoaminoglycans. The torque required to move the knee joint may increase up to ten times the normally required force.

Changes in cartilaginous surfaces and subchondral bone also occur with immobilization. The "chondral unit" requires motion for nutrition and weight bearing stress to maintain biomechanical integrity. If the necessary mechanical stress is prevented, alteration in cartilage fluid dynamics may include a decrease in metachromasia, glucoaminoglycans, and a change in cartilage hydration. Histologically, chondrocyte clumping and subchondral bone atrophy become apparent. These observed changes begin within days of initiation of immobility and can be irreversible after eight weeks. These changes affect both the tibial-femoral and patello-femoral articular surfaces.

Laboratory studies indicate that early ground substance changes can be reversed through initiation of motion. However, overloading through inappropriate rehabilitation
creates disruption of the "chondral unit" followed by irreversible, permanent progressive cartilage degeneration (Woo et al, 1975).

The ligament-bone complex reacts to immobility by a weakening of the bone attachment site and ligament. Tipton (1967) demonstrated loss of ligament strength particularly at the ligament insertion. Ligaments inserting into the bone through a zone of fibrocartilage such as the ACL and proximal portion of the superficial medial collateral ligament (MCL) are affected less by immobilization than are ligaments that insert directly into the bone through periosteum such as the distal portion of the MCL. In such an example, the severe effects of immobilization are related to disuse osteoporosis.

Noyes (1974) determined that following eight weeks of immobilization, the anterior cruciate ligament elongated 40-55 percent greater per unit load than the nonimmobilized anterior cruciate ligament. It was also determined that the maximum load at failure for the ACL was decreased by 39 percent following eight weeks of immobilization. After five months, strength continued to be decreased by 21 percent and by 9 percent at twelve months.

Haggmark and Ericksson (1979) noted peri-articular musculature changes secondary to immobility of five weeks include a decrease of oxidative enzymes including succinodehydrogenase (SDH), selective atrophy of Type I (slow twitch or red) muscle fibers, and a 30-47 percent decrease in total mass. Factors affecting the rate of muscle atrophy include joint position - atrophy occurs more quickly with the muscle in a shortened position. Joint effusion may cause neuromuscular inhibition with an increased rate of atrophy.

ACL reconstruction and immobility

The goal of the sports medicine clinician may be to eliminate the immobility phase through appropriate graft selection, placement, fixation, and rehabilitation. However, a brief period of relative immobilization may be necessary to control forces and prevent disruption of the graft. Some degree of immobility may be necessary especially with multiple ligament and meniscal repairs where the task of reconstruction or repairing multiple ligaments isometrically may be more challenging.

The present post-operative program following ACL reconstruction at the Cleveland Clinic includes range of motion exercise on Day 1 including active knee flexion to tolerance in supine and prone positions and passive extension to 0 degrees. The knee immobilizer is worn at night and a Don Joy 4-point Knee

Orthosis for daily wear.

Similarly, Shelbourne (1990) advocates full knee extension on the first post-operative day and immediate weight bearing according to the patient's tolerance. Emphasis on full extension has been related to observation of athletes through the years experiencing dissatisfaction secondary to extremity pain and fatigue associated with extension loss. Consistent with the protocol practised by this author, Shelbourne (1990), also stresses importance of closed kinetic chain exercises. These exercises are characterized by joint compression associated with weight bearing and consequent reduction of patellofemoral forces compared to those that accompany the traditional open kinetic chain exercises performed in the zone of 30-90 degrees of knee flexion. Closed kinetic chain exercises allow functional stresses to be placed on the joint similar to weight bearing activities. Joint compression can also contribute to stability and reduction of shear forces that occur with open kinetic chain exercises.

Rutherford (1988) points out the importance of taskspecific exercise and task-related practice of movement patterns utilized in daily life and athletic activities rather than emphasis on strength training for isolated muscle groups.

The role of exercise in counteracting the deleterious effects of immobilization was studied by Cabaud (1967). Using a population of rats performing various treadmill protocol, it was determined that endurance exercise performed at low duration and high frequency gave a significant increase in strength and stiffness of the anterior cruciate ligament.

Counteracting the effects of immobility - motion and modalities

Motion has been demonstrated to have the advantages of enhancing joint mobility and preventing contracture, and there is strong experimental evidence indicating that articular cartilage can be preserved through movement. Noyes (1974) demonstrated that primates that had undergone ACL reconstruction had significant articular cartilage degeneration when four weeks of post-operative plaster casts were used. In contrast, with use of continuous passive motion (CPM), the articular cartilage appeared normal without observable gross lesions.

Salter (1984) has observed that CPM facilitated metaplasia from undifferentiated mesenchymal tissue to hyaline articular cartilage and more rapid complete healing of cartilage defects in rabbits. Histological appearance of repaired tissue was maintained for up to one year. Whether there is benefit of CPM on eventual ligament stiffness and strength properties when applied for a few weeks during the initial healing process has been questioned (Butler, 1983).

Following ACL reconstruction, precautions include emphasis on passive motion assuming appropriate substitute selection, graft placement, and fixation have been achieved. Although the composite fibers of the ACL have no single isometric point, isometric placement of the replacement graft is consider substitutes have not duplicated the complex orientation of the normal ACL (Jackson & Drez, 1987). Passive range of motion through full extension is permitted while active knee extension is limited due to the associated anterior drawer forces.

Mobilization has been used as a means to counteract reflex inhibition which may accompany knee joint injury or reconstruction. Major causes of reflex inhibition include joint pain, swelling, and immobilization which lead to generation of afferent stimuli that impede voluntary activation of supporting musculature. This inhibition affects the quadriceps femoris to a greater degree than hamstrings and within the quadriceps group, the vastus medialis is most affected. (Morrisey, 1989).

While controlled motion may be indicated following ACL reconstruction, postoperative pain and effusion may disallow mobilization. Physiotherapy to reduce knee pain may consist of cold, iontophoresis, phonophoresis, and transcutaneous nerve stimulation (TENS). The effectiveness of TENS in increasing quadriceps activation by lessening knee pain has been reviewed by Morrisey (1989). However, the literature remains inconclusive as to the use of TENS, functional electrical stimulation (FES) and CPM. Andersson and Lipscomb (1989) performed a prospective, randomized study of five groups of 20 patients with the same ACL reconstruction. The intent of the study was to determine the effect of TENS, immobilization in extension vs. flexion FES and CPM. It was concluded that TENS did not decrease pain medicine required or improve any parameter of rehabilitative performance. In comparison to immobilization in extension, immobilization in flexion with early limited motion revealed no clear difference in stability. FES did not reduce atrophy, but was effective in minimizing muscle strength decreases that occur with immobilization. CPM reduced the necessity for manipulation compared to immobilization in extension but was not as effective as early limited motion. In summary, the optimal rehabilitation protocol included FES and immobilization in flexion with early limited motion.

Similar conclusions regarding CPM and ACL reconstructions have been drawn by Sachs (1990), who in a prospective randomized study of 50 ACL reconstructions did not find improved range of motion at six months versus controls. Noyes (1987) also studied the initiation of active and passive knee motion in open and arthroscopic ACL reconstructions and found no statistical difference in range of motion, pain medication, or hospital stay. In addition, it was noted that early knee motion did not lead to deleterious effects, such as disruption of ligament repairs or reconstructions. Importantly, it was stated that early motion may potentially aid in aligning collagen fibers and promoting early healing, but it should be realized that soft tissue healing involves a lengthy maturation process as ligament strength and stiffness properties increase over many months. Despite acceleration of rehabilitation, prolonged protection of the graft remains important.

Functional return vs. biological healing

The current trend in sports medicine is to accelerate rehabilitation following ACL reconstruction based on advances in surgical technique and efforts to counteract the effects of immobility. Thus far, there have been few reported failures, but a greater number of cases and longer follow-up need to be considered. The majority of Cleveland Clinic Sports Medicine Staff and all members of the American Academy of Orthopaedic Surgeons ACL Instructional Panel continue to return athletes to competitive sports at approximately one year post reconstruction based on concern for the parameters of biological healing.

References

Andersson AF and Lipscomb AB. (1989) Analysis of rehabilitation techniques after anterior cruciate reconstruction. Amer J Sports Med, **17**, 154-160.

Cabaud WE, Chalty A, Gildengorin V and Feltman RJ. (1980) Exercise effects on the strength of rat anterior, cruciate ligament. Amer J Sports Med, **8**, 79-86.

Haggmark T and Ericksson E. (1979) Cylinder or mobile cast brace after knee ligament surgery: a clinical analysis and morphologic and enzymatic study of changes in the quadriceps muscle. Amer J Sports Med, 7,48.

Jackson DW and Drez, D. (1987) The anterior cruciate deficient knee. The CV Mosby Company, St Louis.

Morrissey MD. (1989) Reflex inhibition of thigh muscles in knee surgery. Sports Med, **7**, 263-276.

Noyes FR, Mangina RE, Barber S. (1987) Early knee motion after open and arthroscopic anterior cruciate ligament reconstruction. Amer J Sports Med, **15**, 149-160.

Noyes FR, Torick PJ, Hyde WB et al. (1974) Biomechanics of ligament failure: an analysis of immobilization, exercise, and reconditioning effec primates. J Bone Joint Surg, **56A**, 1406-1418.

Rutherford OM. (1988) Muscular coordination and strength training: implications of injury rehabilitation. Sports Med, **5**, 196-202.

Sachs R et al. (1990) Complications of knee ligament surgery. In: Daniel D, Akeson W, O'Connor J (eds) Knee Ligaments: Structure, Function, Injury, and Repair, Raven Press, 505-520.

Salter RB, Hamilton WW, Wedge JH et al (1984) Clinical application of basic research on continuous passive motion for disorders and injuries of synovia, joints: A preliminary report of a feasibility study. J Orthop Res, **1**, 325-342.

Shelbourne KD and Nilz P. (1990) Accelerated rehabilitation after anterior cruciate ligament reconstruction. Amer J Sports Med, **18**, 292-298.

Tipton CM, Schild RJ and Tomanek RJ. (1967) Influence of physical activity on the strength of knee ligaments in Rats. Amer J Physiol, **212**, 783-787.

Woo SL-Y, Matthews JV, Akeson WH et al. (1975) The connective tissue response to immobility: a correlative study of biomechanical measurements of the normal and immobilized rabbit knee. Arthritis Rheum, **18**, 257-264.

Hyperbaric oxygen therapy for sports injuries

P.B. James

Abstract. In many countries hyperbaric oxygen therapy is established in the management of problem wounds and soft tissue injuries (Sheffield, 1988). In trauma, tissue injury leads to the release of vasoactive mediators and there is often an accompanying inflammatory response. The increase in microvascular permeability may be so great that proteinaceous oedema occurs, triggering the complement cascade. Despite greatly increased blood flow, hypoxia may develop because oedema limits oxygen transport co-incident with the invasion of cells which have a very high level of metabolic activity. The high dosages of oxygen available under pressure, which cause vasoconstriction and reduce oedema, can assist in healing by generating normal or even supranormal tissue oxygen values.

Keywords: Hyperbaric oxygen, inflammation, hypoxia, sports injuries. non-healing fractures and wounds.

Introduction

With the growth of the diving industry in the development of offshore gas and oil, hyperbaric technology has advanced at a dramatic pace in the UK. Hyperbaric oxygen, or, as it is better termed, high-dosage oxygen, is used routinely both in decompression procedures and to treat decompression sickness. In neurological decompression sickness pressures up to 3 atmospheres absolute are used. The dose time limits in diving have been established for over fifty years and are used as a guide in the use of hyperbaric oxygen therapy. Equally, pressure vessel and breathing apparatus development in diving have provided the basis for the therapeutic chambers used in medicine. The mechanisms involved in decompression sickness are relevant to other conditions. Research into neurological decompression sickness has shown that the mechanism is not simple embolic occlusion such as occurs in arterial gas embolism associated with burst lung. The bubbles arising from decompression are carried in the central venous return to the right side of the heart where they can be detected in the pulmonary artery en route to the lungs. If they pass through the lung filter and reach the brain, they may damage the blood-brain barrier in transit. The increased permeability may allow proteins and even red cells access to the nervous tissue and initiate an inflammatory reaction with complement activation leading to myelin damage. This mechanism is now recognised to be crucial in the demyelination in multiple sclerosis, which may also be due to microembolism (Carnochan et al, 1988).

335

Tissue trauma and inflammation

The disruption of cells from physical injury also releases inflammatory mediators which increase blood flow. There is an invasion of macrophages which are very metabolically active when the supply of oxygen may be severely limited by the increase in tissue water. Using the tuberculin response in Man, it has been shown that in the inflammatory reaction severe hypoxia may result from these mechanisms even when arterial oxygen levels and blood flow in the tissue, assessed by laser Doppler techniques, are well above normal (James, 1982). If this occurs, the central microcirculatory slowing may prevent the delivery of sufficient oxygen and lead to anoxia and tissue necrosis. Although mild hypoxia is a stimulus to capillary neogenesis, a minimum oxygen tension of about 30 mm Hg is required for capillary budding. The optimal tissue oxygen tension for fibroblast cell proliferation is about 80 mm Hg, which is twice the normal value breathing air (Mehm WJ et al, 1988). Hyperbaric oxygen therapy has been found to be effective in the reduction of oedema and necrosis in experimental compartment syndromes (Skyhar et al, 1986).

Haemorrhage often complicates injuries in sport and the release of ferrous ions from the breakdown of haemoglobin may lead to oxygen free radical production and consequent tissue damage. Fortunately, this is a short-lived phenomenon and it is important to relieve hypoxia which, by the formation of intermediate tissue products such as xanthine oxidase, may also potentiate oxygen free radical formation (Misra et al, 1971).

Hyperbaric oxygen in football injuries

An inexpensive monoplace chamber, originally designed in the University of Dundee and now made by Hyox Systems Ltd, has been used in two pilot studies in the treatment of footballers in Scotland. The injuries have involved soft tissue damage and connective tissue tears. In the studies the injured player and the team physiotherapist have been asked independently to assess the time expected for the injury to recover. This was then compared to the actual time taken using the hyperbaric oxygen therapy. In all cases the use of hyperbaric oxygen has more than halved the time taken for the injury to heal. Formal controlled studies are now to be undertaken.

References

Carnochan F, Abbot NC, Spence VA, Beck JS, James PB, Walker WF. (1988) Blood flow and respiratory gas measurements over normal and inflamed skin and their modification by oxygen supplementation. Proc XIVth Annual Meeting of the EUBS Grampian Health Board, Aberdeen, p. 38.

James PB. (1982) Evidence for subacute fat embolism as the cause of multiple sclerosis. Lancet, i, 380-386.

Mehm WJ, Pimsler M, Becker RL, Lissner CR. (1988) Effect of oxygen on in vitro fibroblast cell proliferation and collagen biosynthesis. J Hyp Med, 3, 227-34.

Misra HP, Fridovich I. (1971) The generation of superoxide radical during the autoxidation of ferritins. J Biol Chem, 246, 686-90.

Sheffield PJ. (1988) Tissue oxygen measurements. In: Davis JC, Hunt, TK (eds) Problem wounds: the role of oxygen, Elsevier, Amsterdam.

Skyhar MJ, Hargens AR, Strauss MB et al. (1986) Hyperbaric oxygen reduces edema and necrosis of skeletal muscle in compartment syndromes associated with hemorrhagic hypotension. J Bone Joint Surg, 68, 1218-24.

The effects of non-steroidal anti-inflammatory drugs on cartilage and connective tissue

G. Nuki

Abstract. Nonsteroidal anti-inflammatory drugs (NSAID) are widely used as adjuncts for the management of sports injuries. This paper reviews briefly the mode of action of NSAIDs and their effects on cartilage and the metabolism of connective tissue macromolecules. The clinical use of NSAIDs in patients with soft tissue injuries is also discussed briefly in relationship to their potential risks and benefits.

Keywords: Nonsteroidal Anti-inflammatory Drugs, Sports Injuries, Cartilage, Proteoglycan.

Introduction

In the United Kingdom approximately 8 million people consult general practitioners each year with a broad range of musculo/skeletal symptoms and more than 20 million prescriptions for non-steroidal anti-inflammatory drugs (NSAIDs) are issued. In the United States it was estimated that the number of prescriptions for NSAIDs in 1987 was 70 million and the worldwide market for this class of drugs approached 2 billion dollars (Roth, 1988). Although more than three quarters of those receiving NSAIDs are in the elderly age group the use of NSAIDs for sports related soft tissue injuries in younger people is considerable and increasing. Heere (1988) has suggested that as many as 1 million people in the Netherlands, 6-7% of the entire population, require such treatment for sports related injuries each year.

A recent review of the efficacy of NSAIDs in the treatment of ligament injuries by Almekinders (1990) suggests that the clinical evidence to support the assumption that NSAIDs are effective in speeding and improving recovery following soft tissue injury is by no means uniform or impressive while information on the ways in which NSAIDs may affect the pathophysiology of soft tissue injury and repair is scanty.

This short review includes a brief discussion of the mechanisms of action of NSAIDs and reviews recent experimental work on the effects of these drugs on the metabolism of cartilage.

Mechanism of action

There are 3 lines of evidence to suggest that metabolites of arachidonic acid are key mediators of inflammation (Forrest and Brooks, 1988). Firstly there is a good deal of data from a wide range of experimental animal models and from tissues of human disease associated with clinical inflammation which shows that the cyclo-oxygenase derived metabolites prostaglandins E_2 and F1a and thromboxane B_2; and the lipoxygenase derived arachidonic acid metabolites leucotriene B_4, C_4 and D_4 can be detected in relevant concentrations at the site of inflammation. Secondly there is evidence that these purified metabolites can mimic various aspects of inflammation in suitable models (Table 1).

Table 1.   Pro-inflammatory effects of some relevant arachidonate metabolites.

Metabolite	Proinflammatory effects
PGE_2	Increase vascular permeability, potentiate PGF1a oedema, neutrophil accumulation and prostacyclin hyperalgesia caused by other mediators.
Thromboxanes	Stimulate platelet aggregation and degranulation.
Leucotrienes LTB_4, LTC_4, LTD_4	Chemotactic. Increase vascular permeability.

Thirdly, there is evidence that inhibitors of arachidonic acid metabolism have potent anti-inflammatory effects. In 1971 Vane demonstrated that inhibition of the cyclo-oxygenase enzymes responsible for the metabolism of arachidonic acid to prostaglandins was a property common to all NSAIDs and it was subsequently shown that the rank order of potency of NSAIDs as prostaglandin synthetase inhibitors in vitro roughly reflected their potency as anti-inflammatory agents in vivo (Higgs et al, 1980). However the doses of NSAIDs appear to exceed those necessary for inhibition of prostaglandin synthetase (Abramson and Weissman, 1989) and this has focussed attention on other effects of these drugs which may contribute to their anti-inflammatory action. Notable among these are the capacity of NSAIDs to interfere with a variety of membrane associated processes that result in changes in polymorpho-nuclear leucocyte and monocyte function. These include G protein regulated processes and inhibition of NADPH oxidase in neutrophils and phospho-lipase C in macrophages. The NSAIDs currently available probably do not inhibit lipo-oxygenase enzyme activity significantly in vivo and it is unlikely that secondary effects of NSAIDs on lymphocyte function, such as the "unmasking" of T-cell suppressor activity (Cush et al, 1990) have any relevance to their anti-inflammatory effect in sports injuries where it is assumed that physical damage to cells and collagen lead to an acute inflammatory reaction and subsequently wound healing.

Effects on cartilage and connective tissue metabolism

Tendon and bone

There is rather little published data on the effects of NSAIDs on intact or injured tendons in laboratory animals. Vogel (1977) showed that aspirin, indomethacin and phenylbutazone fed to rats for a 10 day period in doses ranging from 0.03 to 1000mg/kg resulted in significant increases in tensile strength and insoluble collagen content of rat tail tendons and this was attributed to an increase in collagen cross-linking and a decrease in collagen degradation. In muscle-tendon (Almekinders and Gilbert, 1986) and medial collateral ligament injury models in the rat knee (Dahners et al, 1986; 1988) treatment with piroxicam in relatively high doses resulted in an initial decrease followed by an increase in mechanical strength. By contrast the administration of pharmacologically relevant doses of NSAIDs such as indomethacin or ibuprofen inhibits fracture healing in rats (Allen et al, 1968; Ro et al, 1976) and rabbits (Sudmann and Hagen, 1976; Tornquist and Lindholm, 1980) and slows the recovery of bone strength in response to torsional stress following experimental cortical damage (Tornquist et al, 1984). In patients undergoing hip arthroplasty NSAIDs inhibit the formation of heterotopic new bone (Ahrengart et al, 1988).

Cartilage

Because NSAIDs are used widely and for prolonged periods in the management of rheumatoid arthritis and osteo-arthritis there has been a great deal of interest and concern about the possible effects of NSAIDs on the metabolism of articular cartilage (Ghosh, 1988; Brandt, 1991).

At the clinical level there has always been concern that the pain relief obtained from the use of NSAIDs could lead to overuse and accelerated bone and cartilage destruction in patients with arthritis whose joints were already damaged. From clinical anecdotes and small uncontrolled series it has been suggested that the prolonged use of NSAIDs and particularly indomethacin could result in a particular form of analgesic arthropathy ("indomethacin hip") which is characterised by rapid loss of articular cartilage and bone with relatively little osteophyte formation (Coke, 1967; Arora and Maudsley, 1968; Solomon, 1973; Milner, 1973). More recent work has pointed to the fact that rapid destruction of hips in patients with OA is not confined to those using NSAIDs and emphasised the fact that this group of predomiantly elderly female patients are particularly troubled with pain making the overuse hypothesis less plausible (Docherty et al, 1986).

Nevertheless the possibility that NSAIDs and especially indomethacin may have direct toxic effects on cartilage has been kept alive by two clinical studies showing greater radiological destruction in patients with hip OA taking indomethacin (Ronningen and Langelands, 1989) or NSAIDs (Newman and Ling, 1985) when compared with patients not treated with regular NSAIDs. Docherty (1989) criticised these studies on grounds of questionable radiographic assessment and failure to consider other factors which might influence disease progression as well as for their retrospective design and small patient numbers. A more recent randomised prospective comparison of the use of indomethacin and azapropazone (a relatively weak prostaglandin synthetase inhibitor) in patients with hip OA awaiting hip replacement (Rashad et al, 1989) suggested radiological, biochemical and pathological progression was more rapid in the indomethacin treated group who came to hip arthroplasty more quickly, but this study has also been criticised on methodological grounds (Brooks and Ghosh, 1990).

At the laboratory level experiments have been undertaken to examine the effects of a variety of NSAIDs on both the synthesis and degradation of cartilage macromolecules.

In vitro studies on rabbit and bovine articular cartilage have shown that aspirin, diclofenac, indomethacin and phenylbutazone at concentrations of 10^{-4}-10^{-6} M inhibit proteoglycan degradation by inhibiting the release of neutral proteinases from polymorphonuclear leucocytes without having any significant direct effect on the enzymes themselves (Perper and Oronsky, 1974; Kruze et al, 1977). Other studies have shown that the number of NSAIDs or their active metabolites are moderately active in inhibiting purified polymorph elastase and cethepsin G (Stephens et al, 1980; Lentini et al, 1987). Although Shinmei et al, 1985 were unable to demonstrate attentuation of proteoglycan degradation by chondrocyte metalloproteinase in vitro following treatment with aspirin, indomethacin or tiaprofenic acid others have shown dose dependent suppression of cartilage stromolysin activity in vitro by tiaprofenic acid (Martel-Pelletier and Pelletier, 1989) and one clinical study has shown reduction of stromolysin activity in cartilage and synovium from patients with OA coming to hip replacement who were treated with tiaprofenic acid for two months prior to surgery (Vignon et al, 1990).

Oxygen-derived free radicals released from polymorphs or mononuclear phagocytes in inflammatory lesions may lead to direct degradation of matrix macromolecules. In vitro studies have shown that salycylic acid derivatives (Haggag et al, 1986) and NSAIDs (Minta and Williams, 1985) can suppress superoxide anion generation from activated polymorphonuclear leucocytes. Ex vivo studies on polymorphs taken from patients with osteoarthritis and rheumatoid arthritis treated with piroxicam showed evidence of inhibition of superoxide anion generation (Biemond et al, 1986; Van Epps et al, 1987). Cytokines such as interleukin-1 (IL-1) and tumour necrosis factor (TNFa) are currently thought to be important mediators of cartilage destruction in inflammatory joint diseases but NSAIDs could not be shown to have significant chondro-protective action in antigen induced arthritis in mice (de Vries and Van der Berg, 1989). Herman et al (1987; 1991) have however suggested that "catabolin" activity (assumed to be due to IL-1 or related cytokines) in the synovium from patients with OA was suppressed by piroxicam but not by indomethacin or salicylates and this further suggested that this might be due to a selective increase in IL-1 inhibitor production. Pelletier and Martel-Pelletier (1989) also detected IL-1 in OA cartilage and synovium and showed that tiaprofenic acid inhibited proteoglycan catabolism and metalloproteinase activity ex vivo even in the presence of IL-1. These workers (Pelletier and Martel-Pelletier, 1991) and others (Howell et al, 1991) have shown that this NSAID can inhibit proteoglycan degradation and the progression of cartilage defects in the canine model of OA which follows sectioning of the anterior cruciate ligament.

NSAIDs also have variable effects on biosynthesis of cartilage proteoglycans by chondrocytes which appear to be independent of their anti-inflammatory actions.

In vitro studies showed that proteoglycans synthesis was inhibited in human and canine cartilage slices incubated with salicylates (Palmoski and Brandt, 1979) and some other NSAIDs (Palmoski and Brandt, 1980) in a dose dependent manner (Table 2). Indomethacin, piroxicam and diclofenac have not significant effect on proteoglycan synthesis. Sulindac sulphide had a modest stimulatory effect while benoxaprofen, subsequently withdrawn because of hepatotoxicity, was alone in stimulating proteoglycan synthesis significantly (Palmoski and Brandt, 1983a).

The inhibitory effects of salicylate and other NSAIDs were considerably greater in cartilage slices from dogs with experimentally induced osteoarthritis following section of the anterior cruciate ligament (Palmoski et al, 1980). In vivo studies in this dog model showed that degenerative changes were increased in dogs fed with aspirin to maintain serum salicylate concentrations in the 20-25mg/dl range but cartilage from the contra-lateral unoperated joint and from normal control dogs fed aspirin were histochemically and biochemically normal (Palmoski and Brandt, 1983b). Aspirin also decreased proteoglycan concentrations, rates of synthesis and the extractability of proteoglycans from canine articular cartilage in another dog model where articular cartilage atrophy follows immobilisation of a limb (Palmoski and Brandt, 1982). These investigators undertook some further experiments which support the hypothesis that there is an inverse relationship between the proteoglycan concentration in articular cartilage and the uptake of NSAID (Palmoski and Brandt, 1983c). The contrasting effects of different NSAIDs on proteoglycan synthesis and articular cartilage may in part reflect differing binding properties. In this regard it is of interest that the partition coefficient of diclofenac in normal and osteoarthritic

Table 2.   NSAIDs : Effects on chondrocyte proteoglycan synthesis in vitro

Inhibitors
    Salicylates
    Ibuprofen
    Fenoprofen
    Isoxicam
    Tolmetin

No effect
    Indomethacin
    Piroxicam
    Naproxen
    Diclofenac

Stimulators
    Sulindac
    Benoxaprofen
    Tiaprofenic acid

cartilage is threefold higher than that of salicylate and piroxicam (Brandt, 1991). Other workers have shown tiaprofenic acid is another NSAID which does not inhibit proteoglycan synthesis in cartilage in in vitro studies in the concentration range 0.5 micromole-10 micromole (Franchimont et al, 1983; Muir et al, 1988). Recent in vitro work using chondrocyte mono-layer cultures as well as cartilage explants suggested that only diclofenac, from among the NSAIDs examined, stimulated proteoglycan synthesis at physiological concentrations (0.1 micromole/ml) (Coller and Ghosh, 1991). It is interesting that as long ago as 1982 Maier and Wilhelmi reported that oral administration of diclofenac (1-3mg/kg) to C57 black mice would reduce the frequency of occurrence and severity of the spontaneous osteo-arthritis to which this species is prone and Kalbhen (1984) has shown that while the intra-articular injection of most NSAIDs into the joints of chickens induced degenerative arthritis this was not the case following 4 months of weekly intra-articular injection of 2mg of diclofenac.

In summary, although there is a good deal of in vitro and animal experimental data as well as a little preliminary patient data to suggest that individual NSAIDs may differ in their effects on cartilage proteoglycan synthesis, there is insufficient human data at the present time to justify claims that azapropozone, diclofenac, sulindac or tiaprofenic acid have significant clinical "chondroprotective" action.

Clinical use of NSAIDs for the management of sports injuries

Traditionally acute musculo-skeletal sports injuries have been managed with rest, elevation, compression and ice-packs. Increasingly, however, since the early 1970s NSAIDs have been added to the therapeutic regime to counter the symptoms and signs of acute inflammation that follow soft tissue injuries. Reviewing the English language literature in sports medicine in 1990 Almekinders identified 35 clinical reports of trials of NSAIDs for soft tissue injury. Not less than 20 of these were considered scientifically unsatisfactory or inconclusive even though the majority were double-blind prospective comparisons of 2 NSAIDs. It is seldom possible to demonstrate drug efficiency in a comparative trial of 2 NSAIDs in patients with soft tissue injuries unless a placebo group is included because symptoms will improve spontaneously, and usually rapidly, depending on the site and severity of the injury. Because the natural history of recovery is so variable it is very important to try and include large numbers of patients with a single type of sports injury, even in placebo controlled trials, if conclusive evidence of efficacy of an NSAID is to be obtained as one is largely dependent on subjective assessments of outcome (Honig, 1988). Of the 15 placebo controlled trials reviewed by Almekinders (1990) only 8 studied a single type of ligamentous injury (6 ankle, 2 knee) and in only 4 of these was the NSAID clearly better than placebo (Van Heerden, 1977; Viljakka and Rokkanen, 1983; McLatchie et al, 1985; Hutson, 1986). NSAIDs were also shown to be superior to placebo in 4 other trials in patients with a variety of soft tissue injuries (Fitch and Gray, 1974; Krishnan, 1977; Santelli et al, 1980; Lereim and Gabor, 1988). Almekinder's review (1990) showed that the average duration of therapy in these trials was 9.2 days ranging from 4-28 days. No single NSAID is clearly more effective than others and optimal doses have really not been defined accurately for most drugs.

Delayed onset muscle soreness (DOMS) and weakness are separate problems which commonly follow unaccustomed exercise. The soreness and stiffness, which begin typically about 8 hours after muscular exercise, are associated with dramatic rises in plasma levels of muscle enzymes suggesting muscle damage (Newham et al, 1983 and 1987). Frank muscle fibre necrosis has been demonstrated both in marathon runners and following intense eccentric exercise (Hikida et al, 1983; Friden et al, 1983). As the muscle necrosis in marathon runners (Hikida et al, 1983) and in others experiencing delayed onset muscle soreness can be associated with cellular changes of acute inflammation (Smith et al, 1988) it has been suggested that NSAIDs might be effective in reducing symptoms and muscle damage and even allowing increased training loads. Although there is one report of reduction in muscle soreness following treatment with Aspirin (Bansil et al, 1985) the majority of studies found NSAIDs to be ineffective in reducing DOMS (Kuipers et al, 1985; Donnelly et al, 1988; Donnelly et al, 1990). Indeed in one placebo controlled trial anti-inflammatory doses of Ibuprofen not only failed to reduce DOMS but actually appeared to be associated with significantly higher levels of serum creatine kinase, possibly suggesting increased muscle breakdown (Donnelly et al, 1990). In general DOMS is not a serious problem. It usually remits spontaneously in about 72 hours and it can be prevented by prior training (Byrne et al, 1985).

The marginal benefits of using NSAIDs in patients with sports injuries need to be balanced against potential risks. In recent years there has been considerable concern about the risks of this class of drugs. No less than one quarter of all serious adverse reactions reported to the UK Committee on Safety of Medicines were associated with NSAIDs (Committee on Safety of Medicines, 1986). Between 1964 and 1985 the CSM received approximately 3,500 reports of upper gastro-intestinal bleeding or perforation in patients using NSAIDs and 600 of these events were fatal. 90% of these fatalities were however in patients over the age of 60 and it seems that elderly women may be particularly at risk (Mann, 1985). Risks are likely to be much smaller in young and fit people who use NSAIDs for sports injuries, where the drugs are only taken for short periods.

The most important adverse effects of NSAIDs are listed in Table 3.

Table 3.   NSAIDs: potentially life threatening adverse reactions

        Gastric haemorrhage/perforation
        Agranulocytosis/aplastic anaemia
        Stevens-Johnson syndrome
        Toxic epidermal necrolysis
        Asthma/anaphlaxis
        Drug interactions/Warfarin
        Fluid retention/cardiac failure
        Renal failure
        Hepatic failure

Studies have shown that as many as 20% of people exposed to NSAIDs for as little as 1 month have endoscopic evidence of frequently asymptomatic peptic ulceration (Roth et al, 1987) and prospective case control studies have demonstrated a 3.2 risk ratio for serious gastric ulcer complications and death in persons taking NSAIDs (Sommerville et al, 1986). The overall risks to life are however very small. Inman and Rawson (1987) calculated that the incidence of serious upper gastrointestinal tract haemorrhage or ulcer perforation in persons taking NSAIDs was 3-7 per 1,000 years of therapy and the incidence of fatal skin reactions (Wilholm et al, 1987) agranulocytosis and aplastic anaemia (International Agranulocytosis and Aplastic Anaemia Study, 1986) are 0.1-0.21, 0.02-0.05 and 0.01-0.02 per thousand person years of therapy respectively (Henry, 1988).

In the last few years a number of NSAIDs have been marketed as preparations for topical use. Although trials of these gels are characterised by large placebo responses they have been shown to be significantly better than placebo for the management of soft tissue trauma in some studies (McLatchie et al, 1989). As systemic absorption of these topically applied NSAIDs is small it is likely that the risks of serious adverse events will be diminished when compared with NSAIDs taken orally so it seems sensible to consider their use initially in subjects with sports injuries where NSAID therapy is felt to be indicated.

In conclusion one can say that there is some evidence that NSAIDs do have marginal efficacy in relieving symptoms following sports injuries. Although there is some evidence to suggest that NSAIDs may differ in their effects on the metabolism of connective tissue macro-molecules the choice of NSAIDs should not be dependent on such considerations. If NSAID therapy is felt to be indicated because of the intensity of symptoms and signs of local inflammation the choice of NSAID should be based on evidence of clinical efficacy, tolerance and cost.

There is really nothing at present to suggest that the prophylactic use of NSAIDs by sports people is anything other than a form of drug abuse which exposes them to small risks of potentially serious adverse reactions.

References

Abramson SB, Weissman G. (1989) The mechanism of action of nonsteroidal anti-inflammatory drugs. Arthritis Rheum, **32**, 1-9.

Ahrengart L, Lindgren U, Reinhott FP. (1988) Comparative study of the effects of radiation, indomethacin, prednisolone and ethane-1-hydroxy-1, 1-diphosponate (EHDP) in the prevention of ectopic bone formation. Clin Orthop, **229**, 265-273.

Allen HL, Wase A, Bear WT. (1968) Indomethacin and aspirin : effect of nonsteroidal anti-inflammatory agents on the rate of fracture repair in the rat. Acta Orthop Scand, **51**, 595-599.

Almekinders LC, Gilbert GA. (1986) Healing of experimental muscle strains and the effects of nonsteroidal anti-inflammatory medication. Am J Sports Med, **14**, 303-308.

Almekinders LC. (1990) The efficacy of nonsteroidal anti-inflammatory drugs in the treatment of ligament injuries. Sports Medicine, **9**, 137-142.

Arora JS, Maudsley RH. (1968) Indocid arthropathy of hips. Proc Royal Soc Med, **61**, 669.

Bansil CK, Wilson GD, Stone NH. (1985) Role of prostaglandins E and F_{2a} in exercise induced delayed muscle soreness. Med Sci Sports Exerc, **17**, 186.

Biemond P, Swaak AJG, Penders JMA et al. (1986) Superoxide production by polymorphonuclear leucocytes in rheumatoid arthritis and osteoarthritis; in vivo inhibition by the anti-rheumatic drug piroxicam due to interference with the activation of the NADPH-oxidase. Ann Rheum Dis, **45**, 249-255.

Brandt KD. (1991) Pain, inflammation and nonsteroidal anti-inflammatory drugs; the effects of drugs on the metabolism of normal and osteoarthritic cartilage. In: Osteoarthritis current research and prospects for pharmacological intervention (Eds. RGG Russell, PA Dieppe). IBC Technical Services, London, pp. 196-202.

Brooks PM, Ghosh P. (1990) Chondroprotection : myth or reality. Baillieres Clinical

Rheumatology, **4**, 293-303.

Byrnes WC, Clarkson PM, Hsieh SS et al. (1985) Delayed onset muscle soreness following repeated bouts of downhill running. J Appl Physiol, **59**, 710-715.

Coke H. (1967) Long term indomethacin therapy of coxarthrosis. Ann Rheum Dis, **26**, 346-347.

Collier S, Ghosh P. (1991) Comparison of the effects of nonsteroidal anti-inflammatory drugs (NSAIDs) on proteoglycan synthesis by articular cartilage explant and chondrocyte monolayer cultures. Biochem Pharmacol, **41**, 1375-1384.

Committee on Safety of Medicines. (1986) Nonsteroidal anti-inflammatory drugs and serious gastrointestinal adverse reactions. Brit Med J, **292**, 614.

Cush JJ, Lipsky PL, Postlethwaite AE et al. (1990) Correlation of serological indicators of inflammation with effectiveness of nonsteroidal anti-inflammatory drug therapy in rheumatoid arthritis. Arthritis Rheum, **33**, 19-28.

Dahners LE, Phillips HO, Almekinders LC. (1986). The effect of piroxicam on ligament healing in rats. Trans Orthop Res Soc, **11**, 77.

Dahners LE, Gilbert JA, Lester GE et al. (1988) The effect of nonsteroidal anti-inflammatory drugs on the healing of ligaments. Am J Sports Med, **16**, 641-646.

de Vries BJ, Van den Berg WB. (1989) Impact of NSAIDs on immune antigen induced arthritis : an investigation of anti-inflammatory and chondroprotective effects. J Rheumatol, **16** (supp 18), 10-18.

Docherty M, Holt M, MacMillan P et al. (1986) A reappraisal of "analgesic hip". Ann Rheum Dis, **45**, 272-276.

Docherty M. (1989) "Chondroprotection" by nonsteroidal anti-inflammatory drugs. Ann Rheum Dis, **48**, 619-621.

Donnelly AE, McCormick K, Maughan RJ et al. (1988) Effects of a nonsteroidal anti-inflammatory drug on delayed onset muscle soreness and indices of damage. Brit J Sports Med, **22**, 35-38.

Donnelly AE, Maughan RJ, Whiting PH. (1990) Effects of Ibuprofen on exercise induced muscle soreness and indices of muscle damage. Brit J Sports Med, **24**, 191-195.

Fitch KD, Gray SD. (1974) Indomethacin in soft tissue sports injuries. Med J Austral, **1**, 260-261.

Forrest M, Brooks PM. (1988) Mechanism of action of nonsteroidal anti-rheumatic drugs. In: Anti-rheumatic drugs (Ed. PM Brooks). Clin Rheumatol, **2**, 275-294.

Franchimont P, Gysen P, Lecompte-Yerna MJ et al. (1983) Incorporation du souffre radioactif dans les proteoglycans due cartilages in vitro. Effects de certains anti-inflammatoires non steroidiens. Revue du Rheumatism, **50**, 249-253.

Friden J, Sjostrom M, Ekblom B. (1983) Myofibrillar damage following intense eccentric exercise in man. Int J Sports Med, **4**, 1701-1707.

Ghosh P. (1988) Anti-rheumatic drugs and cartilage. In: Antirheumatic drugs (Ed. PM Brooks). Clin Rheumatol, **2**, 309-330.

Haggag AA, Mohamed HF, Eldawy MA et al. (1986) Biochemical studies on the anti-inflammatory activity of salicylates as superoxide radical scavengers. IRCS Medical Science - Biochemistry, **14**, 1104-1105.

Heere LP. (1988) Piroxicam in acute musculoskeletal disorders and sports injuries. Ann J Med, **84** (supp 5A), 50-55.

Henry DA. (1988) Side effects of nonsteroidal anti-inflammatory drugs. In: Antirheumatic drugs (Ed. PM Brooks), Baillieres Clinical Rheumatology, **2**, 425-454.

Herman JH, Appel AM, Hess EV. (1987) Modulation of cartilage destruction by select nonsteroidal anti-inflammatory drugs. Arthritis Rheum, **30**, 257-265.

Herman JH, Sowder WG, Hess EV. (1991) NSAID induction of interleukin-1/catabolin inhibitor production by osteoarthritic synovial tissue. J Rheumatol, **18** (supp 27), 124-136.

Higgs GA, Moncada S, Vane JF. (1980) The mode of action of anti-inflammatory drugs which prevent peroxidation of arachidonic acid. Clin Rheum Dis, **6**, 675-693.

Hikida RS, Staron RS, Hagerman FC et al. (1983) Muscle fibre necrosis associated with human marathon runners. J Neurol Sci, **59**, 185-203.

Honig S. (1988) Clinical trials in acute musculo-skeletal injury states. Am J Med, **84** (supp 5a), 42-44.

Howell DS, Pita JC, Müller FJ et al. (1991) Treatment of osteoarthritis with tiaprofenic acid : Biochemical and histological protection against cartilage breakdown in the Pond-Nuki canine model. J Rheumatol, 18 (suppl 27), 138-142.

Hutson MA. (1986) A double blind study comparing ibuprofen 1800mg or 2400mg daily and placebo in sports injuries. J Internat Res, **14**, 142-147.

Inman WHW and Rawson NSB. (1987) Prescription event monitoring of five nonsteroidal anti-inflammatory drugs. In: Side effects of anti-inflammatory drugs. Part I Clinical and epidemiological aspects. (Eds. KD Rainsford, JP Velo) MTP Press, Lancaster, pp. 111-123.

Kalbhen DA. (1984) Biochemically induced osteoarthritis in the chicken and rat. In: Effects of drugs on osteoarthritis (Eds. E Manthe, A Bjelle), Hans Huber, Berne.

Krishnan A. (1977) A placebo controlled double blind trial of benorylate tablets in the treatment of bursitis and synovitis. Rheumatol Rehab, **16**, 186-189.

Kruze D, Salgam P, Fehr K-L, Boni A. (1977) Degradation of bovine nasal cartilage by a neutral protease from human leucocyte granules. In: Perspectives in inflammation : Future trends and developments (Eds. DA Willoughby, JP Girond, GP Vels). MTP Press, Lancaster, pp. 361-370.

Kuipers H, Keizer HA, Verstappen FTJ et al. (1985) Influence of a prostaglandin-inhibiting drug on muscle soreness after eccentric work. Int J Sports Med, **6**, 336-339.

Lentini A, Ternai B, Ghosh P. (1987) Inhibition of leucocyte elastase and cathepsin G by nonsteroidal anti-inflammatory compounds. Biochem Int, **15**, 1069-1078.

Lereim P, Gabor I. (1988) Piroxicam and naproxen in acute sports injuries. Am J Med, **84** (supp 5a), 45-49.

McLatchie GR, Allister C, MacEwen C et al. (1985) Variable schedules of Ibuprofen for ankle sprains. Brit J Sports Med, **19**, 203-206.

McLatchie GR, McDonald M, Lawrence GF et al. (1989) Soft tissue trauma : a randomised control trial of the topical application of felbinac, a new NSAID. Brit J Clin Pract, **43**, 277-280.

Maier R, Wilhelmi A. (1982) Special pharmacological findings with diclofenac sodium. In: Voltaren - New Findings (Ed. E Kass). Hans Huber, Berne, pp. 11-18.

Mann RD. (1985) The yellow card data : the nature and scale of the adverse drug reactions problem. In: Adverse drug reactions (Ed. R Mann). Parthenon, Carnforth, pp. 5-66.

Martel-Pelletier J, Pelletier JP. (1989) Molecular basis for the action of tiaprofenic acid on human osteoarthritic cartilage degradation. Semin Arthritis Rheum, **18** (supp 1), 19-26.

Milner JC. (1973) Osteoarthritis of the hip and indomethacin. J Bone Joint Surg, **54B**, 252.

Minta JO, Williams MD. (1985) Some nonsteroidal anti-inflammatory drugs inhibit the generation of superoxide anions by activated polymorphs by blocking ligand-receptor interactions. J Rheumatol, **12**, 751-757.

Muir H, Connery SL, Hall LG. (1988) Effects of tiaprofenic acid and other NSAIDs on proteoglycan metabolism in articular cartilage explants. Drugs, **35** (supp 1), 15-33.

Newham DJ, Jones DA, Edward RHT. (1983) Large delayed plasma creatine kinase changes after stepping exercise. Muscle Nerve, **6**, 380-385.

Newham DJ, Jones DA, Clarkson PM. (1987) Repeated high-force eccentric exercise: effects on muscle pain and damage. J Appl Physiol, **63**, 1381-1386.

Newman NM, Ling RSM. (1985) Acetabular bone destruction related to nonsteroidal anti-inflammatory drugs. Lancet, **ii**, 11-14.

Palmoski MJ, Brandt KD. (1979) Effect of salicylate on proteoglycan metabolism in normal canine articular cartilage in vitro. Arthritis Rheum, **22**, 246-254.

Palmoski MJ, Brandt KD. (1980) Effects of some non-steroidal anti-inflammatory drugs on proteoglycan metabolites and organisation in canine articular cartilage. Arthritis

Rheum, 23, 1018-1020.

Palmoski MJ, Colyer R, Brandt KD. (1980) Marked suppression by salicylate of the augmented proteoglycan synthesis in osteoarthritic cartilage. Arthritis Rheum, 23, 83-91.

Palmoski MJ, Brandt KD. (1982) Aspirin aggravates the degeneration of canine joint cartilage caused by immobilisation. Arthritis Rheum, 25, 1333-1342.

Palmoski MJ, Brandt KD. (1983a) Benoxaprofen stimulates proteoglycan synthesis in normal canine cartilage in vitro. Arthritis Rheum, 20, 771-774.

Palmoski MJ, Brandt KD. (1983b) In vivo effect of aspirin on canine osteoarthritic cartilage. Arthritis Rheum, 26, 994-1001.

Palmoski MJ and Brandt KD. (1983c) Relationship between matrix proteoglycan content and the effects of salicylate and indomethacin on articular cartilage. Arthritis Rheum, 26, 528-531.

Pelletier JP, Martel-Pelletier J. (1991) In vivo protective effects of prophylactic treatment with tiaprofenic acid on intra-articular corticosteroids on osteoarthritic lesions in the experimental dog model. J Rheumatol, 18 (supp 27), 127-130.

Perper RJ and Oronsky AL. (1974) Enzyme release from human leucocytes and degradation of cartilage matrix. Effects of anti-rheumatic drugs. Arthritis Rheum, 17, 47-55.

Rashad S, Revell P, Hemingway A et al. (1989) Effect of nonsteroidal anti-inflammatory drugs on the course of osteoarthritis. Lancet, ii, 519-522.

Ronningen H, Langelands N. (1979) Indomethacin treatment in osteoarthritis of the hip joint. Does the treatment interfere with the natural course of the disease? Acta Orthop Scand, 50, 169-174.

Ro J, Sudmann E and Marton PE. (1976) Effect of indomethacin on fracture healing in rats. Acta Orthop Scand, 47, 588-592.

Roth SH, Bennett RE, Mitchell CS et al. (1987) Cimetidine therapy in nonsteroidal anti-inflammatory drug gastropathy. Double blind long term evaluation. Arch Intern Med, 147, 1798-1801.

Roth SH. (1988) Nonsteroidal anti-inflammatory drugs : gastropathy deaths and medical practice. Ann Intern Med, 109, 353-354.

Santelli G, Tuacimei V, Cannistna FM. (1980) Comparative study with piroxicam and ibuprofen versus placebo supportive treatment of minor sports injuries. J Internat Med Res, 8, 265-269.

Shinmei M, Shimada K, Shigeno Y et al. (1985) Effects of anti-inflammatory drugs on proteoglycan synthesis and degradation in rabbit articular chondrocytes in vitro in tiaprofenic acid (Ed. OG Nilsen). Exerpta Medica Amsterdam, pp. 59-68.

Smith LL, McCammon M, Smith S et al. (1988) Leukocytosis: response to metabolic demands or a sign of acute inflammation related to delayed muscle soreness (DMS). Med Sci Sports Exerc, 20, S74.

Solomon L. (1973) Drug induced arthropathy and necrosis of the femoral head. J Bone Joint Surg, 55B, 246-261.

Sommerville K, Faulkner G, Langman M. (1986) Nonsteroidal anti-inflammatory drugs and bleeding peptic ulcer. Lancet, i, 462-464.

Stephens RW, Walton EA, Ghosh P et al. (1980) A radioassay for proteolytic cleavage of isolated cartilage proteoglycan 2. Inhibition of purified leucocyte elastase and cathepsin G by anti-inflammatory drugs. Azneimittel-Forschung, 30, 2108-2112.

Sudmann E and Hagen T. (1976) Indomethacin induced delayed fracture healing. Arch Orthop Trauma Surg, 85, 151-155.

The International Agranulocytosis and Aplastic Anaemia Study. (1986) Risks of agranulocytosis and aplastic anaemia. J Am Med Assoc, 256, 1749-1757.

Tornquist H and Lindholm TS. (1980) Effect of ibuprofen on mass and composition of fractures callus and bone. Scand J Rheumatol, 9, 167-172.

Tornquist M, Lindholm TS, Netz P et al. (1984) Effect of ibuprofen and indomethacin on bone metabolism reflected in bone strength. Clin Orthop Rel Res, 187, 255-259.

Van Epps DE, Grieve S, Potter J et al. (1987) Alterations in neutrophil superoxide production following piroxicam therapy in patients with rheumatoid arthritis. Inflammation, **11**, 59-72.

Van Heerden DJ. (1977) Diclofenac sodium, oxyphenbutazone and placebo in sports injuries of the knee. S African Med J , **27**, 396-399.

Vane JR. (1971) Inhibition of prostaglandin synthesis as a mechanism of action for the aspirin-like drugs. Nature, **231**, 232-235.

Vignon E, Mathieu P, Broquet P et al. (1990) Cartilage degradation enzymes in human osteoarthritis : Effect of a nonsteroidal anti-inflammatory drug administered orally. Semin Arthritis Rheum, **19** (supp 1), 26-29.

Viljakka T, Rokkanen P. (1983) The treatment of ankle sprain by bandaging and antiphlogistic drugs. Ann Chirurg Gynaecol, **72**, 66-70.

Vogel HG. (1977) Mechanical and chemical properties of various connective tissue organs in rats as influenced by nonsteroidal anti-rheumatic drugs. Con Tissue Res, **5**, 91-95.

Wilholm BE, Myrhed M, Ekman E. (1987) Trends and patterns in adverse drug reactions to nonsteroidal anti-inflammatory drugs reported in Sweden. In: Side effects of anti-inflammatory drugs. Part I, Clinical and Epidemiological aspects, MTP Press, Lancaster, pp. 55-70.

Playing quality of natural turf

P.M. Canaway

Abstract. Natural turf is the preferred playing surface for Rugby and related sports. The nature of that playing surface is clearly important to the quality of play and injuries received yet it is often neglected as an area for scientific study and low in priority for improvement. This paper describes how playing quality of natural turf for Association Football can be quantified in terms of: ball rebound resilience, ball roll, player traction and hardness. It describes a project in which standards for these components of playing quality were developed using a combination of field testing and player evaluation work. Standards are given in terms of "preferred" limits and less stringent "acceptable" limits for components of playing quality, for example, players preferred playing surfaces to have ball rebound values between 20% and 50%, the acceptable range being between 15% and 55%. The means of achieving such standards on natural turf playing surfaces through attention to construction and drainage is described using results from a study on the effects of five constructional methods on sports field durability and playing quality. The work showed that vast improvements in natural turf playing surfaces could be achieved and that inappropriate constructional improvements can be a waste of resources.

Keywords: Playing Quality, Ball Rebound, Ball Roll, Player Traction, Hardness, Standards, Construction, Natural Turf.

Introduction

Many sports have their origins on natural turf playing surfaces, for example, Association Football, Rugby, golf, tennis, hockey, cricket and bowls to name but a few. Some of these have moved to man-made surfaces subsequently, e.g. hockey and tennis, but for many players of Rugby and related sports natural turf is still the preferred surface. Although the research and development input into natural turf has probably been small as compared with the technological research on artificial surfaces with a commercial end in sightf steady progress has been made towards understanding the characteristics of a good, natural turf playing surface. In this paper it is my objective to focus on the quality of natural turf for sports such as football and Rugby, especially on playing quality, standards for different components of playing quality and the means of achieving such standards on actual sports fields through attention to their construction and drainage.

Playing quality

Playing quality can be defined in terms of the variables which determine whether a surface is good for the sport in question (Canaway 1985, 1990). For football, components of playing quality include ball/surface characteristics such as ball bounce (rebound resilience) and ball roll (rolling resistance) and player/surface characteristics, such as traction (the amount of "grip" available to the player) and hardness (stiffness and resilience). Other criteria which, although not in themselves components of playing quality, have a direct influence on it include: grass cover; surface trueness and; water infiltration rate (the rate at which incidental rainfall percolates into the surface).

Apparatus and test methods

Ball bounce or rebound resilience.   Ball rebound resilience is measured by releasing the ball from a standard height. For football this height is 3.0 m from the bottom of the ball to the playing surface. The apparatus must release the ball without impulse or spin and a vertical scale must be provided so that rebound height can be measured. It is usual to graduate the vertical scale in terms of % rebound and to arrange the graduations so as to record rebound height, as the maximum rebound height of the top of the ball for ease of recording. The ball must be of a standard size and inflation pressure (FIFA size 5 inflated to 70 kPa) and it should have a rebound resilience of between 56% and 59% when tested on concrete. In practice a number of drops are performed on each test area and the apparatus is moved between drops to avoid successive impacts on the same location.

Ball roll or rolling resistance.   For ball roll the simplest approach is measurement of distance rolled by a ball released from a standard ramp. For measurement of distance rolled an inclined ramp apparatus is used, which consists of two parallel bars mounted on a rigid frame to produce a release "ramp" inclined at an angle of 45°. The foot of the ramp is constructed to a radius of 500 mm to prevent the ball abruptly changing direction and bouncing off the surface. The apparatus is placed so that the ball is released from a height of 1.0 m and allowed to be rolled down the ramp and along the playing surface. The distance rolled by the ball from the end of the ramp to the resting place of the ball is measured. Three observations should be made in two opposing directions on each test area. The greater is the distance rolled by the ball, the lower is the rolling resistance and vice versa. The main drawback of the method is that it is easily influenced by wind and it is not recommended to use the technique if the wind speed exceeds Beaufort Scale 4 (moderate breeze, 5.6-8.1 m s^{-1}). Results are expressed in terms of the mean distance rolled in metres.

Traction. An apparatus for measuring traction and friction on natural and artificial playing surfaces was described by Canaway & Bell (1986). The apparatus (Fig. 1) consists of a mild steel test disc "foot" 145 mm in diameter, centre drilled with 6 football studs arranged in a radially symmetrical manner 46 mm from the centre of the disc. A shaft is screwed in the centre of the disc.

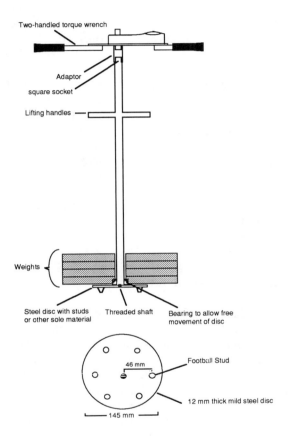

Fig. 1 Apparatus for measuring traction on natural turf.

The shaft incorporates lifting handles and passes through a set of weights to provide a load of 46 kg including the mass of the other components. The weights are supported on a roller bearing to permit free rotation of the disc, whilst the weights remain still. To make the measurements a two-handled torque wrench with a scale up to 80 N m, is attached to the top of the shaft, the apparatus is lifted and allowed to fall on to the turf from a height of 60 mm to ensure the studs penetrate the surface. The torque wrench is then turned without placing any additional vertical force on the handles and torque required to tear the turf is measured. The higher is the value the greater is the traction available to the player. Low values would indicate a surface on which falls are likely and very high values could predispose knee and ankle injuries. After each reading the disc and studs are cleaned of any mud or turf and the measurement repeated on undamaged turf until sufficient data have been collected.

Hardness. Hardness, or more strictly, stiffness and resilience of surfaces, has been measured by a variety of techniques (Baker 1990; Bell et al, 1985) and some of the shortcomings of these methods are discussed by Nigg (1990). However, for rapid evaluation of outdoor sports fields the Clegg Impact Soil tester (Clegg 1976) has been widely used and much experience has been gained with it under a variety of conditions. The apparatus consists of a cylindrical compaction hammer of mass 0.5 kg and a diameter of 50 mm attached to a piezoelectric accelerometer, which feeds into a peak level digital meter. The compaction hammer is released to fall down a guide tube from a height of 300 mm and after impact with the surface, the peak deceleration of the hammer is displayed in gravities on the screen display. After each test the apparatus is moved to a fresh area and the test repeated.

Standards for playing quality of natural turf

The development of synthetic playing surfaces and subsequent criticisms of early versions by players and media alike, encouraged manufacturers to seek methods of quantifying their performance in order to make their characteristics more similar to those of natural turf. This in turn led to an initiative by the Sports Council (London) to develop standards for artificial turf surfaces culminating in the production of "Specifications for artificial turf sports surfaces" (Sports Council 1984a, b). A stage was soon reached where more was known about the playing quality of artificial turf than about natural turf, which the former was supposed to emulate. To rectify this situation, the Sports Council (London) initiated a four year study at the Sports Turf Research Institute on standards for the playing quality of natural turf. This work produced proposed standards for playing quality of football pitches based on a combination of field testing and player evaluation work (Canaway et al, 1990). This work has been supplemented by a further project whose object was to monitor case studies of fields with different construction in order to relate playing quality to levels of use and cost-effectiveness (Baker & Gibbs, 1989). This has provided a "test bed" for the practical application of such standards in the field and has led to some modifications of the original standards. The results of this work, together with additional work needed in some areas not covered previously (e.g. grass length), have now been combined into a forthcoming publication "Specification for natural turf sports areas: Part 1 soccer pitches", which is in the final stages of preparation and will be published in the near future. This document not only contains standards for playing quality tests described above, but also for: surface evenness; grass ground cover; grass sward height; water infiltration rate and gives details of antecedent conditions for testing. Work is to be continued in 1991-1992 to adapt the standards produced to date for use on Rugby and natural turf hockey fields.

Field testing and player evaluation work

The original work has been fully reported elsewhere (Canaway et al, 1990) but a brief summary is given here. The initial phase of the work comprised a review of existing literature (Bell et al, 1985) and development of apparatus and test methods and a pilot study on the use of such apparatus in the field (Holmes & Bell, 1986). Complex electronic apparatus was rejected at an early stage bearing in mind that the tests have to be carried out during the British winter season when adverse weather is prevalent. Apparatus has to be simple, robust, easy and safe to use, portable and above all, reliable. Complex equipment involving computer data capture, whilst suitable for laboratory work was found to be temperamental in the field, with faults due to moisture and power supplies failing in extreme cold, in addition to setting up time and lack of portability on site. Examples of such apparatus include the "Stuttgart Artificial Athlete", the "Berlin Artificial Athlete" and the "impact severity test" referred to by Baker (1990) and by Nigg (1990). Sampling locations in the field testing work comprised six locations on football fields encompassing areas of high wear (goal areas), medium wear (centre circle) and light wear (wings). These are illustrated diagrammatically in Fig. 2.

Playing quality tests were carried out within 2 hours of matches on 49 football fields of different constructional make up. Each field was visited between one and five times during the period of the study and a total of 675 areas measuring 5 m x 5 m was tested. The tests were carried out within 2 hours of matches so that the opinions of players could be sought on the qualities of the surface that the mechnical tests sought to measure. Questionnaires were given out to players after matches and a total of 444 completed questionnaires were returned, which together with the 675 test results, comprised the main data set for the initial formulation of standards for playing quality for natural turf soccer flelds. The questionnaire is given by Canaway et al (1990).

Standards were formulated in terms of "preferred" and slightly less demanding "acceptable" ranges for different tests. As the full set of standards are in preparation in the present paper the standards presented in Table 1 are those referring only to the playing quality tests discussed in detail above: i.e. ball rebound resilience; ball roll; traction and; hardness.

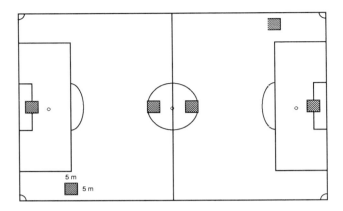

Fig. 2 Location of six test areas on soccer fields

It should be noted that no upper limit for traction is given since traction values in the study were in the low to medium range and players generally did not complain of excessive "grip underfoot". The more likely response was that grip underfoot was poor. The study recorded a maximum traction value of 51.0 N m with mean values of: 27.1 N m (goal areas), 33.0 N m (wing areas) and 27.4 N m (centre circle).

Table 1. Standards for playing quality of natural turf for football

Test	Preferred range	Acceptable range
Ball rebound resilience (%)	20-50	15-55
Ball roll distance (m)	3-12	2-14
Traction (N m)	≥ 25	≥ 20
Hardness (gravities)	20-80	10-120

Construction - the means of achieving standards for playing quality

In cool temperate regions of the world where sports such as football and Rugby are played during the winter months when rainfall is generally high in relation to evapotranspiration, the performance of sports pitches is limited by the inability of most natural soils to transmit water away from the surface at a sufficient rate. This, combined with the detrimental effects of wear on soil structure, leads to the familiar mud baths and poor playing conditions frequently seen during the winter months.

Table 2. Details of the five construction treatments

Pipe drained (PD)	Topsoil was spread over the subsoil formation to a depth of 250 mm. 60 mm perforated plastic drain pipe was introduced at a depth of 600 mm and the drain trench backfilled with gravel to 200 mm from ground level and blinded with 50 mm of coarse sand. Topsoil was placed over the backfill to provide 150 mm firmed depth.
Slit drained (SD)	Topsoil and pipe drainage installed as above. After the sward had established, 50 mm wide slit trenches were excavated at 600 mm centres. These were filled with 125 mm of 6 mm Lytag drainage aggregate topped with 100 mm coarse sand.
Slit drained, sand top (SS)	Initial construction was as the pipe top drained treatment except that the topsoil depth was 225 mm. This was covered with a 25 mm firmed depth of medium-fine sand before sowing. Slit drains were added subsequently to the same specification as the slit drained treatment.
Sand carpet (SC)	Topsoil was spread to a depth of 150 mm. The pipe drainage was installed as above except that the drain trench was only 500 mm deep. The trench was backfilled to 50 mm from the topsoil surface prior to blinding with 50 mm coarse sand. Slit trenches of 50 mm width, 200 mm depth were introduced at 1.5 m centres. These were backfilled with 150 mm of gravel and 50 mm blinding sand. A 100 mm firmed depth of medium-fine sand was then spread over the topsoil surface.
Sand profile (SP)	150 mm of subsoil was excavated from the initial subsoil formation level to give the required depth. The pipe drain was installed at a depth of 250 mm and backfilled with gravel. A 100 mm depth of gravel was then spread over the subsoil formation surface and blinded with 50 mm coarse sand. The rootzone layer of medium-fine sand was then spread to give a 250 mm firmed depth.

In 1986 an experiment was set up to examine the effects of different constructional and drainage techniques on playing quality of football pitches. The methods studied are given in Table 2.

Test plots 13 m x 6 m of each construction type were set up in randomised blocks with two replications. Adjacent plots were isolated using a polythene membrane to avoid lateral water movement and also to allow drain discharge measurements to be made. Once established artificial wear treatments were carried out using a differential slip wear machine (Canaway 1976) to simulate the effects of play. The trial is fully reported by Baker & Canaway (1990a, b, 1991).

The degree to which the different constructions achieved satisfactory playing quality can be determined with reference to the standards given above. In each season, playing quality tests were made on five occasions and the extent to which standards were met by the different constructions is given in Table 3 (Baker & Canaway, 1991).

Table 3. The number of occasions out of 10 (9 for traction) on which 5 different methods of sports pitch construction met standards for playing quality in two seasons of use 1987-1988 and 1988-1989.

Pitch	Ball Rebound Unacc Acc Pref			Ball Roll Unacc Acc Pref			Traction Unacc Acc Pref			Hardness Unacc Acc Pref		
PD	4	-	6	3	-	6	2	1	6	3	4	3
SD	-	2	8	-	2	7	1	1	7	-	1	9
SS	-	-	10	-	-	10	-	1	8	-	-	10
SC	-	-	10	-	-	10	-	1	8	-	-	10
SP	-	-	10	-	-	10	-	1	8	-	-	10

PD = pipe drained, SD = slit drained, SS = slit drained with 25 mm sand top, SC = sand carpet 100 mm thick overlying slit drains, SP = sand profile 250 mm thick over a drainage carpet)

It can be seen at a glance that the three higher specification (and hence more costly) construction methods (SS, SC and SP) gave playing quality in the preferred range for both seasons, except one measurement of traction which fell into the acceptable range. Slit drainage alone (SD) provided better playing quality than the pipe drained areas, but nonetheless failed on traction on one occasion, and was in the acceptable rather than preferred range on a number of occasions. Pipe drainage alone was an unacceptable method of pitch improvement or construction. Since the majority of football and Rugby fields in the UK fall into the pipe drained or even undrained categories it is not surprising that generally poor conditions for play prevail during the wetter months.

Conclusion

The development of standards for the playing quality of Association football pitches has been a slow and difficult process and doubtless further refinements could be devised if funds were limitless. The process to date has enabled us to quantify the characteristics of turf in a meaningful way. It enables us to judge the performance of installations and of experimental treatments in turfgrass research. For example, previously we could only say that a particular treatment increased or decreased traction or ball rebound, but we could not say whether that was good or bad. Now with limits for acceptability we can state positively whether the treatment was beneficial or not. No claim is made that the tests used actually represent what the athlete does, or the potential for injury of the surface. The standards were based on what players preferred, not necessarily what was good for them. These may be the same but we are not qualified to judge, Nigg (1990) quite rightly pointing out the drawbacks of simple tests for prediction of the injury potential of different surface/shoe combinations.

The fact that attention to construction and drainage of fields can so dramatically improve their playing performance is commonly overlooked. In the public consciousness grass is just grass and we have to put up with the surface as we find it. Nothing could be further from the truth. However, on the positive side many of the questions pertaining to sports pitch construction and drainage have now been resolved. The challenge is to raise the awareness level of the need for pitch provision of high enough quality to allow players and spectators alike to reap maximum enjoyment from the game.

References

Baker SW. (1990) Standards for the playing quality of artificial turf for Association Football, in: Natural and Artificial Playing Fields: Characteristics and Safety Features. ASTM STP 1073 (eds RC Schmidt, EF Hoerner, EM Milner & CA Morehouse), ASTM, Philadelphia, pp. 48-57.

Baker SW & Canaway PM. (1990a) The Cost-effectiveness of different construction methods for Association football pitches. I. Soil physical properties. J Sports Turf Res Inst, 66, 8-20.

Baker SW & Canaway PM. (1990b) The effect of sand top dressing on the performance of winter games pitches of different construction types. I. Soil physical properties and ground cover. J Sports Turf Res Inst, 66, 21-27.

Baker SW & Canaway PM. (1991). The cost-effectiveness of different construction methods for Association football pitches. II. Ground cover, playing quality and cost implications. J Sports Turf Res Inst, 67, 53-65.

Baker SW & Gibbs RJ. (1989) Levels of use and the playing quality of winter games pitches of different construction types: case studies at Nottingham and Warrington. J Sports Turf Res Inst, 65, 9-33.

Bell MJ, Baker SW & Canaway PM. (1985) Playing quality of sports surfaces: a review. J Sports Turf Res Inst, 61, 26-45.

Canaway PM. (1976) A differential slip wear machine (D.S.1.) for artificial simulations of turfgrass wear. J Sports Turf Res Inst, **52**, 92-99.

Canaway PM. (1985) Keynote address. Playing quality, construction and nutrition of sports turf. Proc 5th Int Turfgrass Res Conf, (ed F Lemaire), INRA, Paris, pp. 45-46.

Canaway PM. (1990) Golf green agronomy and playing quality - past and current trends, in Science and Golf (ed AJ Cochran), E & FN Spon, London, pp. 336-345.

Canaway PM & Bell MJ. (1986) Technical note: an apparatus for measuring traction and friction on natural and artificial playing surfaces. J Sports Turf Res Inst, **62**, 211-214.

Canaway PM, Bell, MJ, Holmes G & Baker SW. (1990). Standards for the playing quality of natural turf for Association Football, in Natural and Artificial Playing Fields: Characteristics and Safety Features, ASTM STP 1073 (eds RC Schmidt, EF Hoerner, EM Milner & CA Morehouse), ASTM, Philadelphia, pp. 29-47

Clegg B. (1976) An impact testing device for in situ base course evaluation. Australian Road Res Bur Proc, **8**, 1-6.

Holmes G & Bell MJ. (1986) A pilot study of the playing quality of football pitches. J Sports Turf Res Inst. **62**, 74-91.

Nigg BM. (1990) The validity and relevance of tests used for the assessment of sports surfaces. Special Communications, Technical Note. Med Sci Sports Exerc, **7**

The role of the boot in rugby

A. Lees

Abstract. There has been little or no scientific assessment of the design and function of the rugby boot or its ability to protect the wearer. The general principles applying to functions of the boot, based on work undertaken with soccer boots and running shoes, are discussed and appropriate design features are considered in conjunction with highlighting areas for future research.

Keywords: Rugby Boot Design, Rugby Boot Function, Low Cut v High Cut Boots, Ankle and Foot Movements, Research Opportunity.

Introduction

The rugby boot has evolved along traditional lines with features being added gradually to take account of the requirements of players and the trends within the game. Although manufacturers take a systematic approach to boot design, there have been virtually no reported scientific investigations of rugby boot performance which have then been fed back into design. Even in soccer there has been little attempt to apply systematic investigations in order to improve boot performance. Notable exceptions are the work reported by Valiant et al (1988) and Redano et al (1988). Both of these studies have presented data on the vertical and horizontal forces acting on the boot. Essentially the vertical force serves to press the studs into the ground and to compress the sole of the boot, whereas the horizontal forces serve to provide traction and to deform the boot by the action of the foot on the boot leading to deformation of the heel cup, stretching or even splitting of the boot material. In the absence of a substantial body of data on rugby boots, it is necessary to consider general principles extrapolated from other sports footwear studies and then make application to rugby.

General principles

The boot in rugby, as indeed any form of footwear, provides an ergonomic function. It must relate to the demands of the game and provide protection of the foot while at same time enable the foot to perform the functions demanded of it. It must be pleasant to wear and not be an encumberance to the player or the play required of an individual.

The demands of the game

The demands of the game can be established by notational analysis techniques. While these have been conducted in rugby in order to investigate the physiological demands and strategic development (Treadwell, 1987), there is little of this data that can be used for an ergonomic assessment of the requirements of the boot. Therefore the functions that the boot is required to perform are based on anecdotal evidence and the experience of players. In soccer studies such as those by Reilly and Thomas (1976), and Lees and Kewley (1991) provide a suitable model for assessing the demands of the game from the perspective of footwear.

Protection

With regard to the role of the boot for protection, the boot must be comfortable, be a good fit to the foot, protect from external forces, provide a spread the pressures over the sole of the boot, and control foot movement particularly rear foot movement.

Comfort is a difficult term to define objectively. It often relies on subjective experiences of players. It is something that can change with time, or with conditions of play (e.g. wetness, foot microclimate, properties of the boot material). The fit of a boot is related to the type of last and the materials used for its construction. There are substantial ethnic differences in foot shape, and it is unlikely that a boot designed for an American, Italian or oriental foot will fit a British foot well. Manufactures either use standard lasts, or lasts which have been developed for other types of footwear (e.g. running shoes). Certain types of leather have the properties of yielding to accommodate different foot shapes, while still providing a strong material, resistant to splitting. This helps to improve fit and enhance comfort.

The boot should be constructed so as to protect the foot from external forces which may arise from the ground, other players or by contact with the ball. When the foot contacts the ground the typical ground reaction force exceeds 2.5 times body weight. This force can increase as a result of running speed or type of landing action used. The force will also be higher on hard as opposed to soft grounds. The boot should have built into it materials designed to reduce the effect of these forces, but they often do not. In addition the boot should be able to distribute the force so that it is not concentrated in certain areas, such as for example under the heel, or more particularly under the head of the first metatarsal. The positioning of studs is particularly critical in this regard, as well as the method of attachment of stud to the boot. The foot is susceptible to knocking and treading by the feet of other players, and so the material of the boot should be able to provide protection to the foot from this. The use of sound or padded leather is necessary. When the ball is kicked, there is a contact force in excess of 1000 N (1.5 times body weight). This force will deform the foot but could also lead to bruising on the dorsal aspect of the foot. The force can also be a function of ball wetness, ball inflation pressure, and ball construction (Levendusky et al, 1988).

During the game the most frequently used action of the boot is a normal running stride. In such a stride the foot typically contacts the ground on the lateral border of the heel. The foot then rolls over, and goes into a position of pronation. The amount of movement of the rear foot can be affected by the boot. In running shoes the shoe may actually increase this range of pronation, and special construction methods are required to control it. The boot generally does not have these anti-pronation devices, and players with excessive rear foot movement may benefit from some rearfoot control.

Of major interest is the role the boot has for protecting against ankle inversion or eversion sprains. In the past the boot was traditionally made with a high ankle support. The advent of a faster running game has lead to a preference for the low cut soccer-type boot. This boot allows greater movement of the subtalar joint, and may as a consequence lead to more frequent and more severe ankle injuries.

Performance

With regard to the role of the boot for performance, the boot must allow the player to perform without encumbrance and if possible to enhance the playing of the game. The boot must allow the player to run easily, and so lightness is a major consideration. However, there is some incompatibility between the lightness of materials and their ability to protect the foot. The boot must not inhibit the normal joint movement in many phases of the game, particularly running. The lower cut boot has shown itself to allow normal joint function both in terms of plantar and dorsi-flexion, and in supination and pronation. However, the lack of protection against excessive ranges of motion has been indicated above.

The studs are important to provide traction on a variety of surfaces. The grip provided is a function of the depth of penetration of the stud and the firmness of the turf. Very wet turf possibly having a high surface water content will mean that short studs fail to penetrate into the firmer ground underneath. On the other hand very hard turf will not allow good penetration, and lead to pressure areas on the foot at the heel or forefoot of the boot. Studs of varying length help to overcome some of these problems, but studs are also a source of injury to other players. The traction requirements of the game are very different depending on position. The traction needed to push in a scrum is over five times that required in running. However as all players must be reasonably able to apply force in a scrummage, the traction requirement for many playing actions is overspecified.

A point which is little considered is the ability of the boot to provide a sound dorsal surface for kicking. The tendency several years ago for kicking long range balls was with the toe of the foot, and this required a strong toe box construction. With the popularity of round the corner place kicking, the foot is required to impact the ball on its dorsal surface (Asami and Nolte, 1983). The foot as a structure is very deformable under the large force applied during the kick, and this deformation leads to reduced kicking effectiveness. The boot could provide a suitable strengthening of the foot during this action, but to do so would require a high lateral stiffness of the sole. This hiqh lateral stiffness would also inhibit the normal flexion of the foot during the more common locomotor actions. The sole of the boot then should be designed with a hinge locking mechanism, and behave in a similar fashion to the elbow joint, for example.

Results of research on boots

It was noted earlier that there was a dearth of published research reports on the rugby boot. There has been research in other areas which can be documented, and extrapolated to the rugby boot, by way of illustrating the general principles.

In soccer, Lees and Kewley (1991) looked at the physical demand which is placed on the boot during soccer playing anmd training. It did this by identifying the major categories of playing movements made during a game of soccer, and recording their frequency of occurrence during both training and playing. An estimate of the demand put on the boot was obtained by measuring the horizontal force on the boot during each of the categories of movements.The data from these two approaches were then combined to give an overall estimate of the demand on the boot, and related to the problems experienced by the players. The horizontal data were presented as a vector plot together with a 'stress-clock" (Fig. 1). The stress clock was produced by adding up the magnitudes of the force during foot contact which appeared in each of twelve 30 degree or "hourly" segments . The "hour", total stress and number of counts were given on the graphical output, together with their total and the sample rate. The accumulated force was converted to a "severity index" for each of the playing actions. The direction of force was related to the occurrence of splits in the forefront and outside regions correspond very well with the main directions of the stress on the boot. Over a period of 90 minutes playing or training it was estimated that the stress on the boot was three time greater in training than in playing. This has consequences for the type of boots that are used for both types of play. It was concluded that this approach to the assessment of the demand on the boot is useful, and one which has not previously been described in the literature

The ankle joint is one of the most vulnerable joints for a soccer player, and the boot is often relied upon to protect this joint from an inversion/eversion sprain or more serious damage. The role of the boot for protecting the ankle joint was investigated by Johnson et al (1976). They investigated the torsional stiffness of different design boot uppers. They modelled the lower leg by a mass-spring-dashpot system which gave the joint its characteristic features with response to load. The boot added another resistive layer to the outside of the ankle allowing the natural stiffness of the joint to be supplemented by the properties of the boot.

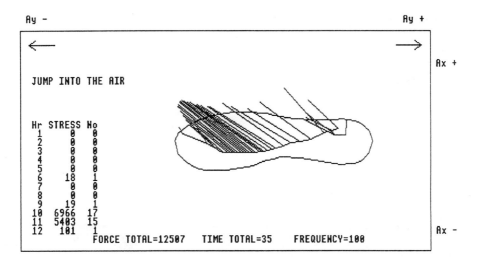

Figure 1. A stress clock for the horizontal friction force vectors acting on the shoe.

The low cut boot protected the subtalar joint, while the higher cut boot protected both this and the ankle joint. In a simulation of the effect of using different stiffness materials, they found that if a low cut boot was used it should be made of low stiffness material. This was because the subtalar joint had a certain amount of mobility, and if the ankle was turned a low cut boot would allow the subtalar joint to accommodate most of the movement. If the low cut boot was of stiff construction, then the boot would transfer some of the load away from the subtalar joint to the ankle joint. As this does not have any degree of flexibility in the inversion/eversion direction the additional load would be taken up by the collateral ligaments, leading to a greater likelihood of ligament damage. On the other hand the high cut boot should be made with stiff material because it already has a protective function with regard to the ankle joint and collateral ligaments. The stiffer the material, the more the load is taken by the boot material rather than the ligaments themselves. It should be noted, however, that the high cut boot with stiff material is only about twice the stiffness of the low-cut, low-stiffness material boot, and that for a severe inversion movement even the high cut boot would be insufficient to prevent damage occurring .

In running shoe design great attention is paid to the reduction of the shock force associated with heelstrike. This force is characterised by a sharp force peak whose magnitude can reach about three times body weight in sprinting (figure 2). This force can also be assessed by the use of acceleration measures on the lower tibia (Lafortune, 1991). In running peak tibial deceleration can be up to 10

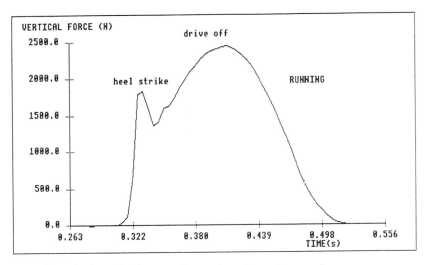

Figure 2. A typical vertical ground reaction force in running.

g (100 m.s^{-2}). While these techniques have not been applied to study field games, the types of boot construction suggest that this is an unimportant factor for players. However, while it may be less important due to the generally softer surfaces that players play upon, nevertheless it is still a feature of any heel contact foot placement. This becomes progressively more important as the ground becomes harder. It is also likely to be more important as players become more used to the softness of everyday shoes and gradually lose the ability to withstand repeated hard heel impacts. The use of shock absorbant materials placed in the heel of the boot is a standard method to reduce the severity of impact, but this is rarely done. In addition, such protective materials would also serve to raise the heel, which would put less stress on the calf muscle tendon complex, as a result of functional shortening from habitual wearing of raised heel footwear in everyday life.

The role of the boot for providing traction with the ground is surprisingly one area which has received little attention. The amount of grip provided by a surface is an important component of playing quality. If there is too little grip the players will slip and fall, while if there is too much there is a danger that players will suffer knee and ankle injuries as their feet become locked during turns and manoeuvres. In a report for the English Football Association, Winterbottom (1985) initiated an investigation into the effects of stud configuration which was later extended by the Football League (Football League, 1989). They found that the relationship of traction between boot and surface was a very complicated one, and identified two categories of movement important to players. These were sliding and turning movements. They tried to establish standardised tests for sliding resistance and torsional traction. The former test measured the distance a boot would slide before coming to a stop when given a known initial velocity. The latter test measured the torque produced when a studded plate was rotated while being subjected to body weight force. The researchers found that the sliding resistance was affected by turf wetness as well as stud configuration. Differences between extreme conditions were as much as 300%. The torsional traction coefficients for different boot sole types ranged from 2.5 at the highest to 1.0 at the lowest. Therefore the type of sole and the stud configuration can lead to a 250% change in the degree of traction offered. This clearly should be matched with the pitch conditions, but is only ever done so subjectively, and is an area which deserves greater research attention.

Conclusions

This paper has sought to focus on the role of the boot in rugby. It has highlighted the dearth of published material on this topic, and indeed the lack of material even applied to other field games. The research base in the area of running shoes is substantial. Many of the general principles which can be stated, are a combination of ideas which apply to footwear generally, and more specifically to the game of rugby. These general principles establish the ergonomic role the boot has to play, and the specific roles for both protecting the foot and enhancing performance. Some specific examples are taken from the literature in order to highlight the general principles. A plea for more rugby specific research concerning the boot is made.

References

Asami T and Nolte V. (1983) Analysis of powerful ball kicking, in Biomechanics VIII-B (eds. H Matsui and K Kobayashi). Human Kinetics, Champaign, Illinois, pp 695-700.

Football League (1989) Commission of enquiry into playing surfaces - Final Report. The Football League, Lytham St Annes.

Johnson G, Dowsonr D and Wright V. (1976) A biomechanlcal approach to the design of football boots. J Biomechanics, 9, 581-585.

Lafortune MA. (1991) Three dimensional acceleration of the tibia during walking and running. J Biomechanics, 24, 877-886.

Lees A and Kewley P. (1991) The demands on the Boot. Second World Congress of Science and Football, Eindhoven, 22-25th May.

Levendusky TA. Armstrong CW, Eck JS, Spryropoulous P, Jeziorowski J and Kugler L. (1988) Impact characteristics of two types of soccer balls, in Science and Football (eds. T Reilly, A Lees, K Davids and WJ Murphy). E & FN Spon, London, pp 385-393.

Redano R, Cova P and Vigano R. (1988) Design of a football boot: a theoretical and experimental approach, in Science and Football (eds. T Reilly, A Lees, K Davids, and WJ Murphy). E & FN Spon, London, pp 416-425.

Reilly T and Thomas V. (1976) A motion analysis of work rate in differential roles in professional football match play. Journal of Human Movement Studies, 2, 87-97.

Treadwell PJ. (1987) Computer aided match analysis of selected ball games (soccer and Rugby union) in Science and Football (eds. T Reilly, A Lees, K Davids and WJ Murphy). E & FN Spon, London, pp 282-287.

Valiant GA. Ground reaction forces developed on artificial turf,in Science and Football (eds. T Reilly, A Lees, K Davids and WJ Murphy). E & FN Spon, London, pp. 406-415.

Winterbottom Sir W. (1985) Artificial, grass surfaces for Association Football - Report and Recommendations. London, The Sports Council.

The role of orthoses in minimising injury in rugby

J.A. Black

Abstract. The role of orthoses in minimising injury is based on the ability of an orthotic insert in a shoe or boot to correct an improperly balanced foot with a view to reducing the biomechanical stresses on the lower limb thus easing the frequency and severity of overuse injuries such as plantar fasciitis, anterior knee pain, knee medial collateral ligament sprain and ilio tibial band or groin strain.

Keywords: Orthoses, Subtalar Joint Movement, Gait Analysis, Forefoot Varus, Forefoot Valgus, Calcaneal Varus, Calcaneal Valgus, Relief of Overuse Injury, Design of Orthoses.

Introduction

To understand the role of orthoses in minimising injury in sport it is necessary to review the basic principles of podiatric biomechanics and, in particular, the influence of the subtalar joint in the mechanics of running. D'Ambrosia (1985) states that, "orthotic devices are a means of aligning an improperly balanced foot by controlling the subtalar joint".

Hicks (1954), Mann (1982), Inman (1976) and Manter (1941) all describe the anatomy and function of the subtalar joint and the biomechanics of running. Black (1986) demonstrated that runners with biomechanically abnormal feet were much more likely to suffer overuse injuries of the lower limb than runners who had normal feet.

In describing orthotic function it is necessary to appreciate the variations of gait caused by abnormal motion in the subtalar joint and the effects that this will have on the lower limb. The foot is the primary contact with the ground and acts as an effective shock absorption system as well as distributing load and smoothing out the effects of irregular ground surface.

Each foot strikes the ground, on average, 800 times per mile. Mann (1982) quantified the load each limb absorbs in an eleven stone man running a mile at 110 tons per limb. In adult rugby most players weigh over eleven stone, run approximately four miles and generate significant extra forces while jumping in the lineout, scrummaging and tackling. Accordingly, it is clear that the loads absorbed at the foot/ground interface by a rugby player are colossal and it is surprising that there are not more overuse injuries.

Supination and pronation of the subtalar joint while running are complex but normal physiological movements enabling the foot to adapt to an even terrain,

371

absorb shock and assist propulsion.

The examination of the patient's foot is done with the patient lying in the prone position, feet extended beyond the end of the examination couch. The head of the talus is palpated about an inch anteriorly to the lateral and medial maleolli. The foot is then dorsiflexed to resistance using pressure on the plantar aspect of the 4th and 5th metatarsal heads, maximally pronating the midtarsal joints. This position mimics the position of the foot at the midpoint of stance and, in this position, it is possible to assess the relationship of the forefoot to the hindfoot and the foot to the leg. In the normal foot the plantar aspect of the forefoot and hindfoot are parallel in the transverse plane. The calcaneum will lie at right angles to the transverse plane, aligned with the leg.

This examination is critical if the practitioner is going to recognise those feet which have biomechanical discrepancy and require the prescription of a functional orthoses. The most common variations are:

forefoot varus - the forefoot is inverted to the hindfoot when the subtalar joint is in its neutral position

forefoot valgus - the forefoot is everted to the hindfoot and there is a plantar flexed first ray.

The equivalent hindfoot variations are calcaneal varus and calcaneal valgus. In those feet where compensation occurs, excessive pronation or supination results. Hyperpronation produces internal rotation of the leg, which unlocks the knee joint and allows it to become unstable in a valgus position. Oversupination on the other hand externally rotates the leg, producing a limb with very little capacity to absorb shock and all the concomitant problems associated with a rigid limb.

How then do orthoses minimise injuries? The original statement by D'Ambrosia (1985) describes orthoses as re-aligning improperly balanced feet and Cavanagh et al (1978) demonstrated that 9.5mm of material placed along the medial border of the foot not only decreased the degree of pronation but markedly reduced the angular velocity at which pronation occurred. Using the dynamic pedobarograph it is possible to demonstrate that functional orthoses reduced pressure in forefoot varus by 13% and in forefoot valgus by 46%.

What then is the application to rugby? Most coaches, physiotherapists and doctors associated with rugby have noticed a change in injury patterns with an increasing number of overuse injuries. These injuries have been attributed to changes in training routines with increasing use of grids, shuttles and ball work, all of which involve the players in more repetitive turning and running and a higher intensity of training. Orthoses are applicable for most overuse injuries where foot discrepancy is identified. Forefoot varus tends to produce midfoot strain, plantar fasciitis and heel bumps, while in the lower limb posterior tibial tendonitis, posterior tibial subluxation, posterior compartment syndrome, anterior knee pain and medial ligament sprain are most common. Forefoot valgus, on the other hand, provokes different symptoms such as inversion ankle sprains, achilles tendonitis, Robert Jones fracture of the base of the 5th metatarsal in the foot and anterior compartment syndrome, peroneus longus strain, lateral knee pain, lateral hamstring strains and ileotibial band problems in the leg and groin strain in the thigh.

When providing orthotics for sport there are a number of factors which must be taken into consideration such as whether it is for training or participating in the game, the weight of the patient, the footwear being worn, the playing surface and whether the orthosis is for correction of a deficiency or protection of the foot. These factors will determine the choice of materials used. The quality of the negative cast taken from the patient's foot is critical if effective orthoses are to be prepared.

In conclusion, top class athletes are extremely self motivated and rightly critical of inadequate treatment modalities. The athlete has to have confidence in the practitioner and it is essential that the patient fully understands the principles behind the treatment and agrees with them. The athlete must be given quite specific instructions with regard to the use of the orthoses, what problems may be encountered and what prognosis can reasonably be expected.

References

Black JA. (1986) The Influence of the Subtalar Joint in Running Injuries of The Lower Limb. Sport and Medicine, E & FN Spon.

Cavanagh PR et al. (1978) An Evaluation of the Effects of Orthotics on Force Distribution and Rearfoot Movement During Running. American Orthopaedics Society Sports Medicine Meeting, Lake Placid, New York, June.

D'Ambrosia RD. (1985) Clinics in Sports Medicine, 4, 4

Hicks JH. (1954) The Mechanics of the Foot. J Anat, 88, 25.

Inman VT. (1976) The Joints of The Ankle. The Williams and Wilkins Co, Baltimore.

Mann RA. (1982) Biomechanics of Running. In American Academy of Orthopaedic Surgeons: Symposium on the Foot and Leg in Running Sports. CV Mosby, St Louis.

Manter JT. (1941) Movements of the Subtalar and Transverse Tarsal Joints. Anat Rec, 80, 397.

The body clock: jet-lag, physical and psychological rhythms

D.S. Minors, J.M. Waterhouse and L.R. Smith

Abstract. Many physiological and psychological variables exhibit circadian rhythmicity which arises from an endogenous timing mechanism, the biological clock. This paper will consider how a knowledge of the properties of the biological clock and circadian rhythmicity may be of relevance to sports performance. In addition, the elite sports performer involved in international competitions is increasingly exposed to the rigours of transmeridian jet-travel and its detrimental effects upon well-being and performance, commonly termed jet-lag. Such symptoms arise, at least in part, from a lack of immediate adjustment of the biological clock to the new time zone, as well as from physiological and psychological variables adjusting at different rates. Ways in which the re-adjustment of the biological clock can be hastened, and thus the duration of performance decrements minimised, will be discussed.

Keywords: Jet-lag, Circadian Rhythms, Physical Performance, Psychological Performance

Introduction

Man is a diurnal creature, that is, his natural habits and social history indicate that he is used to daytime activity and work, and sleep at night. Physically and mentally, his body is more efficient by day and recuperates metabolically during the night. Sports events also reflect the diurnal nature of Man, being arranged during the daytime, this being a time of day which is not only socially acceptable but also when exercise performance is at its crest (see Section 3).

However, elite sports performers are increasingly required to travel worldwide to compete. Air travel to such competitions often involves the rapid crossing of several time zones with the consequence that the natural sleep/activity schedule has to be changed to coincide with new local time. Such a change in sleep/activity schedules leads to the disruptive effects upon physical and psychological well-being and performance, collectively known as jet-lag. Jet-lag manifests itself as a variety of psychophysiological symptoms which include gastrointestinal disorder, insomnia, headaches, dizziness, irritability, general feelings of weakness and fatigue, and poorer mental agility.

This paper will consider the effects of jet-lag upon the physical and psychological aspects of sports performance. In addition, consideration will be given to how our understanding of the body clock, and of the mechanisms which control and adjust it, enables us to offer advice on how best to ameliorate the difficulties associated with jet-lag.

Circadian rhythms - the basics

An important principle in physiology is that of homeostasis and the mechanisms whereby a relative stability is maintained in the body's internal milieu. Such stability is not absolute, however, and fluctuations in many physiological processes occur. In many cases the fluctuations show a marked rhythmic component. The cycle lengths (or periods) of these rhythms cover our every division of time but predominant are the circadian rhythms - rhythms which oscillate once per 24 hours. Circadian rhythms have been demonstrated in a wide range of physiological variables including sleep, metabolism, heart rate, blood pressure, urinary excretion and hormonal output (Minors and Waterhouse, 1981a) as well as psychological variables (Colquhoun, 1982; Folkard, 1990). Several of these rhythms are likely to affect exercise performance and thus have implications for sports performance at different times of the day (see Section 3).

In humans, overt circadian rhythmicity has two components. First, and most obviously, there is an exogenous component due to the rhythmic changes in our behaviour over the 24 hours; for example, the alternation between diurnal wakefulness and activity, and nocturnal sleep and inactivity. In addition, however, circadian rhythms have an endogenous component as evidenced by the fact that rhythmicity continues even if an individual remains awake and at about the same level of activity (e.g. sedentary) for 24 hours or more. The endogenous timing mechanism responsible for this component of circadian rhythms is often colloquially referred to as the body or biological clock.

Evidence accumulated over the past 20 years (see, for reviews, Minors and Waterhouse, 1986; Rosenwasser and Adler, 1986) has indicated that, in several mammalian species, a circadian clock which controls behavioural rhythms (drinking, activity patterns) resides in the paired suprachiasmatic nuclei (SCN) of the ventral hypothalamus, and more recent experiments have indicated that circadian rhythmicity can be reinstated by transplantation of fetal SCN tissue into an animal previously made arrhythmic by removal of its SCN (Silver et al, 1990).

The biological clock and its entrainment
The inherent properties of the biological clock in humans have been investigated by the use of specially constructed units in which an individual can be isolated from all external time cues. When placed in such conditions, it is found that circadian rhythms in the individual continue oscillating with a period deviating from an exact 24 hours; on average, in humans, it is 25 hours (Wever, 1979). It

is for this reason that the rhythms are termed **circadian** (**circa diem:** about a day).

Although inherently the biological clock has a period deviating from 24 hours, when we live in a normal environment exposed to all the rhythms, external and social, associated with the solar day, the biological clock (and hence the rhythms it controls) is synchronised (entrained) to keep exact 24-hour time. The external time cues responsible for this entrainment are referred to as **zeitgebers** (German: time givers). For most species, it is well established that the most important zeitgeber is the light/dark cycle associated with the solar day. However, in humans the situation appears more complex. Thus, originally Wever (1979) advanced the view that the rhythmic cues provided by social influences were of greater importance as a zeitgeber than the alternations of light and dark. However, more recent work has demonstrated that light, provided it is of sufficient intensity might act as a zeitgeber in humans (for further details, see Section 8.2.2).

It is our view that, for humans in a normal environment, entrainment of the biological clock is brought about by a group of zeitgebers acting simultaneously, some derived from our social behaviour and some directly from the environment. The recognition of these zeitgebers is important since it provides a means of promoting adjustment of the biological clock after time-zone transitions.

Not only the identification of the zeitgebers, but also the mechanism through which they act can be of importance. The action of a zeitgeber is to induce a phase shift of the biological clock, the size of which is equal to the difference between the inherent period of the clock and the period of the zeitgeber. The phase shift induced by light is dependent upon where, in the circadian day, the light falls; in most species studied thus far, exposure to light in the hours around dawn advances the clock, whereas in the late evening/early night light exposure delays the clock. During most of the day, light has no effect. This relationship between the phase at which light is given and the phase shift it evokes is called a phase-response curve (PRC). The recognition of such a PRC allows us to predict the effect of a zeitgeber on the biological clock and to produce phase shifts of the biological clock preferentially in one direction. This has proven to be an important strategy in hastening re-entrainment of the biological clock after a time-zone transition (See Section 8).

Circadian rhythms and physical performance

Physical responses to exercise

In view of the ubiquitous nature of circadian rhythms in physiological systems, it is no surprise to find that there is circadian variation in physical performance. Many of the factors which might affect or limit physical performance, - for example, heart rate, blood pressure, catecholamine secretion, muscle strength, joint flexibility, airway resistance - show circadian variation (for full reviews of these factors, see Shephard, 1984; Winget et al, 1985). Many of these rhythms parallel the rhythm of body temperature to a large extent, showing a peak during the late afternoon/early evening. It might be predicted, therefore, that physical performance would be best at this time of day. This view seems to be confirmed by the observation that most world records in athletic events have been achieved at this time of day. Interpretation of such an observation, however, is complicated by the fact that this is the time of day when most top class athletic events and finals are scheduled. Nonetheless, when athletic performance has been assessed at different times of day under controlled conditions, an evening performance is found to be better than that in the morning. These aspects have been covered in detail in several reviews (Reilly, 1987; 1990; Winget et al, 1985).

Psychological factors underlying performance

In addition to physiological factors, exercise performance is also determined by psychological factors. Thus the performance of complex sports skills draws on several fundamental psychological resources and capacities. These include various cognitive processes such as information processing and memory. For example, the athlete processes sensory information which involves perceiving, making decisions about and organising responses to immediate demands. There is a low memory requirement if a rapid response is needed; conversely, there is a high memory load when spatial information about people and objects, and their direction of movement has to be stored briefly in order to decide upon a suitable action. These processes show different patterns of activation depending on the experience of the performer, the nature of the sport and/or performance demands at a particular point within a sport.

In addition to these cognitive aspects, it is also well recognised that exercise performance, particularly when
maximal exertion is involved, is determined by perceptual and motivational factors such as mood, well-being, vigour, alertness and perceived exertion. Like physiological processes, many of these psychological processes exhibit circadian variation. For example, Reilly (1990) reported a circadian rhythm in the rating of perceived exertion associated with steady intense exercise. This was reflected in higher work rates being sustained for a longer period in the evening. Furthermore, a rhythm in self-chosen work rate similarly has been found to be at a maximum in the evening (Coldwells et al, 1992).

What this section has shown is that the circadian variations in physiological and psychological variables lead to a predictable increase in athleticism later in the day. Thus, the scheduling of most sports events in the afternoon or evening is not only socially convenient but also at a time which is most biologically advantageous to the sports performer and, indeed, at a time when athletes prefer to make record attempts (Reilly, 1987).

Advantages and disadvantages of a circadian timing system

The advantages of possessing a circadian clock is that it enables the individual to adjust better to a rhythmic world. The circadian clock provides the individual with a form of **predictive** homeostasis (Moore-Ede, 1986). That is, the biological clock prepares us for the regularly recurring challenges which occur, or are likely to occur, day-by-day by activating physiological responses ahead of the perturbation so that at the time of the perturbation we can respond with maximum efficiency. For example, the circadian timing system enables the body to prepare for waking - by increasing blood pressure, plasma cortisol and adrenaline levels, and body temperature towards the end of the night - and to prepare for sleep by enabling us to "tone down" in the evening.

If the evolutionary value of such a circadian system is clear, then its disadvantages must be considered also (Minors et al, 1986). The biological clock is slow to adjust to changed schedules of sleep and activity. Under most circumstances this inertia is advantageous insofar as that it prevents inappropriate adjustment of the circadian timing system by capricious events, such as an accidental nocturnal wakening. It is disadvantageous, however, when time-zone transitions are considered. The sudden translocation across time zones leads to a sudden change in the phase relationship between external (solar) and internal (biological clock) time. It is during such a mismatch of the biological clock and environmental rhythmicity that the symptoms and inconvenience of jet-lag arise.

Jet-lag effects and performance

The mismatch between external and internal time (termed **external desynchronisation**) following the rapid movement from one time zone to another, results in the temporary malaise colloquially referred to as jet-lag. Individuals may experience fatigue and sleepiness at inappropriate times of the day, and yet may have difficulty in initiating and maintaining sleep through the night. They may lose their appetite, might suffer from gastrointestinal disorders, irregular bowel movements, increased irritability, emotional lability and generally feel "below par". Not unexpectedly, the symptoms tend to increase with the number of time zones crossed, as the degree of external desynchronisation increases, and is generally perceived to be worse after a flight to the east than after one to the west (for reviews, see Comperatore and Krueger, 1990; Winget et al, 1984). The explanation of this asymmetry effect of flight direction is that it reflects the inherent period of the biological clock which, in humans, is greater than 24 hours (see Section 2.1). As a result the resynchronisation of the biological clock which requires a lengthening of period or phase delay, as after a westward flight, is easier to achieve. Of course, jet-lag is a temporary complaint because, with continued time in the new time zone, the biological clock is gradually resynchronised to the local time as it is exposed to the zeitgebers phased appropriately for the new time zone. However, within an individual, the overt rhythms in different variables appear to re-adjust at different rates (Aschoff et al, 1975; Klein et al, 1972; Winget et al, 1984). As a result the normal phase relationship between different rhythms is disrupted, a condition referred to as **internal dissociation,** and this too probably contributes to the symptoms of jet-lag.

Psychological performance decrements

Although fatigue and sleep disturbances are the most frequent complaints associated with jet-lag, the external desynchronisation and internal dissociation associated with transmeridian travel also result in decrements in various aspects of psychological performance (for review, see Winget et al, 1984). The general trends are:

a.   Relatively simple performance, such as reaction time, adapts more rapidly to time-zone shifts than does performance on more complex tasks and those involving dynamic muscle strength, vigilance and endurance.

b.   As with physiological rhythms, phase adjustment is more rapid in the first few post-flight days and adjustment occurs more quickly following westward than eastward flights.

In addition, motivation may be affected. For example, Davis (1988) reported that some athletes have shown an increased failure to comply with team schedules following time-zone transitions.

Physical and sports performance

The general disruption of internal temporal order in physiological systems following a time-zone transition leads to decrements in physical performance. For example, Wright et al (1983) reported about 10% decrements in dynamic arm strength and elbow flexor strength for up to 5 days after a 6-hour time-zone change. In this same study, 270m sprint times and endurance running were also adversely affected 2 to 3 days after the time change. In a further study, decrements were found in international volley-ball and ice hockey competition (Sasaki, 1980). Thus, it is likely that the internal dissociation of rhythms following a time-zone shift will to lead to an athlete being unable to show peak performance, as confirmed in a study of French fencers competing at the Los Angeles Olympics (Reinberg et al, 1985). Even if there is no decrement in sports performance, there is the added complication that, due to the external desynchronisation, peak performance might be found at an inappropriate time of day. For example, Reilly and Mellor (1988) found that following an eastward flight across 9 time zones, grip strength in a group of Rugby League players showed a higher morning value than in the evening and that only by the fourth day after arrival had it reversed to the normal evening peak.

There is a further way in which jet-lag might affect optimal sports performance. A team can also be considered a complex performance system of interacting components, namely the players; individual team members may be differentially affected by jet-lag and show variation in rates of adaptation to a new time zone. Thus, if one or two players in a team have not adjusted to the same extent as the other team members, team performance may be compromised. Overall, the disruptive effects of jet-lag could well be reflected by decrements in psychological performance and ultimately problems in the smooth execution of complex skills. It only takes reaction times to be slightly slower, working memory functioning to be marginally below par, or for there to be a small fault in motor programming, for sport performance to be affected. In addition, it is reasonable to suggest that elevated injury rates may result from reduced functional competence due to jet-lag stress.

Moderating factors

Not all individuals are affected equally by jet-lag and the time necessary for resynchronisation varies between individuals. Winget et al (1985) reported that 25-30% of travellers report only minor or no difficulties adjusting to a new time zone, whilst about an equal proportion reported considerable difficulties. It should be noted, however, that there is a clear dissociation between the subjective complaints associated with jet-lag and objective deficits recorded. People who feel worst do not necessarily perform worst; conversely, and perhaps more importantly, people who report few subjective complaints may show largest objective deficits.

What factors may contribute to the differences in both the objective and subjective deficits reported between individuals?

Age and experience

Age or experience may play a part. It has been reported that following an eastward flight older individuals realistically perceived and rated the gradual improvements in their overall level of performance compared to younger individuals who, despite demonstrating very similar levels of proficiency, rated their performance in a far more negative light (Graeber, 1982). This has obvious implications for the self-confidence, attitude and morale of teams having to compete after rapid time-zone transitions.

Motivation and psychological skills

A highly motivated, cohesive and highly trained team who have wide experience of international travel may well be more resistant to jet-lag effects on performance (see, for example, McFarland, 1975). At one level the activation pattern for extremely well-learned and practised skills may be harder to disrupt. At another level, successful, elite performers tend to possess a highly developed repertoire of psychological skills such as concentration, anxiety control and motivating techniques (Mahoney et al, 1987) which operate to maintain or regain the necessary pattern of psychological processes for performance to proceed relatively smoothly (Hardy and Fazey, 1988; Jones and Hardy, 1989). The sports psychology literature is increasingly reporting the vital role played by such psychological skills (Hardy, 1990). Their significance in the context of performance following transmeridian flight remains to be investigated.

Personality differences

Personality differences, such as introversion-extraversion and neuroticism have also been suggested to influence tolerance to circadian disruption (Colquhoun and Folkard, 1978), especially that related to shiftwork schedules which require regular bouts of night duty. Similarly, circadian type characteristics based upon features of circadian rhythms such as rhythm stability, amplitude, or phase, could theoretically moderate the degree to which a person feels jet-lagged. For example, flexibility of sleeping habits, described as the ability to sleep at unusual times and in unfamiliar locations (Folkard et al, 1979), or morningness-eveningness (Horne and Ostberg, 1976) which relates to the degree to which a person is a "lark" (morning active) or an "owl" (evening/night active) could influence the experience of malaise and debilitation. Colquhoun (1979), for example, reported that evening types showed a greater shift (resynchronisation) in their circadian temperature phase compared to morning types, and noted that this difference persisted for at least 12 days post-flight.

Flight stress, sleep disturbance and fatigue

Despite the evidence presented in the preceding sections, not all of the stress effects associated with rapid time-zone transition can be laid at the door of disturbed circadian rhythms. Having to fly itself, fly long distances for extended periods of time in the confined space of an aircraft, and negotiate the procedures at airports may be a stressful process which has particular physical and psychological consequences for the individual (Monk, 1987).

Sleep deprivation and fatigue

Nevertheless, relative sleep deprivation and degradation of sleep quality stemming from a phase shift of the sleep/wake cycle may well impact on performance by contributing to the experience of fatigue which is possibly the most frequently reported complaint connected with transmeridian flight. It is well established that fatigue as a result of partial sleep deprivation can affect performance on tasks tapping underlying cognitive abilities as well as on more complex skills. As fatigue increases, skilled individuals appear to lose the smooth coordination and organization of parts of a task, and concentration tends to falter.

Thus, performance patterns may lose cohesion, timing may be put out, responses may become more variable and distractibility can increase (Boff and Lincoln, 1988). There may thus be a combined detrimental effect since sports performers become fatigued anyway, as a result of their exertions in their sport.

Alleviation of jet-lag

As indicated in previous sections, immediately following a flight across several time zones an individual is likely to suffer the symptoms of jet-lag, and for the sportsperson this is likely to result in decreased performance and athleticism. Therefore, it is advised that the individual should arrive several days early at the site of competition. (If for some reason the rules of competition forbid this, then arrival at a place nearby, in the same time zone or a neighbouring time zone, is recommended.) The number of days required, as indicated previously, is dependent upon the direction and number of time zones crossed. As a "rule of thumb", about 0.75 day for each time zone crossed in a westward direction and at least one day per time zone crossed in an eastward direction, is recommended. In addition, several ways of assisting and even accelerating the adjustment of the biological clock during these days have been suggested.

Pre-adaptation
It has been suggested that an individual can attempt to pre-adjust the biological clock prior to a flight across time zones. This would involve adjusting the time of sleep to correspond to that in the destination time zone. This could be achieved by changing the time of sleep by 1 or 2 hours each day for several days before the flight, advancing them in the case of an eastward flight or delaying them before a westward flight. However, in addition to possibly interfering with a training schedule, such a change is difficult to achieve since the individual is having to live at variance with the zeitgebers in the environment around him and the rest of society. As a result adjustment of the body clock is difficult to achieve; this is a problem faced by the nightworker, who also has difficulty shifting his biological clock (for review, see Folkard et al, 1985). Indeed, in one study in which athletes attempted to preadapt (Sasaki, 1980) it was concluded that the effort involved made it unsatisfactory.

Nevertheless, the process of resynchronisation of the biological clock should be attempted as soon as possible, even starting during the flight. This involves resetting one's wristwatch to the destination time immediately upon boarding the plane and, particularly if a long flight is involved, attempting to sleep at the time appropriate for the destination.

Strengthening zeitgebers
The sleep/wake cycle, social behaviour and activity
On arrival in a new time zone an individual should adopt a sleep/wake cycle appropriate for new local time. Thus, even if it is difficult to initiate sleep after an eastward time-shift, or there is premature awakening after a westward time-shift, the individual should remain lying in bed attempting to sleep. The practice adopted by some athletes of having early morning training session and then an afternoon nap is likely to hinder resynchronisation in the first few days after a flight, particularly after one in an eastwardly direction. This is because the afternoon will correspond to night-time by pre-flight time and so a portion of sleep is being anchored at a time which will hinder resynchronisation to the new time zone (Minors and Waterhouse, 1981b).

In addition, an individual should develop local social contacts, participate in outdoor activity and take meals at an appropriate time of day. (Although it might be tempting to try the local specialist menus, an individual should attempt to take meals of habitual composition since sudden changes in diet are likely to lead to gastrointestinal upset.) Thus, when a group of subjects was transported across 6 time zones and restricted to their hotel rooms, adjustments to the new time zone took 5-6 days longer than in a group who performed regular exercise and were allowed outdoor activity on alternate days (Klein and Wegmann, 1974). It should be noted, however, that the group restricted to their hotel rooms, would be more restricted in their access to daylight (see Section 8.2.2), as well as being more isolated socially and restricted in their physical activity. That physical activity itself might accelerate resynchronisation of the biological clock is indicated by observations on hamsters. Thus, it has been possible to produce phase shifts of the biological clock in this species by forcing them to exercise (in a running wheel) at certain times of the day (Mrosovsky and Salmon, 1987). Furthermore, the size and direction of the phase shift produced was dependent upon the time of exercise; that is, a PRC (see Section 2.1) to exercise exists in this species (Reebs and Mrosovsky, 1989). Whether or not exercise **per se** can induce such phase shifts in humans has yet to be tested.

More recently there has been the attempt to identify which component of the environment and/or social behaviour might act as a zeitgeber in humans and thus might be used to hasten re-entrainment of the biological clock after a time shift. In particular, the role of the light/dark cycle has been investigated.

Light
Originally it was believed that, although an important zeitgeber in most species, the light/dark cycle associated with the solar day was relatively unimportant in the human since artificial light enabled us to develop independent of the solar day. However, the experiments which indicated little role for the light/dark cycle as a zeitgeber in humans (Wever, 1979) used light of normal artificial domestic intensity (about 300-500 lux). Relatively recently it has been shown that man **does**

respond to light provided it is of sufficient intensity. Thus, work by several groups has shown that exposure to bright light at specific times of the day can phase-shift the human circadian clock (for review, see Minors, and Waterhouse, 1990) and recently a phase-response curve to light in humans has been demonstrated by two groups (Czeisler et al, 1989; Minors et al, 1991). Both these groups have shown that exposure to bright light (>8000 lux) for 3-5 hours will produce a phase shift of the biological clock provided that exposure occurs near the time of the body temperature minimum (normally about 0500); a light pulse centred just prior to the body temperature minimum produced a phase delay of the biological clock, whereas when the light exposure was centred just after the body temperature minimum, a phase advance was produced. Based on these findings, the following recommendations can be made:

a   In the first few days after a time-zone transition an individual should attempt to be outdoors in natural daylight at some times of day, but avoid exposure to daylight at others.

b   After an eastward flight when an advance of the biological clock is required, exposure to daylight (bright light) should take place, if possible, for at least three hours, starting about one hour ahead of 0500 on the time of the point of departure (that is, 0400 plus the number of time zones crossed, by local time). In addition, the individual should try to relax indoors (in dim light) in the four hours prior to the above time.

c   After a westward flight, exposure to daylight, of at least three hours duration, should terminate at about 0600 on the time of the point of departure (that is, 0600 minus the number of time zones crossed, by local time). Outdoor light exposure should then be avoided for the next five hours.

Meals

The evidence that regular **times** of meals can act as a zeitgeber is contentious and has been summarised elsewhere (Minors and Waterhouse, 1986). However, there remains the possibility that the **composition** of meals might affect the biological clock, perhaps by changing the availability of the precursors of certain neurotransmitters. Based on earlier experiments in rats, Ehret and Scanlon (1983) devised a regimen for combatting jet-lag which involved modifications of meals. Briefly, the regimen consists of alternating days when heavy meals are taken with days of light meals for four days prior to the day of travel. Both on days before and after the flight the composition of meals is controlled. Breakfast and lunch are high protein/low carbohydrate meals (which, in theory, results in increased brain uptake of the amino acid tyrosine, the precursor of catecholamines - the mediators of wakefulness) and a low protein/high carbohydrate meal is taken in the evening (which leads, in theory, to an increase in brain uptake of tryptophan, the precursor of the neurotransmitter 5-HT, which may mediate drowsiness). In addition, the intake of caffeine is encouraged at certain times of day. Whether or not the changes in diet bring about the proposed changes is contentious (for critique, see Redfern, 1989). The efficiency of the regimen has been tested by Graeber (1982) on military personnel. After a westward flight over 6 time zones, subjects adhering to the regimen reported less subjective fatigue, fewer sleep disturbances and increased cognitive performance, compared with control subjects who did not use the regimen. However, it is to be noted that the regimen not only used changed meals but also rigorous adoption of sleep/wake schedules (and thus social contacts, etc. - see Section 8.2.1). Thus, it is unclear to what extent the benefit to be gained by the regimen results from these latter factors rather than by altered meals. In addition, the regimen is unacceptable to many sports performers who have rigorous training diets.

Chronobiotics

In addition to manipulation or reinforcement of environmental and/or social zeitgebers, acceleration of the resynchronis-ation of the biological clock after a time-zone transition by the use of drugs or other substances has been investigated. Substances which are able to induce phase shifts or changes in period of the biological clock are referred to as **chronobiotics.**

Although in other species several chronobiotics have been identified, here we will concentrate on two, those where most advance in the potential for amelioration of jet-lag has been made.

Melatonin

The hormone melatonin is secreted by the pineal gland and controls many photoperiod responses (e.g. seasonal breeding) in several non-human species. Its role in man is more controversial. Nevertheless there is a close functional and anatomical relationship between the biological clock in the suprachiasmatic nuclei and the pineal gland (for review, see Armstrong, 1989).

The potential use of melatonin to alleviate jet-lag in humans was first tested by Arendt et al (1986). In a double-blind study, a group of 8 subjects who took melatonin in the evening for several days before and after a flight across 8 time zones in an eastward direction, subjectively rated almost no jet-lag, whereas 6 of a group of 9 subjects taking a placebo reported quite severe jet-lag. That melatonin can decrease the **subjective** feeling of jet-lag (mostly sleep disturbance) has also been reported subsequently by others (see, for example, Petry et al, 1989). However, the evidence that melatonin accelerated resynchronisation of the biological clock was less clear (Arendt et al, 1987).

More recently, the experiments of Arendt et al have been repeated to assess whether or not melatonin can indeed

accelerate resynchronisation of the biological clock (Samel et al, 1991). Results gave some evidence that resynchronisation of circadian rhythmicity after a simulated eastward flight across 9 time zones was more rapid in a group receiving melatonin than in a control group. An explanation to these results has been provided recently by the findings of Lewy et al (1991) who have described a PRC to melatonin. They report that administration of melatonin in the afternoon/evening causes phase advances of the biological clock (required after an eastward flight), whereas a phase delay results following administration in the late night/morning (required after a westward flight).

Thus, the potential use of melatonin for alleviation of jet-lag is clear. However, two further points need be made. First, possible toxic side effects of this hormone cannot yet be excluded. Second, whether or not the governing bodies of various sports allow the use of this hormone is still to be resolved.

Hypnotics

One of the most frequently reported symptoms of jet-lag is the inability to take a full night's sleep and then a consequent fatigue at an inappropriate time of day. The initiation of sleep by hypnotics may be beneficial not only in reducing the amount of fatigue as a result of improved sleep, but also the regular sleep induced at an appropriate time of day might act as a zeitgeber (see section 8.2.1) and thus hasten resynchronisation of the biological clock. (Note, however, that if physical and psychological decrements are to be avoided, the hypnotic used should be short-acting and for many athletes there are likely to be competition drug restrictions which bar the their use.)

Anecdotal evidence suggests that many individuals who frequently undergo time-zone transitions often use alcohol to induce sleep. Use of alcohol is not recommended, however, since although it induces slow wave sleep, it leads to disturbances of REM sleep and sleep fragmentation. Furthermore, its diuretic effect is likely to lead to an awakening to empty a full bladder.

In addition to induction of sleep, there is another way in which hypnotics might be useful in the treatment of jet-lag. It has been shown in hamsters that the short-acting benzodiazepine, triazolam, can phase-shift the biological clock and hasten resynchronisation following a phase shift of the external light/dark cycle (see, for reviews, Turek and Van Reeth, 1988;l989). Furthermore, a phase-response curve to this hypnotic was described; a phase advance of the biological clock being obtained when triazolam was administered 3-6 hours before the normal time of the animals' activity onset and a phase delay when it was administered 6-12 hours after the activity onset.

Whether or not these hypnotics can phase shift the human biological clock remains to be thoroughly investigated. It is noteworthy that, in hamsters, the effect of triazolam is to **increase** activity, indicating that it may not be possible to extrapolate from animal experiments to human.

Concluding remarks

Today's frequency of sport-related international jet travel suggests that elite competitors are increasingly exposed to the experience of jet-lag and that their overall performance may suffer, possibly for a week or more, following transmeridian flight. Although such conclusions seem reasonable in the light of existing research, there have been only few scientific studies which have systematically examined the relationships between sport-specific performance and the effects of rapid travel across time zones. Such research would have the dual benefits of helping improve sporting achievement as well as contributing to the knowledge base and understanding of jet-lag which, of course, has implications for a much wider population. When the means of alleviating jet-lag are considered, it is likely that the drug restrictions imposed by many sports governing bodies will make many of the potential chronobiotics unavailable to the sports performer. Thus, those methods using naturally available zeitgebers are likely to prove the most effective way of ameliorating jet-lag for the sports performer.

References

Arendt J, Aldhous M and Marks V. (1986) Alleviation of jet-lag by melatonin: Preliminary results of a controlled double blind trial. Br Med J, 292, 1170.

Arendt J, Aldhous M, English V, Marks M and Folkard S. (1987) Some effects of jet-lag and their alleviation by melatonin. Ergonomics, 30, 1379-1393. Armstrong SM. (1989) Melatonin: the internal zeitgeber in mammals? Pineal Res, 7, 157-202. Aschoff J, Hoffman K, Pohl H and Wever R. (1975) Re-entrainment of circadian rhythms after phase shifts of the zeitgeber. Chronobiologia, 2, 23-78.

Boff KR and Lincoln JE. (1988) Fatigue, Section 10-8, Engineering Data Compendium: Human Performance and Perception. Vol III, Harry G Armstrong Aerospace Medical Research Laboratory, Wright-Patterson Airforce Base, Ohio.

Colquhoun WP. (1979) Phase shift in temperature rhythm after transmeridian flight, as related to pre-flight phase angle. Int Arch Occup Environ Hlth, 42, 149-157.

Colquhoun WP. (1982) Biological rhythms and performance, in Biological Rhythms, Sleep and Performance (ed WB Webb), Wiley, London, pp. 59-86.

Colquhoun WP and Folkard S. (1978) Personality differences in body temperature rhythm, and their relation to its adjustment to night work. Ergonomics, 21, 811-817.

Coldwells A, Atkinson G, Reilly T and Waterhouse JM. (1992) Self-chosen work-rate determines day-night differences in work capacity. Ergonomics, In Press.

Comperatore CA and Krueger GP. (1990) Circadian rhythm desynchronosis, jet-lag, shift-lag and coping strategies. Occupational Medicine: State of the art reviews, Vol 5(2), (ed A Scott), Hanley and Belfus, Philadelphia, pp. 323-341.

Czeisler CA, Kronauer RR, Allan JS, Duffy JF, Jewett ME, Brown EN and Ronda JM. (1989) Bright light induction of strong (type O) resetting of the human circadian pacemaker. Science, 244, 1328-1333.

Davis JO. (1988) Strategies for managing athlete's jet lag. Sport Psychologist, 2, 154-160.

Ehret CF and Scanlon LW. (1983) Overcoming Jet-Lag. Berkley Publishing Corp, New York.

Folkard S. (1990) Circadian performance rhythms: some practical and theoretical implications. Phil Trans R Soc B, 327, 543-553.

Folkard S, Minors DS and Waterhouse JM. (1985) Chronobiology and shift work: current issues and trends. Chronobiologia, 12, 31-54.

Folkard S, Monk TH and Lobban M. (1979) Towards a predictive test of adjustment to shiftwork. Ergonomics, 22, 79-91.

Graeber RC. (1982) Alterations in performance following rapid transmeridian flight, in Rhythmic Aspects of Behaviour (eds FM Brown and RC Graeber), Erlbaum, Hillsdale NJ. pp. 173-212.

Hardy L. (1990) Sport psychology, in Psychology Survey 7 (eds AM Coleman and JG Beaumont), BPS and Routledge, London, pp. 73-92.

Hardy L and Fazey J. (1988) Mental Preparation for Performance, National Coaching Foundation, Leeds.

Horne JA and Ostberg O. (1976) A self-assessment questionnaire to determine morningness-eveningness in human circadian rhythms. Int J Chronobiol, 4, 97-110.

Jones JG and Hardy L. (1989) Stress and cognitive functioning in sport. J Sport Sci, 7, 41-63.

Klein KE and Wegmann HM. (1974) The resynchronization of human circadian rhythms after transmeridian flights as a result of flight direction and mode of activity, in Chronobiology (eds LE Scheving, F Halberg and JE Pauly), Igaku Shoin, Tokyo, pp. 564-570.

Klein KE, Wegmann HM and Hunt BI. (1972) Desynchronization of body temperature and performance circadian rhythm as a result of outgoing and homegoing transmeridian flights. Aerospace Med, 43, 120-132.

Lewy AJ, Sack RL and Latham JM. (1991) Melatonin and the acute suppressant effect of light may help regulate circadian rhythms in humans, in Advances in Pineal Research 5, (eds J Arendt and P Pevet), John Libby, London, pp. 285-293.

Mahoney MJ, Gabriel TJ and Perkins TS. (1987) Psychological skills and exceptional athletic performance. Sport Psychologist, 1, 181-189.

McFarland RA. (1975) Air travel across time zones. Amer Sci, 63, 23-30.

Minors DS, Scott AR and Waterhouse JM. (1986) Circadian arrhythmia: shiftwork, travel and health. J Soc Occup Med, 36, 39-44.

Minors DS and Waterhouse JM. (1981a) Circadian Rhythms and the Human. Wright-PSG, Bristol.

Minors DS and Waterhouse JM. (1981b) Anchor sleep as a synchronizer of rhythms on abnormal routines. Int J Chronobiol, 7, 165-188.

Minors DS and Waterhouse JM. (1986) Circadian rhythms and their mechanisms. Experientia, 42, 1-13.

Minors DS and Waterhouse JM. (1990) The influence of light on the entrainment of the circadian system: an introduction, in Shiftwork: Health, Sleep and Performance (eds G Costa, G Cesana, K Kogi and A Wedderburn), Peter Lang, Frankfurt, pp. 235-240.

Minors DS, Waterhouse JM and Wirz-Justice A. (1991) A human phase-response curve to light. Neurosci Lett, In Press.

Monk TH. (1987) Coping with the stress of jet-lag. Work and Stress, 1, 163-166.

Moore-Ede MC. (1986) Physiology of the circadian timing system: predictive versus reactive homeostasis. Am J Physiol, 250, R735-R752.

Mrosovsky N and Salmon PA. (1987) A behavioural method for accelerating re-entrainment of rhythms to new light-dark cycles. Nature, 330, 372-373.

Petry K, Conaglen JV, Thompson L and Chamberlain K. (1980) Effect of melatonin on jet-lag after long haul flights. Br Med J, 297, 705-707.

Redfern PH. (1989) "Jet-lag": strategies for prevention and cure. Hum Psychopharm, 4, 159-168.

Reebs SG and Mrosovsky N. (1989) Effects of induced wheel running on the circadian activity rhythms of syrian hamsters: entrainment and phase response curve. J Biol Rhythms, 4, 39-48.

Reilly T. (1987) Circadian rhythms and exercise, in Exercise: Benefits, Limits and Adaptations. (eds D Macleod, RJ Maughan, M Nimms, T Reilly and C Williams), E & FN Spon, London, pp. 346-364.

Reilly T. (1990) Human circadian rhythms and exercise. Crit Rev Biomed Eng, 18, 165-180.

Reilly T and Mellor S. (1988) Jet lag in student Rugby League players following a near-maximal time-zone shift, in Science and Football (eds T Reilly, A Lees, K Davids and WJ Murphy), E & FN Spon, London, pp. 249-256.

Reinberg A, Proux S, Bartal JP, Levi F and Bicakova-Rocher A. (1985) Circadian rhythms in competitive sabre fencers: internal desynchronisation and performance. Chronobiol Int, 2, 195-201.

Rosenwasser AM and Adler NT. (1986) Structure and function in circadian timing systems: Evidence for multiple coupled circadian oscillators. Neurosci Behav Rev, 10, 431-448.

Samel A, Wegmann H-M, Vejvoda M, Maass H, Gundel A and Schutz M. (1991) Influence of melatonin treatment on human circadian rhythmicity before and after a simulated 9-hr time shift. J Biol Rhythms, 6, 235-248.

Sasaki T. (1980) Effect of jet-lag on sports performance, in Chronobiology: Principles and Applications to Shifts in Schedules (eds L Scheving and F Halberg), Sijthoff & Noordhoff, Rockville, MD, pp. 417-431.

Shephard RJ. (1984) Sleep, biorhythms and human performance. Sports Med, 1, 11-37.

Silver R, Lehman MN, Gibson M, Gladstone WR and Bittman EL. (1990) Dispersal cell suspensions of fetal SCN restore circadian rhythmicity in SCN-lesioned adult hamsters. Brain Res, 525, 45-58.

Turek FW and Van Reeth O. (1988) Altering the mammalian circadian clock with the short-acting benzodiazepine triazolam. Trends Neurosci, 11, 535-541.

Turek FW and Van Reeth O. (1989) Use of benzodiazepines to manipulate the circadian clock regulating behavioural and endocrine rhythms. Horm Res, 31, 59-65.

Wever R. (1979) The Circadian System of Man. Springer-Verlag, New York.

Winget CM, DeRoshia CW, Markley CM and Holley DC. (1984) A review of human physiological performance changes associated with desynchronosis of biological rhythms. Aviat Space Environ Med, 55, 1085-1096.

Winget CM, DeRoshia CW and Holley DC. (1985) Circadian rhythms and athletic performance. Med Sci Sports Exerc, 17, 498-516.

Wright JE, Vogel JA, Sampson JB, Knapik JJ, Patton JF and Daniels WL. (1983) Effects of travel across time zones (jet-lag) on exercise capacity and performance. Aviat Space Environ Med, 54, 132-137.

Heat acclimation

M.A. Kolka

Abstract. The international nature of sport, with athletes of all ages moving between different climatic conditions and across time zones is associated with impaired performance of intense exercise as the result of failure to make appropriate arrangements for heat acclimation, failure to allow adequate time to overcome jet-lag and inadequate hydration.

Keywords: Heat Acclimation, Intense Exercise, Hydration, Avoidance of Cardiovascular Strain.

Weekend, collegiate or world class sportsmen all face similar difficulties when travelling to different climates or different time zones for competition, much like businessmen who travel around the world to close important business deals. It is essential that changes in climate are fully considered before the actual competition begins, or the sportsman starts the competition at a decided disadvantage.

Recently, our laboratory reviewed problems associated with different environmental and physiological challenges such as heat acclimation, sleep loss or circadian period on exercise performance (Pandolf et al, 1988). This paper will address issues associated with heat acclimation, as problems associated with jet lag and biological rhythms are discussed elsewhere in this conference.

The International Union of Physiological Sciences Thermal Commission has defined heat acclimation as adaptive changes which occur in response to experimentally induced changes in climatic factors in a controlled environment, and has defined heat acclimatization as those adaptive changes which occur in response to changes in the natural environment (Pflugers' Glossary of terms, 1987). Before specifically addressing physiologic issues associated with heat acclimation, I would like to introduce some basic tenets of heat exchange and temperature regulation.

Body temperature regulation in humans is based on a proportional control svstem (Figure 1), in that, a thermoregulatory response, i.e. sweating or dilation of blood vessels near the skin surface (to dissipate heat) occurs proportionally to increases in core temperature (Boulant et al, 1980). Furthermore, higher skin surface temperature can also stimulate sweating or cutaneous vasodilation, but only about a tenth as effective as increasing core temperature (Bullard et al, 1970).

In looking at Figure 1, it is important to understand how the terms "threshold" and central thermosensitivity are used in thermoregulatory control theory. The threshold is the core or skin temperature above which the thermoregulatory effector response (R, sweating or cutaneous vasodilation for heat loss) is greater than the response observed at rest in a thermoneutral environment. A change in the thermoregulatory effector threshold is often referred to as a change in the "thermoregulatory set point". Threshold changes occur during the circadian period, with menstrual cycle phase, as a result of fever, and after heat acclimation (Stephenson et al, 1988). The slope or thermosensitivity is the difference in thermoregulatory effector response (R), usually per °C change in core temperature. Slope changes can be indicative of peripheral changes at the effector or central alterations in effector response. Slope changes occur after sleep loss, during exposure to hypobaria or following dehydration (Stephenson et al, 1988).

Heat exchange can be expressed by a series of equations, the most common is the heat balance equation, which is consistent with the First Law of Thermodynamics.

$$S = M - (\pm W_k) \pm E \pm R \pm C \pm K [W \cdot m_{.2}]$$

where: S = heat storage; M = internal heat production, or metabolism; Wk = work; E = evaporation or insensible (wet) heat exchange which is set by the environment, and is influenced by the sweating rate; R = radiation; C = convection; K = conduction, R and C combine as sensible (dry) heat exchange which is determined by the environment. Heat exchange via K is minimal during upright exercise. All parameters are expressed in W·m-2.

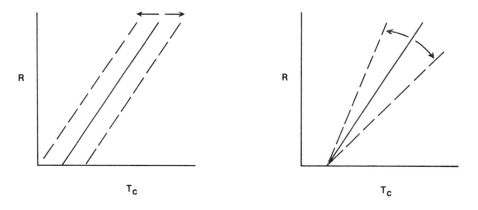

Fig. 1 Graphic representation for proportional control of human body temperature. R is an effector response, such as sweating or vasodilation and T_c is the body core temperature. Movement along the X axis indicates a threshold change in the effector response. A slope change indicates alteration in the sensitivity of the effector response to a given change in T_c.

Heat exchange from the body core to the skin surface and from the skin surface to or from the environment is shown in Figure 2. Metabolic heat production (H) shown in Figure 2, is metabolism - work. Upon exposure to a hot environment, radiative and convective (R+C, dry) heat loss is less than during exposure to a comfortable environment, as the temperature gradient between the skin surface and the ambient temperature determines dry heat loss. At 27°C, skin temperature averages 30-31°C, therefore a favorable gradient exists for heat loss via R+C. However, at 36°C, skin temperature (T,) averages 35°C and little heat exchange is possible. If the ambient temperature is higher than skin surface, R+C will be negative, indicating heat gain. If the ambient temperature is warm and has a high water vapor content, heat loss will be compromised by both inefficient evaporation of secreted sweat, and by an unfavorable gradient for dry heat loss from the skin surface to the environment.

A sportsman not acclimated to the heat cannot sustain performance in the heat at the same level as in a cool or temperate environment. For example, at 40°C (T, = 36°C) compared to 27°C (T, = 31°C), although metabolic heat production from the sport may be similar in the two environments, the sportsman will be gaining heat from the environment (R+C) instead of losing heat from the body as was the case at 27°C. Higher core and surface temperatures at 40°C increase sweating rate (proportional control, Figure 1) leading to increased water loss primarily from extracellular compartments.

Additionally, a greater proportion of blood is directed to the skin vascular beds for heat dissipation from core to skin and from skin to the environment thereby increasing cardiovascular strain. However, heat from the body core cannot be effectively dissipated through increasing skin blood flow, and the cardiovascular system becomes compromised.

In 1943, Adolph identified various physiologic effects upon acclimation to desert heat (Adolph, 1943). Among these physiologic changes were lower heart rate, lower pulse pressure, lower core temperature, lower basal oxygen consumption, decreased sweat concentration (electrolytes), increased sweating rate, increased endurance and increased work output (Adolph, 1943). Regular heavy exercise in the heat is the best method to promote the physiologic changes necessary for heat acclimation. However, moderate exercise for ~1 hour/day will result in some heat acclimation, as will resting in a hot environment (Wenger, 1988).

Cardiovascular changes that decrease the heart rate, such as increased plasma volume are observed in the first few days of heat acclimation. In addition higher sweating rates are seen early in the acclimation process. Sweating starts at a lower core temperature (lower threshold), and the sensitivity to increasing core temperature may be higher after heat acclimation (Wenger, 1988). That is, the sweat glands become more responsive to stimulation from core and skin inputs. Secreted sweat becomes more dilute as sodium is reabsorbed and the sweat glands become more responsive to aldosterone which is releassd in response to heat exposure or exercise. These higher sweating rates can be maintained for longer

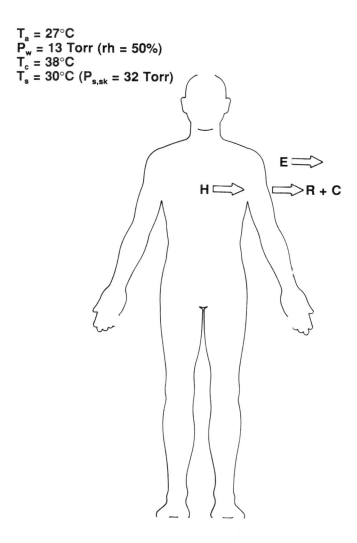

$T_a = 27°C$
$P_w = 13$ Torr (rh = 50%)
$T_c = 38°C$
$T_s = 30°C$ ($P_{s,sk} = 32$ Torr)

Fig. 2   Basic pathways for heat loss in an upright human.

Table 1. Physiologic changes which occur with acclimation to dry or wet heat which assist in decreasing physiologic strain associated with heat exposure.

DRY HEAT	WET HEAT
sweating rate	sweating on limbs
plasma volume	plasma volume
heart rate	heart rate
core temperature	core temperature

periods of time after heat acclimation without additional cardiovascular strain (Wenger, 1988).

The decrease in heart rate may be due to decreased circulatory strain from increased plasma volume (same plasma protein concentration), increased venous tone, decreased peripheral pooling, and lower core and surface temperatures (Wenger, 1988). Heat acclimation decreases the core temperature threshold for skin blood flow which parallels the effect seen for eccrine sweating (Wenger, 1988).

Possible changes ((Wenger, 1988) in blood flow to the skin which occur during heat acclimation include: 1) longer residence of blood in the skin vascular beds as more vessels are opened; 2) routing of blood through vessels which may be more advantageous for heat loss; or 3) preferentially increasing blood flow to specific vascular beds in the skin, such as the arms or legs. At present, there is little experimental evidence to support any of these possibilities.

Acclimation to humid heat can pose different problems to the sportsman than acclimation to dry heat. Evaporation of sweat is the primary mode of heat loss in any environment in which the ambient temperature is equal to, or higher than the temperature of the skin surface and is limited by the ambient water vapor pressure. Therefore, in hot, humid environments, limited evaporative cooling results in higher heat storage, greater cardiovascular strain and decreased performance. It has been suggested that there must be a gradient between saturated vapor at the skin surface and the ambient air of approximately 18-20 Torr for adequate evaporative heat loss (Gonzalez et al, 1974).

Eccrine sweat glands are distributed over the entire body surface. The density of sweat glands ranges from 270 glands cm^{-2} on the face to 160-185 glands cm^{-2} on the trunk and arms to 130 glands cm^{-2} on the legs (Szabo, 1962). During acclimation to humid heat, whole body sweating rate increases and the proportion of sweat secreted is redistributed toward limbs to increase the surface area for heat exchange (Hofler, 1968). This allows more efficient use of the wetted surface for evaporative heat loss. In humid environments, skin blood flow is crucial for heat exchange. Increased blood flow to the skin not only transfers heat from the core, but increases skin temperature slightly so a more favorable gradient for dry heat loss occurs. In addition, increasing skin temperature can raise the saturated vapor pressure at the skin surface thereby establishing a more favorable gradient for evaporative heat loss. Acclimation to humid heat requires substantial circulatory adaptation (Wenger, 1988).

To show the difference between unacclimated and partially acclimated subjects, the physiologic responses to two different heat acclimation regimens (dry heat) are presented in the following paragraphs. In the first study, eight young healthy men walked at 30% of their maximal aerobic power for two, fifty minute periods separated by a ten minute rest period. The environmental conditions were 49°C and 20% relative humidity. The acclimation period lasted nine days. The results of heat acclimation to a very hot, dry environment are shown in Figures 3-5.

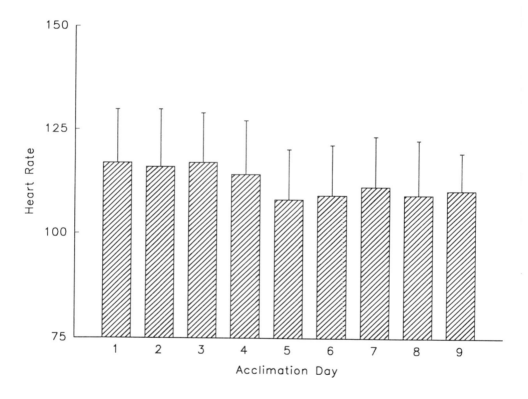

Fig. 3   Heart rate responses to a 9 day heat acclimation program at 49°C/20%rh.

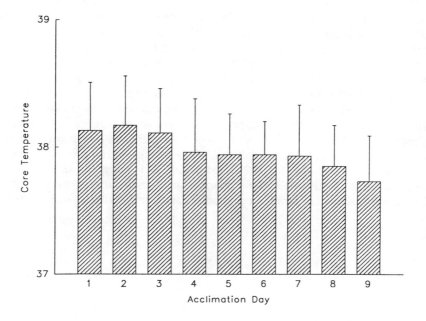

Fig. 4   Core temperature responses to a 9 day heat acclimation program at 49°C/20%rh.

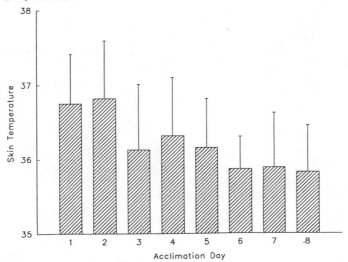

Fig. 5   Skin temperature responses to a 9 day heat acclimation program at 49°C/20%rh.

Heart rate decreased with heat acclimation, showing the biggest effect after day 4. Core and skin temperatures were lower after heat acclimation. The lower skin temperature shows that sweating and skin blood flow adapted to increase heat dissipation. In fact, the sweating rate was 10-15% higher during exercise in the heat on day 9 of heat acclimation compared to day 1.

In a second study, eight young healthy men walked at 30% of their maximal aerobic power for 100 minutes. The environmental conditions were 42°C and 20% relative humidity. This study was run in the spring and the subjects were already partially acclimated to the heat. These results are shown in Figures 6-8. Heart rate was approximately 10 beats per minute lower on day 5 than day 1 with the most dramatic change after day 3. Core and skin temperatures were fairly stable during heat acclimation decreasing 0.1-0.2°C from day 1 to day 5. Although these physiologic changes were small, these changes are beneficial as greater heat loss with lower cardiovascular strain occurs after heat acclimation which increases performance.

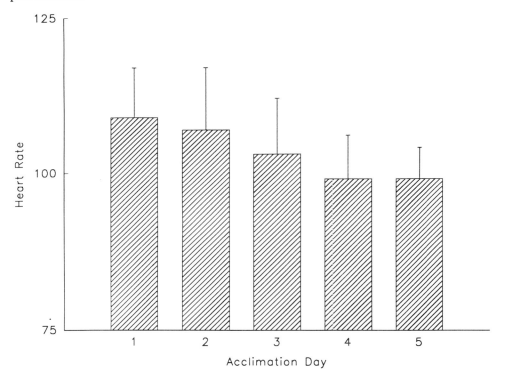

Figs. 6   Heart rate responses to a 5 day heat acclimation program at 42°C/20%rh.

Damage limitation

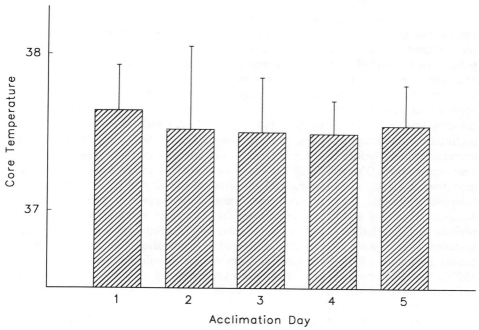

Fig. 7 Core temperature responses to a 5 day heat acclimation program at 49°C/20%rh.

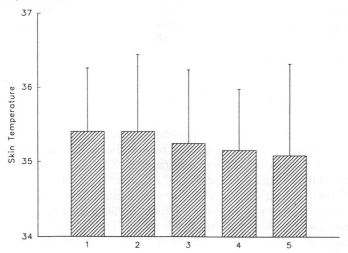

Fig. 8 Skin temperature responses to a 5 day heat acclimation program at 49°C/20%rh.

The effects of exercise training are similar to those seen after heat acclimation. Among the physiologic changes observed after exercise training are lower heart rate, higher stroke volume, lower core and skin temperatures, decreased core temperature threshold for sweating and skin blood flow, increased aerobic power, and increased work performance. In some studies the effects of exercise training and heat acclimation cannot be distinguished as subjects "train" during a heat acclimation protocol (Wenger, 1988). This commonly occurs when untrained subjects are used. To avoid possible confounding effects of training and heat acclimation, investigators 1) choose to use highly trained subjects, 2) institute exercise training before heat acclimation, 3) or use low exercise intensities during heat acclimation. Gisolfi (1977) has reported that work in the heat, by previously untrained subjects, can be enhanced by physical training in a cool environment. However, physical training does not completely replace a program of heat acclimation as core and skin temperatures do not remain elevated for long enough periods to fully challenge the cardiovascular system. Subjects with long training histories, that is years of physical training at high metabolic work intensities, can readily perform light work in very hot, dry or hot, humid environments (Gisolfi, 1977). However, performance of intense exercise in warm and hot environments remains compromised. Again, the best method for heat acclimation is regular, heavy exercise in the heat.

In summary, exposure to hot environments, whether dry or humid, puts additional cardiovascular and thermal strain on the body. When core and skin temperatures remain elevated, when increased sweating causes progressive dehydration and when perfusion of skin vascular beds is increased, heat loss and cardiovascular stability may be compromised. The physiologic changes associated with acclimation to a hot environment, allow more efficient heat loss without additional cardiovascular strain.

Practical implications

In preparing for the 1990 Race Across America, Nancy Raposo visited our laboratory in the fall of 1989 to discuss tactics she might use in the upcoming Race Across America to better her performance. The Race Across Amenca is a bicycle event which starts in California and ends two weeks later in New England. After a brief discussion, it was clear that her third place finish, in fact finishing the 1988 Race Across America (13 days, 18 hours and 30 minutes), was an incredible athletic achievement. When she started the race in 1988, Raposo was not adapted to west coast time, she was not acclimated to the desert heat, she became severely dehydrated the first day biking through the Mohave, and she slept very little during the 12-13 days of the race. We 1) suggested that she artificially acclimate to the heat of the Southern California desert while still in New England, 2) stressed hydration, especially early in the race to prevent a substantial total body water deficit over days which would severely affect her performance, 3) asked her to arrive in California with enough time before the start of the Race Across America to shift her biological timing to the west coast, 4) required 4-5 hours of sleep each night to insure a period of slow wave or restorative sleep, and 5) asked that she wear clothing that would minimize heat gain. From her 1988 results, we determined that her daily milage was low for an athlete of her caliber during the Race Across America, probably due to lack of heat acclimation, chronic dehydration and little or no sleep. At minimal cost, Raposo was able to prepare for the Race Across America by training in a greenhouse, stressing fluid intake, and arriving in California two weeks before the race. After following the suggestions outlined above, Nancy Raposo won the 1990 Race Across America by a significlant margin.

References

Adolph EF. (1943) Physiological fitness for the desert. Federation Proceedlngs, 2, 158-164,

Boulant JA. (1980) Hypothalamic control of thermoregulation. In: PJ Morgane, J Panksepp (eds.) Handbook of the Hypothalamus Vol 3, Part A, Behavioral Studies of the Hypothalamus, New York, Marcel Dekker, 1-82.

Bullard RW, Banerjee MR, Chien F, Elizondo RE, MacIntyre. (1970) Skin temperature and thermoregulatory sweating: a control systems approach. In: JD Hardy, AP Gagge, JAJ Stolwljk (eds.) Physiological and Behavioral Temperature Regulation, Springfield II: Thomas, 597-610.

Gisolfi CV, Wilson NB, Claxton B. (1977) Work-heat tolerance of distance runners. In: P Milvy (ed), The Marathon: Physiological, Medical, Epidemiological, and Psychologlcal Studies, 139-150.

Glossary of terms for thermal physiology. (1987) Pflugers Archiv, 410, 567-587.

Gonzalez RR, Pandolf KB, Gagge AP. (1974) Heat acclimation and decline in sweating during humidity transients. Journal of Applied Physiology, 36, 419-425.

Hofler W. (1968) Changes in regional distribution of sweating during acclimatization to heat. J Appl Physiol, 25, 503-506.

Pandolf KB, Sawka MN, Gonzalez RR (eds.). (1988) Human Performance Physiology and Environmental Medicine at Terrestrial Extremes, Indianapolis, Benchmark Press.

Stephenson LA, Kolka MA. (1988) Effect of Gender, Circadian Period and Sleep Loss on Thermal Responses during Exercise. In: KB Pandolf, MN Sawka, RR Gonzalez (eds.) Human Performance Physiology and Environmental Medicine at Terrestrial Extremes, Indianapolis: Benchmark Press, 267-304.

Szabo G. (1962) The Number of Eccrine Sweat Glands in Human Skin. In: W Montagna, RA Ellis, AF Silver (eds.) Advances in Biology of the Skin Vol 3, Eccrine Sweat Glands and Eccrine Sweating, New York, Pergamon Press, 1-5.

Wenger CB. (1988) Human Heat Acclimation. In: KB Pandolf, MN Sawka, RR Gonzalez (eds.) Human Performance Physiology and Environmental Medicine at Terrestrial Extremes, Indianapolis, Benchmark Press, 153-197.

PART FOUR

Epidemiology of injury

Introduction   Epidemiology of injury

The prevention of sports injuries must be based on accurate reproducable data which can readily be interpreted by the Governing Body of the sport concerned. The lack of comparability of results between most sports injury surveys is a continuing problem – consistency is a problem when defining injury and no universally accepted way exists to identify the number of participants at risk in most sports.

The International Rugby Football Board and its members, such as the Scottish Rugby Union and South Africa, have undertaken a series of studies into the incidence of rugby injuries and these studies are reported in the following section of the Congress Proceedings. The need for an internationally agreed definition of a rugby injury is emphasized, as well as greater uniformity in classifying injuries.

The vagaries in comprehensive reporting remains a handicap in most prospective studies. The problem of shortfall in recording injuries could be minimized by improved contact between the responsible Governing Body, survey co-ordinators and club respondents. The level of co-operation would be improved with the establishment of a Rugby Injuries Case Registration Scheme (Garraway et al, 1991)*.

The incidence and nature of injuries in sport, especially a contact sport, are greatly influenced by the psychological preparation of individuals and teams for competitions. The rules or laws governing a sport must also be designed to minimize injury without detracting from the nature of the activity.

J.C.M. Sharp

* Garraway W.M., Macleod D.A.D. and Sharp J.C.M. (1991) *Rugby Injuries*. British Medical Journal, **303**, 1082.

Epidemiology of rugby football injuries

W.M. Garraway

Abstract. Rugby injuries are frequent occurrences which produce substantial periods of temporary disability, but fortunately, permanently disabling events are rare. Injuries increase with increasing age, are more frequent in the forward positions and evenly distributed amongst the different parts of the body, divided into upper limb, lower limb, trunk, head and neck. Tackling and being tackled are where most of the damage is done. Soft or muddy rather than hard ground favours injuries. Hard, competitive play at a senior level produces more injuries than social games. Practice games are relatively benign as far as injuries are concerned. Before these broad conclusions can be dissected out to address more detailed issues, more accurate ways of collecting information about rugby injuries need to be devised. This could be done by setting up rugby injury registers, based on the development of chronic disease registers which epidemiologists have developed over the past fifty years in seeking to establish the underlying causes of our chronic diseases such as ischaemic heart disease, stroke and cancer.

Keywords: Rugby Injuries, Sport, Case Definition, Epidemiology, Case Register.

Introduction

People play sport with varying degrees of enthusiasm in order to keep fit, look good, reduce weight, leave the strains and stress of life behind for a while as well as a whole variety of other reasons. Players who participate in contact sports such as rugby football, soccer, hockey and its Gaelic variant, shinty, accept and expect to suffer knocks and bruises at some point in the playing season. Several comparisons of the relative frequencies of injury occurring in different sports have been made. For example, a survey of public hospital admissions carried out in New Zealand in 1981-82 found that rugby provided more than half the total number of hospital admissions and at 13.2 per 1000 estimated participants, had the highest admission rate of all sports and nearly double that for soccer (McKenna, Berman, Findlay et al, 1986). Although rugby players would not be surprised to know that their sport was at the top of this particular list, fewer would appreciate that at a senior level, they are almost certain to be injured at least once in the season and that once injured, that four in every ten players would have to miss at least three concurrent weekly matches during the season because of injury (Sharp & Macleod, 1981; Dalley,

Laing, Rowberry et al, 1982). Even fewer would relish the prospect of being permanently disabled through sports injury as a result of sustaining a fracture of the cervical vertebra and many rugby players must feel a great deal of concern about reports that such devastating injuries may be increasing over time.

So rugby injuries are common and are of concern to players, coaches and referees. Through media attention which tends to concentrate on the few tragic and emotionally charged incidents which result in permanent handicap, the importance of injuries occurring in rugby is also being brought to the attention of the general public. So perhaps it is not surprising that there has been increasing interest amongst the medical fraternity in recording the origins, frequency and distribution of rugby injuries. As Figure 1 shows, there has been a marked rise in the number of medical articles written about rugby injuries in recent years (Coleman & Nicholl, 1988).

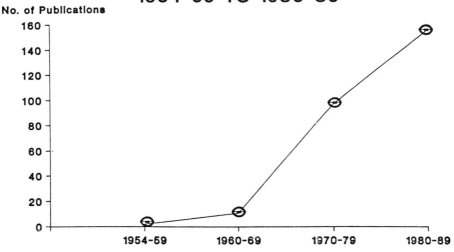

OUTPUT OF RUGBY INJURY ARTICLES IN MEDICAL JOURNALS 1954-59 TO 1980-89

Source: derived from Coleman and Nicholl. University of Sheffield. 1988

Fig. 1 Number of medical articles written about rugby injuries over time.
Source: derived from Coleman and Nicholl. University of Sheffield, 1988

Interpreting existing data

What limitations influence our understanding of the facts which have emerged about rugby injuries over the years? First of all, what is the definition of a rugby injury? The answer depends on which source has been consulted. Virtually every survey reported in the medical literature used its own definition and at least 10 different sets of criteria used to define rugby injuries in previous surveys can he identified.

Table 1. Examples of criteria used to define a rugby injury

"Causes at least a temporary interruption of a player's contribution to a game or impaired his subsequent ability to train or play" Davies & Gibson, 1978

"Prevents the player from returning to rugby for at least seven days after injury" Nathan, Goedeke & Noakes, 1983

"Presence of pain, discomfort or disability arising during and as a result of playing in a rugby match" Addley & Farren, 1988.

Injury graded as ...
severe:	if two or more games are missed
moderate:	if one game is missed
mild:	requiring attention but was fit to play again next month.

Dalley, Laing, Rowberry et al, 1982

Table 1 illustrates four ways in which this has been tackled in surveys reported from four different countries (Davies & Gibson, 1978; Dalley, Laing, Rowberry et al, 1982; Nathan, Goedeke & Noakes, 1983; Addley & Farren, 1988). So like cannot be compared with like when looking at the findings of different studies. A second major limitation in the interpretation of previous findings is that they have been derived from different sources.

Table 2 provides examples from studies where different people have completed the abstracts on which the information derived from the surveys was based (Archibald, 1962; Durkin, 1977; Davies & Gibson, 1978; Myers, 1980; Sparks, 1981; Weightman & Browne, 1984; Watters, Brooks, Elton et al, 1984). Clearly, differences in perception, experience, motivation, accuracy and interpretation of the nature, extent and severity of injuries recorded will be present, according to the person recording the information. A degree of self-

409

selection as to which injuries are included in surveys will also occur. So not all injuries may be accounted for. Surveys based on attendances at hospital accident and emergency departments are possibly the best example of this.

Table 2. Sources of information about rugby injuries

Honorary Medical Officer of a senior rugby club.
Medical Officer of a public school.
Panel of referees.
Medical staff of Hospital Accident and Emergency Departments. General practitioner in a University Health Centre. Physiotherapist attached to senior rugby clubs.
Team coaches of school rugby.
Rugby players themselves.

Figure 2 demonstrates the extent to which injuries which would have been missed in a survey carried out in Brisbane if the data gathered had been limited to those players who attended accident and emergency departments or were admitted to hospital (Myers, 1980).

The self selection factor in reporting rugby injuries

Ballymore, Brisbane

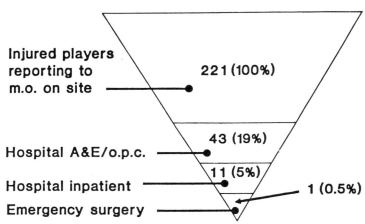

Injured players reporting to m.o. on site — 221 (100%)

Hospital A&E/o.p.c. — 43 (19%)

Hospital inpatient — 11 (5%)

Emergency surgery — 1 (0.5%)

Source: derived from Myers. Med. J. Aust. 1980.2.17-20

Fig. 2   Self selection in the reporting of rugby injuries. Source: derived from Myers. (1980) Med J Aust, 2, 17-20

A further limitation is the difference in ways in which "exposure" to rugby injuries has been documented. The denominator population exposed or at risk to being injured has not always been expressed in a universally accepted way. Table 3 provides some examples of what has been reported in calculating rates of rugby injury. Other studies have made no attempt to estimate rates of "exposure" to injuries but have limited their analyses to the number of injuries recorded.

Finally, no standardised format for describing the nature or site of rugby injuries or any of the circumstances concerning the occurrence of rugby injuries has been adopted. Each survey has been carried out using its own questionnaire, many of which have not been published in detail or included as appendices to papers published in the medical literature. Given these limitations, what is already known about the frequency, distribution and factors associated with the occurrence of rugby injuries?

Table 3. Different ways of expressing exposure to rugby injuries

Exposure to injury of the population of rugby players has not been expressed uniformly

per player hour
per 100 player appearances
per 100 player games
per 100 boy hours of rugby play or practice
per 10,000 man hours of play
percentage of players injured per season

Frequency of rugby injuries

Using data collected on behalf of the Scottish Rugby Union, Sharp & Macleod (1981) estimated that the frequency of rugby injuries was 1.45 per 100 player appearances; of whom 0.72 per 100 left the field permanently, 0.26 per 100 were temporarily absent from the field of play and 0.47 per 100 remained on the field despite being injured (Sharp & Macleod, 1981). In this survey, no life threatening or permanently disabling injuries were found. A New Zealand survey carried out in Christchurch reported that 18% of injuries were recurrences of previous injuries (Dalley, Laing, Rowberry et al, 1982). It is impossible to be sure whether or not overall rugby injuries are on the increase over time. There are virtually no long-term trends in rugby injuries from one particular source which could provide us with a clue to the answer to this important question. A comparison has been reported between a large French survey carried out in 1968-69 and one conducted in Christchurch in 1980 (Dalley, Laing, Rowberry et al, 1982).

Although the criteria used were probably not identical in these surveys, the data presented suggest that injuries may be getting more frequent over time (Table 4). They increase from 1 per 256 player exposures in 1969 in France to 1 in 191 player exposures in 1980 in New Zealand.

Table 4. Frequency of rugby football injuries. Source: Dalley, Laing, Rowberry et al, 1982

FRANCE 1969 COMPARED WITH NEW ZEALAND 1980

	France 1969	New Zealand 1980
Players surveyed	75,338	5,000
Injuries reported	11,349	1,002
Average number of games/ practices p.a.	40	38
Injury rate per player exposure	1:256	1:191

Interpretation of these data is made more difficult by the fact that in 1969, a change in the Laws occurred whereby a direct kick into touch outside the 22 metre line was no longer permitted. In practice, this had the effect of actually increasing the playing time in which players were exposed to injuries. What has also been reported from a number of sites, in both adult and schoolboy rugby, is an apparent increase in the 1970s of the number of spinal cord injuries (Taylor & Coolican, 1987; Williams & McKibbin, 1987; Hoskins, 1979). But these reports must be treated with caution because they are based on rather small numbers of cases and the changes may be due sometimes to an increase in the number of participants in the sport over these time periods. Others have concluded that the incidence of cervical spinal injuries is probably not going up over time or may actually be declining (Silver & Gill, 1988; Burry & Calcinai, 1988). Figure 3 illustrates the findings of Burry and Calcinai who reviewed the number of spinal injuries occurring in New Zealand rugby and related them to the introduction of changes in the Laws. This suggests that these Law changes may have contributed to a reduction in such catastrophic injuries in that country.

Factors associated with injury

What is not in doubt is the increase in the rate of rugby injuries with increasing age. This has been demonstrated by several authors, including Dalley and his colleagues in Christchurch (Dalley et al, 1982). There is a steadily increasing gradient of injury from under 14 to the senior level (Table 5).

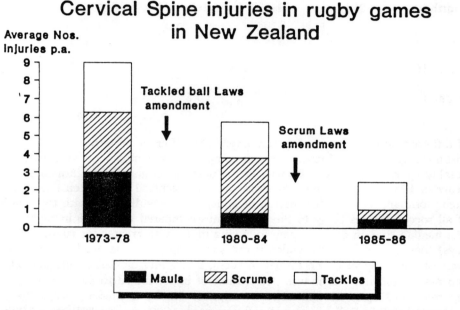

Fig. 3 Cervical spine injuries in rugby games in New Zealand. Source: adapted from Burry and Calcinai. (1988) Brit Med J, 296, 149-150

It has been suggested that this pattern is present because with increasing age, players become physically more developed but are not yet hardened to the game as regards their mental attitude. Comparison of the nature of injuries sustained shows broad similarity in surveys carried out in different parts of the world. There is also broad agreement on the site of such injuries if the findings

Table 5. Rugby injury rates according to grade of play: Christchurch survey, 1980. Source: Adapted from Dalley, 1982

Level/age range of play	No of players	No of injuries	Injuries per 100 players during season
Senior	271	275	101.5
Second XV	308	84	27.3
Fourth XV	216	21	9.7
Under 19	275	78	28.4
Under 16	238	33	13.9
Under 14	33	34	10.2

of different authors are roughly compared. The different pattern of injuries sustained by soccer and rugby football competitors has also been compared, notably by Weightman and Browne in the north of England (Weightman & Browne, 1984). They found that soccer injuries occurred more often than in rugby football, that the distribution of injury sites was different with two-thirds of all soccer injuries being to the lower limbs compared with 36% in rugby. The median time in days off play following injury was greater for rugby (12 days) than soccer (6 days), which is not surprising given the much greater force of body impact in the former of rucks, mauls and tackles. Illegal play also appears to contribute to injuries, with rates of injury linked to illegal play reported to be up to 30% of all rugby injuries. (Davies & Gibson, 1978; Sharp & Macleod, 1981; Dalley, Laing, Rowberry et al, 1982; Addley & Farren, 1988). Illegal play is a factor implicated in a considerable proportion of line-outs (where presumably players are often off-balance and sudden elbow or knee movements can give injury if collisions occur). Overall, the ruck is the area of play which produces the greatest number of injuries due to illegal play. What is needed in order to complete the picture is what proportion of illegal play does not result in injury. And whether or not, over the next few years, we will see a reduction in the proportion of injuries associated with illegal play as the influence of touch judges in bringing episodes of such play to the attention of referees grows. It is difficult to make any meaningful comparisons about the severity of injuries reported because different criteria of severity have been adopted by different studies. Finally, the position which a player holds on the field appears to have a bearing on the probability of his being injured. Forwards and flankers have the highest probability of injuries (Myers, 1980; Dalley, Laing, Rowberry et al, 1982; Nathan, Goedeke & Noakes, 1983). In an Irish survey, carried out in Dungannon, 87% of injuries were sustained in player-to-player contact, limiting non-bodily, running/walking/standing injuries to 13% (Addley & Farren, 1988). Being tackled and tackling accounted for the highest proportion of injuries in this survey and in a South African survey (Roy, 1974). In Christchurch, the tackle was by far the most likely situation for a severe injury (subsequently resulting in missing two or more games), or for the player requiring to leave the field (Dalley, Laing, Rowberry et al, 1982). Overall, backs and forwards had a similar risk of being injured in Scotland (Sharp & Macleod, 1981). Backs were more likely to be involved in high-speed collisions during a tackle, whereas forwards are more frequently involved in close contact during mauls and rucks. One must remember in putting forward these figures that confusion may arise amongst players in some circumstances as to exactly what happened in a ruck, maul and pile-up. So they should be treated with caution. The line-out is comparatively safe, presumably because of the upright position of the players and the lack of momentum. Senior games are presumably more competitive, they tend to produce more injuries than those involving second, third or fourth fifteens, confirmed by Dalley in Christchurch (Table 5) and by Myers in Brisbane (Myers, 1980; Dalley, Laing, Rowberry et al, 1982). Myers found more than three times the injury rate in international or interstate representative matches compared with fourth team outings. The state of the pitch can also have an impact on the prevalence of injuries during a game, soft or muddy pitches contributing a higher proportion of injuries than hard surfaces, particularly for head and neck injuries found in the Guy's Hospital survey (Davis & Gibson, 1978). Injuries during rugby games as opposed to practice sessions are also very much higher; in a Capetown schools survey, eight times the rate of injury occurred in senior school and over six times the rate in the junior school (under 14 years) in matches compared with practices or practice games (Nathan, Goedeke & Noakes, 1983). As regards associations of time, there is no clear indication of what stage in the game produces the highest proportion of injuries. In Ireland, it was the first and third quarter, whereas in Stellenbosch, South Africa, the opposite was reported (Roy, 1974; Addley & Farren, 1988). All one can conclude is that injuries occur throughout the game. There is some evidence from another South African survey and from a survey carried out by Durham RFU Referees Society, that a higher proportion of injuries occur at the beginning of the season and mid-way through the season compared with other times (Archibald, 1962; Nathan, Goedeke & Noakes, 1983). Davies and Gibson reported that the highest proportion of injuries occurred in the final quarter of the game (Davies & Gibson, 1978). The peak at the beginning of season may be related to a lack of fitness (players may actually be playing games in order to get fit), just as reports of increased proportion of injuries occurring in the fourth quarter of a game could represent the influence of fatigue on the occurrence of these injuries.

Out of these associations of rugby injuries between time, place and person certain conclusions emerge. Rugby injuries are frequent occurrences producing substantial periods of temporary disability, but permanently disabling events are rare. Injuries increase with increasing age, are more frequent in the forward positions and evenly distributed amongst the different parts of the body, divided into upper limb, lower limb, trunk, head and neck. Tackling and being tackled are where most of the damage is done. Soft or muddy rather than hard grounds favour injuries. Hard, competitive play at a senior level produces more injuries than social games. Practice games are relatively benign as far as injuries are concerned.

The way forward

Despite the best intentions of many investigators over the past few decades, there are major gaps in knowledge about rugby injuries. There are difficulties in reaching firm conclusions about the size, distribution and pattern of injuries which occur in rugby union football. Several authors have commented on the inadequate provision of statistical information about rugby injuries. One medical practitioner writing in the British Medical Journal recently stated "that ... until the Rugby Football Union retains a department of epidemiology and social medicine to conduct a large prospective study of rugby injuries), it has failed in its duty to all who play the game. It would be expensive but not impossible. Those of us who have sons who play rugby would, I am sure, support such an initiative" (Porter, 1984). If such a large prospective study were to be monitored, it would not only be able to describe more accurately the frequency and distribution of rugby injuries, but to begin to carry out studies to provide firmer aetiological evidence of the causes of rugby injury. This could be achieved by undertaking case control studies which would give us an estimate of the relative risk of injury which an individual player who is "exposed" to a particular factor has in comparison to players who are not exposed. This would bring to rugby one of the basic tools which epidemiologists have developed over the past 50 years in seeking to establish the underlying causes of most of our chronic diseases such as ischaemic heart disease, stroke, peptic ulcer, lung cancer and so on. Only when such studies have been carried out can causal mechanisms for rugby injuries begin to be understood and the most effective ways of preventing such injuries be implemented.

Case registers

What is needed is for the rugby football unions of participating countries in the World Cup to establish case registers of rugby injuries, either on a national or a regional basis. A register of this kind was set up by the National Football League in the United States some years ago, in response to growing concern about cervical spinal injuries in American football players and was a key feature in identifying the impact which "spearing" tackles and the use of the head and helmet as a battering ram in blocking, tackling and butting had on cervical spinal injuries (Torg, Truex, Quedenfeld et al, 1979). The essential ingredients which would go into the formation and maintenance of a rugby injuries register would include the need to achieve complete case ascertainment which would identify all rugby injuries which occurred in the "population" of rugby players who were being included in the survey. An accurate denominator of all those "exposed" to the risk of injury, in terms of the number of players and duration of play would be required. Agreement would need to be reached on the use of a universally acceptable definition of rugby injury. A standard explicit abstract would need to be designed to record primary details of the injury. This should be set out in such a way that it could be easily administered by a lay person. A linkman would need to be identified in each club or school, responsible for completion and collation of information. Methods of providing regular contact between the central data processing and analysis centre which would collect and collate the returns from the linkmen based in rugby clubs and schools would need to be devised. The analysis of the data contained in the case register should lead to annual reports to the Rugby Football Union on trends in injuries and regular feedback to participating clubs and schools. An important facet of the work of the investigators responsible for the organisation and running of the case register would be to monitor completeness of injury and player coverage throughout the survey, as well as establish that the criteria which have been adopted were being applied uniformly by all participants.

What advantages would accrue from the establishment and maintenance of such rugby injury register? First of all, it would provide true incidence rates of injury, and thus identify absolute risk of different kinds of injuries which occur in rugby matches. The description of accurate associations of time, place and person would be possible and a build-up of information on trends in the frequency, distribution and nature of injuries over time could take place. A rugby injuries register would enable the impact of Law changes on patterns of injury to be maintained over time. It would allow us to build up an accurate picture of the rugby "playing" population which is not available anywhere else at present. Monitoring the outcomes of injury, e.g. injury recurrence rates, would become possible. The Register would give each club/school a summary of their players' injury profile in comparison with their country or region as a whole. This could act as an aid to coaching and player selection at club or school level. Finally, it would allow case control studies to be organised quickly and easily to enable relative risks of different factors associated with rugby injuries to be estimated.

References

Addley K, Farren J. (1988) Irish Rugby Injury Survey: Dungannon Football Club (1986-87). Br J Sports Med, 22, 22-24.

Archibald RMcL. (1962) An analysis of rugby football injuries in the 1961-1962 season. Practitioner, 189, 333-334.

Burry HC, Calcinai CJ. (1988) The need to make rugby safer. Br Med J, 296, 149-150.

Coleman P, Nicholl J. (1988) Bibliography on Rugby Injuries. Medical Care Research Unit, University of Sheffield. Private printing.

Dalley DR, Laing DR, Rowberry JM, Caird MJ. (1982) Rugby Injuries, An Epidemiological Survey, Christchurch 1980. NZ J Sports Med, 10, 5-17.

Davies E, Gibson T.(1978) Injuries in Rugby Union Football. Br Med J, 2, 1759-1761.

Durkin TE. (1977) A survey of injuries in a 1st class rugby union football club from 1972-1976. Br J Sports Med, 11, 7-11.

Hoskins T. (1979) Rugby injuries to the cervical spine in English schoolboys. Practitioner, 223, 365-366.

McKenna S, Berman B, Findlay J, de Boor M. (1986) Sports injuries in New Zealand. NZ Med J, 31, 899-901.

Myers PT. (1980) Injuries presenting from Rugby Union Football. Med J Aust, 2, 17-20.

Nathan M, Goedeke R, Noakes TD. (1983) The incidence and nature of rugby injuries experienced at one school during the 1982 rugby season. S Afr Med J, 64, 132-137.

Porter A. (1984) Injuries of the spine sustained in rugby. Br Med J, 288-400.

Roy SP. (1974) The nature and frequency of Rugby Injuries. A Pilot Study of 300 injuries at Stellenbosch. SA Mediese Tydskrif, 48, 2321-2327.

Sharp JCM, Macleod DAD.(1981) Injuries in Competitive Rugby Football in Scotland. Update, 7, 1355-1361.

Silver JR, Gill S. (1988) Injuries of the spine sustained during rugby. Sports Med, 5, 328-334.

Sparks JP. (1981) Half a million hours of rugby football. Br J Sports Med, 15, 30-32.

Taylor TKF, Coolican MRJ. (1987) Spinal-cord injuries in Australian footballers 1960-1985. Med J Aust, 147, 112-118.

Torg JS, Truex R Jnr, Quedenfeld TC, Burstein A, Speakman A, Nichols C. (1979) The National Football Head and Neck Injury Registry. Report and Conclusions 1978. JAMA, 241, 1477-1479.

Watters DAK, Brooks S, Elton RA, Little K. (1984) Sports injuries in an accident and emergency department. Arch Emergency Med, 2, 105-112.

Weightman D, Browne RC. (1984) Injuries in Association and Rugby Football. B J Sports Med, 8, 183-187.

Williams P, McKibbin B. (1987) Unstable cervical spine injuries in rugby - a 20 year review. Injury, 18, 329-332

The epidemiology of schoolboy rugby injuries

C.E. Roux and T.D. Noakes

Abstract. A prospective study, which documented all injuries that prevented schoolboy rugby players at 26 high schools from participation for at least one week, was conducted over a two year period. The study showed that rugby injuries show specific trends with age, team level, playing position, time of season, anatomical site, type of injury and phase of play. Monitoring injuries through correspondence also resulted in underreporting of injuries. Speed and the competitive level of play may be the most important aetiological factors in the majority of rugby injuries.

Keywords: Schoolboy Rugby, Injuries.

Introduction

Rugby injuries are a cause for concern in medical and non-medical circles, but few scientific investigations into their nature and frequency have been undertaken. Our understanding of such injuries is hampered by a lack of adequately controlled, prospective epidemiological surveys in well-controlled rugby-playing communities. The majority of reported rugby injury surveys are retrospective, have considered only specific injuries or have reported only those seen at one location. Also, most studies have not distinguished between minor and major injuries.

A pilot study, conducted at one school during one season showed clear patterns of injury (Nathan et al, 1983). In this report we used similar survey techniques to study rugby injuries in a much larger number of high schools over a two-year period.

Materials and methods

The 26 high schools selected for the study were divided into two groups. The first group, consisting of 20 schools, were monitored through correspondence. Instruction, weekly report and injury questionnaire forms were sent to these schools and the teacher/coach of each team were required to assist injured players with the completion of injury questionnaire forms. The weekly report form recorded the total number of participants and injured players for the preceding week. Injury questionnaire forms contained the injured player's personal data (age, team-level, playing position, etc.) and injury data (date of injury, site and type of injury, phase of play, etc.). Completed questionnaire forms were attached to the school's weekly report and returned. Schools which either failed to return a form any week during the season or returned inadequately completed forms were contacted immediately.

The second group consisted of six schools. The forms and data collection processes were similar, except that the schools were personally monitored by two researchers. This survey technique was used in order to establish the accuracy of the mail survey technique used in the other twenty schools.

All results were computerised using programmes specifically designed for the project. At the end of the project, the complete data were made available on computer printouts which were analysed manually to determine the overall number and incidence of injury, the age-group and playing level (team) of injured players, the incidence of injury during different 4-week periods of the season, the injured player's position, the phase of play at the time of injury and the nature and anatomical site of injury. Finally, data from the two different groups of schools were compared to determine whether injury reporting was the same for both groups of schools.

Definition of an injury

For the purposes of this study an injury was defined as one severe enough to prevent the player from returning to rugby for at least seven days. All concussion injuries had to be reported even if the player continued to play.

Results and discussion

Overall injury incidence - evidence for underreporting

During the two years that the study was conducted, the 26 high schools fielded an average of 317 teams, involving approximately 4750 players. A total of 6496 matches were played over the two-year period and 905 players, who sustained 1068 specific injuries, were injured. Thus, with an average of 452 players being injured each year, one out of every ten high school rugby players was likely to sustain an injury that will prevent him from participating for at least one week.

Of the 905 players that reported injuries, 617 (68%) were injured during matchplay and 288 (32%) during practices. Nathan et al (1983) reported that 63% of schoolboy players were injured during matchplay and 37% during practices. A similar trend was found by Sparks, 1985), who reported 60% of all injuries as match injuries.

The overall injury incidence, which was calculated as previously described (Nathan et al, 1983), was one injury for every 679 boys-hours of rugby (Fig.1. The incidence of injury for matches was one injury for every 158 boy-hours of matchplay and that of practices one injury for every 1795 boy-hours of practice. These figures are all lower than those found by Nathan et al (1985) and Sparks (1985).

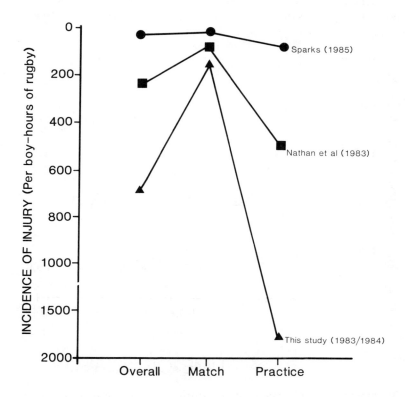

Fig. 1 The overall, match and practice incidences of injury for three schoolboy rugby injury studies which used similar definitions for an injury.

When the results were separated into those for the six schools monitored personally by the researchers and the 2 schools monitored only through correspondence there was a clear difference. The overall incidence of injury for the six closely monitored schools was one injury for every 42 boy-hours of rugby and that of the 20 schools monitored through correspondence one injury for every 736 boy-hours of rugby, a percentage difference of 43%. This suggests that underreporting of injuries had occurred in the schools monitored through correspondence and may explain the lower incidences found in this study when compared to other schoolboy studies.

Incidence of injury during the different periods of the season

Injuries were more likely to occur at the beginning of the season and again after the mid-year vacation (Fig. 2). This clearly suggests that players are not physically wellconditioned at the beginning of the season and do not maintain their fitness during the mid-year vacation. Nathan et al (1983) and Sparks (1985) reported similar findings.

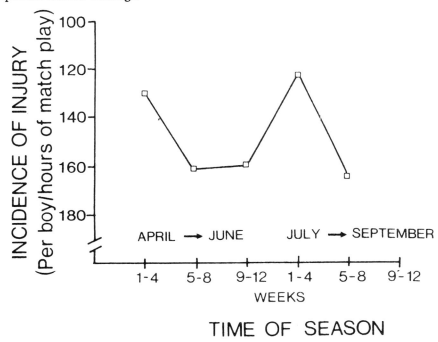

Fig. 2 The matchplay incidence of injury during different four-week periods of the season.

Age and level of play

Figure 3 shows the relative number of injuries sustained by players in the different age-groups and playing levels during matches and practices. Expressed as an incidence, the results showed a low incidence at U/14 level, rising through U/15 and U/16 to a high incidence at U/19 level. At all ages A-team players sustained the most injuries. Under-19 A-team players were especially injury-prone and sustained 20% of all injuries, as was also found by Nathan et al (1983).

The most probable reason for the high injury incidence at higher levels of competition is that players in A-teams are likely to be bigger, faster and more competitive than players in the lower teams.

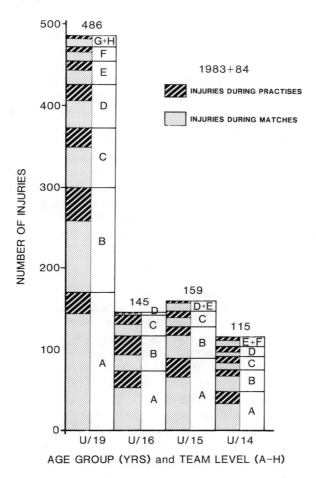

Fig. 3 The relative number of injuries in the different age-groups and team levels during matches and practices.

Incidence of injury in different playing positions

Eighthmen (13%) sustained most injuries during both years that the study was conducted. Wings and full-backs (12% each) were also at high risk followed by centres (11%) and fly-halves and scrum-halves (10% each). The safest positions were those of the tight-forward players. Locks and hookers each reported 7% and props 8% of all injuries.

Thus the tight forwards, which represent a third of the 15 players in the team, contributed only 22% of all injuries. The remaining three forward players (loose-forwards) sustained 23% of all injuries and this indicates, as was the case with most backline positions, that players involved in the tackling phases of play and play executed at speed are at greater risk of being injured.

Incidence and nature of injury during the different phases of play

More than 50% of all injuries reported occurred during the two tackling phases of play. Thirty percent of these injuries occurred to the player being tackled and 23% to the tackling player. A further 20% of injuries were sustained during the loose-scrum/maul, bringing the total for all injuries sustained during the above three phases of play to 73%. Almost all previous schoolboy studies have identified these phases of play as the major causes of injuries. Nathan et al (1983) reported that 47% of all injuries occurred during the tackling phases of play. They did, however, report a much higher percentage of injuries occurring in the scrum (18% vs 8% in this study) but this may be due to the unusually high injury incidence reported by hookers in that study. Sparks (1985) who separated all injuries into two groups found that 40% of all minor and 53% of severe injuries occurred to players whilst tackling or being tackled.

Incidence of injury at different anatomical sites

Most injuries occurred to the lower limb (32%) followed by the head and neck (33%) and upper limb (26%). The trunk (11%) was the anatomical site to which the fewest injuries occurred. Neck injuries represented 37% of head and neck injuries, a figure similar to the 33% found by Nathan et al (1983). Sparks (1981) reported that only 17% of all injuries sustained by players at Rugby School over a period of 29 years (1950 to 1979) occurred to the head and neck. Lower limb (47%) and upper limb injuries (26%) were the commonest injuries reported. In a further study (1980 to 1983) Sparks 1985) reported figures for all four anatomical sites which were remarkably similar to the findings of this study. He noted that there had been an increase in the number of head and neck injuries (from 17% - 27%) at Rugby School during these years. A similar finding was made by Briscoe (1985), who noted that the incidence of minor head injuries caused by contact sports at Eton School had risen fourfold during the period 1977 to 1982 when compared to the period 1965 - 1977.

Incidence of different types of injury

Fracture and ligament injuries were the most commonly reported injury types and accounted for almost 60% of all injuries. A further 19% were muscle and 13% concussion injuries.

Findings from the studies of Sparks (1985) and Nathan et al (1983) differ significantly when the incidences for different injury types were compared with those of this study. Particularly interesting was the reported incidences for concussion, dislocations and fractures. In the study of Sparks (1985), the incidences for these types of injury accounted for only 6%, 3% and 10% of all injuries respectively. All were significantly lower than incidences found for these injury types in this study.

The reason for these lower incidences is not clear. In both this study and that of Sparks (1985), most injuries occurred during the two tackling phases of play. Since more than 50% of concussion, and 60% of fracture injuries, were reported during these phases of play in this study, the findings by Sparks are indeed strange. The only probable explanation may be that playing fields are softer in England, thereby lessening the impact of players falling to the ground after being tackled or whilst tackling.

In the study of Nathan et al (1983), concussion and muscle injuries (each 22%) were the most commonly reported injury types. Fracture and ligament injuries accounted for only 33% of all injuries, compared with 59% in this study. As the Nathan et al study was conducted for only one season and at only one school, it is likely that the high percentage reported for concussion was an unusual occurrence and therefore influenced the overall percentages reported for other injury types. That this may have been the case, seems highly probable when the results from each of the two seasons in this study are examined. Very little difference between the percentages for the different injury types reported was found.

Conclusions

The principal conclusions of the study are as follows:

a. There was underreporting of between 40 to 50% of rugby injuries by schools monitored through correspondence. It appears that the most accurate method of data collection is direct personal contact between the researcher and the injured player.

b. Schoolboy rugby injuries are more common during the early season and after the mid-year winter vacation.

c. More than two-thirds of all injuries occurred during matchplay and the incidence of injuries rises with age and competitive level.

d. The majority of injuries occurred while the players were tackling or being tackled.

e. Eighthmen and backline players sustained most injuries, whereas the tight-forwards were the least frequently injured.

The two major aetiological factors in rugby injuries would appear to be the speed and competitive level at which the game is played or a combination thereof.

Evidence for these conclusions is:

a.   The greater incidence of injury among the fast, mobile players playing in the best teams.

b.   The high prevalence of injuries that occurred during the tackling and being-tackled phases of play, both of which occur at speed.

c.   The greater incidence of injury amongst players in the older age-groups, playing in the best teams.

d.   The very significant difference in incidence between matchplay and practice injuries.

The similarities which were found when this study, and those of Nathan et al (1983) and Sparks (1985) were compared, have been discussed. With particular reference to the last three points above, these similarities indicate that the major aetiological factors, as suggested by the findings of this study, may be common in schoolboy rugby players across the world. However, this will only be confirmed once more studies, using similar definitions and survey methods, have been conducted.

References

Briscoe JHD. (1985) Sports injuries in adolescent boarding school boys. Brit J Sports Med, 19, 67-70.

Davidson R, Kennedy M, Kennedy J, Vanderfield G. (1978) Casualty room presentation and schoolboy rugby union. Med J Australia, 1 , 247-249.

Davidson RM. (1987) Schoolboy rugby injuries. Med J Australia, 147, 119-120.

Nathan M, Goedeke R, Noake TD. (1970) The incidence and nature of rugby injuries at one school during the 1982 rugby season. S Afr Med J, 64, 132-137.

Sparks JP. (1981) Half a million hours of rugby football. Brit J Sports Med, 15, 30-32.

Sparks JP. (1985) Rugby football injuries: 1980- 1983. Brit J Sports Med, 19, 71-75.

The Scottish Rugby Union data collection systems

J.C.M. Sharp

Abstract. A review is presented of the several data collection systems developed by the SRU since 1978 towards obtaining better clinical and epidemiological information on the incidence and causes of injuries (and illnesses) arising out of participating in rugby football in Scotland. The advantages and disadvantages of the respective systems are discussed.

Keywords: Rugby Injuries, Scottish Rugby Union, Data Collection Systems.

Introduction

During the 1970s competitive rugby became increasingly widely criticised in the media based on an alleged increase in aggression and deliberately dangerous play. Since the mid-1970s following the introduction of competitive club rugby in 1973, the Scottish Rugby Union (SRU) has taken an active interest in the treatment and prevention of rugby injuries at all levels of the game throughout Scotland. Towards this end, it became apparent that in order to promote more prevention, that better information was required regarding the frequency, nature and causes of rugby injuries in Scotland.

Epidemiological studies of various aspects of rugby injuries have been undertaken over the past 20 years or so by several interested individuals in the British Isles (Durkin, 1977) (Davies & Gibson, 1978) (Addley & Farren, 1988) and overseas (Dalley et al, 1982). Among the four Home Unions the SRU led the way in an effort to obtain better data in initiating the first nationally co-ordinated survey of competitive rugby injuries in the British Isles. Only France had a more comprehensive system, based on the FFR insurance scheme.

League Championship Injuries Survey

The SRU League Championships were introduced in 1973, this being the first structured form of competitive club rugby in the British Isles, involving 84 clubs divided into seven divisions (I to VII). During 1978-79, 26 clubs participated in a pilot study of injuries occurring in league matches in Scotland that season, the findings of which provided a practical definition of injury.

Before the start of the following season (1979-80), all 84 clubs involved in the Championship were invited to participate in a prospective study of injuries sustained in a league match; 44 of the 84 clubs co-operated, including all 12 clubs in Division I, 9 from Division II and 23 from the other five divisions. Each club participating designated a "link man", usually although not invariably the club doctor or physiotherapist, who was responsible for completing and returning a standard pre-coded questionnaire relating to any player who was "injured during a league match and had to attend hospital on the same day or was unable to play rugby within 7 days of being injured", i.e. was unfit to play the following Saturday.

A total of 103 injuries sustained during competitive league matches that season were reported by 34 clubs, with 10 clubs reporting no relevant injuries in the form of "Nil returns". The results of this study (Sharp & Macleod, 1981), highlighted amongst other findings, that:

a.   One injury occurred for every 69 player appearances or 1 every 2.3 matches.

b.   Backs and forwards were equally at risk, although the cause and nature of the injuries sustained differed. Certain playing positions, in particular scrum-half,hooker, wing forward and centre were the most vulnerable.

c.   The tackle, followed by the ruck and maul were the most dangerous phases of the game.

Four players were injured while playing in other than their normal positions, viz. 2 at scrum-half and one each at hooker and full-back.

Table 1. League Championship Injuries Survey

Advantages	Disadvantages
Competitive league matches	1st XV league matches only
Nature of injuries	Dependent on interest and goodwill of clubs
Phase of match	? Excess information sought
Follow-up of injuries	

The survey was repeated over the next few seasons, with similar findings. Despite continued efforts to expand the study by promoting more comprehensive reporting by clubs, the response became increasingly sluggish. In part this was due to some difficulties in completion of the questionnaire such as in the local follow-up of those players who gave up playing as a consequence of their injury compounded by the variabilities in the interest and enthusiasm of individual "link-men" among the clubs. By and large only a relatively small cadre of clubs, mainly although not exclusively in the top three divisions, remained reliable responders. Despite further urgings from the SRU for improved co-operation, the response continued to be erratic and in consequence the survey was discontinued at the end of season 1986-87.

Serious Injuries Survey

In 1984-85, a survey of "Serious Injuries" embracing rugby at all levels in Scotland was implemented in parallel with the "League Championship" study, using a simpler one-page questionnaire. All clubs affiliated to the SRU, including London Scottish, districts and rugby playing schools were asked to report any serious injury or illness that occurred during, or as a result of training or playing rugby.

The definition of a "serious" injury or illness being any player who required "admission to hospital". It was accepted that such a definition would preclude many important injuries (e.g. some fractures, most lacerations, etc.) where the player returned home on the same day following treatment.

Analysis of the data obtained over the seven seasons since the study began, further emphasised the importance of the tackle as the most dangerous phase of the game and the vulnerability of centre and wing-threequarters among backs, along with flanker and prop of the forwards. The tackle was the cause in 70 per cent of all injuries recorded, with over 60 per cent featuring the tackled player. Other important phases of the game included the ruck and maul (13%), scrummaging (5.5%) and sundry other causes (11.5%) such as punching, tramping, careless and illegal play. Pitch problems also contributed with two players being badly injured as a result of hitting boundary fences. Concussion featured in 17 per cent of injuries, while other common injuries involved the lower limbs (fractures/knee ligament damage) and the face (fractures and eye injuries).

An integral feature of the survey has been the highlighting of several life-threatening injuries and deaths, arising out of participation in rugby football in Scotland, viz.

a. Deaths
    Four deaths were reported, all of which occurred between seasons 1984-85 and 1986-87. Of these, three were due to previously unknown cardiac conditions. The fourth involved a 19-year-old prop forward whose neck was

broken when a scrum collapsed, becoming quadriplegic and dying three days later. In the subsequent four seasons since 1987 to date, no deaths have been reported.

b. Quadriplegia

Three other seriously injured players developed quadriplegia. All were young players; a 16-year old schoolboy was playing out of position in the second row in an adult match when a disrupted scrum went to the ground with the opposition continuing to push; collapsing of a scrum also led to the injury of an 18-year-old tight head prop; and a 16-year old schoolboy centre-threequarter was injured after a tackle when a ruck formed and his own team drove over him.

c. Other Life Threatening Injuries

Several other life-threatening injuries were recorded. These related to:-

A 20-year-old wing-threequarter whose spleen was ruptured when another player's head struck him heavily in the lower rib-cage in a maul;

A 27-year-old wing threequarter who acquired a deep cut to a finger, apparently from a stud, while tackling an opponent. Despite receiving immediate hospital treatment he developed tetanus one week later;

A 19-year-old centre-threequarter who sustained a fractured skull with cerebral laceration leading to partial motor, sensory and expressive brain damage, as the result of an opponent's knee striking his head, while attempting a "head-on" tackle;

A 33-year-old second row forward whose ribs were broken by a tackle from behind, ruptured an artery resulting in a haemopneumothorax;

A 36-year-old prop forward who ruptured a kidney following a heavy tackle, requiring emergency surgery.

Other life-threatening injuries known to have occurred since 1984 for which no reports were received, were an extradural haematoma and a pneumothorax.

Table 2. Serious Injuries Survey

Advantages	Disadvantages
All levels of rugby	Hospital admissions only
Nature of injuries	Dependent on interest and goodwill of clubs
Phase of match	Limited follow-up
Simple questionnaire	

The "Serious Injuries" survey has continued to date, although problems continue to be experienced in the response rate, despite all clubs being reminded at the beginning of each season of the on-going need to report such injuries. Whereas the more interested clubs continue to report regularly, the overall response has varied considerably each year.

A separate survey of schoolboy injuries was undertaken by the Scottish Schools Rugby Union during seasons 1988-89 and 1989-90, relating to players taken off the field of play and unable to return whether or not hospital admission was required. Co-operation from the majority of the ca. 174 rugby-playing schools in Scotland, was extremely patchy with only 15 per cent (23/174) responding over the two seasons. In consequence, the study was discontinued (EI Adam - personal communication).

Referee Replacement Reports

Another invaluable source of epidemiological information introduced in 1988-89, is the weekly reporting by referees to the SRU of all replacements which have been made for injured players requiring to leave the field during League Championship matches in Scotland. Details reported relate to playing position and time of injury within the match for all seven divisions of the Championship over a period of 13 weeks viz. 637 matches, giving a further insight into injury rates and the vulnerability of particular playing positions. This study is also unique amongst national injury surveys with 100 per cent reporting, it being incumbent on referees to make weekly returns to the SRU.

Table 3.   Referee Replacement Reports

Advantages	Disadvantages
Routine weekly reports	1st XV league matches only
Simple to operate	Phase of match
Time of injury	Nature of injuries

During season 1990-91, a total of 412 replacements were made involving 284 (45%) of the 637 matches played, an average of 32 replacements per week or 2 per cent of 19110 player appearances. Forwards (60%) were replaced more often than backs (40%), with flanker, the front row and scrum-half featuring most frequently. The frequency of replacements increased as matches progressed with

37 (9%) taking place during the 1st quarter, 108 (26%) in the 2nd, 132 (32%) in the 3rd and 135 (33%) in the last quarter of matches.

Hospital records

The heartland of rugby in Scotland traditionally has been in the Border country, in particular in the towns of Hawick, Galashiels, Melrose, Kelso, Jedforest and Selkirk, whose club sides have been in the forefront of Scottish rugby for over 100 years. The acute general hospital which services the district, viz. the Borders General Hospital, receives virtually all acute rugby injuries requiring hospital treatment in the South of Scotland.

Throughout the playing season of 1990-91 from September to May, a computerised record was maintained of every acute rugby injury attending the hospital's Accident & Emergency (A&E) Unit, representing all levels of rugby from Division I down through lower club XVs and schools (HJ van der Post - personal communication).

Table 4 Hospital Records (Borders General Hospital)

Advantages	Disadvantages
All A&E attendances	GP orthopaedic referrals
Known no. of matches	Cottage hospital referrals
Defined population	Injuries attended to by club doctors
Phase of match	Direct admissions to specialist unit in Edinburgh
Time of injury	

Nature and treatment of injuries - routine records

A total of 292 injuries, 18 of which required to be admitted to hospital for treatment or observation, were recorded during the season. Of the 292 injuries treated, 214 related to players from local teams playing matches in the South of Scotland, representing 1.2 injuries per 100 player appearances. Amongst the 78 other injuries treated, 39 (13%) were training injuries and 13 (4%) were associated with 7-a-side tournaments, a popular sport in the Borders.

The tackle accounted for over half (58%) of injuries followed by the ruck and maul (28%), with prop forwards, centre three-quarters, number 8s and wing-forwards most frequently injured. Full details of the nature and anatomical site of all injuries were recorded, along with temporal features such as the quarter of the match and stage of the season.

Omissions from the study included injured players who were attended to by club doctors at match venues, those referred to one or other of the two cottage hospitals in the district, those referred by their general practitioner direct to the orthopaedic clinic and also potentially any serious head injuries which may have required direct admission to the specialist unit in the Royal Infirmary, Edinburgh. Nevertheless a comprehensive epidemiological picture of all acute rugby injuries attending a hospital accident & emergency unit for investigation or treatment in a defined population over one complete season has successfully been documented.

Discussion

Few, if any, individual data collection systems are capable of providing sufficiently comprehensive information over an adequate period of time to enable trends of rugby injuries to be measured meaningfully. Among the studies undertaken in Scotland, each differed to a greater or lesser extent in the type of information obtained and also in their respective merits and demerits. The "Replacement Reports" by referees for example, although comprehensive in reporting, do not identify the nature of the injuries sustained nor the phase of the match in which injuries occurred. Nevertheless all four systems highlighted the vulnerability of certain playing positions, in particular wing forward and the front row.

Epidemiological surveys, in particular prospective studies, are frequently dependent on the goodwill and ongoing interest of colleagues in the "field" collecting and forwarding relevant information. Whereas simple questionnaires will be unable to provide information on every facet of rugby injuries, many details may be superfluous to basic needs. More sophisticated "questionnaires" ("League Championship Injuries") may be counter-productive by seeking too much information from respondents. In addition to under-reporting problems, a feature of the simpler "Serious Injuries" survey was the accepted omission of those players "failing" to be admitted to hospital i.e. being discharged home after treatment. In surveys, whose success is dependent on the continuing interest and goodwill of respondents, on-going contact and regular feed-back to the clubs and "linkmen" is critical for continued co-operation.

Of the four systems, the hospital-based study provided the most comprehensive data, detailing a wide range of clinical and epidemiological factors of all A & E attendances at the principal hospital in the district.

The prime purpose of any epidemiological survey is the collection and analysis of data in order to identify contributory factors. The information obtained can then be utilised for the purposes of intervention and thereby enhancing prevention, in the case of rugby injuries by improving awareness among a) players, club officials and coaches (Health Education) and b) administrators and lawmakers leading to the introduction of legislative control measures relating to the laws of rugby football (Legislation).

The data collected in rugby (or other) injury surveys, must therefore be used to prevent, or at least minimise the occurrence of serious injury as well as enabling players and officials to be better prepared to cope with injury.

References

Addley K & Farren J. (1988) Irish rugby injury survey: Dungannon football club, 1986-87. Br J Sports Med, 22, 22-24.

Dalley DR, Laing DR, Rowberry JM & Caird MJ. (1982) Rugby Injuries: an epidemiological survey, Christchurch, 1980. NZ J Sports Med, 10, 5-17.

Davies JE & Gibson T. (1978) Injuries in rugby union football. Br Med J, 2, 1759-61.

Durkin TE. (1977) A survey of injuries in a first class rugby union football club from 1972-76. Br J Sp Med, 11, 7-11.

Sharp JCM & Macleod DAD. (1981) Injuries in competitive rugby football in Scotland. Hospital Update, 7, 1355-61

Psychological preparation for physical contact in rugby football

R.L. Cox

Abstract. This paper outlines a number of techniques that can be employed by rugby players to prepare themselves psychologically for the moments of impact. Individual and team preparations and the balance between them are considered, as is the balance between physical and mental preparation. Recommendations are made for certain behaviours to be enacted during the final sixty minutes before kick-off.

Keywords: Visual Specificity, Mood Words, "As If", Mental Rehearsal, Performance Goals, Pre-Competition Strategies, "What If?", Coping Strategies.

Introduction

Since physical contact is an integral part of the game of rugby football and is the cause of most injuries, it makes sense for players to prepare themselves for it, both physically and psychologically.

The first important point to highlight is the fact that psychological preparation for playing rugby is, in general, inextricably linked to physical, technical and tactical preparation. For instance, when a player is technically proficient in all the skills demanded by his position on the field, is sufficiently aware tactically to execute these skills at the right moment in time and physically fit enough to demonstrate them as and when required for the full eighty minutes, then he will have little need to improve his self-confidence. More specifically, if he has mastered the correct techniques for enjoying physical contact with the opposition then he should have little to be concerned about.

Each of the fifteen players involved has a specific role to fulfil and, in some ways, each is like no other. Thus, the work done in preparing for a match should be tailored to the demands of each position and should reflect each individual's particular strengths and weaknesses. By way of example, let us examine how a wing-threequarter might spend the final sixty minutes before kick-off. Assuming he is changed and in full track-suit by this stage, he should go out onto the field with the rest of his team mates and begin his warm-up. For the first ten minutes he would work through a programme designed to raise core body temperature and gently mobilise joints. Thereafter, he would need to reproduce some of the physical demands of his particular position and this would necessitate building up his running to full sprinting speed. By the end of this period he should have experienced short but intense periods of breathlessness. It is important here to note that, as reported by Rushall (1979), elite players are likely to want some time to themselves for a variety of reasons before a game begins. The latter stages of this warm-up phase provide an opportune moment for this to happen.

The second phase of preparation should involve skill routines in small groups. For our winger, this might involve him working with the outside centre and full-back through various passing, reverse-passing and loop-passing routines, some of which might involve physical contact to some degree. The final routines of this phase might well involve a more committed form of physical contact. For instance, the three players involved could take it in turn to either throw or gently kick the ball into the air for one of the other two to field and set as though for a maul before the thrower, or kicker, can tackle him. Initially, this would be done at jogging pace but should graduate to half-speed at least. Done properly, the risk of injury is minimal and would go a long way towards preparing both body and mind for an all out tackle which one might have to make or receive in the first minute of the game.

Visual specificity

Two important features of these types of practice must be rehearsed at the conscious level. The first is what might be termed "Visual Specificity". This involves narrowing one's focus of attention at the point of contact between either man and ball or man and opponent to a particular part of the target. (For a detailed discussion of different foci of attention see Nideffer (1978). Thus, the catcher might focus on the inscription on the ball or on the stitching between its panels rather than on the ball as a whole. Similarly, the tackler might focus on pinning the target's arms to his torso so that he cannot pass the ball or on hitting him at the point where his legs become visible below his shorts rather than on his whole body. The point here is that many errors are made at crucial moments in a game because the player in question is focussing too broadly to execute a skill that requires fine precision.

Mood words

The second important feature that must be rehearsed is the thought content at the most crucial point of the movement or skill. Meichenbaum and Turk (1975) and Suinn (1977) demonstrated that the quality of skilled movement can be modified and enhanced if the participants use a "Trigger" or a "Mood" word coincidently with the movement. In making contact in rugby, therefore, a player should be focussing his eyes on a particular part of the target and, at the point of impact, be thinking of nothing more than a single word. Possible examples are "crush", "through" and "power". Whatever the choice of Mood word, however, three points must be borne in mind. First, every Mood word must be chosen by the player concerned and no-one else because it is the quality of his own performance he is trying to govern. Secondly, he must associate each Mood word chosen directly with a particular skilled movement, or part thereof, and he must practise this association until it becomes automatic. Thirdly, how he says the Mood word to himself is crucially important. For example, if he wanted to use the word "crush" to govern the quality of his tackles then he would need to think of the word as he would shout it out loud.

Mood words must either immediately precede a particular movement or be coincident with it but they must never be allowed to lag behind - hence the need to practise them regularly.

"As if"

If our wingers has difficulty in using Mood words then he might do better to try the "As If" technique which was recommended by Syer and Connolly (1984). This technique would involve him in pretending he is a player whom he admires and trying to play "As If" he were that player. For this techique to work properly three factors, at least, must pertain. First, the model player's performance must be very familiar to the would-be imitator. This means that the latter must have studied the role model's performance many times previously, either in real life (preferably) or on videotape. Secondly, the performance to be modelled must be better than his own but not so far removed from it as to be beyond the latter's capabilities. Thirdly, he must have rehearsed playing like the model player many times to the point where he takes on what he believes to be the same attitude and emotions as the model player portrays at these crucial moments in a game.

Whichever of these two mental strategies our winger adopts one thing is common to both. Whilst he is occupying his thoughts with either strategy he cannot be entertaining negative thoughts about his ability to cope with the situation and therefore he is preventing himself from becoming anxious. He is also raising the probability of a successful outcome to whatever he is trying to accomplish which will provide him with instant, positive reinforcement from his own actions and delayed, positive reinforcement from the comments made by his team mates and the crowd. In keeping with the principles of operant conditioning, explained by Skinner (1969) and applied to sporting context by Dickinson (1976), this will go a long way towards ensuring a positive attitude towards the next physical encounter with the opposition.

For our winger, it is now approximately 2.30pm and the next five to ten minutes should be spent with the rest of the team, working unopposed through some of the well-established set moves developed in practice sessions. This not only helps relieve any anxiety that might be developing but also contributes to the corporate identity which, in turn, helps develop team spirit. Thereafter, the team should return to the dressing room for final preparation.

Mental rehearsal of performance goals

Having retired to the dressing room with about twenty minutes to go before kick-off the next ten minutes might be most usefully spent in mentally rehearsing one's own Performance Goals. Performance goals refer to desired, or intended targets, concerning actual phases of play. Thus, skills, tactics and strategies are suitable subject matter for performance goals whereas winning and scoring so many points are not. The latter are outcome goals which cannot be controlled by the players concerned. Some examples of performance goals for our winger might be as follows:

a. To prevent my opposite number from passing me on the outside (at least!).
b. To position myself correctly for any kicks from the opposition's fly-half.
c. To catch all kicks to my wing cleanly.
d. To position myself such that I take all passes while accelerating ("on the burst").
e. To cover for our full-back whenever he is drawn to the opposite wing from mine.
f. To make the ball available at all times when tackled (or held).

Three performance goals should be enough for any one game providing they involve the most important aspects of wing play as perceived by the player concerned. Performance goals should also be negotiated initially between player and coach and never imposed on a player.

In mentally rehearsing any of these performance goals our winger should always visualise a successful performance; he should always rehearse at the correct speed and never in slow motion; he should rehearse as he has actually experienced the performance and not as if he were watching himself on a videotape recording and he should have rehearsed them many times previously as well as practised them on the training ground. Thus, this ten minute period of mental rehearsal would be an effective means of continuing the preparation begun earlier on the field. It is also an opportunity for players to have a second, short period of time to themselves even though they may be in each other's presence physically. For the majority of elite rugby players this is likely to be welcomed for the reasons identified earlier.

The final phase of preparation should be devoted to orienting each individual's thinking towards the team effort and his role in it. This is probably best conducted by the team captain although it is a widely held belief that the club coach should have the final word. Whoever it is would do well to begin by inviting each player in turn to declare one of his performance goals to the rest of his team mates (stating goals publicly is known to raise commitment to them) and then to say how he intends helping one or more of them to fulfil their particular role. Having done this the leader should finish with a short exhortation, perhaps along the following lines:

"Work for each other, support each other, take on your opponent and aim to get the better of him but, as you do so, be aware of the support available - your team mates will ensure that it is available! Enjoy the game and keep your mind on the objectives you have set for yourselves and for one another. If you get the performance right we'll get the result we deserve. **MAKE THINGS HAPPEN**. Now shake hands with every one of your team mates before you leave this dressing room and wish him luck".

This example is sufficient, for few players want to hear a long-winded speech at this late stage. Besides which, the players' levels of arousal are likely to be high by now and typically this will impair their ability to attend to any information and particularly so if it requires them to think analytically. It is also important to point out here that the recommendation to shake hands is based on the psycholigical knowledge that physical contact of one kind or another between people with a common objective helps raise their individual commitment to that common objective. It is a form of **BONDING** and this knowledge is obviously now seeping into the game of rugby for many teams are known to indulge in it and particularly so just before a match is due to begin. Moreover, this form of behaviour is no longer confined to simply shaking hands nor to the privacy of the dressing room. A number of international teams, for instance, have been seen, on the field of play, to bond by linking arms to body at either the shoulder or waist and thus to form a circle and to sing, or chant in unison, while doing so.

The players are now ready to take the field and, once out there, they should engage in nothing more than maintenance activities. These would include modified versions of the routines worked through earlier in the warm-up. Thus, the programme for the final sixty minutes before the game begins can now be set out in timetable fashion as illustrated below:

Preparation behaviours during the final sixty minutes before kick-off.

2.00 - 2.15 pm	Physical warm-up - stretching, running, sprinting with team mates and ending with solo work.
2.15 - 2.30 pm	Skill routines in small groups, including some which involve various forms of physical contact.
2.30 - 2.40 pm	Whole team in unopposed practice of pre-planned moves from set piece play and a sample of loose play situations.
2.40 - 2.50 pm	In dressing room - mental rehearsal of personal performance goals.
2.50 - 2.55 pm	Team orientation - public declaration of ONE performance goal from each player followed by captain's (or coach's) final words.
2.55 - 3.00 pm	On the field - keep active through a variety of suitable maintenance activities.
3.00 pm	Kick-off.

Pre-competition strategies

The timetable shown above amounts to what the present author (1986) described as a "Pre-Competition Strategy" which is a plan of all the behaviours that are to be enacted before a particular event begins. Having a detailed and well-planned pre-competition strategy is important because when a player works through a schedule of familiar routines he feels confident that his preparation is thorough and, as a result, he is less likely to develop anxiety.

In developing a pre-competition strategy one should always begin with the start of the event and work backwards. This is to ensure that enough time is made available to complete every behaviour thought necessary. The one illustrated above is for sixty minutes only and would be a useful start for a team that has only recently adopted this approach. However, pre-competition strategies should be developed by each player back to breakfast time at least on the day of the match. A pre-competition strategy should be negotiated between each player and his coach and completed in writing. It should be more detailed the nearer to the start of a match one gets and should include considerations of the criteria outlined below. Each player's pre-competition strategy will differ slightly from one game to the next in accordance with contingencies of travelling arrangements and the distance involved, location of match venue and idiosyncrasies of different changing rooms and practice grounds. When an overnight stay is necessary then a twenty-four hour, pre-competition strategy should be devised.

Criteria to be considered when devising a pre-competition strategy

1. What and when to eat and drink.
2. When to rest and when to engage in light activity.
3. The form of such rest and light activity.
4. When to check equipment and what to look for.
5. When one should be alone and when with other people.
6. Who these "other people" should be.
7. When to report to either the coach, physiotherapist or manager.
8. When to travel to the match venue and by what means.
9. When and how to check for arousal and anxiety levels.
10. When and how to warm-up, both physically and mentally.

"What if?" and Coping Strategies

An important feature of any pre-competition strategy is a set of "coping strategies" to fall back on if the primary strategies cannot be enacted for any reason. This is where the coach can be most useful for he is well placed to view each behaviour in the primary strategy and ask the player concerned the question "Ah, but what if ....?"

The details of the pre-competition strategy outlined above for the final sixty minutes before kick-off are not likely to be affected markedly by external influences. The "what if" question applies more to what each player wants to do and thinks he ought to do before the final sixty minutes. A pro-forma for recording all the details of a pre-competition strategy, including the post-event evaluations should be prepared.

Pre-competition strategies will also change slightly over time in accordance with post-match evaluations between player and coach. For instance, one particular behaviour might have proved inhibiting for some reason on an occasion or be deemed to have been ill-timed in relation to other behaviours. However, the major part of the strategy (including coping behaviours), once refined, will be repeated from one match to another. Not only will this degree of routine and familiarity result in feelings of security and confidence but also of control which is vital for any player to experience before a game begins. The more he feels in control of himself and his own destiny in the game the more he will feel he can influence it directly. This, in turn, will create a positive frame of mind which is more easily associated with attacking play. Since players can only feel either positive (attacking), neutral (fatalistic) or negative (defensive) most people concerned with and for the game of rugby would prefer players to feel positive and particularly so in those phases which involve them in physical contact.

References

Cox RL. (1986) Psychological preparation of elite athletes for high level competition. Self-learning packages produced by the Scottish Sports Council, Edinburgh.

Dickinson J. (1976) A Behavioural Analysis of Sport. Lepus Books, London.

Meichenbaum D and Turk D. (1975) The Cognitive-behavioural management of anxiety, anger and pain. Paper presented at the Seventh Banff Internatioal Conference on Behaviour Modification.

Nideffer R. (1978) The Inner Athlete: Mind plus Muscle for Winning. TY Crowell, New York.

Rushall BS. (1979) Psyching in Sport, Pelham Books, London.

Skinner BF. (1969) Contingencies of Reinforcement: A Theoretical Analysis. Appleton-Century-Crofts, New York.

Suinn R. (1977) Easing athletes' anxiety at the Winter Olympics. Physician Sports Med, 5, 88-92.

Syer J and Connolly C. (1984) Sporting Body, Sporting Mind. Cambridge University Press, London.

Injury prevention and the laws of rugby football

I.R. Vanderfield

Abstract. The Laws of Rugby Football are laid down by the International Rugby Football Board which was formed in 1887. Over the following ninety years the Laws were designed to make rugby an enjoyable game at all levels both for players and spectators. Over the years the nature of the game changed significantly and in 1977 the first law changes were introduced specifically designed to ensure player safety. This coincided with the development of a Medical Advisory Committee working with the International Rugby Football Board. Since that time player safety is one of the major factors under consideration with any law changes applying to the game.

Keywords: Injury Prevention, Contact Sport,Laws and Regulations, Role of the Coach, Role of the Administrator, Role of the Medical Advisor.

Injury prevention

"Injury Prevention" in a body contact sport is an unattainable ideal but it is essential to pursue the concept. This paper will outline important factors which contribute to a reduction in the number and severity of injuries, emphasising the significance of the Laws of Rugby Football. Many of the points raised will apply to all team games or contact sports (Table 1).

Injury Prevention hinges on an appropriately skilful and fit group of players combining together as a team to enjoy the game of Rugby Football, adopting a positive attitude to their opponents and the on-field officials. This positive attitude will ensure respect for the Laws of the Game and minimise injury in a sport such as Rugby Football where there is an element of physical danger and body contact.

Coaching and playing attitudes exemplified by the "win at all costs" approach adopted by some coaches and club officials in which they make every effort to get round the laws to suit a style of play will increase injuries. Club or Representative Teams who consistently select players who persistently and deliberately do not respect the laws, the on-field officials or their opponents will inevitably lead to increased injury risks. The Club Doctor who injects a painful injury or allows a player to return to the game a week after concussion is not adopting good standards of clinical practice as well as contravening the spirit of the game and increasing the risk of injury.

Table 1

INJURY PREVENTION

THE PLAYER	Selection of Appropriate Position
	Fitness
	Development of Skills
	Equipment
THE COACH	
THE ON-FIELD OFFICIALS	The Referee
	The Touch Judges
ADMINISTRATION	Selection Policies
	The Laws of the Game
MEDICAL	Management of Injured Players
	Anti-Doping Policies
	Data Collection and Research

Referees must not opt out and "do their own thing" when interpreting the laws, particularly those laws specifically designed to minimise the risk of injury.

The administration of the game at club, national and international levels must ensure that safety standards are maintained and enhanced by constant evaluation of the injuries that are occurring and the level of fitness among players leading, where appropriate, to changes in the laws. The Medical Officer or Club Doctor has an increasingly important role to play in this context.

A century of changes

Law changes for better rugby

The original Laws of Rugby Football were formulated at Rugby School and by the Rugby Football Union. In 1884 a dispute arose following the match between England and Scotland and, after three years' discussion, the International Rugby Football Board was formed in 1887. The first major review of the laws took place in 1892 and they have been subsequently revised on a regular basis trying to ensure that the balance of advantage is given to the team which wishes to attack, making rugby an open, running game.

Law changes for safer rugby

During the 1970s serious injuries which had not previously been encountered in rugby were noted to be occurring with greater frequency. This was noted throughout the rugby playing world and resulted in the International Rugby Football Board adopting a policy whereby it hoped to minimise the possibility of unintentional injury, remove aspects of potential danger and deal more strongly with foul play. Player safety had not been mentioned as the reason for law changes prior to 1977. Since that date the majority of changes are made with safety as one of the primary considerations.

In addition the International Rugby Football Board was becoming increasingly concerned about public allegations that sportsmen were using drugs. The International Board had already issued a statement to the effect that the use of drugs to enhance performance or to allow a player to play contravened the spirit of the game but the Board recognised that it had an increasing need to obtain medical advice on this aspect of modern sport (Table 2). Accordingly the International Board established, in 1977, a Medical Advisory Committee.

The International Board has modified laws dealing with the tackle and lying on the ground, as well as scrums, rucks and mauls in which player safety has been given major consideration. In addition to changes in these technical aspects of the game player safety has been enhanced by enforcing laws on foul play where any deliberate action has endangered the safety of other players. In 1988 it was made mandatory for touch judges to report foul play to the referee.

Detailed studies have taken place with regard to the design and safety features of the equipment used by players, such as mouthguards, boots and studs. The International Board financed a research project by SATRA (Shoe and Allied Trade Research Association) conducted over three years and this resulted in an international standard of design of studs which has subsequently become mandatory.

The replacement of two injured players has been allowed in representative rugby since 1971 and this has subsequently been extended to include competition and other domestic matches as determined by each individual national rugby union. More recently the number of replacements has been increased to three and up to six replacements are permitted in Under-21 rugby.

One of the most important advances made allowed the referee, upon receiving appropriate medical advice, to require injured players to leave the field if for any reason it would be harmful for the player to continue. This is particularly important with regard to concussion and the International Rugby Football Board, on the basis of medical advice, has issued a series of directives on this particular topic designed to enhance player safety and minimise the risk of a second injury or the accumulative effects of repeated concussion (Table 2).

The International Board could not have developed the concept of a Medical Advisory Committee or received appropriate advice from its member unions if all the rugby playing countries had not been able to recruit the enthusiastic support of interested doctors, chartered physiotherapists, sports scientists and other health care professionals to work with the game of rugby football at club, representative and international level.

Table 2.

International Rugby Football Board Resolutions of the Council

5. MEDICAL

5.5	**Use of Drugs:** The use of drugs by participants in Rugby Football, other than for therapeutic reasons in accordance with medical advice, is regarded by the Council with disapproval and is contrary to the spirit of the game. Any player unable to participate without the administration of drugs or injections to relieve pain or acute illness must be considered unfit to play in a game. The taking of drugs by players to enhance performance is forbidden. The Council supports the principles outlined in the Declaration on "Anti-doping in Sport", issued following the World Conference in Ottawa, Canada, in June 1988.
5.6	**Drug Testing:** All players participating in the game of Rugby Football may at any time be subject to a drug test.
5.7	**Concussion:** A player who has suffered definite concussion should not participate in any match or training session for a period of at least three weeks from the time of injury, and then only subject to being cleared by a proper neurological examination.

LAW 3. NUMBER OF PLAYERS

(6)	If the referee is advised by a doctor or other medically trained person or for any other reason considers that a player is so injured that it would be harmful for him to continue playing, the referee shall require the player to leave the playing area. For this purpose the referee may also require a player to leave the field to be examined medically.

What of the future?

So far as the laws are concerned, there is a need to evaluate what has been done in the perceived interests of safety as well as to improve the game ensuring that it remains enjoyable for the players and entertaining for the spectators.

The laws play an important part in injury prevention in any contact sport, but I believe there are and always will be a number of equally important aspects which must contribute to this goal based on player fitness; appropriate selection and coaching; and replacement of injured and unfit players. Foul play must be consistently condemned by players, coaches, on-field officials and both club and representative administrators. There is a continuing role for medical support and advice in monitoring injury patterns to evaluate the effect of law changes as well as to help look after the interests of the individual player and ensure the continuing development of the role of sports medicine in rugby football.

Dr Vanderfield's paper has been abbreviated by the editor.

PART FIVE

Clinical aspects of injuries in contact sports

Introduction
Clinical aspects of injuries in contact sport

Injuries in contact sport are being documented with increasing accuracy. The majority of injuries affect the lower limb and the opening paper of this section of the Proceedings gives an overview of the common problems. This review is followed by a series of papers highlighting areas of controversy – compartment compression syndromes, groin strain and knee injuries, with particular emphasis on the repair and rehabilitation of the ruptured anterior cruciate ligament. The experience of treating serious injuries in professional footballers in the USA has acted as a stimulus to world wide interest in Cruciate Ligament injuries.

Upper limb injuries in contact sport have tended to receive less attention because they are relatively infrequent. Injury to the shoulder girdle is reviewed in detail, highlighting the emerging role of arthroscopy in the management of the unstable shoulder and some rotator cuff lesions. The significance of injuries to the hand, thumb and fingers in contact sport is frequently underestimated. The importance of an early and accurate diagnosis of tendon and colateral ligament injuries is stressed if definitive treatment is to be effective.

Concussion is another common, underdiagnosed and potentially serious injury occurring in all contact sport and guidelines are offered on the assessment of the condition. The paper draws attention to the exaggerated effects of a second concussion, which requires careful specialist assessment and a prolonged period of rest.

The rare but catastrophic sports injury of quadraplegia is reviewed in detail, concentrating on the injuries occurring in rugby football. The less serious but more common problems of the early onset of degenerative disease of the cervical spine and spinal concussion are also discussed.

R. Nutton

The lower limb

The pattern of lower limb injuries in contact sport

L.J. Micheli

Abstract. The lower extremity sustains the highest portion of injuries seen in contact sports. The most obvious type of injury sustained in body-contact sports is that of acute traumatic injury. The second, more general mechanism of injury in sport is that of repetitive micro-trauma. The pattern of lower extremity injuries will be detailed by anatomic site, including a discussion of current methods of orthopaedic treatment.

Keywords: Contact Sports, Acute Traumatic Injury, Repetitive Microtrauma, Lower Limb.

Mechanism of injury

Contact sports, in which direct body contact occurs between opponent players, is subject to a variety of types of injury. The most obvious type of injury sustained in body-contact sports is that of acute traumatic injury, in which there is injury to tissue as a result of 2 single application of force or impact. These acute traumatic injuries, however, can be further subdivided into extrinsic and intrinsic injuries. Extrinsic injuries are the direct effect of the application of external force, such as the blow from the shoulder or limb of an opponent or their equipment, while intrinsic injury is the result of sudden application of force by the player's own muscle-tendon units.

A simple example of this would indeed be the tackling injury in which a contusion is sustained from the driving force of an opponent's shoulder, but at the same time, in an attempt to avoid the tackle, a sudden cutting motion by the ball carrier results in acute strain of the hamstring musculature on the opposite extremity.

The second, more general mechanism of injury in sport is that of repetitive microtrauma, resulting in overuse or training injury. This type of injury is common to all sports in which there is repetitive training to perfect fitness or playing technique. These injuries are the result of repetitive exposure to relatively small trauma, such as the foot-fall of running or the twisting of overhand throwing; the cumulative effect of these small forces is to cause tissue damage to muscle-tendon, bone, or ligament. These injuries include the tendinitises, bursitises, and stress fractures seen in athletes. They occur in a rather predictable fashion and are generally the result of the interaction of a number of risk factors. (Table 1) While a number of these risk factors may interact to result in injury, often an increase in the intensity of training will be the most obvious explanation for the occurrence of these injuries.

Types of injury

Acute traumatic injuries sustained in contact sports include fractures to the bones, dislocations of the joints, strains or avulsions of the muscle-tendon units, and contusions of the soft tissues. In addition, and as a result of excessive forces, particularly about the joints, neurovascular injury may result directly from the acute traumatic episode or be seen as a complication after the initial injury.

Sites of injury

The lower extremity sustains the highest proportion of injuries seen in contact sports; in some sports, as high as 70-80% of all injuries wlll be sustained in the lower extremities. These sites include the hip and pelvis, upper leg, including the thigh in front and the hamstring compartment behind, the knee, lower leg, ankle and foot. The knee wlll be discussed in another chapter and will not be discussed in our present review.

Hip and pelvis injuries

Injuries about the hip and pelvis in athletes, although relatively less common than other lower extremity injuries, can be extremely devastating.

Pelvic rim fractures are relatively rare. Frank avulsions of the muscles of the hip or the abdomen are, however, encountered in athletes. They may sometimes be associated with a small bony rim which is diagnostic. In addition, contusions of the pelvic rim, entitled "hip pointers" in athletic circles, can be extremely debilitating and may result in weeks or even months of debilitation. In some instances, drainage of the blood in association with these contusions may be necessary.

In younger athletes, apophyseal avulsions of the insertions of the sartorius, rectus femoris, or ischial spine may be encountered.

Table 1. Overuse injury risk factors

Training error	Muscle-tendon imbalance
Anatomic malalignment	Footwear
Playing surface	Associated disease state
Nutritional factors	Cultural deconditioning

In general, these apophyseal avulsions are treated conservatively in this younger athletic population. The one exception to this is the cases of extended displacement; these may be best treated by early reduction and internal fixation.

Injuries to the hip joint themselves are not rare in this group. Frank dislocations of the hip joint are a true athletic emergency. The athlete is totally disabled. The most common dislocation is superior anterior dislocation, a result of posturing of the hip into a shortening, internally rotated position.

Immediate reduction of this injury is necessary in order to limit the compromise of the blood vessels of the femoral head. Late reduction may result in avascular necrosis. Another associated injury or complication of hip dislocation is injury to the sciatic nerve.

It is our policy to obtain immediate reduction of this injury. This approach is facilitated by the practice common now in North America of having nitrous oxide analgesia available in the operating room setting.

Following this immediate reduction, CAT scans should be obtained to ensure that there are no associated fractures of the acetabular rim or displacement of fracture fragments into the joint.

Fractures of the hip may also be encountered in this population. They are usually of the base of the neck in the young athletic population and are best treated by immediate reduction and internal fixation. Once again, complications of this injury include avascular necrosis or non-union.

Contusions to the gluteal musculature, either of the gluteus maximus or the abductors, can be painful and debilitating in the athlete. These generally result from a direct blow or kick to the gluteal musculature. These contusions of the gluteal abductors must be treated immediately with icing and general compression to eliminate the further spread of bleeding and tissue injury. This should then be managed by crutch gait ambulation until the player can ambulate without limp and without pain. Physical therapy to restore the full range of motion and strength of the extremity is mandatory. These injuries may result in absence of play for as long as six weeks.

Upper leg

The anterior musculature of the upper leg is subject to both contusions and strains which can dramatically limit further competition. Contusions of the quadriceps may be of variable severity. The lowest in severity is designated grade I in which there is full range of motion of the knee into flexion actively and passively, but obvious pain and tenderness in the quadriceps with this movement. Grade II is an injury in which there is obviously an injury to the quadriceps musculature and the knee can be flexed to at least 90°, but not beyond. In grade III or severe injuries, there is less than 90° of active or passive knee flexion. In addition, dramatic swelling of the thigh may occur with associated extreme pain. As with any such injury, immediate icing, immobilization, and rest are required. Hospitalization may also be required and relatively strong analgesics may be necessary to aid in comfort of the athlete.

We favor a period of relative rest for this extremity until the swelling and the size of the extremity approaches that of the opposite side. The dreaded complication of this injury is myositis ossificans. This formation of bone in the injured muscle may take up to a year to resolve. In addition, this thigh is at increased risk of re-injury. There is some evidence in the literature that too early and aggressive return to physical therapy, and in particular the use of heat modalities and ultrasound, may increase the chance of myositis occurring.

Once the initial injury and inflammatory phase has passed, and this may take as long as three to four weeks, well directed physical therapy to restore the motion and the strength of the quadriceps is indicated.

In the event that myositis ossificans has occurred, it is our feeling that the therapy should be rather dramatically decreased and only done within the range of comfort, allowing the myositis to migrate to the femur and then become reattached to it, at which time progressive restoration of strength and motion may be pursued more aggressively.

If the athlete has good resolution of symptoms and restoration of motion and strength after a quadriceps contusion, it is our feeling that it is still important to protect this structure for at least the next twelve months in order to prevent re-injury, which, again, seems to carry an increased risk of myositis ossificans occurrence. The use of soft padding in rugby football, of course, is necessary, whereas in association football or gridiron football, more rigid padding taped directly under the thigh is allowed.

Injuries to the posterior musculature or hamstrings of the leg usually consist of muscle-tendon strains. These, of course, can also occur to the quadriceps musculature, but are less common and debilitating. The functional problem presented by hamstring strains is the potential for recurrence and the potential for persistent tightness or weakness of the musculature. Whereas in the past rehabilitation has consisted primarily of restoration of the range of motion and flexibility of these injured muscles, much more emphasis is now put upon restoration of both the dynamic concentric and dynamic eccentric strength of these structures. This type of rehabilitation is particularly important following hamstring injuries, since the hamstrings function in an eccentric contraction mode in sports activities.

Recent work on muscle-tendon strains, particularly of hamstrings, by Garrett and associates has shown that these injuries always occur at muscle-tendon junctions. Further research has shown that there are muscle-tendon junctions at every level of the hamstring musculature from the very proximal site of attachment, the ischium, down to the attachment at the posterior aspect of the tibia, both medially and laterally, as well as over the fibular head.

A symptom of upper leg pain in the contact sport athlete must be assessed very carefully. In addition to direct injuries to the tissues of this structure, this can be a common site of referred pain. Injuries or derangements about the hip, including slipping of the capital femoral epiphysis in the prepubescent or pubescent adolescent athlete, as well as stress fractures of the hip or femur, can express themselves as leg pain. On occasion, these injuries may suddenly displace and become complete fractures.

Knee pain

Pain about the knee will be noted in this section only insofar as it may be a referred pain from structures above or below. We have seen an athlete complain of knee pain as a result of stress fractures of the distal femur, sciatica from a herniated nucleus pulposus of the lumbar spine, tumor of the proximal tibia, and chondroblastoma of the distal femur. A careful assessment of the athlete complaining of knee pain must include not only the structures of the knee, including the extensor mechanism, but also careful examination of the hip, upper leg, and proximal lower leg.

Lower leg

Acute traumatic injuries to the lower leg are relatively uncommon. These obviously can be the result of direct blows from opponents, including tackles, kicks, and other impact. In addition, strains of the musculature of this compartment are relatively common. Both the tibialis anterior and tibialis posterior can be strained in the mid and distal portions of the lower leg, resulting in difficulty in performance and running. Contusions of the tibialis anterior, in particular, can be quite debilitating. The athlete should be monitored carefully and attention should always be given to the possibility of development of late acute traumatic compartment syndrome.

Activity or performance related lower leg pain is relatively more common. The differential diagnosis of leg pain developing in association with protracted running activities includes that of tibial or fibular stress fractures; periostitis, particularly of the insertion of the tibialis posterior musculature around the posterior and medial margin of the tibia; compartment syndrome, particularly of the anterolateral compartment of the leg, but occasionally of the posterior compartment: and tendinitis of the muscles of these compartments. New imaging techniques, including magnetic resonance imaging and bone scan, have been particularly useful in making a correct diagnosis. In assessing lower leg pain, it has been our practice to obtain initial plain radiographs and, depend on the suspected origin of the pain, whether bone or soft tissue, to then proceed to either a bone scan or a magnetic resonance imaging.

There are two acute traumatic injuries of the muscle-tendon structures of the lower leg which merit special mention. The first is an acute avulsion of the medial head of the gastrocnemius, sometimes dubbed "tennis leg", which can be very specifically diagnosed by careful physical examination. This is an injury which is invariably treated effectively by relative rest and immobilization. Symptomatic improvement can be helped simply by giving a heel lift followed by gentle restoration of range of motion and strengthening of gastrocnemius. Return to activity may be expected within three to six weeks, depending on the severity of injury.

Unfortunately, this relatively minor injury can be confused with or mistakenly diagnosed as a rupture, complete or total, of the tendo-Achilles.

Ruptured tendo-Achilles in athletes is generally relatively easy to diagnose. Quite interestingly, it is often the result of intrinsic overload to the structure. The athlete will describe a sudden attempt to accelerate followed by acute onset of pain and a sense that something has struck him in the back of the leg.

The management of this injury in athletes remains somewhat controversial. There are two alternative treatments, that of immobilization in the equinus position versus that of direct surgical repair. Both have proponents. In one widebased study in Scandanavia, it was shown that the restoration of strength was very similar using the two techniques. The only difference was a higher incidence of re-rupture in the cast-treated patients. Of course, the potential complications of surgical intervention are greater than of the casting technique. This does not mean that the casting technique is without its complications as rehabilitation for an ankle after cast-immobilization may take the same period of time. In addition, there are other risks of casting these extremities, including phlebitis. Whether surgical or cast immobilization treatment is elected, it will generally take the athlete between nine and twelve months to resume full safe sport participation in a contact sport setting.

Ankle injury

Injuries about the ankle in the contact sport player are relativelv common. In some sports such as association football, they rank closely after knee injuries in prevalence as the site of injury. Fractures or fracture dislocation of the ankle are the most severe of acute traumatic injury to be sustained at this site. Inability to sustain weight on the extremity and gross deformity make the diagnosis obvious. However, the ability of the athlete to run or even cut on the injured extremity by no means eliminates the possibility that the injury is a fracture. Careful physical examination with exact localization of the site of maximal tenderness or pain is imperative. It is particularlv useful to do this examination as soon as possible after injury in order to minimize the resultant distortion of anatomy and the spread of pain and swelling in this area. As with any acute traumatic injury, immobilization and icing, as well as gentle compression with elastic bandages, is useful to prevent any further swelling and derangement.

In the event that there is gross deformity of the extremity and in some cases of fracture dislocation of the ankle or fracture dislocation of the subtalar joint, immediate reduction of the deformity should be done at field-side in order to prevent neurovascular compromise or development of late compartment syndrome, particularly that of the foot, which is not often appreciated following such injuries.

Following the immediate reduction of the deformity, immobilization, icing, and gentle compression can then be instituted.

Sprains of the ankle may involve any of the ligamentous structures at the talotibial and talofibular joints. The most commonly injured ligaments of this joint are the lateral ligament structures of the ankle. In one series in North America, these ligaments were sprained in 85% of the cases of acute traumatic ankle injury.

Further studies have demonstrated that these ligaments appear to be torn in a sequential fashion beginning at the anterior tibial talar joint; secondly, the lateral tibiocalcaneal; and, finally, the posterior ligaments. the management of injuries to the lateral ligament structures of the ankle has remained controversial. There is general agreement that grade I or grade II derangements of this ligamentous complex can be treated quite satisfactorily by relative rest, immobilisation, and then progressive restoration of strength and function. This approach is further facilitated by the easy availability of certain splinting techniques, such as the Aircast, which gives good early comfortable stabilization and allows rehabilitation while stabilization is maintained in the early and subacute phases of this injury. There is, however, controversy regarding management of grade III sprains of these ligament complexes. It is really quite rare now in North America to have an acute ligamentous repair of these structures. It has been demonstrated that conservative management can result in full functional recovery. An initial seven to ten day period of complete immobilization with casting or removable boot immobilization is followed by progressive functional restoration of motion and strength while protecting these structures. There has been some question in certain activities, such as ballet, or by certain authorities dealing with high performance cutting sports, such as association football in particular, as to whether better results are obtained by early direct repair of the ligamentous structures. Cox has hypothesized that in a certain small portion of athletes with this injury, who are having symptoms ten to twelve weeks after injury, there is still a place for subacute repair and direct suturing of these structures. In general however, in North America, there is a tendency now to go to early rehabilitation or functional restoration of these injuries and to reserve surgical intervention to reconstruction of a very small number of individuals who have persistent symptoms. This approach has been further supported by recent observations that a certain number of these injuries are accompanied by intra-articular injury. Intra-articular injury may actually be the source of subsequent symptoms and swelling and not the associated ligamentous injury. Magnetic resonance imaging in association with CAT scan arthrograms and, on occasion, arthroscopy of the ankle, has made this approach much more plausible and the diagnosis of the ankle derangements much more specific in this group of athletes.

While the tendency to remain more conservative with lateral ligamentous injuries about the ankle has now become widespread in North America, there is also a consensus that injuries to the syndesmotic ligament of the ankle must now be treated very specifically either with immobilization and complete non-weight bearing casting or early use of a syndesmotic screw for immobilization, followed by early removal of this screw fixation and then restoration of function. Once again, this diagnosis can be made most easily by early, very careful physical examination in which there is discrete pain localized to the anterior tibiofibular structures with pressure, or in which there is severe pain with dorsiflexion and/or external rotation of the foot in the ankle mortise localized to the syndesmotic joint.

Injuries to the medial ligamentous complex are relatively rare as isolated injuries. They can certainly be seen in conjunction with distal fibular injuries in an abduction external rotation injury about the ankle joint. They are often treated indirectly by reduction of the ankle joint and internal fixation of the fibular injury. On relatively rare occasions, direct surgical repair of the injured ligament may be required.

As noted above, new imaging techniques have made it possible to diagnose intra-articular injuries of the joint surface at the time of the acute traumatic insult to the ankle joint. Baker et al have documented at least nine cases which were treated successfully by arthroscopic intervention and debridement where ankle injury was followed by chronic pain and recurrent swelling, despite apparent healing of the ligaments.

Hindfoot pain

Hindfoot pain in the contact sport athlete is rarely the result of direct trauma. Nonetheless, it can be a very debilitating injury. In our experience, this pain may be the result of injury at three different sites. Certainly, retrocalcaneal bursitis or insertional tendinitis of the tendo-Achilles can account for pain at this site. This can often be treated by relative rest in association with a heel lift, use of an anti-inflammatory medication, and careful physical therapy. An additional site of hindfoot pain is at the base of the heel and reflects a bursitis of the os calcis. This pain can be associated with training on very hard ground or in stiff boots. It can be alleviated to some extent with heel inserts or rubber cups on the heel and sometimes changing the boot to a more multi-cleated type. Anti-inflammatory medication and, on occasion, direct corticosteroid injection at this site may relieve symptoms.

The third injury which can occur in contact sport players and which, again, can be very debilitating is a chronic or an acute rupture of the plantar fascia. Pain and tenderness is localized anteriorly and medially to the os calcis. Treatment is often dependent on severity of symptoms. We will often use a heel cup, anti-inflammatory medication, and, on occasion, corticosteroid treatment. Additional therapeutic modalities such as ultrasound and gentle stretching of the plantar fascia may be instituted. On relatively rare occasions where an athlete does not respond to this conservative management, we have successfully treated this group with complete surgical division of the plantar fascia. This approach is supported by several reports in the literature of plantar fasciitis being totally relieved by a late complete rupture of the plantar fascia.

Midfoot injuries which can occur in the contact sport athlete include the devastating injury of pantalar dislocation. This is truly an athletic emergency. The dislocation must be reduced to avoid neurovascular complications and development of compartment syndrome of the foot. As with other ligamentous injuries, the newer approach to this type of injury is to begin gentle early mobilization of the injured ligament while providing support of the extremity. The newer commercially available removable boots of the bivalved plastic type have facilitated this approach. It has been our experience that this early mobilization approach is preferable to complete immobilization as recommended in the older orthopaedic literature. Often, the athlete will never have a return to full mobility and motion of the foot after immobilization treatment, and will often remain mildly symptomatic thereafter. Additional injuries of the midfoot include a fracture of the navicular which is usually an overuse stress fracture injury. However, the onset of pain can be quite acute after one particular episode, such as a cut.

Initial diagnosis of this condition can be difficult. This has been greatly aided by the use of new diagnostic tests such as bone scanning or MRI imaging. On occasion, CT tomograms will help in making the diagnosis.

The accepted treatment for this condition is immobilization for six to eight weeks using non-weight bearing technique. This can be a very difficult fracture indeed to obtain healing. On occasion, internal fixation and screw fixation may be required to obtain healing in this lesion.

An additional midfoot injury which merits discussion is that of injuries to the fifth metatarsal. Avulsion injury of the peroneus brevis muscle are well known in athletes. This can be the result of direct or indirect trauma. Most commonly the athlete will attempt to stand up after a fall and their own musculature will do the avulsion from the site of insertion.

While the general orthopaedic literature sometimes suggests that this injury can be treated symptomatically, it has been our own experience that an athlete who obtains a fibrous union of this injury wlll often remain symptomatic and limited in athletic function. We will often give the athlete the alternative of either open reduction and internal fixation, depending on the size of the fragment, or cast immobilization. We do not treat this with simply soft dressings and elastic bandages as has been advised by some authorities.

Once union has been obtained and the patient has developed good eversion strength, he may successfully return to sports activities; but, once again, it has been our experience that this may take up to twelve to sixteen weeks to occur.

Another fracture which can be seen in contact sport athletes at this site is the so-called "Jones fracture" which is a metaphyseal fracture of the proximal fifth metatarsal. As with navicular stress fractures, this is most commonly a stress fracture which has often an acute component resulting in pain.

This is a slow healing difficult fracture. It is most successfully treated by internal fixation with an intramedulary screw with or without bone grafting. The essential point about this fracture is that it must be taken very seriously and not be confused with the avulsion fracture of the peroneal which is a much more readily healing fracture.

Forefoot injuries in contact sport athletes are not uncommon. One of the very common injuries is a sprain of the first MP joint. This injury can be quite debilitating. We once again take this injury quite seriously. We will put the athlete in a rigid-soled shoe or sometimes even a plastic slipper, and then commence supervised non-weight bearing range of motion and strengthening exercises under the direction of a physical therapist. It has been our experience that this injury may remain symptomatic for months and may actually result in early arthrosis and spurring of the joint with hallux rigidus as a late result.

Additional injuries of the forefoot in contact sports include subungual hematomas of the toe which can be quite painful. As with similar injuries in the fingers, these are often best treated by drainage of the entrapped blood. The toenail may be lost and every attempt should be made to keep the toenail in place as long as possible as a protector for the more sensitive tissue underneath.

Fractures of the metatarsals and metatarsophalangeal joints can occur and are the result of either direct or indirect trauma in contact sport athletes. As with any significant injury, careful diagnosis, including AP, lateral, and oblique x-rays, of the foot should be obtained. These fractures might sometimes be initially missed and may remain symptomatic in the forefoot with localized tenderness. Additional x-rays may be required. A relatively unusual injury, but one which may be missed for some time, is a fracture of the proximal metaphysis of the second metatarsal. Again, a bone scan or CT may be required to make this diagnosis accurately. In the athlete in particular, exact reduction of these fractures is often indicated; whereas in the general, relatively sedentary population, the attitude towards metatarsal fractures is relatively sanguine. One may hear the adage, as long as they are "in the same room", they will heal and be fine. It has been our experience that anatomic reduction is the best rule of thumb for the athlete. Fortunately, this can often be obtained quite easily by open reduction and intramedulary pinning, followed by relatively early removal of the pins.

Recommended Reading

Cantu RC and Micheli LJ. (1991) ACSM's Guidelines for the Team Physician. Lea & Febiger, Philadelphia, PA.

Micheli LJ. (1984) Pediatric and Adolescent Sports Medicine. Little, Brown, Boston, MA.

Micheli LJ and Jenkins MD. (1990) Preventing Rugby Injuries. Proceedings of the International Conference on Rugby Injuries, US Rugby Football Foundation, Boston, MA.

Nicholas JA and Hershman EB. (1986) The Lower Extremity and Spine in Sports Medicine. CV Mosby, St Louis, MO.

Chronic compartment syndrome

L.H. Boobis

Abstract. Chronic compartment syndrome is a relatively infrequent cause of exercise induced leg pain that limits performance. It is usually encountered in young athletes involved in endurance sports and there is often a long delay prior to the correct diagnosis being made. The anterior and lateral compartments are more often involved than the posterior ones and a clinical diagnosis is made by the exclusion of other causes and an awareness of the clinical features associated with the syndrome. A definitive diagnosis is made by measurement of intramuscular pressure by a catheter technique, infusion techniques being more suitable for measurements made during exercise. The use of ultrasound may aid catheter placement in the deep posterior compartments. A resting pressure >15 mmHg, a mean exercise pressure of >50 mmHg, a muscle relaxation pressure >35 mmHg, a post-exercise pressure >35 mmHg with a delay in return to normal of more than 15 minutes, or a post-exercise pressure of >25 mmHg persisting for more than five minutes have all been reported as diagnostic of the condition. Conservative treatment is only of value in those patients who have decided to abandon their previous lifestyle. Subcutaneous fasciotomy offers a complete cure in 75% of patients and fails to help less than 10%. Operative complications can be reduced by careful surgery. A small proportion of patients may develop a recurrence but they invariably respond to a further operation.

Keywords: Chronic Compartment Syndrome, Athletes, Exercise, Intramuscular Pressure. Fasciotomy

Introduction

Acute compartment syndrome was first described by Volkmann in 1881 (Amendola et al, 1990) but it was not until three quarters of a century later that the first account of chronic compartment syndrome was published (Mavor, 1956). Since then much has been written about the diagnosis and management of the problem although there is still some controversy concerning its pathogenesis. The condition can be defined as recurring exercise induced leg pain, confined to a specific muscular compartment, that limits performance and subsides with rest. A number of different terms have been given to this condition and these include; recurrent compartment syndrome, subacute compartment syndrome, chronic exertional compartment syndrome and chronic compartment syndrome, as well as the non-specific term of "shin splints". This latter term includes other conditions which must be considered in the differential diagnosis.

Patients presenting with the syndrome are typically in their early twenties and involved in endurance running although it has been reported in a wide variety of activities including skating, skiing, golf, fencing, dancing, boxing, ice hockey and football as well as in non-athletes. (Detmar et al, 1985; Puranen and Alavaikko, 1981; Styf and Korner, 1987). Pain is invariably well localised and the condition is frequently bilateral with males and females being equally affected (Lutz et al, 1989).

Anatomy

Anatomically there are five osteofascial compartments of the leg (Grant, 1962); anterior (containing the extensors, tibialis anterior and the deep peroneal nerve); lateral (containing the peronei and the superficial peroneal nerve), superficial posterior (containing the superficial calf muscles and the sural nerve), deep posterior (containing the flexors and the tibial nerves) and an autonomous tibialis posterior compartment (Fig 1). Some authors however, include the tibialis posterior compartment as part of the deep posterior one (Allen, 1990; Amendola et al, 1990; Martens et al, 1984).

Pathophysiology

The osteofascial compartments are tight envelopes of connective tissue enclosing the muscles of the leg and have a limited ability to accommodate changes in volume which may increase by as much as 20% during exercise (Matsen, 1980). Alterations in the compliance of the fascial envelope by its thickening or as a result of injury, or increases in the volume of its contents by muscle hypertrophy or swelling may increase tissue pressure to a level that will compromise tissue perfusion. Exertion, trauma and venous diseases appear to be important aetiological factors (Styf, 1989).

During muscular contraction, as in cardiac muscle, skeletal muscle perfusion is thought to occur during relaxation (Folkow et al, 1980). This is consistent with the finding that muscle contraction pressures exceed 120 mmHg in normal persons whereas relaxation pressures are normally <15 mmHg (Styf and Korner, 1987). Patients with compartment syndrome appear to be involved in a higher level of physical activity than those with leg pain due to other reasons. It has been postulated that this leads to microtrauma to the muscle cells and damage to the capillary and lymphatic bed. This results in an inflammatory reaction with a resultant increase in capillary filtration of up to five fold (Rippe et al, 1978). In susceptible persons continued exercise will result in a progressive increase in intercompartmental volume with a concomitant rise in pressure so that muscle relaxation pressure exceeds the level at which muscle perfusion can occur between contractions. Muscle ischaemia will then result and the pain thus produced will prevent the athlete from continuing with his exercise (Fig 2).

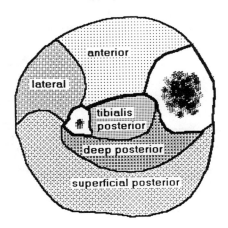

Fig. 1   Osteofascial compartments of the leg

There is little information about the histological and biochemical changes that occur in the muscle of these patients. Hoffmeyer et al (1987) have described accumulation of lipid droplets in the myofibrillar space together with ragged slow twitch fibres (which they felt predominated) and an increased number of abnormally large mitochondria. These changes are similar to those seen in patients with intermittent claudication due to peripheral vascular disease. Variation in fibre size with oedema and fibre destruction together with widespread intracellular nuclei has also been reported (Detmer et al, 1985).

Clinical features

History
Patients with the syndrome tend to be young and involved in endurance sports. The initial complaint is of tightness, cramping, or discomfort in the leg brought on by exercise and relieved by rest, although it may persist for several hours or more. The pain which may also be described as stabbing or sharp is invariably well localised to a specific muscular compartment and the level of activity required to produce pain can be remarkably constant. An attempt to resume exercise before

the pain has fully settled is unsuccessful and patients find that they are unable to run through the pain. Athletes often report a decrement in performance and the cessation of exercise improves symptoms in the majority. Typically symptoms worsen slowly over many months and have often been present for a year or more prior to seeking medical advice. The patient may have had multiple consultations prior to a diagnosis being made. Additional symptoms include an awareness of muscle weakness or alteration in gait and well localised areas of paraesthesia which resolve with rest. Often the leg feels tender and

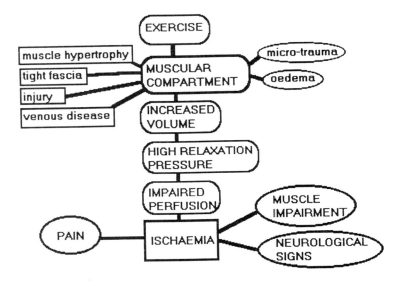

Fig. 2 Proposed mechanism for chronic compartment syndrome (after Styf, 1989)

stretching is uncomfortable. Occasionally the athlete may notice a lump on the muscle due to herniation and bilateral symptoms are present in up to 90% (Detmer et al, 1985; Martens et al, 1984; Lutz et al, 1989; Bouche, 1990).

Examination

Examination of the patient at rest will often reveal no obvious abnormality although muscle herniae are present in 30% to 60% of patients. A careful examination is made for other disorders. Peripheral pulses are palpated and if there is any doubt about their integrity then doppler ankle pressures should be recorded. Venous abnormalities are sought and the presence of a popliteal cyst is excluded. Tenderness along the medial border of the tibia should raise suspicion of the Medial Tibial Syndrome particularly if the patient is able to exercise through the pain (Allen and Barnes, 1986).

After exercise Bouche (1990) has described specific signs that point to involvement of a particular compartment. Paraesthesia in the first interspace with weakness on ankle dorsiflexion, pain on ankle plantarflexion and tenderness in the anterior leg suggests anterior compartment syndrome. Sensory loss on the dorsum of the foot, weakness on dorsiflexion and foot eversion, pain on plantarflexion and inversion with lateral leg tenderness is indicative of lateral compartment syndrome. Neurological signs on the sole of the foot, weakness in plantarflexion, inversion and toe flexion, pain on the opposite range of movement and tenderness in the medial calf is diagnostic of the deep posterior compartment. The superficial posterior compartment is characterised by hypoaesthesia on the dorsal-lateral foot, weakness on ankle plantarflexion, pain on dorsiflexion and tenseness in the calf. The tibialis posterior compartment is difficult to diagnose clinically and may be confused with cortical causes of the medial tibial stress syndrome, although tenderness tends to lie deep to the medial border of the tibia (Lutz et al, 1989). In all cases there is preservation of the peripheral pulses during and after exercise.

Differential diagnosis

As well as a variety of soft tissue injuries, there are a number of conditions which can mimic the symptoms of the chronic compartment syndromes.

Stress fractures are usually associated with localised tenderness over the bone and the diagnosis is confirmed by an isotope bone scan and an interval plain radiograph.

Although peripheral vascular disease is uncommon in this population intermittent claudication does occur in association with the popliteal entrapment syndrome as well as being more rarely due to atherosclerosis. The diagnosis should be easily made by measurement of pre- and post-exercise doppler ankle pressures.

Nerve entrapment syndromes (deep and superficial peroneal) cause sensory changes in association with point tenderness over the point at which the nerve leaves the fascia (anterior aspect of the ankle and middle third of the medial aspect of the leg respectively).

Medial tibial syndrome or shin splints is associated with localised tenderness over the medial border of the tibia. It is a hetrogeneous condition due variably to chronic periostealgia, stress fracture or microfracture ((Lutz et al, 1989).

Other medical conditions including diabetic neuropathy, spinal disease, osteo-arthrosis, infection and neoplastic disorders should be excluded by means of a thorough physical examination.

Diagnosis

Although the history and clinical findings before and after exercise allow a tentative diagnosis of chronic compartment syndrome to be made it can only be confirmed with certainty by the measurement of intracompartment pressure (Puranen and Alavaikko, 1981; Martens et al, 1984; Detmer et al, 1985; Allen and Barnes, 1986; Styf and Korner, 1987; Styf, 1989; Pedowitz et al, 1990; Bouche, 1990). Other less reliable tests have included ultrasound, venography, radionucleotide blood flow measurement, electromyography and nerve conduction studies (Bouche, 1990). More recently magnetic resonance imaging has been reported as being helpful in the diagnosis, there being a correlation between prolongation of the relaxation constant T1 (an index of an increase in hydrogen ion density) and intramuscular pressure (Amendola et al, 1990) and this tool may prove useful in the future.

Pressure measurement

Pressure measurements allow a reproducible and quantitative means of establishing the diagnosis of the condition and of assessing the effectiveness of any treatment.

There are a number of different techniques for recording intramuscular pressure which can variously measure pressure at rest, before and after exercise, and dynamically during exercise. These include injection techniques, infusion techniques, non-infusion techniques and micro-tip transducer techniques. Most of the devices that have been described are satisfactory for pressure recordings at rest but if it is intended to measure pressure during or immediately after exercise, then it is important that the appropriate technique is chosen. Of these methods only infusion techniques appear to offer sufficient sensitivity and accuracy to allow pressure measurements to be made during exercise (Allen and Barnes, 1986; Styf and Korner, 1987; Styf, 1989) and if an estimate of muscle contraction and relaxation pressures is desired then the microcapillary infusion method has been demonstrated as having the required characteristics (Styf and Korner, 1986 & 1987).

Normal intramuscular pressure

Normal resting intracompartment pressure is in the order of 5 mmHg [although values as high as 15 mmHg have been reported (McDermott el al, 1982; Allen and Barnes, 1986; Rorabeck et al,1988)] and there seems to be close agreement between the different muscular compartments (Styf and Korner, 1987; Styf, 1989; Pedowitz et al, 1990; Bouche, 1990) . During muscular contraction, pressures as high as 250 mmHg have been recorded (McDermott et al, 1982; Styf and Korner, 1986) but this falls to between 15 and 25 mmHg during relaxation (Styf and Korner, 1986). Immediately after exercise pressure remains at the level of the relaxation pressure but returns to normal pre-exercise values within a few minutes

(McDermott el al, 1982; Styf and Korner, 1986 & 1987; Styf, 1989).

Intramuscular pressure in compartment syndrome

Although some authors have described elevated resting pressure as being an inevitable finding (Lutz et al, 1989), others have found it of no diagnostic value (Allen and Barnes, 1986). Resting pressures do appear variable and the values recorded are dependent on the depth of the catheter in the muscle, the position of the ankle joint and an increased muscle tone due to apprehension or pain (Styf, 1989; Bouche, 1990). However a value greater than 15 mmHg should be considered as abnormal (Detmer et al, 1985; Pedowitz et al, 1990; Bouche, l990). Of more diagnostic value, however is the pressure immediately post-exercise and the time for the pressure to return to the resting level. Styf (1989) feels that a post-exercise pressure exceeding 30 or 35 mmHg which does not normalize within 15 minutes is pathognomic of the syndrome, whereas Pedowitz et al (1990) feel that a 5 minute post-exercise pressure greater than 25 mmHg is diagnostic. Pressures during exercise are difficult to measure (Styf and Korner, 1986 & 1987) and it must be recognised that mean pressures are dependent on both contraction and relaxation pressures and changes in both these variables have been reported. Allen and Barnes (1986), using a static slit catheter technique [which Styf (1989) considers an injection technique by virtue of the need for frequent flushing to prevent tip occlusion] have reported exercise pressures for the anterior compartment of >50 mmHg and the deep posterior compartment of >40 mmHg as diagnostic which compares quite well with the values of between 50 and 85 mmHg reported by other authors (McDermott et al, 1982; Styf and Korner, 1986 & 1987; Styf, 1989). However Styf (1989) considers mean pressure less suitable than muscle relaxation pressure and he feels that a value for this in excess of 35 mmHg correlates very well with the development of the clinical signs and symptoms of the syndrome.

Involved compartments

In an early study (Puranen and Alavaikko, 1981) in which they examined only the lateral and "medial compartment" in 32 patients almost 70% were in the medial (deep posterior) group. Martens et al (1984) studied all four major compartments in 29 patients and found 43 involved compartments of which 60% were deep posterior, 30% anterior, 7% lateral and one was a superficial posterior. A different distribution has been reported by Detmer et al (1984) who have published their findings of 233 compartments in 100 patients. They found that 40% of their patients had involvement of the anterior compartment, 12% of the lateral, 32% the deep posterior (which they subdivided into proximal and distal) and 17% superficial posterior (which they again subdivided into medial, lateral and distal). By contrast Allen and Barnes (1986) noted that the anterior compartment was affected in 75% (together with the deep posterior in 15% of these) in the 118 compartments that were involved in the 82 patients with the syndrome. In 14%

the deep posterior alone was affected but they do not report on the lateral or superficial posterior compartments. A similar distribution is reported by Pedowitz et al (1990) who diagnosed chronic compartment syndrome in 80 compartments of 45 patients of which the majority affected the anterior compartment (56% anterior, 20% lateral, 5% superficial posterior and 19% deep posterior). From these studies it appears that the most frequently involved compartments are the anterior and lateral ones.

Catheter placement

The anatomy of the anterior and lateral compartments allow easy and safe catheter placement and as a consequence these compartments appear to have been better studied than the deep posterior compartment (Styf and Korner, 1987; Styf, 1989; Wiley et al, 1990). Because of the proximity of the neurovascular bundles some observers are reluctant to perform blind catheter insertion of the deep posterior compartment (Detmer et al, 1985) and in addition the variability of the anatomy makes correct catheter placement less reliable. Real-time ultrasound is now universally available and Wiley et al (1990) have demonstrated the usefulness of this in the identification of the anatomy of the deep posterior compartment including visualisation of the tibialis posterior muscle compartment, thus allowing correct, safe and accurate placement of catheters for pressure measurement.

Treatment

Although some authors have advocated conservative treatment for this condition (Stefl and Gudas, 1981) there is more or less universal agreement that it is of little benefit (Martens et al, 1984; Styf, 1987; Lutz et al, 1989; Bouche, 1990). Patients must choose between living with the problem or accept the need for operative intervention. If conservative treatment is chosen then it should include prolonged rest and then avoidance of the type of strenuous exercise that precipitated the problem. Additional therapy in the form of physiotherapy, non-steroidal anti-inflammatory drugs, alterations in shoe wear and diuretic therapy have been described (Bouche, 1990) but if patients try to resume their previous level of exercise they invariably develop a recurrence of their symptoms unless their original problem was due to a cause other than compartment syndrome. Some authors (Allen and Barnes, 1986) advocate a six month period of conservative treatment to screen out those patients who do not have the syndrome prior to undertaking intracompartment pressure measurements. If non-operative treatment is chosen then it must be explained to the patient that if they do not modify their activity then they are at risk of developing acute exertional compartment syndrome (Bouche, 1990).

Operative treatment

The decision to operate must be considered entirely an elective one as surgical intervention will only be undertaken in those patients who are unwilling to accept a change in their desired lifestyle. As such if the operative results were poor or the risks of surgery substantial then it would be difficult to justify surgery. Fortunately this is not the case and the majority of patients are able to return to their former level of exercise.

Fasciotomy

The operative treatment for chronic compartment syndrome is fasciotomy. Unlike acute compartment syndrome it should never be necessary to perform an open fasciotomy nor should such radical measures as excision of the fibula be required (Detmer et al, 1985). In the majority of cases subcutaneous fasciotomy of the involved compartment is curative (Bouche, 1990; Lutz et al, 1989: Detmer et al, 1985; Allen and Barnes, 1986). There are a number of different techniques described for the procedure but an excellent description of the surgical technique is given by Detmer et al (1985). All but release of the deep posterior compartments can be carried out under local anaesthesia. Care should be taken to avoid damage to superficial nerves and the saphenous veins. Release of the deep posterior compartment involves dissection in close proximity to the posterior tibial vessels which can be at risk of injury. Fasciotomy of the anterior compartment should not be carried out in isolation but should be combined with release of the lateral compartment to prevent a superficial peroneal nerve entrapment syndrome. If fascial defects are present then it is advisable to include the defect in the fasciotomy being aware that defects often occur at the point of exit of a peripheral nerve. No attempt should be made to close these defects for fear of inducing an acute compartment syndrome.

Post-operatively patients should retain some form of compression bandage and keep their leg elevated for two or three days. Following this early mobilisation is encouraged with return to running within two to three weeks although return to maximal activity is quite variable. Post-operative reactive oedema appears most marked in high class athletes and can be controlled with a graduated compression support stocking.

Complications of surgery include arterial injury, haematoma, superficial wound infection, peripheral nerve injury, nerve entrapment syndromes and deep venous thrombosis. Although in theory some muscle weakness as a result of the division of the fascia could be expected, this is not borne out in clinical practice.

Results of fasciotomy

Detmer et al (1985) have published the largest series of fasciotomy for compartment syndrome and reported that 91% of their patients were functionally improved and 93% relieved of pain. Of these 73% were described as being completely cured. No patient was functionally worse and only four patients out of their series of 100 were unimproved. They described a recurrence rate of 3.4% in five patients involving eight compartments all of whom were cured by further surgery. These results compare favourably with those of Pedowitz et al (1990) and Martens et al (1990) who reported that 60% and 80% of their patients respectively were able to return to the highest level of activity post-operatively. Functional results appear to correlate well with a normalization of exercise compartment pressure post-operatively (Puranen and Alavaikko, 1981; Allen and Barnes, 1986, Bouche, 1990).

References

Allen MJ.(1990) Compartment syndromes of the lower limb. J R Coll Surg Edinb, **35** (Suppl), S33-S36 .

Allen MJ and Barnes MR. (1986) Exercise pain in the lower leg. Chronic compartment syndrome and medial tibial syndrome. J Bone Joint Surg, **68B**, 818-823 .

Amendola A, Rorabeck CH, Vellett D, Vezina W, Rutt B and Nott L. (1990) The use of magnetic resonance imaging in exertional compartment syndromes. Am J Sports Med, **18**, 29-34

Bouche RT. (1990) Chronic compartment syndrome of the leg. J Am Podiatr Med Assoc, **80**, 633-648.

Detmer DE, Sharpe K, Sufit RL and Girdley FM. (1985) Chronic compartment syndrome: diagnosis, management, and outcomes. Am J Sports Med, 13, 162-170, Physician, **39**, 191-196.

Folkow B, Gaskell P and Waaler BA. (1980) Blood flow through limb muscles during sustained contraction. Acta Physiol Scand, **80**, 61-72.

Grant JCB. (1962) An Atlas of Anatomy. The Williams & Wilkins Co, Baltimore.

Hoffmeyer P, Cox JN and Fritschy D. (1987) Ultrastructural modifications of muscle in three types of compartment syndrome. Int Orthop, **11**, 53-59.

Lutz LJ, Goodenough GK and Detmer DE. (1989) Chronic compartment syndrome. Am Fam Physician, **39**, 191-196.

Martens MA, Backaert M, Vermaut G and Mulier JC. (1984) Chronic leg pain in athletes due to a recurrent compartment syndrome. Am J Sports Med, **12**, 148-252.

Matsen FA (1980) Compartment Syndrome. Grune & Stratton, Inc, New York.

Mavor GE (1956) The anterior tibial syndrome. J Bone Joint Surg, **38B**, 513-517.

McDermott APG, Marble E, Yabsley RH and Pillips B. (1982) Monitoring dynamic anterior compartment pressure during exercise; a new technique using the STIC catheter. Am J Sports Med, **10**, 83-89.

Pedowitz RA, Hargens AR, Mubarak SJ and Gershuni DH. (1990) Modified criteria for the objective diagnosis of chronic compartment syndrome of the leg. Am J Sports Med, **18**, 35-40.

Puranen J and Alavaikko A. (1981) Intracompartmental pressure increase on exertion in patients with chronic compartment syndrome in the leg. J Bone Joint Surg, **63A**, 1304-1309.

Rippe B, Kamiya A and Folkow B. (1978) Simultaneous measurements of capillary diffusion and filtration exchange during shifts in filtration-absorption and at graded alterations in the capillary permeability surface area product (PS). Acta Physiol Scand, **104**, 318-336.

Rorabeck CH, Bourne RB, Fowler PJ, Finlay JB and Nott L. (1988) The role of tissue pressure measurements in diagnosing chronic anterior compartment syndrome. Am J Sports Med, **16**, 143-146.

Stefl DJ and Gudas CJ. (1981) Subacute anterior tibial compartment syndrome. J Foot Surg, **20**, 258-261.

Styf J. (1989) Chronic exercise-induced pain in the anterior aspect of the lower leg. An overview of diagnosis. Sports Med, **7**, 331-339.

Clinical aspects of injury

Styf JR and Korner LM. (1986) Microcapillary infusion technique for measurement of intramuscular pressure recordings during exercise. Clin Orthop, **207**, 253-262.

Styf JR and Korner LM. (1987) Diagnosis of chronic anterior compartment syndrome in the lower leg. Acta Orthop Scand, **58**, 139-144.

Wiley JP, Short WB, Wiseman DA and Miller SD. (1990) Ultrasound catheter placement for deep posterior compartment pressure measurements in chronic compartment syndrome. Am J Sports Med, **18**, 74-79.

"Gilmore's groin": a previously unsolved problem in sportsmen

O.J.A. Gilmore

Abstract. Groin injuries are a common problem in Sports Medicine. They frequently prevent sportsmen from playing, often for many months and in professionals may lead to a permanent loss of employment. In the past many such problems were diagnosed as osteitis pubis or pelvic instability and treated by a prolonged rest or pubic symphysis fusion (Harris and Murray, 1974). Gilmore's Groin constitutes a newly recognised syndrome of groin disruption which is readily treated by the surgical restoration of normal anatomy. During the decade 1980-1989, 313 sportsmen were treated surgically of whom 46 were internationals.

Keywords: Groin Injury, Sportsmen, Conjoined Tendon, Inguinal Ligament, Surgical Repair.

Recognition of Syndrome

The syndrome was recognised following the successful treatment of 3 professional footballers who each presented with similar symptoms, signs and operative findings between 1980 and 1982.

Symptoms

CASE 1:   Full Back. 27 (Tottenham Hotspur FC) presented 28.8.80 with pain in the right groin for 17 weeks following an external rotation injury and had not played since. The pain in the groin was exacerbated by sprinting, kicking, coughing and sneezing.

CASE 2:   Midfield player. 24 (Aberdeen and Scotland) presented 16.3.81 complaining of pain in the right groin for 15 weeks following hyperextension. He was unable to run and had not played football since the injury. The pain was increased by jogging, kicking, sudden movement, coughing and sneezing.

CASE 3:   Central defender. 29 (Tottenham Hotspur FC and Wales) presented 10.6.82 with pain in the left groin for 72 weeks. There had been no specific injury and he had been unable to play football for 12 weeks. Again, pain was increased by running, kicking, coughing and sneezing.

Previous Investigations & Treatment

All 3 players had been extensively investigated (X-rays, ultrasound and CT scans) and each had consulted at least 3 different specialists. All had been subjected to prolonged rest and various forms of treatment, including local steroid injection, without improvement. One player had received acupuncture and another non-steroidal anti-inflammatory drugs.

Physical Signs

There were no external physical signs. Palpation with the little finger via an inverted scrotum, however, revealed a dilated superficial inguinal ring, a cough impulse and marked tenderness on the affected side.

Operative Findinqs

At operation, through an inguinal skin crease incision, all 3 players were found to have:

* torn external oblique aponeurosis
* torn conjoined tendon
* a dehiscence between the torn conjoined tendon and the inguinal ligament.

In no cases was an inguinal hernia present, either direct or indirect.

Treatment

Consisted of restoring normal anatomy and by using a 6 layered surgical repair as described later.

Results

All 3 players were running at 3 weeks. Case 1 played football at 6 weeks, case 2 and 3 at 7 weeks - both returning to their international squads at this time.

Professional Association Football

The cases of the first 65 consecutive professional footballers treated between 1980 and 1987 have been analysed. These players constitute a uniform group with a minimum of 2 year follow-up.

Presentation

All players presented with chronic pain in the inguinal region, right sided in 27, left sided in 30 and bilateral in 8 (12%). Twenty-five also had pain in the adductor origin region and 4 in the perineal region.

The duration of symptoms and the length of time since the patient last played a game of football are shown in Table 1.

TABLE 1

GROIN DISRUPTION:
DURATION OF SYMPTOMS IN 65 PROFESSIONAL FOOTBALLERS
1980 - 1987

PAIN IN INGUINAL REGION

RANGE: 1 week to 8 years
MEAN: 22 weeks

TIME SINCE LAST GAME

RANGE: 1 to 57 weeks
MEAN: 8 weeks

Pain was usually increased by:
*   sudden movement
*   sprinting
*   kicking
*   coughing
*   sneezing
*   getting out of bed (especially the day after a game).

The players' other symptoms varied according to their position on the field (Table 2). All goalkeepers had ceased taking goal kicks because of pain caused by kicking a dead ball. Full backs found long ball kicking particularly troublesome. In central defenders sudden turning was inhibited. Midfield players were usually small, busy players whose game slowed in the second half and especially during the last 20 minutes. Strikers and wingers complained of slowness off the mark and diminished acceleration.

Aetiology
In 47 patients (72%) the onset of symptoms was gradual. In only 18 player

TABLE 2

POSITION ON FIELD

%

Goalkeeper	4	6
Full-back	10	15
Central defender	11	17
Midfield	27	42
Striker	10	15
Winger	3	5
	65	100

(28%) was there a specific injury (Table 3). Eight players, in whom there was no specific injury, blamed hard pitches encountered while playing abroad - mainly in the World Cup in Mexico in 1986 after a long domestic season.

TABLE 3

AETIOLOGY OF GROIN DISRUPTION
IN PROFESSIONAL ASSOCIATION FOOTBALL

No Specific Injury:	47 Players (72%)
Specific Injury:	18 Players (28%)

OVERSTRETCHING	9
KICKING	4
ABDUCTION	3
EVERSION	2

TOTAL   65

Physical Signs

There were no visible or palpable physical signs in any patient. Diagnosis was made by inverting the scrotum, and placing the examining little finger in each superficial inguinal ring in turn. On the affected side the ring was dilated, there was a cough impulse and the patient was tender, sometimes exquisitely, so. Tenderness was absent in 25% of patients and diminished with increasing rest.

Patho-physiology

The essential pathology in Gilmore's Groin is groin disruption due to:

1. torn external oblique aponeurosis causing dilatation of the superficial inguinal ring
2. torn conjoined tendon
3. a dehiscence between the inguinal ligament and the torn conjoined tendon: this constitutes the major injury.

The patients' tenderness diminishes with increasing rest as the inflammation and oedema at the injury site subsides.

Diagnosis

Gilmore's Groin is a clinical diagnosis based on symptoms and physical findings. Pelvic instability must be excluded by stork views of the pelvis. Movement at the symphysis should be less than 3 mm.

Treatment

The principal of surgical treatment in Gilmore's Groin is restoration of normal anatomy. Following the plication of transversalis fascia, the torn conjoined tendon is repaired with vicryl. The repaired conjoined tendon is then approximated to inguinal ligament using a nylon darn. This constitutes the vital element of the repair. If the darn is too tight the player is unable to sprint and if too loose the repair is ineffective. The torn external oblique is then repaired reconstituting the superficial inguinal ring before the wound is closed carefully in layers.

Patients are admitted the morning of surgery and remain in hospital from 1 to 3 days depending on domicile, domestic conditions and insurance cover. A standard rehabilitation programme is given to all players (Table 4).

Results

Surgery was successful in 63 of 65 players (97%). The criteria for success being a return to training within 3 weeks and first team professional football within 10 weeks. The average time between surgery and return to playing was 6 weeks. All patients were playing professional football at more than 2 years after surgery. One player returned for further surgery to the same side 5 years later.

Three players subsequently required contralateral repair having recognised the symptoms of groin disruption themselves. Of the 2 failures, 1 required symphysis fusion for pelvic instability and the other adductor muscle surgery to free

TABLE 4

REHABILITATION PROGRAMME

WEEK 1: Essential to stand upright and walk 20 minutes first day after operation.
Thereafter walk gently 4 times a day

WEEK 2: Walk for 30 minutes 2 times a day for 4 days
Jogging and gentle running for rest of the week

WEEK 3: Running in straight lines
Gentle sit-ups

Adductor Exercises

WEEK 4: Sprinting in straight lines
Increase sit-ups
Swimming (crawl)

WEEK 5: Kick
Play

adhesions from a previous adductor muscle tear. The 25 players with combined groin disruption and adductor weakness proved the most refractory. Experience has shown that full recovery can only be obtained by surgical repair of the groin disruption followed by intensive post-operative adductor exercises.

There were no complications, no haematomas and no wound infections. All patients were given 500 mgs of Flucloxacillin i/v at the time of induction of anaesthesia.

Other sportsmen and women

Surgery was undertaken in 248 other sportsmen between 1987 and 1989 (Table 5).

Rugby Union
Gilmore's Groin is less common in Rugby Union than in professional Association

TABLE 5

GILMORE'S GROIN:
ALL SPORTSMEN OPERATIONS 1987-1989

ASSOCIATION FOOTBALL	Professional	139
	Semi-professional	19
	Amateur	37
RUGBY UNION		12
RUGBY LEAGUE		12
ATHLETES		7
RACQUET GAMES		6
CRICKET		3
HOCKEY		3
MARTIAL ARTS/GYM		3
OTHER		7
TOTAL		**248**

Football because the game is less demanding on the groin, both in terms of training and the number of games played. The majority of patients requiring surgery were back row forwards and scrum halves; players whose work rate and involvement in the game is usually greater than that of players in other positions.

The aetiology and symptoms of groin disruption are similar to those found in soccer players. In addition all complained of pain on striding out and sprinting away from the base of the scrum and on side-stepping.

Rugby League
Players from all positions except wing have been successfully treated, indicating the difference between Rugby League and Rugby Union in terms of mobility and involvement in the game. In Rugby League, half of the patients gave a history of a specific injury compared to only one-third in soccer and Rugby Union.

Combined groin disruption and adductor lesions were more common in Rugby League players and were often bilateral, especially in those Internationals playing back-to-back seasons between Great Britain and Australia. Continuous professional sport appears to significantly increase the rate of wear and tear in such players.

Athletes

All athletes presenting were middle, long distance or marathon runners in their late twenties or older, again suggesting an overuse injury. The operative findings were similar to those found in footballers and rugby players. The symptoms in one amateur marathon runner (aged 40) started after undertaking vigorous sit-ups. As a result he was unable even to jog for 8 weeks. Following surgery, he was running 20 miles a week at 3 weeks, did a half-marathon at 10 weeks (in 1 hour 19 minutes) and a full marathon at 17 weeks in (2 hours 30 minutes!)

Racquet Games

In squash and racquets, twisting and turning were especially painful and thus the players' game was slowed and inhibited. In addition, in tennis, the patients complained of pain in the groin on their serving side.

Cricket

The majority of cricketers were fast bowlers who complained of pain in the inguinal region of the leg that they landed on when bowling, not the drag leg. As a game progressed, the duration of each bowling spell had to be reduced because of increasing pain. The other cricketers requiring surgery were busy batsmen/fielders, whose agility in the field suffered due to their groin disruption.

Hockey

The majority of patients requiring surgery were midfield players, playing hockey 2 or 3 times a week on artificial surfaces. History of a specific injury was rare. As each game progressed, the player slowed; twisting, turning and striding out were especially painful and acceleration was diminished.

Sportswomen

Five women have also been treated successfully. One athlete, one ballet dancer, one professional modern dancer, a tennis player and a karate international. The diagnosis in women is made difficult by the absence of a scrotum and is based on the history and the presence of tenderness at the superficial inguinal ring externally. Surgical repair in women is similar to that in men, except that the round ligament is excised and the inguinal canal closed completely.

International sportsmen

During the first decade, 31 international soccer players were successfully treated and 15 other international sportsmen (Table 6). It is of interest that of the 14 English soccer internationals requiring surgery, 9 had played for England at under-21 level, again suggesting wear and tear as the main aetiological factor.

TABLE 6

OPERATIONS ON
INTERNATIONAL SPORTSMEN 1980-1989

ASSOCIATION FOOTBALL	31
RUGBY LEAGUE	6
RUGBY UNION	2
HOCKEY	2
CRICKET	2
HANDBALL	2
RACQUETS	1
TOTAL	46

Confirmation that a return to sport at the highest level after Gilmore's Groin repair is possible, is indicated by the fact that the England World Cup squad in Italy in 1990 included 3 postoperative patients, while the Great Britain Rugby Squad which beat the Australians in the First Test at Wembley in 1990 contained 4 post-operative patients.

The ratio of presentation to operation was studied in 1989. Surgery was necessary, most frequently, as one would expect, in professional sportsmen whose livelihood is jeopardized by their absence from their game. 91% of Rugby League, 79% of Football League and 75% of professional cricketers presenting required surgery; compared with 65% in non-league football and Rugby Union, and 50% in athletes and racquet game players. Overall 68% of patients presenting with groin pain required exploration and repair for disruption.

Discussion

Gilmore's Groin is not a hernia. A hernia is a protrusion of viscus beyond its normal confines. In Gilmore's Groin there is disruption of the groin musculature but no visceral protrusion. If it were a hernia, the diagnosis would be simple and the treatment established years ago.

The incidence of diagnosis of Gilmore's Groin is increasing as more sports clubs, their doctors and physiotherapists become aware of the syndrome and its surgical treatment. Prior to this, many sportsmen were subject to long periods of rest. Some were given local steroid injections, others systemic anti-inflammatory drugs, both of which may mask the patients symptoms.

Rest and careful rehabilitation is effective in some sportsmen, especially younger players with lesser acute injuries. Many, however, do not make a complete recovery even with prolonged rest. In severe chronic cases healing will not occur because the main injury is the inguinal ligament-conjoined tendon dehiscence. No amount of rest will result in the approximation of these 2 structures, thus healing is unable to occur, just as a fracture will not heal unless the 2 bone ends are approximated and stabilised.

The recognition and surgical treatment of Gilmore's Groin, a previously unrecognised syndrome has resulted in the rapid restoration of many a sportsman's career, as demonstrated by the 97% cure rate achieved in Professional Association footballers.

Reference

Harris NH & Murray RO. (1974) Lesions of the Symphysis in Athletes. Br Med J, **4**, 211-214.

The knee

North American experience of knee injuries in the professional athlete

T.E. Anderson

Abstract. The experience of managing acute knee injuries in professional and high level amateur athletes is presented. An emphasis is placed upon surgical reconstruction of ligaments injuries with autograft augmentation of anterior cruciate ligament tears, particularly when combined with collateral ligament injuries. Carefully monitored physiotherapy after surgery is an integral part of the treatment programme.

Keywords: Knee Injuries, Anterior Cruciate Ligament, Collateral Knee Ligaments, Primary Surgical Repair, Rehabilitation.

Knee injuries in the professional athlete do not differ greatly from those seen in recreational sports. As the saying goes "common things occur commonly". There are indeed the usual variety of anterior cruciate, posterior cruciate, medial collateral and occasional lateral collateral ligament injuries. Additionally, there are also meniscal tears. There do however, seem to be a higher number of chondral injuries and the actual extent of the so-called bone-bruise as noted on MRI scans, has yet to be determined. Certain professional sports in North America do have their distinct problems. In professional basketball, the nemesis is the anterior cruciate ligament tear with subsequent anterior lateral rotatory instability. Basketball being a jumping activity, this can be a devastating injury. In my opinion, the best treatment is an autograft using patellar tendon with bone-tendon-bone through drill holes in the bone, there is concern for increased risk of patellar tendinitis at the donor site. With gradual increase in training, and avoiding too abrupt a return to full play, the problems with the patellar tendon donor site can be minimized. The reconstruction itself is much less of a problem. The knee following the anterior cruciate ligament reconstruction, will continue to improve for up to a year and a half. During this time however, the player has a somewhat symptomatic knee, the extent of which varies from player to player. This takes some getting used to the new knee, and the player frequently has a difficult time the first year back. This coupled with professional sport being extremely competitive, may cut short that individual player's return to play at a similar level.

In professional American football, the anterior cruciate ligament is also a problem. There is a considerably higher percentage of meniscal pathology associated with the ligament tear, as the majority of these tears occur in the full weight position and it is not infrequent that both menisci are torn along with the anterior cruciate ligament. Similar problems with patellar tendinitis also exist with football as with basketball.

Professional North American football also involves considerable weight lifting. These individuals are lifting excessive amounts of weight in order to condition, gain strength and weight for competition. Occasionally, strength coaches will consider a deep squat to be beneficial in building up the thigh and buttock musculature. These deep squats however, put the menisci, as well as the chondral surfaces at risk. Indeed, even in the off-season, we have seen a number of injuries from deep squats with meniscal pathology and indeed an occasional articular surface shear injury, all of these necessitating arthroscopy for treatment.

Another professional sport in North America is downhill skiing. The anterior cruciate ligament is particularly at risk for this group, as they are often skiing barely in control and, not infrequently, out of control. With downhill skiing a sudden torque on the ski tip will tear the anterior cruciate ligament without being full with weight bearing. This group tends to have a fairly low incidence of meniscal pathology associated with their anterior cruciate ligament tear. The majority of these skiers, however, function quite well with downhill skiing as they are often in the flexed knee position that is moderately stable. If, however, they continue to have problems with instability of their knee, these can be reconstructed later. The reconstruction is at a high risk if the individual continues racing, and it is not infrequent for a person to have had bilateral anterior cruciate ligament tears with anterior cruciate ligament reconstruction, both of which have failed due to new injuries.

Knee injuries in professional baseball are relatively uncommon, however, due to twisting and pivoting on the knee, meniscal pathology is generally the rule. There is an occasional anterior cruciate ligament tear as well, but almost as frequently as the posterior cruciate ligament tear this is "isolated". The posterior cruciate ligament tears are often experienced in going down for the ball quite rapidly and impacting the tibial tubercle onto the surface of the playing field. Most of these are regarded as relatively minor injuries at the time. Frequently we have treated these with physical therapy. Maintenance of a good quadriceps strengthening program is important for the longevity of this individual's career. They respond quite well to this usually with only minimal symptoms through the remainder of their career, and these often being treated with ice following workouts or competition. I feel that injuries to the posterior cruciate ligament when coupled with additional injuries to the other ligaments, is an indication for reconstruction. In my experience, if both cruciate and lateral collateral are torn, there is also frequently a stretch injury to the peroneal nerve. These combined injuries are usually seen primarily in football.

Reconstruction of the cruciate ligaments as well as repair of the collateral ligaments and posterior lateral corner of the knee, done acutely, is often satisfactory. They, however, need to be protected from going into varus in the eight weeks following this repair, in order to keep the posterior lateral corner from stretching out. Peroneal nerve injuries, when they occur, will often take four to five months before they resolve. During that time the patient is in a dorsiflexion assist brace. It is not uncommon for the individual to go a full three months with no evidence of any reinnervation of the muscle, to come back one month later with only a flicker, and another month later with full muscle bulk and power.

With the advent of the MRI in evaluating meniscal and ligamentous pathology of the knee pre-operatively, there is a group of injuries referred to as bone bruise that has now been identified. The natural history of this bone bruise, whether this is an incidental MRI finding, or a significant long-term prognostic factor, remains to be determined. It appears that, when associated with the anterior cruciate ligament tear, the bruising is on the posterior aspect of the tibia and the anterior aspect of the femur in the lateral compartment. There may or may not be gross articular surface changes associated with this at the time of arthroscopy. Again, the significance needs to be determined. The majority of these ligamentous injuries in professional athletes can be treated quite aggressively. Additionally, the physical therapy can be performed quite aggressively as the patients themselves are extremely well monitored with a number of trainers and coaches involved as well. This aggressive treatment has led to a number of advances.

Reconstruction of the anterior cruciate ligament

M.F. Macnicol

Abstract. Anterior cruciate ligament ruptures occur relatively frequently but are often missed by the inexperienced clinician. A significant proportion of knees fail to compensate after this injury, and bracing rarely offers adequate support in the knee with a positive pivot shift. Therefore surgical treatment remains the only solution in many elite athletes, although the timing of surgery and the details of operative technique remain controversial.

Keywords: Anterior Cruciate Ligament, Ligament Rupture, Acute Repair, Chronic Repair, Ligament Grafts, Prosthetic Ligaments.

Introduction

Injuries as a result of sporting activities account for between 5 and 10% of all referrals to Accident and Emergency Departments in the UK. Approximately one-quarter of the sports injuries involve the knee joint and these principally soft tissue problems account for 10% of all time lost from work. In the context of the professional athlete, and the rugby player in particular, a rupture of the anterior cruciate ligament of the knee may spell the end of a promising career and is known to lead on remorselessly to osteoarthritis if the joint fails to compensate for the lost constraint.

The anterior cruciate ligament functions as one of the more obvious components of the knee, controlling forward subluxation of the tibia during quadriceps contraction and weight bearing. This demanding role should not, however, overshadow its responsibilities towards proprioception and the helical movement of the tibia under the femur during flexion and extension, both of which are central factors in the rapid and precise movements which characterize the healthy knee.

Although the mechanism of injury is not always clear from the description afforded by the patient, three classic stresses during sport are recognized: (1) hyperextension; (2) hyperflexion with the tibia internally rotated; (3) forced valgus, often associated with rotation when the foot is firmly planted. Complex rotational stresses particularly when there is no protective muscle guarding, impart great strain through the ligament. Rupture of the anteromedial fascicle of the anterior cruciate ligament generally occurs first, but the rest of the ligament is involved to a greater or lesser degree.

It is now accepted that ruptures of the anterior cruciate ligament are both common and disabling. A full realisation throughout the medical profession that the ligament is regularly torn in sporting accidents has only been appreciated in the last two decades. It is still evident from the later referral of these symptomatic cases that the significance and regularity of anterior cruciate ligament rupture is poorly understood by the personnel who attend to younger subjects with problem knees.

The ligament is also centrally concerned with knee proprioception and its provision of an efficient feedback loop is as important as its function as a constraint. Gold chloride stains of the ligament demonstrate the neural elements which are as follows (Schutte et al, 1987) (1) true nerve endings responsible for pain perception; (2) slow-adapting Ruffini nerve endings sensitive to speed and acceleration (3) a rapidly-adapting Pacinian corpuscle which detects motion. The reflex arc triggered by these nerves is an essential mechanism in recruiting muscle contraction which in turn protects the knee. This compensates in large measure for the skeletally vulnerable design of the joint which cannot depend solely upon its passive restraints and its relatively planar surfaces as a means of preserving normal articulation.

Reasons for knee decompensation

After complete rupture of the ligament the knee usually becomes symptomatic, yet in the longer term some knees eventually compensate and others do not. Factors that influence the recovery include (1) the extent of other soft tissue injuries such as a medial collateral ligament rupture, meniscal tears, patellar instability, chronically weakened muscles and unrelenting synovitis; (2) intrinsic ligament laxity in each individual affecting collateral ligament tension, the posterior capsule and posterior cruciate ligament, the alignment of the leg and other collagen-related characteristics; and (3) the bony morphology of the knee joint, particularly the shape of the lateral tibial condyle which will tend to sublux forwards in a more obvious way proportional to its convexity (Macnicol, 1986).

Undoubtedly the chosen sport of the individual is important since skiers, cricketers and other non-contact sportsmen are more likely to return to their chosen activity than soccer, rugby or basketball players. Nevertheless, certain top-class players do return to competitive league football despite the presence of a proven rupture of the anterior cruciate ligament and it is instructive to note how many professional soccer players present with asymptomatic knee laxity particularly of the dominant kicking leg.

Treatment

The initial management of symptomatic chronic antero-lateral laxity relies upon physiotherapy and re-education of the patient. Emphasis is placed upon hamstring tone and the general development of thigh muscle strength, which can do so much to minimize the effects of anterior cruciate ligament rupture. While derotation braces provide some degree of support, particularly in skiers and in certain racquet sports, these appliances are unsafe for use in contact sport and often limit the use of the leg unacceptably. Surgical intervention is therefore considered to be the only option for many athletes, despite our uncertainty about the techniques and results of the endeavour. In a paper such as this details about surgical management cannot be covered fully, but the principles are of interest and will be dealt with briefly.

Acute repair

Direct suture of the acutely torn ligament is fruitless (Odensten et al, 1985), but re-attachment of avulsed femoral or tibial bone is worthwhile. In many cases there is slackening also of the ligament which partially ruptures prior to the bony attachment yielding. Nevertheless, re-attachment with sutures, wires or a small screw is usually effective. The results of early repair of mid-substance tears with the complemetary use of a stent is valid experimentally and possibly clinically (Sandberg et al, 1987). However the concern is that the material used, if derived from the patient in autogenous graft form, may produce its own separate trauma when being harvested, and therefore the debits may outweigh the gains. The use of some form of augmentation device is therefore exciting interest, both in acute and chronic repairs. Long-term results are unavailable as yet, and further comment about this approach is unwarranted.

Chronic Repair

Patients whose knees fail to compensate after the ligament disruption are referred for surgical review, usually 1-5 years after the injury, with poorer results occurring after undue delay (Zarins & Rowe, 1986). Surgeons have exercised their ingenuity in deciding which ligament or tendon to use as a means of secondary repair and these autogenous materials are rarely as strong as the anterior cruciate ligament when tested in the laboratory (Fig. 1). The limiting factors in vivo are not so much to do with the basic connective tissue strength of the structure, but the integrity of the anchor points of the graft and the weakening effects of revascularization which become pronounced at the sixth week and persist for up to 1 year (Clancy et al, 1981) (Fig. 2). A chronic reactive synovitis will also imperil the axial strength of the graft.

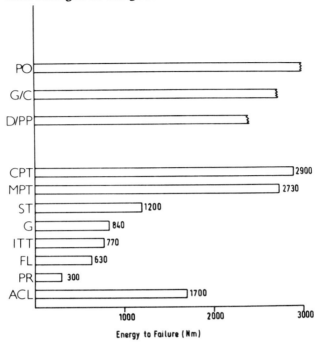

Energy to Failure (Nm)

Fig. 1 Relative "bench" strengths of various autogenous grafts and artificial fibres. The width of the material used and the strength of fixation will obviously influence these data. ACL, anterior cruciate ligament; PR, patellar retinaculum; FL, fascia lata; ITT, iliotibial tract; G, gracilis; ST, semitendinosus; MPT, medial strip of patellar tendon; CPT, central strip of patellar tendon; D/PP, Dacron^R/polypropylene; G/C, GORE-TEX^R/carbon fibre; PO, polyolefin. D/PP, G/C and PO all exceed natural fibres in strength and are ranked in approximate order.

Artificial materials such as Dacron (du Pont), polypropylene and Gore-Tex (W.L. Gore and Associates, USA) are in common use, but these tend to rupture since they do not have the elasticity or long-term resilience of a living anterior cruciate ligament. Attempts at producing a more compliant material have yet to produce a prosthesis which mimics the natural elasticity of the human anterior cruciate ligament.

Combinations of an artificial material and a natural substance, such as part of the patellar tendon or the semitendinosus tendon are widely favoured and the

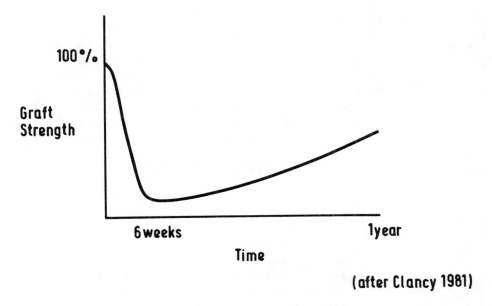

Fig. 2 In vivo an autogenous graft weakens rapidly owing to the effects of revascularization and local inflammation.

Kennedy LAD (ligament augmentation device) (3M Health Care, Loughborough, UK) has now been in use for over 10 years. McPherson et al (1985) reviewed the histological reaction associated with the implant of this polypropylene splint in the goat. An inflammatory foreign-body reaction develops locally within the knee, and the presence of eosinophils and lymphocytes suggests a low-grade immunological response. This may be secondary to the material itself, or produced by friction between the braided fibres and the normal tissues of the knee.

Placement and fixation

There has been a proliferation of operative techniques, with greater emphasis now upon an atraumatic approach, possibly limited to arthroscopic portals and one or two stab wounds. Fixation of the ligament needs to be strong and as near to the isometric position of the ligament as possible. The "over the top" method which places the prosthesis over the upper posterior aspect of the lateral femoral condyle requires that the ligament should stretch up to 10 mm during the last 10 or 20° of knee extension. While this attachment site offers a technically easy solution this is a serious drawback and may result in early rupture or elongation of the ligament. Equally, the use of bony tunnels through the tibia and femur may cause fraying of the ligament, particularly if the tunnels are angled in relation to the chosen route of the intra-articular prosthesis, which subtends an angle of approximately 30° to the femur when the knee is flexed to a right angle.

Lastly, abrasion between the ligament and the femoral notch, which is often narrowed in the chronically lax knee, will also result in a chronic synovitis and a likely early rupture. Therefore, an adequate "notchplasty" may be necessary if the ligament is to move freely within the knee, and a tensioning device is recommended by some surgeons, attempting to ensure that the inserted ligament is sufficiently tight. Whether this improves matters in the longer term is open to doubt in view of the biological factors mentioned previously.

Post-operative recovery

Ideally, there should be a restriction of knee movement after surgery. Some degree of support is advisable when the knee wounds are healing, and the postoperative haemarthrosis inevitably triggers a short-lived synovitis. However, if the anchorage of the substitute ligament is secure, flexion and extension of the joint can be permitted within certain limits. The insertion of interference fit screws into the bone plug-tunnel site, or fixation of an augmentation device with staples or screws, allows this rapid return of movement with reasonable safety. But the ligament does require protection for up to 6 months at the time when it is most vulnerable to stretch. Some form of femoral cast brace or commercial derotation brace with stops is therefore recommended after the second week and weight-bearing must be guarded. Anti-inflammatory medication is advisable, and the patient should be closely supervised by a physiotherapist with a special interest in this form of treatment so that hamstring and quadriceps power is progressively developed. If a synovitis persists or effusions become recurrent, the speed of rehabilitation must be reduced.

Generally speaking, there is a 10-15° flexion deformity at the third month which should reduce to approximately 5-10° 6 months postoperatively. A minor flexion deformity in the longer term is often therapeutic, since a recurrence of hyperextension indicates that the new ligament restraint is incompetent. Most knees regain full movement by 18 months.

Results of artifical ligament replacement

A series of Leeds-Keio open-weave polyester ligament (Howmedica, UK) replacements were recently reviewed clinically, arthroscopically and histologically after two to four years (Macnicol, Penny and Sheppard, 1991). The prosthesis is biologically inert when intact and its strength is considerably greater than the natural ligament. Fujikawa et al (1989) have claimed that the structure of the artifical ligament allows a significant ingrowth of longitudinally aligned collagen, resulting in the progressive development of a "neoligament" during the first 24 months post-operatively. Rupture of the polyester would then allow the natural fibres to operate as a competent ligament.

Macnicol et al (1991) found that the collagen response was unpredictable, although collagen bundles did appear to be arranged longitudinally (Fig. 3). The artifical fibres of dacron broke up into small fragments, demonstrated by their birefringence under polarised light. Multinucleate giant cells formed in response to the particulate material, and a synovitis was evident at sites along the implanted fibres, similar to that reported by McPherson et al (1985) when they evaluated the Kennedy ligament augmentation device (LAD). The concern about the inflammatory response evoked by these breakdown products is that capsular fibrosis and articular cartilage degeneration may be promoted. Thus the same pathological changes that occur secondary to chronic knee instability may accompany the use of artificial ligaments, even if the initial clinical results are satisfactory in terms of knee stability.

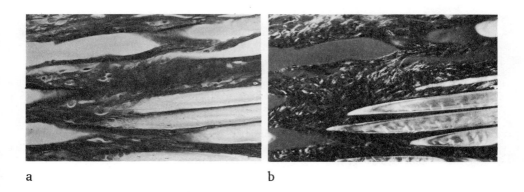

a   b

Fig. 3 Living and apparently thriving collagen-secreting fibroblasts lie alongside the implanted fibres (Haematoxylin and eosin; conventional illumination (a), polarised light (b) x 320).

The comparable long-term results of bone-patellar tendon-bone and other autogenous replacements of the anterior cruciate ligament are awaited with interest. Valid assessment must ensure a postoperative review period of two years minimum, and preferably the findings at 5-10 years. The arthroscopic and histological appearances should be described, in addition to the clinical findings using standard systems of grading (Lysholm and Gillquist, 1982; Tegner and Lysholm, 1985). Prospective comparative trials will also provide better information, and currently a semitendinosus graft, augmented with either an absorbable stent of PDS (polydioxanone, Ethicon) cord or the Kennedy LAD (3M Health Care), is under review in Edinburgh.

References

Clancy WG, Narechania RG, Rosenberge TD, Gmeiner JG, Wisneske DD and Lange TA. (1981) Anterior and posterior cruciate ligament reconstruction in rhesus monkeys. J Bone Joint Surg, 63A, 1270-84.

Fujikawa K, Iseki F and Seedhom BB. (1989) Arthroscopy after anterior cruciate reconstruction with the Leeds-Keio ligament. J Bone Joint Surg, 71-B, 566-70.

Lysholm J and Gillquist J. (1982) Evaluation of knee ligament surgery results with special emphasis on use of a scoring scale. Am J Sports Med, 10, 150-4.

Macnicol MF. (1986) The Problem Knee. London, William Heinemann Medical Books.

Macnicol MF, Penny ID, Sheppard L. (1991) Early results of the Leeds-Keio anterior cruciate ligament replacement. J Bone Joint Surg, 73B, 377-380.

McPherson GK, Mendenhall HV and Gibbons DF et al. (1985) Experimental, mechanical and histologic evaluation of the Kennedy ligament augmentation device. Clin Orthop, 196, 186-95.

Odensten M, Hamberg P, Nordin M, Lysholm J and Gillquist J. (1985) Surgical or conservative treatment of the acutely torn anterior cruciate ligament. A randomised study with short term follow-up observations. Clin Orthop, 198, 87-93.

Sandberg R, Balkfors B, Nilsson B and Westlin N. (1987) Operative versus non-operative treatment of recent injuries to the ligaments of the knee. J Bone Joint Surg, 69A, 1120-6.

Schutte MJ, Dabezies EJ, Zimmy ML and Happel LT. (1987) Neural anatomy of the human anterior cruciate ligament. J Bone Joint Surg, 69A, 243-7.

Tegner Y and Lysholm J. (1985) Rating systems in the evaluation of knee injuries. Clin Orthop, 198, 43-9.

Zarins B and Rowe CR. (1985) Combined anterior cruciate ligament reconstruction using semitendinosus tendon and ilio-tibial tract. J Bone Joint Surg, 68A, 160-77.

Rehabilitation of the knee following anterior cruciate ligament injury and reconstruction - considerations for rugby football

J.P. Long

Abstract. Rugby football is a contact-collision sport with consequent risk to its participants. One of the most severe disabling injuries to the knee is that of the anterior cruciate ligament. Reconstructive procedures are followed by comprehensive rehabilitation. Guidelines for rehabilitation are based on stages of biological healing and protocols are individualized for each athlete. Emphasis is placed on task-specific or functional training as the athlete progresses through the program. Assessment is undertaken at regular intervals to provide the athlete with physical and psychological reinforcement.

Keywords: Knee, Anterior Cruciate Ligament, Reconstruction, Rugby Football, Rehabilitation, Functional Assessment.

Introduction

The literature regarding injuries and treatment in rugby football remains less than prolific. In the United States, modifications of rugby led to the evolution of American football with the first rugby style game being played in the United States between Harvard and McGill University in Boston in 1874. A number of differences continue to exist between the two games: rugby football prohibits the use of sophisticated protective equipment characteristic of American football. Tackling is a feature of rugby football but blocking as in American football is prohibited. The allowance of the "cross-body" block prior to reform of playing rules was consistent with the higher incidence of knee injuries in American football, and although rugby football has been given the distinction of being a more dangerous sport, the use of protective equipment for the head, shoulders, and forearms allows the tackler or blocker to deliver impact at a greater velocity and higher level of kinetic energy with resultant damage in American football.

Micheli and Riseborough (1974) cite a 9.8 percent rate of injury for seven Boston area rugby clubs which appears to be lower than comparable surveys of American football. The
authors point out, however, that such comparisons are difficult based on accuracy of data available and interpretation thereof.

Silver and Gill (1988) pose several important thoughts related to injuries in rugby football, specifically of the spine. They contend that a majority of the injuries they observed were not attributed to bad luck but rather to irresponsible actions. It was suggested that existing regulations were adequate, but being broken or not enforced by officials. The recommendations through Rugby Union meetings of physicians, physiotherapists, players, coaches, and administrators have encouraged changes in the laws to keep players on their feet in both set scrums and in rucks and mauls with shoulders to remain waist high in scrummage. Discontinuance of the ruck and maul in rugby league was not an obvious factor in reducing these injuries at the time of the study. Injuries cited in their work occurred in relationship to second rows continuing to push following collapse of the scrum; players being pushed to the ground while stooping to pick up a loose ball with players then piling on top, and players being inexperienced and not having played in their position or being overmatched. Situations associated with the incidence of injury that seem to reflect the traditional disarray associated with rugby football included unfit or retired players coming off the sideline with little intent to play but deciding "to have one more go at it" or the player who had been assigned to referee a match but later persuaded to play. Have you not as a player or spectator given an accepting nod to such gallant displays ... and observed associated injuries as well? The authors point out the importance of continued investigation to determine mechanisms of injury and refer to the use of video analysis in American football as a model to correlate mechanism with clinical findings in rugby football. The authors cite a Rugby Football Union study using video which attributed 19 percent of all injuries to foul play with the referee being unsighted during these incidences.

Roy (1974) through previous work analyzed 300 injuries at the University of Stellenbosch and stated that many injuries were found to be unnecessary and related to foul play. Mechanism of injury categories, e.g. tackled without the ball, loose scrum, and foul play accounted for 35 percent of ankle injuries and 29 percent of knee injuries. His study concluded that knee injuries were the most common disabling injury and 35 percent were operated upon, most for definitive third degree ligament tears.

The author related knee injuries to force being applied to the knee with the foot firmly fixated by boot studs being locked in the thick and tough grass at Coetzenburg during March, April, and May. It was determined that the knee injury rate dropped as the grass became softened by rain. Based on these findings, recommendations were made to modify the conventional boot. These included a synthetic molded sole with a minimum of 14 studs per boot, a minimum stud diameter of one-half inch and a maximum stud length of three-eight inch.

Similar considerations were made in the United States with development of synthetic playing surfaces and their relationship to injuries of the knee and ankle. The author also noted that boot revisions would not protect the knee against injury in a loose scrum where a player falls on the outstretched leg of another. Seventeen percent of the knee injuries observed occurred as a result of late or early tackles. Recommendations at the time of the study included dismissal of players for repeated offences such as two late tackles in one match and revisions in tackling methods to avoid trauma just above or below the knee joint, e.g. tackling the opponent at the waist level with one arm above the ball.

Injuries are often thought to be associated with match play, but 31 percent of the injuries occurred during practice sessions. Roy suggested increasing emphasis on skills, coordination, how to tackle and how to fall. It was also stressed that a well trained physician with experience in rugby football could pick up on minor strains and sprains, treat them at the time of occurrence aggressively, and prevent them from becoming major chronic conditions. In short, the physician and physiotherapist could serve as advisors to mold the attitudes of coaches, referees, and players as well as establishing health standards and providing pre-season and in-season screenings for players.

Certainly, it has become commonplace in the United States for athletic trainers and team physicians to provide day to day coverage for other scholastic and collegiate sports. Rugby football players continue to have less structured care.

A related paper (Roy, 1975) described a survey of 115 acutely injured knees and pointed out the importance of an accurate history from the player especially when related to mechanism of tackling. The classic rugby injury described was that of being hit from the lateral side while pushing off with the foot fixed in external rotation with valgus force leading to rupture of the MCL, posterior oblique ligaments, then medial meniscus and the anterior cruciate ligament (O'Donoghue's triad). It was noted that 15 percent of the knee injuries in this series were related to subluxation or dislocation of the patella and sometimes mistaken for injury to the medial meniscus. Failure to diagnose this properly could lead to a chronically unstable patella.

The physician of first contact was described as the "king pin" for establishing a definitive diagnosis. Unfortunately, as noted, presence of a competent physician, physiotherapist, or athletic trainer at rugby football matches and practices appears to be the exception rather than the rule although tournament play is usually staffed with identified individuals to assess and treat casualties.

Kaufman (1985) surveyed injuries during tournament play in Lancaster, PA, U.S.A. and determined climatic conditions to be the most important cause for requesting one minute or leaving the match. Heat related casualties accounted for 29 percent of serious injuries. Suggested guidelines for play were based on the temperature-humidity index with changes in water policy. Based on the relatively low incidence of musculoskeletal injury, the author concluded that the reputation of rugby being a brutal sport was not justified.

A survey of 1000 rugby football injuries by Adams (1977) described an 11.3 percent incidence of complete ligamentous tears of the knee compared to Roy (1974) with a reported 43 ligamentous injuries of the survey's 300 injuries. Variance was attributed to difference in injury, orthopaedic practice, playing surface, or footwear. Other players who had appreciable ligamentous laxity upon exam were viewed as candidates for comprehensive rehabilitation prior to return to play, but it proved difficult to restrain these players long enough to achieve this end.

The issue of compliance of rugby players to follow-up after initial evaluation and suggested rehabilitation was alluded to by Dineen and Gallagher (1981). In their survey of rugby injuries, it was determined that 68 percent of the players with injuries classified as mild did not return for re-evaluation and clearance to return to play. Several players who had wrists immobilized by casting for suspected fractures did not return as well. Certainly, the misperceptions held by outside observers of rugby football may be reinforced by behavioral traits of some of its participants.

Ligamentous injuries to the knee

The most frequent severe ligament injury and most disabling is that to the anterior cruciate ligament (ACL). Although assumed to be related to contact/collision events in rugby, isolated ACL tears can often occur with deceleration-valgus-external rotation or hyperextension-internal rotation forces. The injury is usually associated with severe swelling within the first 1-2 hours. On the field management including assessment, ice, and immobilization with mild compression can be critical in stabilizing the condition. Players may describe feeling or hearing a "pop" in 30-50 percent of ACL injuries.

Physical examination of the player on the field should include the Lachman test which is performed with the knee in approximately 20 degrees of flexion. Anterior translation of the tibia upon the femur particularly with a soft endpoint is highly suggestive of ACL insufficiency. It has been recognized that the acutely torn anterior cruciate ligament not surgically repaired will not heal and when surgically repaired without reconstruction, may stil] heal. For the aggressive player involved in contact collision sports such as rugby, resultant instability is unacceptable.

Anterior cruciate reconstruction and rehabilitation

There continues to be discussion related to functional and biological return associated with reconstruction of the anterior cruciate ligament. The majority of this author's experience has been with rehabilitation following patellar tendon autografts with bone to bone fixation and interference fit by Kurosaka screw. Accelerated protocols as noted by Shelbourne (1990) have emerged in an effort to minimize the effects of immobility and disuse such as joint contracture, alteration in cartilaginous surfaces and subchondral bone, decreased strength of normal ligament bone units and dramatic changes in periarticular musculature. Quadriceps performance loss related to reflex inhibition following ACL reconstruction is highly advanced as compared to hamstring loss. Deliberate de-emphasis of isolated quadriceps exercise to minimize anterior tibial translation may confound the problem (Morrissey, 1989).

Recovery has been accelerated by advancement of surgical instrumentation and technique and rehabilitative methods including use of cast and functional braces, neuromuscular stimulators, dynamometers, and aggressive return to activity programs. Of concern with these advances is opportunity for functional return to precede biological healing. As a result, mechanical failure related to excessive overload, cyclic forces, or overelongation may occur (Jackson & Drez, 1987).

Rehabilitation and physiology of ligament healing

The basis for pursuing treatment of severe injuries of the ACL through reconstruction is reflected in the outcome of the ligament if it is left to heal on its own. The first week is characterized by hematoma formation and infiltration of inflammatory cells followed by fibroblastic proliferation during the second week. The third to sixth week is characterized by collagenization and decreasing populations of fibroblasts. Organization may take six to twelve weeks (Ewen, 1950). The outcome of ligament healing is directly contingent upon the apposition of torn ligament ends, local blood supply, effects of surgery, and local environmental factors. For instance, it has been determined in tissue culture studies that the growth rate of fibroblasts from the anterior cruciate ligament was slower than that of the superficial medial collateral ligament. Also, when the ACL is torn, the ligament ends are exposed to synovial fluid with resultant diminished growth of those cells exposed.

Cell populations treated with synovial fluid resulted in aggregation clumping, and cell death (Andrish, 1980). Surgical primary repair of the anterior cruciate ligament has yielded to reconstructive procedures which have been deemed more effective and physiologically compatible (Jackson & Drez, 1987).

Variables influencing the rehabilitation prescription

There are a number of variables associated with reconstruction of the anterior cruciate ligament that influence development of prescription and protocol. Consideration of these variables illustrates the necessity of approaching each case individually (Drez & Jackson, 1987).

The first consideration relates to the substitution for the anterior cruciate ligament. Was the procedure performed intra-articular, extra-articular or a combination thereof? What are the mechanical properties of the substitute graft e.g. patellar tendon, iliotibial band, semitendinosus, or fascia lata? Was the substitute tissue allograft or autograft?

Secondly, what was the manner of fixation? Various methods have been utilized with varying results including sutures and buttons, staples, and bone-to-bone attachment with or without interference bone screws.

Thirdly, consideration should be given to the substitute placement and tension as well as measures taken to reduce opportunity for graft impingement such as notchplasty. The stages of substitute tissue transition including avascular necrosis, revascularization, cellular proliferation, and remodelling are also important to consider when establishing timelines for implementation of various exercises.

Fourthly, associated concomitant surgical procedures may be considered such as repair or removal of menisci, patellofemoral involvement and other ligamentous involvement (medial collateral ligament, posterior cruciate ligament, and lateral collateral ligament).

Finally, variations in patients, namely size and somatotype, age, intended use of the limb and most importantly, compliance with the treatment plan can be reason to structure rehabilitation programs on a per individual basis.

Guidelines for rehabilitation following ACL reconstruction

A representative protocol following ACL reconstruction would be initiated by an morning bedside physiotherapy visit on the first post-operative day. The athlete is then seen in the sports medicine department during the afternoon for heel to toe touch down weight bearing as tolerated. Exercises include ankle pumps, quad and hamstring isometrics and assisted straight leg raising in a knee immobilizer. The knee immobilizer is worn at night and a Don Joy 4-Point knee orthosis for daily wear. Range of motion exercise includes active knee flexion to tolerance in supine and prone position and passive extension to zero degrees with a towel roll supporting the ankle in supine position. The patient is discharged with home instructions for exercise and returns at one week for a post-operative check by the surgeon.

At two weeks, the athlete returns for a second postoperative check and is instructed in performing mini-dips and hamstring progressive resistance exercises. Mini-dips are performed by balancing on the involved leg with trunk slightly flexed. The knee is flexed to approximately 10 degrees and returned to full extension. The role of the hamstrings in rehabilitation has been described to include reduction in ACL strain as opposed to isolated quadriceps contraction which through the last 60 degrees of extension may increase strain within the ACL 5 - fold. The contribution of the hamstring toward increased knee stiffness and reduction of laxity at 90 degrees of flexion may result in reduction of total laxity to 24 percent of that of passive laxity (Solomonow, Baratta & D'Ambrosia, 1989). At approximately four weeks, leg presses from 90 degrees of flexion and to 30 degrees of extension, begin with stationary cycling and progressive ambulation to wean the athlete off crutches. As the athlete moves off crutches, aquatic exercise including use of the Aquajogger or Wet Vest flotation devices for deep water running begins.

At six weeks, the athlete returns for evaluation by the surgeon and quadriceps knee extension exercises are initiated from 90 to 40 degrees. Use of the Sport Cord begins with the cord secured at waist level. Emphasis is placed on maintaining flexion of the knees. Exercises include mini-dips, forward, backward and side walking, and side hop. Proprioceptive exercises continue tnroughout rehabilitation and include balancing on the involved extremity with eyes open or eyes closed, balancing while catching a ball, use of the B.A.P.S. board (biomechanical ankle platform system) and theraband resisted balancing.

The slideboard apparatus is used to assist in developing balance, coordination, muscular power and endurance, and to enhance co-contraction. The exercise consists of performing a skating motion over a gliding surface with cushioned bumpers at each end of the board. This mode of training has been used in the past by speedskaters and has become an integral part of our rehabilitation program. Running in a controlled fashion may begin at five months provided other aspects of rehabilitation are progressing at an acceptable rate.

Isokinetic testing may be performed at six months to assist in quantifying recovery. Although there continues to be value in acquiring isokinetic information, our experience

has been that closed kinetic chain exercises and functional assessment may be a more accurate measure of successful rehabilitation. Depending on the variables aforementioned, the athlete may return to activity at 10-11 months postoperative.

Closed kinetic chain exercise

The term closed kinetic chain refers to the distal limb segment being fixed in a weightbearing or loaded posture e.g. leg press, Sport Cord exercise, or slideboard. Open kinetic chain refers to the distal limb segment being free as with a conventional leg extension exercise. Rutherford (1988) summarizes the importance of task specific training which requires learning relevant movement patterns and notes that strength training for isolated muscle groups may not increase functional ability effectively.

Other features of closed kinetic chain exercise include movement proximal and distal to the joint axis. Movement in open kinetic chain occurs distal to the joint axis. Closed kinetic chain exercise is characterized by concentric, eccentric, and isometric contraction through the limb while open chain features primarily concentric contraction proximal to the joint axis. Joint stabilization in closed kinetic chain exercise is provided by normal physiologic means through muscle co-contraction. Stresses of exercise are distributed through the entire limb while compression of the joint decreases shear force following ACL reconstruction. Closed kinetic chain activities provide us with a functional method of rehabilitation which assists the athlete with redevelopment of proprioceptive and motor skills while strengthening the joint.

Functional assessment and return to activity

One of the areas of greatest interest in sports rehabilitation has been that of functional assessment and structuring of an athlete's formal transition back to activity. Functional progression has been defined as an ordered sequence of activities enabling the acquisition or re-acquisition of skills for safe effective performance of athletic endeavors. Functional training has a number of purposes including reinforcement of motor pathways through simulation of sports-specific situations and minimizing anxiety often associated with anterior cruciate ligament reconstruction. Periodic assessment through task-specific exercises can provide positive reinforcement by acclimatizing to demands of the sport.

Procedures for functional assessment

The functional assessment of the athletes following ACL reconstruction at the Cleveland Clinic begins at three months, is repeated at six months and at regular intervals thereafter. Athletes are evaluated using a rating scale from 1 to 5 for various activities with (1) designating no deficiency and (5) designating great difficulty with the task. The scale is based on motor control, speed, capability, confidence in movement, endurance and accuracy of performance.

Examples of manoeuvres performed include static balance with arms crossed in front of the body with the unaffected leg not touching the affected and flexed behind the individual between 30 and 90 degrees. At three months, the athlete must maintain balance for 15 seconds with eyes open and closed to pass the test. At six months, the athlete must maintain balance for 60 seconds to pass.

Dynamic balance requires standing on the involved leg. The tester begins by throwing 30 seconds of warm-up tosses to the athlete with a rugby ball. The tester then varies the throws to different areas, requiring the athlete to respond but maintain position. Ratings are determined by the number of times the uninvolved leg touches the ground during a 30 second period for athletes 3 months post-operative and 60 seconds for athletes 6 months postoperative. Touching down five times or more indicates deficiency or great difficulty. Similar procedures are undertaken for one-legged hop, sport-cord balancing, leg press, retro step-ups, lateral shuffle, and Figure of 8s. Data is recorded on a form which becomes part of the athlete's clinical record. Our experience has been that creation of new challenges and changing the stimulus of training through functional exercise and assessment can provide a refreshing approach for the athlete both physically and psychologically.

Conclusion

Rehabilitation following anterior cruciate ligament reconstruction is based on sequencing functional return in accordance with biological healing. Accelerated programs have evolved in an effort to return athletes to competition as quickly as possible. Clinical judgement must be exercised based on the individual. Return to activity is allowed only upon completion of functional assessment and sports specific drills as well as incorporation of cardiovascular conditioning with attention to aerobic and anaerobic components.

References

Adams ID. (1977) Rugby football injuries. Br J Sports Med, 11, 4-6 .

Andrish JT. (1980) Effects of synovial fluid on fibroblasts in tissue culture. CORR, 147, 258-261. Clinical Orthopaedics and Related Research. (1983) (ed MR Urist), JB Lippincott Company, Philadelphia, 172.

Dineen PF and Gallagher JE. Survey of rugby injuries. Ir Med J, 75, 137.

Ewen JA. (1950) Experimental rupture of the medial collateral ligament of the knee. JBJS, 32, 396-402.

Jackson DW and Drez D. (1987) The Anterior Cruciate Deficient Knee. The CV Mosby Company, St Louis.

Kaufman T. (1985) Rugby injuries sustained during tournament play. J Orthopaed Sports Phys Therapy, 16-19.

Micheli LJ and Riseborough ED. (1975) The incidence of injuries in rugby football. Sports Med, 2, 93-98.

Morrissey MC. (1989) Reflex inhibition of thigh muscles in knee injury. Sports Med, 7, 263-276.

Rothwell AG. (1982) Quadriceps hematoma . A prospective clinical study. Clin Orthop, 171, 97-103.

Roy S. (1975) The diagnosis and initial management of the acutely injured knee with particular reference to sport injuries. S Afr Med J, 49, 363-367.

Roy SP. (1974) The nature and frequency of rugby injuries: a pilot study of 300 injuries at Stellenbosch. S Afr Med J, 48, 2321-2327.

Rutherford OM. (1988) Muscular coordination and strength training. Implications for injury rehabilitation. Sports Med, 5, 196-202.

Shelbourne KD and Nitz P. (1990) Accelerated rehabilitation after anterior cruciate ligament reconstruction. Am J Sports Med, 18, 292-298 .

Silver JR and Gill S. (1988) Injuries of the spine sustained during rugby. Sports Med, 5, 328-334.

Solomonow M, Baratta R and D'Ambrosia R. (1989) The role of the hamstrings in the rehabilitation of the anterior cruciate ligament-deficient knee in athletes. Sports Med, 7, 42-48.

The upper limb

Shoulder injuries in rugby

T.L. Wickiewicz, J.C. Edwards, R.F. Warren and S. Scarangella

Abstract. Rugby is a fast paced contact sport played with minimal protective gear and as such is associated with a high number of injuries, Over the past several years there have been a number of studies that have appeared in the literature attempting to chronicle these injuries. Clark et al followed eight adult club rugby teams prospectively during the 1988 season and found a total of 114 injuries sustained by 78 players; Sparks has reported an injury rate of around 195 per 10,000 player hours in two separate studies. Both authors agree that tackling is the activity associated with the highest incidence of injury, and it follows that the shoulder is the site of a high percentage of these injuries. An unpublished study from our institution that dealt with rugby in the state of New York was in basic agreement with these other studies, and added that those who were recently introduced to the sport in the United States had an even higher percentage of shoulder injuries than those who were more accustomed to playing without pads. This paper will discuss the shoulder, its anatomy, and how this anatomy can be affected by both the repetitive microtrauma and acute macrotrauma that is associated with the sport of rugby.

Keywords: Shoulder Injuries, Acromioclavicular Separation, Glenohumeral Dislocation, Rotator Cuff Impingement.

Introduction

Rugby is a fast paced contact sport played with minimal protective gear and as such is associated with a high number of injuries. A prospective study was undertaken at the Hospital for Special Surgery in an attempt to evaluate the incidence and type of injuries that occurred in the New York Metropolitan rugby league during the 1980-1981 spring season. Nine teams in two divisions were followed for the season by either a physicain or medical student who kept track of any injury that caused a player to be removed from a game. These injuries were tabulated at the end of the season disclosing several trends. Of note was the fact that the level of experience and expertise rather than lowering the injury rate actually increased it. This was felt to be secondary to the increased level of intensity that was present in the more advanced divisions. However, the percentage of injuries that occurred in the shoulder was actually higher in the less experienced division. It was postulated that this was the result of the players changing their technique from tackling with pads, as in American football, to tackling without them in rugby.

In our study, as in several other studies from around the world, the activity that was most associated with injury was the tackle. Over 50% of the injuries occurred either in the player who was being tackled or the player doing the tackling. follows that a high percentage of the injuries will occur in the shoulder, and this was borne out in our study with the shoulder being the anatomic site most frequently injured. After an overview of the pertinent anatomy, this paper will discuss those injuries that occur in the shoulder in rugby or any contact sport.

Anatomy

In order to allow motion in different planes, the shoulder requires its anatomy to strike a delicate balance between motion and stability. This balance is accomplished through the interactions between the static stabilizers, shoulder capsule and ligament structures, and the muscles about the shoulder. They are integrally involved in movement and support of the inherently unstable glenohumeral joint throughout its range of motion.

There are three major bones that combine to form two functional joints within the shoulder. The scapula essentially sits free on the posterior thoracic wall and is balanced by periscapular musculature. It articulates with the distal end of the clavicle through its anteriomedial edge or acromion to form the acromioclavicular (AC) joint, and it articulates with the humerus via the glenoid fossa to form the glenohumeral joint. In addition, a joint exists between the scapula and thoracic wall known as the scapulothoracic joint.

The AC joint is stabilized by two major ligamentous complexes, the acromioclavicular ligament running between the acromion and the clavicle, and coracoclavicular ligament complex. The latter is comprised two ligaments that run from the inferior surface of the clavicle to the corocoid process in the scapula and is essential for holding the distal end of the clavicle in proper position for its articulation with the acromion.

The glenohumeral joint is stabilised by both the static ligament stabilizers (the inferior, middle, and superior glenohumeral ligaments, the posterior capsule, and the anterior and posterior labrum) as well as the dynamic stabilizers, specifically the muscles of the rotator cuff.

Glenohumeral and scapulothoracic motion occur in ratio of approximately 2:1 with the first 30 degrees of abduction in the plane of the scapula essentially being all glenohumeral motion (Poppin and Walker, 1976). It is facilitated by the muscles of the rotator cuff, the deltoid and the biceps brachii. The biceps act as an accessory elevator of the shoulder in the forward flexion plane as well as playing an integral role in the deceleration of the arm during the throwing motion in sport.

Impingement syndrome

Impingement syndrome is a term which was coined by Dr Charles Neer (Neer, 1972) and refers to a phenomenon of mechnanical impingement of the rotator cuff tendons, particularly the supraspinatus tendon against the overlying coracoacromial arch when the arm is brought into forward flexion, its functional motion plane. This is classified as being present in 3 stages from stage 1 being a reversible process involving the supraspinatus tendon and sub-acromial bursa, through stage 2 where changes become irreversible and finally to stage 3 where full thickness rotator cuff tears are present. With the advent of increased participation in throwing sports, it has become known that not all painful shoulders, especially in the young thrower, are representative of this mechanical process. Subtle instabilities of the shoulder will often lead to a cuff tendonitis with clinical symptoms that mimic impingement. It is important to make the proper diagnosis as classical impingement operations often will prove to be of no benefit to the shoulder with microsubluxation as the etiology of their symptoms.

Clinically the patient with impingement will present with a history of repetitive overuse in the overhead plane. Ultimately they will develop pain with this motion which may eventually persist even after the activity has been discontinued. The patient with microsubluxation may be able to relate the point in the throwing motion when the pain starts, with the pain being primarily located on top of the shoulder and occasionally radiating to the mid-brachium. Night pain also becomes a common complaint of people with impingement. Although thought of as an inflammatory condition, pathology has never yielded evidence of an acute inflammatory response but rather that of degeneration with the tendinous structure.

Physical examination should begin with an inspection of the individual viewed from behind looking specifically for asymmetry of scapulothoracic and glenohumeral motion when the shoulder is elevated both in the forward flexion and abduction planes, as well as for evidence of muscle wasting about the shoulder. In addition, it is essential to assess motion of the shoulder specifically for internal and external rotation both with the arm at the side and in the overhead plane. Often individuals will present with contractures, for example, a thrower will have increased compensatory external rotation at the expense of internal rotation. Physical examination also includes the performance of one of the impingement maneuvers either with forced forward flexion or forced internal rotation of the shoulder. The second method starts with the shoulder being held at 90 degrees of abduction in the plane of the scapula. A positive test with either maneuver consists of reproduction of the patient's symptoms as the supraspinatus or greater tuberosity impinge on the coracoacromial arch. An impingement test involves the installation of local anesthesia in to the sub-acromial space with the elimination of the symptoms. Care should be taken in the interpretation of this test as it will render painless both impingement conditions.

Radiographically, rotator cuff pathology is diagnosed by means of an arthrogram. Recently the MRI has gained popularity offering the benefit of a non-invasive method of gathering information on the soft tissues about the shoulder. Its accuracy with regards to being able to predict full thickness cuff tears still needs to be established.

The treatment of stage I consists of rest, NSAID's and occasional sub-acromial injections, followed by rotator cuff rehabilitation with emphasis on elimination of contractures of motion prior to the individual returning to his or her sport.

Stage II impingement is more common in individuals in the fourth and fifth decade. The process has now advanced to where the sub-acromial structures start showing changes specially on the acromial side of the rotator cuff and bursa. Often there is thickening of the bursa causing sub-acromial crepitus. Initial conservative treatment is similar to that of stage I but often will be more protracted. At times, the individual may be rendered asymptomatic until he or she returns to the same activities that initially brought their condition to light. At this point activity modification may be required. If the symptoms persist the patient may be a candidate for an acromioplasty performed as either an open or arthroscopic procedure.

In stage III impingement the process has progressed to the point of a full thickness rotator cuff tear. Although the symptoms may mimic the earlier stages, the physical examination will demonstrate weakness of the supraspinatus muscle when tested for external rotation or resistive abduction strength. In individuals in whom continued sports participation is important surgery may be required in the form of either open or arthroscopically assisted decompression and rotator cuff repair.

Instability

Shoulder instability is a common sequel to a traumatic anterior dislocation of the glenohumeral joint. However, it can also occur in a posterior direction or have an inferior component and be considered a multi-directionally unstable shoulder. In addition, shoulder instability may be both traumatic or atraumatic in its onset. Shoulders with atraumatic instability often have inherent capsular looseness that when superimposed with the trauma of sports will lead to a symptomatic instability. It is important for the examiner to classify instability thus allowing more accuracy of diagnosis, prognosis and treatment. (See figure 1).

As stated above, the most common dislocation associated with athletic participation is the acute traumatic anterior dislocation. The mechanism of injury is usually forced abduction, external rotation and extension of the shoulder. Clinically these patients present with intense pain located at the shoulder and will often be seen holding the arm off to the side attempting to immobilize it. The physical examination should include a detailed neurologic examination of the

CLASSIFICATION OF SHOULDER INSTABILITY

A.	DEGREE	Microsubluxation
		Subluxation
		Dislocation

B.	DIRECTION	Anterior
		Posterior
		Inferior
		Multi-Directional

C.	ONSET	Acute
		Chronic
		Fixed

D.	ETIOLOGY	Traumatic
		Atraumatic	- Voluntary
			- Involuntary

Fig. 1   A classification scheme for shoulder instability.

involved extremity paying particular attention to the distribution of the axillary and musculocutaneous nerves, which are vulnerable to injury in anterior dislocation of the shoulder.

If witnessed by a physician at a sporting event the acute dislocation can often be reduced on the playing field. This may allow the joint to be reduced before muscle spasms make relocation more difficult. Methods of reduction using both humeral and scapular positioning have been described. However, if the patient is seen in the emergency room radiographs should be obtained before a reduction is attempted. Three views are needed to define the dislocation and rule out concomitant fractures, particularly in the older patient: a true AP of the glenohumeral joint, a transcapular or "Y" view, and an axillary view of the shoulder. The latter two views are important to establish the position of the head of the humerus relative to the glenoid.

The initial treatment consists of reducing the humeral head back on to the glenoid. If the shoulder has been out for a significant period of time either analgesics or sedation may be required to relax the muscle spasm and allow the reduction to take place. Most of the techniques used to relocate the shoulder employ a period of traction to help relieve muscle spasm followed by manipulation of either the humerus or the scapula into a position that facilitates relocation. Reduction of the joint is usually accompanied by a distinct sense to the practitioner and immediate relief of the patient's pain.

Following the initial dislocation, some evidence exists that immobilization for a period of 6 weeks in a sling may reduce the incidence of recurrent instability. However, in young athletic individuals an untreated primary anterior dislocation has a greater than 90% likelihood of developing recurrent instability with continued sports participation. As individuals become older this likelihood of recurrence diminishes but does so primarily because the older individual tends to put fewer demands on their shoulder. In individuals over the age of 20 who have primary dislocations and who persist in having an inordinate degree of pain in the first few weeks following the dislocation, suspicion should be aroused that a concomitant rotator cuff injury may have occurred, especially if the individual exhibits weakness of elevation or external rotations. In this setting an arthrogram should be performed early to make the diagnosis.

In individuals in whom the likelihood of recurrence and dislocation is high, such as high school and collegiate athletes, consideration should may be given to primary stabilization of the shoulder followed by a period of immobilization. In recent years arthroscopic techniques have been developed to facilitate such surgery. However, at the present time it is fair to say that recurrence rates following arthroscopic stabilization will be higher than with traditional open surgical techniques.

Acromioclavicular (AC) joint dislocation

Acromioclavicular joint dislocations, commonly referred to as shoulder separations, can be categorized into six groups (Neer and Rockwood, 1984). The groups are based on the anatomy of the AC joint and its supporting structures (See Figure 2). This paper will deal with the first three types which are the most common in athletic participation. Type 1, sprain of the AC joint and coracoclavicular ligaments without anatomic disruption. Type 2, partial displacement less than half the width of the distal clavicle on the acromion. A Grade II soft tissue injury of AC and coracoclavicular ligaments is necessary to allow the displacement. Type 3, total disruption of the AC and coracoclavicular ligaments allows complete separation of the clavicle from the acromion.

In taking the history the patient will often state that the mechanism of injury was a fall directly on the tip of the shoulder followed by immediate pain. Physical examination of all three types will reveal pain to direct palpation of the acromioclavicular joint and prominence of the clavicle with Types 2 and 3 injuries

CLASSIFICATION OF ACROMIOCLAVICULAR DISLOCATION

TYPE I   Sprain of the AC joint
          AC joint intact

TYPE II   AC joint is disrupted
          AC joint wider and slightly displaced upward as compared to the
          normal shoulder
          Sprain of the coracoclavicular ligaments

TYPE III AC ligaments disrupted
          AC joint dislocated with clavicle displaced upwards
          Corcoclavicular ligaments disrupted

TYPE IV   AC ligaments disrupted
          AC joint dislocated with the clavicle displaced posteriorly through
          the trapezius muscle
          Coroclavicular ligaments partially or completely disrupted

TYPE V   AC ligaments disrupted
          AC joint dislocated and clavicle displaced superiorly towards the
          base of the neck
          Coroclavicular ligaments disrupted

TYPE VI   AC ligaments disrupted
          AC joint dislocated and clavicle displaced inferiorly
          Coracoclavicular ligaments either intact or disrupted

Fig. 2   Classification of acromioclavicular dislocations based upon the
          anatomic structures affected (Neer and Rockwood, 1984).

will be present.   Often acute swelling will obscure the clavicular prominence
especially in Type 2 injuries. The patient will usually exhibit a decreased range
of motion of the shoulder and pain with adduction in the forward flexion plane.
   The AC joint can be visualized by most standard AP views of the shoulder but

clavicular views which angle the x-ray tube cephalad should be obtained. With Type 1 injuries the x-ray appearance is normal. In Type 2 and 3 there is a range of partial to complete displacement of the clavicle in a cephalad direction. If a Type 2 or 3 injury is suspected from the history or the physical examination, a stress view of the shoulder should be obtained. This is accomplished by shooting the x-ray with the patient holding a weight of approximately 10 to 15 pounds in both hands and thereby accentuating the deformity.

Treatment of AC separation is controversial. Most authors agree that symptomatic treatment consisting of a short period of sling immobilization until the pain settles followed by an early return to activities is sufficient for Type 1 injuries. Although consensus is not quite as strong, most authors suggest surgical repair of grossly displaced type 3 injuries, particularly if the patient participates in active overhead sports. Type 2 injuries promote most of the controversy. Although operative intervention may be a reasonable choice, the authors prefer conservative management consisting of sling immobilization until pain subsides and then mobilization of the shoulder. Overhead rehabilitation is delayed for about 6 to 8 weeks to allow tissue healing. More restrictive immobilization such as utilizing a Kenny Howard splint do not offer any advantage over conservative treatment in our opinion.

Fractures of the proximal humerus

Fractures of the proximal humerus have historically been an injury of elderly people that was usually treated conservatively with acceptable symptomatic results, but at times less than optimal functional outcome with many patients having a decreased range of motion. Unfortunately this attitude has at times carried over into the treatment of similar fractures in the younger population who place higher demands on their shoulders and who do not tolerate a major decrease in the range of motion of this joint. In an attempt to differentiate between those fractures that could be treated conservatively and those that would be better served with operative intervention, a classification was proposed by Dr Neer based on the anatomy of the fracture. These fractures are divided into two major groups, nondisplaced/minimally displaced and displaced, with displaced being defined as a fracture with a fragment that is either displaced more than one centimeter or angulated greater than 45 degrees. The fracture fragments are the greater and less tuberosities, the head, and the shaft, with the displaced fractures being divided according to the number of these fragments seen on the x-ray.

As stated above, this type of fracture in the younger population, is of high energy, and therefore the mechanism of injury is one where the athlete suffers a severe impact or twisting force to the shoulder. The initial physical examination is particularly important in this injury because the practitioner must distinguish between a fracture and any of the other possible injuries to the shoulder. The upper humerus will obviously be painful to palpation with crepitus or gross movement between the fracture fragments in those injuries that are displaced and unstable. As with an acutely dislocated shoulder, it is extremely important to perform a thorough neurovascular check of the affected extremity, paying particular note to the axillary and musculocutaneous nerves.

The acute treatment of these injuries consists of immobilization until radiographs can be obtained. Normally plain x-rays are sufficient to make the diagnosis, but since the treatment of these fractures is based on the radiographs, it is important that adequate images be obtained showing both AP and lateral views of the proximal humerus.

If the fracture fulfills the criterion for being minimally or non-displaced, the treatment is immobilization in a sling until clinical union appears to have taken place at which time physical therapy can be advanced until the patient once again returns to full activity. If the fracture is displaced, then treatment is determined by the anatomy of the fracture. In younger individuals most fractures, particularly if they are unstable, need to be operatively stabilized in order to achieve the best possible result. In order to accomplish this it is important to have a thorough understanding of the anatomy of the different fragments, their attachments and their blood supply. Any of the many different techniques that have been described for fixation of these fractures will be successful if they restore normal anatomy.

References

Clark DR, Roux C, Noakes TD. (1990) A prospective study of the incidence and nature of injuries to adult rugby players. S Afr Med J, 77, 559.

Hawkins RJ, Kennedy JC. (1980) Impingement syndrome in athletes. Am J Sports Med, 8, 151.

Iannotti JP, Ziatkin MB et al. (1991) Magnetic resonance imaging of the shoulder: Sensitivity, specificity, and predictive value. J Bone Joint Surg, 73-A, 17.

Nathan M, Goedeke R, Noakes TD. (1983) The incidence and nature of rugby injuries experienced at one school during the 1982 rugby season. S Afr Med J, 64, 132.

Neer CS. (1972) Anterior acromioplasty for the chronic impingement syndrome in the shoulder. J Bone Joint Surg, 54A, 41.

Neer CS, Rockwood CA. (1984) Fractures and dislocations of the shoulder. In Rockwood CA and Green DP (eds) Fractures in adults, vol 1, Philadelphia, J Lippincott Co.

Neer CS II. (1970) Displaced proximal humeral fractures: Part I. Classification and evaluation. J Bone Joint Surg, 52A, 1077.

Neer CS II. (1970) Displaced proximal humeral fractures: Part II. Treatment of three-part and four-part displacement. J Bone Joint Surg, 52A, 1090.

Poppin NK, Walker PS. (1976) Normal and abnormal motion of the shoulder. J Bone Joint Surg, 58A, 195.

Sparks JP. (1985) Rugby football injuries, 1980-1983. Br Sports Med, 19, 71.

Warren RF, Scarangella S, Wickiewicz TL. Rugby injury study. Unpublished study from the Hospital for Special Surgery.

Management for acute injuries around the shoulder

S.A. Copeland

Abstract. Management for acute injuries around the shoulder.
Acute shoulder injuries occur commonly in sport either by direct injury in contact sports or by overuse of the arm. The acromio clavicular separation seen so commonly in rugby can be managed conservaitvely in most cases with expectation of an excellent outcome. Rotator cuff injuries can arise from a fall or more commonly by overtraining placing a stress on the rotator cuff tendons; in the younger sportsman the injury can be treated conservatively but in older invividuals (over 40) degenerative changes can supervene resulting in a tear of the rotator cuff and a loss of shoulder function. These individuals more often require surgical treatment.

Keywords: Shoulder, Sports Injury, Acromio Clavicular Joint, Sterno Clavicular Joint Rotator Cuff.

Introduction

Acute injuries around the shoulder area are extremely common in all the contact sports. They can present in two separate ways (1) direct injury sustained in the procedure of the sport and (2) overstrain/overuse injuries caused by training for the sport.

Diagnosis of site of injury

Approximately one third of shoulder girdle problems presenting at a sports injury clinic arise from the acromio clavicular joint. The history may be of a direct fall onto the point of the shoulder or sometimes onto the outstretched hand. The pain is acute and easily localised by the patient who points with a finger to the site of injury. Confirmation of the site of injury is made by local tenderness and by stressing the AC joint. When asked to abduct the arm as high as possible, a painful arc will be induced which is increased from approximately 150° to 180° with increasing pain on increasing abduction. This is evident both actively and passively because the clavicle rotates through 60° in the coronal plane above 90° of elevation, hence stressing the AC joint. The joint may also be stressed by pulling the arm forward across the front of the body and by straining both elbows together behind the chest. If the clinical state of pain is with the acromio clavicular joint itself, then special X-ray views should be requested and not just straight AP views of the shoulder which do not show the AC joint clearly. In the standard AP view of the shoulder the lateral end of the clavicle is seen to overlap the acromium. The AC joint may be viewed tangentially by a 25° upshot view. Traditionally acromio clavicular joint injuries are divided into three types:

Type 1   Sprain only of the acromio clavicular ligament.

Type 2   Subluxation of the joint with some disruption of the intrarticular meniscus and tearing of joint capsule with stripping of periosteum.

Type 3   Complete dislocation of the joint with instablity and disruption of the coroclavicular ligaments.

Type 1 and Type 2 injuries are always treated conservatively. This injury may be acutely painful such that relief of pain is the very first priority. Local ice packs, oral analgesics, anti-inflammatories and rest in a sling are all helpful. The most comfortable position for the joint is with the arm abducted to approximately 50° in neutral rotation. This may be achieved by lying flat with a pillow over the chest, or lying flat on the back with a rolled pillow between the shoulder blades to allow the shoulder girdle to fall back. This may certainly be the most comfortable position to achieve sleep at night or even sitting up. Occasionally Type 2 subluxation may require surgical treatment at a much later date when secondary degenerative changes may supervene, but this is unusual, the majority becoming pain free within weeks. As there is no one muscle that crosses the acromio clavicular joint, active physiotherapy is really unhelpful, but passive mobilising and pain relieving techniques are all helpful to speed recovery from this painful injury.

The sterno clavicular joint

Injuries to this joint represent about 3 per cent of injuries to the shoulder girdle in contact sports. Usually this is an indirect rollover injury sustained while the player is on the floor and other players are forced on top of him. An anterior subluxation may be induced and he may complain of pain directly after the match but the swelling may take several weeks to present, such that a rather florid swelling over the sterno clavicular joint can cause some concern as to its nature some weeks after the original injury. Again, pain is induced by work above shoulder height. Rarely, this may develop into an habitual, painful subluxation of the joint each time the arm is elevated. If allowed to rest properly in the early stages the joint can spontaneously stabilise and the anterior sterno clavicular ligaments may heal. If it is pushed too early, then painful repetitive subluxation may be induced requiring either stabilisation or excision surgery at a later date.

Rotator cuff injuries

Pain arising in the rotator cuff is poorly localised. The patient may often indicate a site on the upper outer aspect of the arm associated with night pain. The pain is rather generalised and indicated with the flat of the hand and tenderness does not correspond to the site of the perceived pain. In the acute injury pain may be severe and all movements are difficult, but after a short time it can be demonstrated that the pain is within a painful arc from approximately 60° to 120° of elevation. The site of the tear within the rotator cuff could be further delineated by testing for power of external rotation in abduction and internal rotation in abduction, to decide whether the site of injury is posterior, central or anterior rotator cuff as these sites carry a different prognosis after injury. Diagnosis may be confirmed by injection into the subacromial bursa of local anaesthetic although often in the acute injury this is not necessary.

Because these acute injuries are painful they can lead on to a spectrum of rotator cuff disability and it is the timing along this clinical pathway which determines the symptoms of presentation. Pain leads to disordered humeral and scapulo thoracic rhythm which upsets the very delicate relationship between the power of deltoid and the rotator cuff muscles to centralise the humeral head in the glenoid. If this relationship is disturbed then progressive disability may ensue. Pain leads to weakness of the cuff muscle, the cuff is then weak in relation to deltoid: the head rises up in the glenoid and painful impingement ensues.

The shoulder is the most mobile joint in the body and there are several force vectors which stabilise it such that if any one muscle is affected, it must have an equal and opposite effect on its antagonist. The rotator cuff contributes approximately 90° of the power of external rotation and the cardinal sign of rotator cuff function is loss of power in external rotation and this must always be tested in an individual with a suspected rotator cuff injury. It is often assumed that sports injuries only occur in the young and fit, but the incidence of rotator cuff injury dramatically increases with age presenting a spectrum of injury ranging from acute rotator cuff tear to degenerative change. In the young, what might be considered to be a reversible acute injury, in those over forty may be the beginning of a progressive disability unless it is treated at an early stage.

Rotator cuff failure

A sprain may be considered a disruption of some fibres of a muscle. If this occurs in the rotator cuff it leads to an increasing load on the neighbouring non-disrupted fibres. This results in a decrease in the force of that muscle and a loss of power to depress the humeral head. There is distortion of local vascular anatomy along with blood vessel rupture. Haematoma is washed away by joint fluid and hence progressive devascularisation can occur. With loss of power of depression of the humeral head, the deltoid elevates the head and causes a secondary mechanical impingement causing the cuff to mechanically impinge on the corocoacromial arch. Mechanical wear may then lead to further rotator cuff tearing and secondary boney change on the anterior aspect of the acromium and overloading of the corocoacromial ligament. This spectrum may take several years to occur and can be stopped at any stage by adequate treatment.

In the young acute injury, rest and pain relieving measures such as ice and gentle passive mobilisation is all that is required. Having relieved the pain the rotator cuff must then be re-strengthened to restore its function with a static exercise regime.

With those beyond the first flush of youth presenting a little later, then chronic changes may already have developed. Night pain may be a feature and Neer (1972) has described three stages of impingement:

Stage 1   Those under 25 years of age, with pain brought on by either acute injury or overuse, settling completely with rest and conservative measures.

Stage 2   Pain in shoulder usually presenting under the age of 40 years which occurs each time repetitive use is made of the shoulder above shoulder height, but which settles with conservative measures and may require injection therapy.

Stage 3   Mechanical changes are established and the rotator cuff is scarred, there may be spur formation and possibly a rotator cuff tear. These degenerative changes are not reversible by conservative methods of treatment and may well require surgery to relieve symptoms.

Injection of Shoulder

Injection therapy around the shoulder is a useful adjunct to treatment as long as it is used with caution and discretion. It is rarely required in the young acute injury as they will almost certainly settle by other conservative means, ie anti-inflammatory medication, physiotherapy, rest and a sling. Injection of local anaesthetic alone may be helpful in making the diagnosis (see above). If the clinical diagnosis has been made and the pain is arising the subacromial region, then it is reasonable to inject the subacromial bursa with local steroid. My own preference is to use a large volume of local anaesthetic, i.e. 10mls of 0.25% bupivacaine and a local steroid e.g. methyl prednisolone 40mg or triamcinalone.

The easiest way to enter the subacromial bursa is one thumb's breadth medial to the posterior angle of the acromion. The needle is then aimed at 45° medially and caudally to enter the subacromial bursa. A slight 'give' is felt as the needle enters the bursa and then the whole volume is injected into the bursa. There should be little resistance felt as the fluid enters the bursa. Within minutes of giving the injection the discomfort should be abolished or greatly reduced and the painful arc diminished. I do not give two separate injections, but give the two together both as a test and a treatment to save two injections. It is advised that no more than three injections are given at three weekly intervals. It is advisable not to repeat the injections within one year.

References

Neer CS II. (1972) Anterior acromioplasty for the chronic impingement syndrome in the shoulder. J Bone Joint Surg, **54a**, 41.

Common hand injuries in contact sports

M.G. Hullin

Abstract. This paper presents some of the commonest sports related injuries of the hand and wrist with special emphasis on the initial assessment of the injury to prevent the development of late deformity and functional impairment.

Keywords: Hand Injuries, Mallet Finger, Boutonniere Deformity, Carpal Fractures, Wrist Instability.

Introduction

The true incidence of hand injuries in contact sports is unknown. A study of American college athletes showed that those sports at greatest risk were football, gymnastics, wrestling and basketball (Posner, 1990). However, there are no uniquely sports-related injuries of the hand and wrist and the number of non-athletic injuries far outweigh those related to contact sports.

Athletes have high expectations and are often reluctant to take medical advice if it interferes with their sporting ambitions. This is particularly true of injuries to the hand most of which can be treated conservatively though they may require prolonged periods of sporting abstinence. Surgical intervention to appease the unrealistic desire of an athlete should be avoided. There are very few instances in which early surgery should be recommended on the grounds that the patient is a sportsman. Conservative treatment does not mean neglect and all hand injuries must be promptly and carefully assessed to allow the earliest return of normal hand function whilst avoiding long term deformity or instability. The period of rehabilitation is as important and often more demanding in the conservatively treated athlete as in a patient upon whom surgery has been performed.

Assessment of hand injuries

As in all branches of sports medicine the initial assessment of the injury is critical in ensuring the best possible outcome. The history and in particular the examination of the hand is of most importance. There are few investigations required apart from good quality plain radiographs including true lateral views of the injured part. For this reason it should be possible to make an accurate diagnosis and plan of management very soon after the injury. An awareness of the essential points of the examination of the injured hand should prevent missed diagnoses and prevent both over treatment and neglect of potentially serious injuries leading to a permanent disability.

An acute hand injury is characterised by pain, swelling and often deformity which may make the diagnosis apparent immediately, However, the absence of deformity does not exclude a very significant injury. Superficial inspection must be avoided and a detailed history of the injury obtained and a careful examination carried out to ascertain the site of maximum tenderness and any underlying instability. A chronic injury usually presents as deformity, muscle contracture or instability. There is usually a history of acute injury which received little attention and often the athlete had not sought advice at the time of the original injury.

Mallet finger deformity

The commonest sports related injury is the "mallet" finger deformity. There is rupture of the insertion of the extensor tendon into the distal phalanx which may be associated with a fracture at the base of the distal phalanx. The commonest mechanism of injury is a blow to the extended finger causing forced flexion at the distal interphalangeal (DIP) joint. The joint is held flexed by the unopposed action of the flexor tendon and active extension is lost. A secondary hyperextension deformity may occur at the proximal interphalangeal (PIP) joint. Treatment is by continual splinting of the joint in slight hyperextension for at least six weeks. The PIP joint must not be immobilized. Surgery has been advocated in the presence of a distal phalangeal fracture but even displaced intra-articular fractures will heal and remodel. Surgery is reserved for cases in which the DIP joint is subluxed.

Mallet finger deformity often presents at a late stage because no attention is sought at the time of injury. If there is no functional disability then no treatment is required. Results of late splinting or surgery are unpredictable, though treatment by splinting even 18 weeks after injury has proved effective (Patel et al, 1986). Late surgical reattachment of the tendon may be effective but involve splinting for six to eight weeks and this may explain the success rather than the surgery itself. Alternatively division of the central slip of the extensor tendon at the middle phalanx may improve DIP joint extension at the risk of a flexion deformity at the PIP joint. Arthrodesis of the DIP joint is reliable and effective.

Rupture of flexor digitorum profundus

Avulsion of the flexor profundus tendon is typically associated with "jersey pulling" incidents when the DIP joint is forcibly extended. The ring finger is most commonly involved. This diagnosis is frequently missed as no deformity is present and superficial examination will not reveal the underlying serious pathology. The athlete presents with pain and swelling along the tendon sheath but in the acute stage the inability to flex the DIP joint is not recognised unless specifically tested for. All acute ruptures should be repaired surgically. The tendon usually retracts to the level of the PIP joint but may retract into the palm or remain at the level of the DIP joint if there is an associated bony avulsion.

If the diagnosis is missed or the patient presents late then a secondary contracture of the muscle belly will have resulted. The possibility of direct repair depends upon the time from injury, the degree of muscle and joint contracture and the distance of retraction of the tendon. If the athlete presents late then if the flexor digitorum superficialis is not adherent and there is no hyperextension at the DIP joint, no treatment may be necessary. DIP joint fusion is a reliable and effective method of treatment. The only way to restore DIP joint movement if direct repair is not possible is a one or two stage tendon graft, but scarring may inhibit PIP joint function and the value of late reconstruction is doubtful.

Injuries around the proximal interphalangeal joints

The extensor apparatus and the volar plate associated with the PIP joints are complex structures of great functional importance. Their injury is common and can lead to some of the most difficult problems of management if unrecognised or inadequately treated. At this level the extensor tendon consists of a central slip which provides dorsal stability to the joint and two lateral slips which distally join to form a single tendon inserting into the distal phalanx. Lateral joint stability is provided by the collateral ligaments. The volar plate through its two lateral attachments to the middle phalanx prevents hyperextension at the PIP joint.

A boutonniere deformity will result if the central slip of the extensor tendon is avulsed from its insertion into the middle phalanx. The dorsal restraint is lost and the head of the proximal phalanx "buttonholes" through the extensor mechanism. The lateral bands of the extensor apparatus are displaced volarward and act to flex the PIP joint and extend the DIP joint. With time this deformity becomes fixed. Injury to the central slip of the extensor tendon results from direct trauma or from sudden forced flexion of the extended joint. Early diagnosis is essential for best functional outcome and a high index of suspicion for this injury is needed. Often there is little to find on inspection apart from slight swelling at the joint. Maximum tenderness over the dorsum of the middle phalanx at the point of insertion of the tendon is of greatest importance. Initially almost full extension may be possible. The range of flexion of the DIP joint should be assessed with the PIP joint splinted in full extension. Loss of flexion may occur early in the development of the deformity. Treatment consists of immobilising the PIP joint in extension while encouraging a full range of active and passive DIP joint movement. The joint is immobilised for at least six weeks and then the joint is protected during sporting activities for a further six weeks.

Late presentation with an established deformity may present a considerable problem. Presentation up to six weeks from injury may be treated successfully by immobilisation for eight weeks (Souter, 1974). After this time if there is minimal deformity and functional impairment the situation should be accepted as the risks of operative surgery are significant and may lead to a stiff extended finger. Surgical techniques differ but a staged approach should be adopted with more radical surgery reserved for severe deformity (Curtis et al, 1983). A pseudoboutonniere deformity can occur if a hyperextension injury leads to volar plate damage and a late flexion contracture develops. This condition is characterised by a normal range of DIP joint movement.

Hyperextension injuries and dorsal dislocations of the PIP joints are common. Often the central portion of the volar plate alone is disrupted and the joint remains stable. Early mobilisation is recommended. A more severe injury leads to tearing of the lateral] attachments of the volar plate and the joint may dislocate. The collateral ligaments remain intact but the joint is susceptible to hyperextension following reduction. Splintage in slight flexion is recommended to prevent chronic volar plate instability which may cause the joint to become intermittently locked in hyperextension.

Intra-articular fractures at the base of the middle phalanx comprising a third or more of the articular surface may render the PIP joint unstable and early recognition and internal fixation is needed to allow full functional recovery. A severely comminuted fracture precludes fixation and excision of the fragments and reattachment of the volar plate may be needed. Most other fractures of the phalanges can be treated conservatively but attention to rotational deformity of the fingers is important.

Thumb injuries

Two important injuries to the thumb are commonly encountered and if untreated can lead to instability. Fractures of the base of the first metacarpal if intra-articular (Bennet's fracture) can lead to subluxation of the trapezio-metacarpal joint. Treatment consists of reduction of the subluxation by pronation and flexion of the metacarpal and not by extension. Once reduced the position is maintained by percutaneous K wires which should avoid the small volar fragment.

Damage to the ulnar collateral ligament of the first metacarpo-phalangeal joint is common in skiers but can be seen in contact sports after falls causing forced abduction of the joint. Diagnosis is by a stress test with the joint in full extension after radiographs have excluded associated fractures. Partial ruptures with pain on stressing but no instability are treated by immobilisation for 4 to 5 weeks. The treatment of complete ruptures is controversial but many surgeons recommend immediate surgery. The rationale is that early repair provides a greater likelihood of a stable pain free joint than immobilisation alone since if the ligament lies external to the adductor aponeurosis (the Stener lesion) chronic instability will result. The Stener lesion is estimated to occur in about 50% of ruptures (Green and Rowland, 1984) and can only be diagnosed at surgery.

Assessment of carpal injuries

Careful assessment and investigation of all wrist injuries is essential. The term "wrist sprain" is a diagnosis of exclusion. A careful history of the mechanism of injury may reveal a chronic underlying instability or an overuse syndrome. Careful examination with comparison to the other wrist should include inspection, palpation and measurement of active and passive ranges of movement. A painful click on palmar flexion and radial deviation may indicate scapho-lunate disassociation. Routine radiographs (Posterio-anterior and lateral) are of great value but in the wrist further investigations such as specialised X-ray views, cine radiographs, arthrograms and arthroscopy should be considered.

Fractures

70% of carpal fractures involve the scaphoid (Borgeskov et al, 1966). These fractures are difficult to diagnose and often must initially be treated on clinical grounds and repeat radiographs taken at two weeks. X-rays taken in radial and ulnar deviation and clenched fist views as well as the standard four scaphoid views are often helpful. The method of treatment is controversial. Most fractures can be treated conservatively but there is growing enthusiasm, particularly in the U.S.A., for internal fixation of displaced fractures to attempt to reduce the high rate of non-union (Cooney et al, 1980). Conservative management is also open to debate. Some recommend the use of an above elbow cast for fractures of the proximal two thirds (Melone, 1990). Immobilisation for up to two months and sporting restriction for six months may be necessary.

Fractures of the hook of hamate are associated with sports involving holding sporting equipment. Diagnosis requires special radiographs including carpal tunnel views, oblique views in radial deviation or lateral views with the thumb abducted. Undisplaced fractures require immobilisation for up to three months. Surgical excision is recommended for displaced fractures (Bishop and Beckenbaugh, 1988).

Ligament injuries

Ligamentous disruptions may lead to carpal instability which may be static or dynamic. Static instabilities can often be identified on posterio-anterior (PA) and true lateral radiographs. PA x-rays may reveal an increased scapholunate interval (Terry Thomas sign). On lateral radiographs the scapholunate angle can be measured. Angles greater than 65° indicate scapholunate disassociation and angles less than 30° may mean ulnar instabilities.

Dorsal Intercalated Segmental Instability (DISI) exists if the capitolunate angle measures more than 15° (normal - zero degrees). This is associated with palmar subluxation and dorsiflexion of the lunate. The radiolunate angle is more than 30°. Volar Intercalated Segmental Instability (VISI) exists if the capitolunate angle is greater than -15° and the lunate is palmarflexed more than 30°. Dynamic deformities may require videofluorography and arthrography for their diagnosis.

Acute instability, when diagnosed, is probably best treated by percutaneous pinning and immobilisation though some recommend open repair. Most patients present with chronic instability and a localised intercarpal fusion may be beneficial if no secondary degenerative changes are present.

Disruption of the distal radioulnar joint may cause pain and instability. The triangular fibrocartilage complex (TFCC) acts as the major stabiliser of the radioulnar joint, serves as a cushion to the transfer of axial loads and stabilises the carpus on the forearm. In the acute injury if the ulnar head is unstable or painful to stressing, the arm should be immobilised in full supination with the elbow at 90°. CT scanning has been suggested to ensure accurate closed reduction of the joint. Tears of the TFCC may be diagnosed and even treated arthroscopically in skilled hands. Chronic instabilities of the distal radioulnar joint may require excision of the ulnar head and possible permanent wrist weakness.

Conclusion

Most hand and wrist injuries can be managed conservatively but the outcome is dependent on early and accurate diagnosis. The results of treatment for chronic deformity or instability are unpredictable and often lead to permanent impaired function. It behoves all persons involved in the management of hand and wrist injuries to be aware of the importance of careful examination and assessment of all injuries. Full restoration of function should be the aim though a realistic time scale should be given to the athlete at the start of treatment to prevent disregard of the advice, a premature return to sporting activities and a disappointing end result.

References

Bishop AT and Beckenbaugh RD. (1988) Fracture of the hamate hook. J Hand Surg, 13A, 135-139.

Borgeskov S, Christiansen B, Kjaer A and Balsey L. (1966) Fractures of the carpal bones. Acta Orthop Scand, 37, 276-287.

Cooney WP, Dobyns JH and Linscheid RL. (1980) Fractures of the scaphoid: a rational approach to management. Clin Orthop, 149, 90-99.

Curtis RM, Reis RL and Provost JM. (1983) A staged technique for the repair of the traumatic boutonniere deformity. J Hand Surg, 8, 167-171.

Green DP and Rowland SA. (1984) Fractures and Dislocations in the Hand, in Fractures in Adults (eds CA Rockwood and DP Green), JB Lippincott, Philadelphia, p. 388.

Melone CP. (1990) Fractures of the wrist, in The Upper Extremity in Sports Medicine (eds JA Nicholas and ER Hershman) The CV Mosby Company, St Louis, pp. 428-429.

Patel MR, Desai SS and Bassini-Lipson L. (1986) Conservative management of chronic mallet fingers. J Hand Surg, 11A, 570-573.

Posner MA. (1990) Hand Injuries, in The Upper Extremity in Sports Medicine (eds JA Nicholas and EB Hershman), The CV Mosby Company, St Louis, p. 496.

Souter WA. (1974) The problem of the boutonniere deformity. Clin Orthop, 104, 116-131.

The head, face and neck

Concussive injuries in rugby and their management

G.K. Vanderfield

Abstract. A modern definition of cerebral concussion is given after discussion of some earlier views. The value of grading to guide management and subsequent discussion is indicated. Return to competition should only be permitted after an appropriate examination by a doctor. Complications of the head injury must be suspected if a player is not recovering progressively afterwards and should be treated accordingly.

Keywords: Cerebral Concussion, Definition, Diagnosis, Management, References.

Introduction

The nature and implications of cerebral concussion often do not seem to be clearly understood by many involved in hard contact sport today. Accordingly, I believe the injury and its management are of considerable importance and warrant special attention.

For a long time concussion was explained as a result of sudden deformation of the skull; this either produced a sudden anaemia of the brain or possibly created a pressure wave transmitted by the cerebro-spinal fluid to the floor of the ventricles.

Following work by Denny-Brown and Richie Russell published in 1941 on "Experimental cerebral concussion" it was considered to be due to a sudden change in the velocity of the head rather than increase in intracranial pressure.

At that stage Jefferson and Symons had also reached the conclusion that concussion was neurogenic not vascular in origin and was essentially due to the alteration in neurophysiological activity in neurones in the hypothalamus or brainstem.

These views were consistent with the work of Magoun published in 1951 on the ascending reticular activating system in the brainstem and which indicated that this region was the site of the primary disturbance in concussion.

Definition

In 1964 a committee of the Congress of Neurological Surgeons headed by ES Gudjian proposed the following definition of concussion:
"A clinical syndrome characterised by immediate and transient impairment of

neural function, such as alteration of consciousness, disturbance of vision, motion, sensation, due to mechanical forces."

This definition has since been widely adopted.

It has further been considered that the depth of the initial disturbance and the rate of recovery may depend on such factors as the situation and number of neurones involved. With mild concussion the effects are transient and recovery follows. If the physical forces acting on the head are sufficient to cause loss of consciousness, then there is a risk that they may cause other injuries including fracturing of the skull, cerebral contusion and intracranial bleeding. Accordingly, if recovery of consciousness is delayed or there is deterioration then complications have to be suspected.

Thus there are good clinical reasons to stop a player returning to the game without an adequate medical examination, even if his early recovery appears good.

To guide further management on the field and subsequent decisions, the level of concussion should be graded according to severity as soon as first aid has been instituted.

It has become expedient to establish sub-divisions based on the duration and severity of the findings in order to enhance their practical application to injured footballers. In this regard Richard Schneider in 1969 recommended a classification into three grades as follows:

1   Mild - with little, if any, loss of consciousness.
2   Moderate - loss of consciousness with mild retrograde amnesia and a short period of post-traumatic amnesia.
3   Severe - unconsciousness longer than five minutes and a lengthier amnesia.

Field testing

Assessment on the field will be assisted by tests such as those shown in this Table 1.

Mental dullness and confusion can be judged by answers to questions such as "what is the score?" and "which half is it?" - if he answers "when is the game starting?" all concerned will realise his state.

If the pulse is weak and the colour pale he may have suffered an injury elsewhere and be suffering from syncope or surgical shock. These in some ways are similar but in concussion the initial loss of consciousness is the characteristic feature and effects are usually of shorter duration. Inequality of the pupils and diplopia or nystagmus may be evident. Signs of inco-ordination may be detected by the usual clinical tests.

Table 1   Field Testing in Concussion

Lying down	Conscious level
	General condition and pulse
	Eye movements and pupils
	Co-ordination - finger/nose, heel/shin
Standing	Balance
	Romberg's test
	Tandem walk
	Short run

If the player is well enough to get to his feet then his balance and co-ordination can be examined more adequately. If concussion has been severe and the player is still unconscious then he should be treated as if he may also have suffered a fractured cervical spine and be moved accordingly. A player should not be allowed to resume after a definitive concussive injury and, if he has sustained a severe concussion, he should not be allowed to play for at least three weeks. This recommendation is clearly put in the following Resolution of the International Rugby Football Board:

> "A player who has suffered definite concussion should not participate in any match or training session for a period of at least three weeks from the time of injury, and then only subject to being cleared by a proper neurological examination."

Return to game

This is an area in which it is important that coaches and officials exercise their discretion to protect the players and prevent them returning too soon. They will recover well usually, if given sufficient time. But it has to be remembered that even with simple concussion there has been evidence that neural changes might occur, and if further blows are sustained before recovery these will have a cumulative effect. An appropriate clinical examination is the best way to assess fitness to return to competition.

If there has been a previous concussion then return to contact sport should be delayed or possibly not permitted till the following season depending on the time and severity of each injury.

In my opinion the player cannot be cleared to return to sport just by negative CT scan of the brain. This is because the usual cuts taken are often not good enough to demonstrate fine changes such as petechial haemorrhages in the relevant regions. MRI will have more to offer when it becomes readily available but really all that CT scanning can do in most cases is to exclude complications such as supratentorial bleeding and haematomas.

Complications

Complications of the head injury associated with concussion should be suspected if a player is not recovering or is deteriorating, as it then usually means more than concussion and he should be taken straight to hospital.

Investigations

The following are suggested guidelines for the care of the player on arrival at hospital after a recent head injury.

Criteria for CT scan of the head

1   Slowness to recover consciousness
2   Neurological symptomatology
3   Severe local injury to the head
4   The occurrence of epileptic seizure

Criteria for Admission to hospital

1   Persistent confusion or deterioration of consciousness
2   Neurological symptoms or signs
3   Fracture of the skull
4   and/or an abnormal CT scan

In conclusion then I would point out that the assessment and management of concussive injuries is essentially clinical and I hope that these views gained from practising neurosurgery and treating rugby players over the years will be of assistance to those actively concerned in the management of the players who suffer such injuries.

References

Denny-Brown D and Russell R. (1941) Brain, **64**, 273.

Glossary of Head Injury including some definitions of injury of the Cervical Spine. (1986) Clin Neurosurg, 12, 388.

Gurdjian ES and Voris HC. (1966) A Glossary of Head Injury Nomenclature. Clin Neurosurg, The Williams & Wilkins Co, Baltimore, **12**, 388.

Jefferson G. (1944) The nature of concussion. Br Med J, **1**, 31.

Jefferson Sir G. (1955) Changing views on the Integration of the Brain. Clin Neurosurg, **1**, 1-10.

Magoun HW. (1951) The alerting system of the brain. CC Thomas, Springfield, Illinois.

Schneider RC and Kriss FC. (1969) Decisions Concerning Cerebral Concussion in Football Players. Med Sci Sports, **1**, 112.

Symonds CP. (1940) Concussion and contusion of the brain. In Brock's Injuries of the Skull, Brain and Spinal Cord, Baltimore.

The consequences of injuries to the spine and spinal cord in contact sports: the South African experience of rugby injuries

A.T. Scher

Abstract. A retrospective study was undertaken to determine aetiological factors for 117 catastrophic neck injuries in rugby players admitted to the Spinal Cord Unit, Conradie Hospital, Cape Town, South Africa between 1963 and 1989. The findings of this study were analysed in conjunction with the findings of an on-going research study commenced in 1977 into the mechanisms of rugby spinal injuries. The mechanisms of rugby injuries to the spine are briefly reviewed. Two other findings of interest that have emanated from the on-going research study were the identification of the entity of spinal cord concussion in rugby and the observation that rugby players are prone to premature onset of degenerative disease of the cervical spine. These observations are briefly reviewed. The results of the retrospective study demonstrate a dramatic increase in the number of injuries after 1976. This sustained increase has continued to date and contrasts with a falling incidence of these injuries in Britain, Australia and New Zealand. The principal risk factors identified for spinal cord injuries in rugby players were: the phase of play, match play, age, level of play, playing position and time of season. This study confirms that spinal cord injuries in rugby occur under predictable circumstances and are therefore foreseeable and preventable.

Keywords: Sports Medicine, Spinal Cord Injuries, Spinal Injuries, Spondylosis.

Introduction

Of all the sporting injuries, those to the spinal cord are the most tragic, leading, as they frequently do, to permanent quadriplegia with loss of bowel, bladder and sexual function (Scher, 1985).

Since the mid-1970s, increasing concern has been expressed about the incidence of catastrophic neck injuries in rugby (Walkden, 1975; Scher, 1977, 1978). The incidence of such injuries appears to have increased in all rugby playing countries in recent years (Williams and McKibbin, 1978; Hoskins, 1979; O'Carrol, Sheehan and Gregg, 1981; McCoy et al, 1984, Taylor and Coolican, 1987). In an attempt to identify the mechanisms of rugby injuries to the cervical spine and ultimately to arrive at preventive measures, I have been analysing these injuries since 1977 and the mechanisms of injury will briefly be reviewed.

During the course of this on-going research into rugby spinal injuries, two other findings of interest have been made. A group of players who have suffered spinal cord concussion (neurapraxia) in association with cervical spinal stenosis have been identified (Scher, 1991b) and will be discussed. Further, the suspicion that rugby players are prone to premature development of degenerative osteoarthrosis of the cervical spine has been confirmed in a study (Scher, 1990b) and the findings of this study will also be briefly presented.

South Africa has been no exception to the experience of other countries as regards the increase in incidence of rugby spinal cord injuries. Indeed, it has been stated that "in South Africa, rugby is associated with the highest incidence of spinal cord injury of all organised sports" (Tomasin, Martin and Curl, 1989). Yet the particular reasons why this should have occurred in South Africa are not known.

Accordingly, a retrospective study of 117 spinal cord injuries in South African rugby players was undertaken in collaboration with colleagues from the Spinal Cord Injuries Unit at Conradie Hospital and from the Department of Physiology at the University of Cape Town (Kew et al, 1990. This study has been done in order to determine whether factors to explain the increase in incidence of spinal injuries in rugby in South Africa could be identified.

Materials, subjects and methods

This study was conducted primarily from the Spinal Unit at Conradie Hospital in Pinelands, Cape Town. This is the only specialised spinal unit in the Cape Province and receives all spinal cord injuries occurring from whatever cause in the Cape Province, Namibia, Ciskei and Transkei.

We used three different methods to collect data: (i) admission files for 1963-1989 were accessed to determine the names of all persons admitted to the unit between 1963 and 1989 as a result of a spinal cord injury incurred while playing rugby; (ii) the medical files of these patients were accessed and all relevant information retrieved - this included length of hospital stay, radiological findings, final outcome, and most recent address; and (iii) a simple 7-page questionnaire was mailed to the last known address of the patients identified by (i) and (ii) above.

Results

One hundred and seventeen players with spinal cord injuries were admitted to the unit between 1963 and 1989, Fig. 1.

Fig. 2 compares the injury frequency by month for all schoolboys and adults.

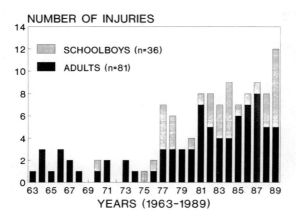

Fig. 1 The annual number of rugby players admitted to the Spinal Cord Unit at Conradie Hospital between 1963 and 1989. Adults and schoolboys are indicated separately.

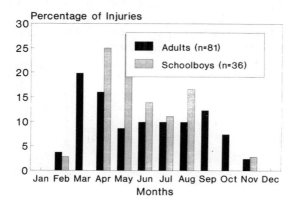

Fig. 2 Percentage of spinal cord injuries occurring in the different months of the year in adult and schoolboy rugby players. (Kew et al, 1991)

Table I lists the number of injuries in the different playing positions for the 76 players injured before 1989 who could be traced. When corrected by the uneven number of players in the different positions, Table I shows that hookers, centres and flyhalves were at the greatest risk of injury, whereas flanks, fullbacks and scrumhalves were at the least risk. Eighty-three per cent of players indicated that they were playing in their normal positions at the time of their injury.

Table I.   Percentage of spinal cord injuries in the different playing positions

	No. of injuries	Corrected %
Hooker	14	26.1
Centre	14	13.1
Flyhalf	6	11.2
Lock	10	9.4
Eighth man	5	7.5
Wing	8	7.5
Prop	7	6.5
Flank	6	5.6
Fullback	3	5.6
Scrumhalf	3	5.6
Total	76	100

Of the 52 injured players for whom the data were available, 36 (69%) were playing either in the first team (adults) or in the age-group A team (schoolboys). Only 2 players indicated that they were playing out of their usual teams. Fifty-one of these 52 injuries (98) occurred during matches.

The phase of play during which injury occurred for all 117 injuries is shown in Fig. 3.

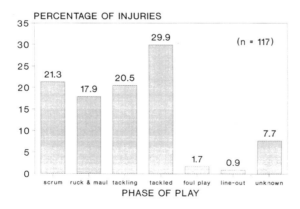

Fig. 3 Percentage of spinal cord injuries occurring in the different phases of play. (Kew et al, 1991)

Table II shows that the majority (85%) of the scrummaging injuries occurred in the front row forwards, whereas the majority (67%) of tackling-related neck injuries occurred to backline players. Sixty-five per cent of the injuries occurring during rucking and mauling were incurred by the forwards.

Table II.   Percentage of 76 injuries occurring in the different phases of play in the different playing positions

Phase of play

Position	Scrum	Ruck and maul	Tackling	Being tackled	Foul play	Line-out	Total
Front row	17	5	0	4	1	0	27
Forwards	3	8	8	7	1	1	28
Halfbacks	0	4	1	7	0	0	12
Backline	0	3	16	14	0	0	33
Total	20	20	25	32	2	1	100
	40		57		3		

Fig. 4 shows the number of injuries by year that occurred either during tackling or the scrum, rucking and mauling.

Fifty-two per cent of players reported that they were injured while playing on level fields; 25% felt that the field was uneven; another 10% reported that potholes were present on the field. Eight per cent of injuries occurred on fields that were not grassed. Only 6% of injuries occurred in wet playing conditions.

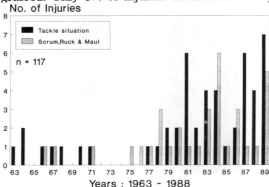

Fig. 4   The annual number of spinal cord injuries that occurred in three different phases of play. (Kew et al, 1991)

Table III lists the radiological level of the cervical injury and the corresponding phase of of play in which the injury occurred. The majority (81% of injuries occurred at spinal levels C4/C5 and C5/C6. There was no relationship between the level of injury and the phase of play in which the injury happened.

TABLE III. PERCENTAGE OF INJURIES OCCURRING AT DIFFERENT SPINAL LEVELS AND THE PHASE OF PLAY IN WHICH THE INJURY OCCURRED

| | | | Spinal level | | | |
Phase	C3/C4	C4/C5	C5/C6	C6/C7	T1-T8	>T8
Tackled	3	11	14	3	4	0
Tackling	0	11	9	2	0	0
Scrum	1	13	9	4	2	1
Ruck & maul		0	6	5	2	00
Foul	0	1	1	0	0	0
Line-out	0	1	0	0	0	0
	–	—	—	—	–	–
Total	4	43	38	11	6	1

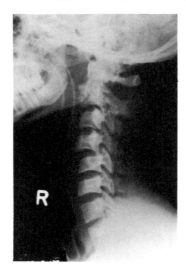

Fig. 5   Unilateral facet dislocation at the C4/C5 level. Fatal injuries sustained by hooker in scrum. (Courtesy South African Medical Journal)

Mechanisms of injury

I have been analysing the mechanisms of rugby spinal injuries since 1977 and have reported my findings in a series of papers (Scher, 1977, 1978, 1979, 1980, 1981a, 1981b, 1982a, 1982b, 1983a, 1983b, 1985, 1987, 1989, 1990a, 1990b, 1991a, 1991b).

These analyses have consisted of a careful correlation of the history of injury, neurological deficit on admission to the Spinal Injuries Centre and analysis of the admission x-rays of the cervical spine. These surveys have led to the conclusion that spinal cord injuries in rugby players are due to the same mechanisms responsible for spinal cord injury due to other trauma. These mechanisms of injury are consistent, predictable and correlate well with the circumstances of injury as described by the players. The mechanisms of injury as revealed by the previous studies mentioned will briefly be reviewed. The phases of the game that have been identified as being responsible for the majority of these injuries are the tight scrum, the tackle, rucks and mauls.

Scrum injuries

Analysis of the orthopaedic injuries sustained after the collapse of the scrum have consistently shown a similar pattern of injury, allowing two important conclusions to be made. Firstly, the common mechanism of injury is hyperflexion trauma as the major injuring force, with a rotational component in cases of unilateral facet dislocation, Fig. 5. Secondly, a striking majority of players suffered anterior dislocation with bilateral locking of facets, Fig. 6.

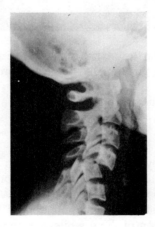

Fig. 6   Anterior dislocation of C4 on 5 with bilateral locking of facets. Injuries sustained after collapse of the scrum. (Courtesy South African Medical Journal)

This marked preponderance of one particular type of orthopaedic injury is of considerable importance because it is indicative of the mechanism of injury, and because of all the orthopaedic injuries to the cervical spine, it is the one with the most grave prognosis regarding paralysis and death, Fig. 7.

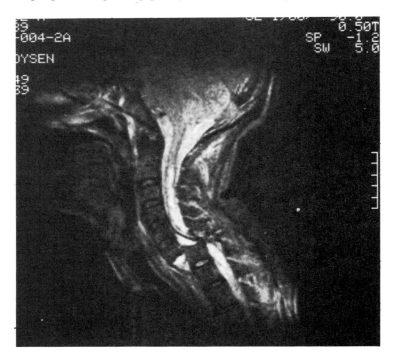

Fig. 7   Sagittal Magnetic Resonance image showing anterior dislocation of C6 on C7. Note the pinching of the spinal cord at the level of dislocation. There is a high intensity (white) signal in the spinal cord from C2 to T1 indicating haemorrhage of the cord.

The collapsing scrum

The collapsing tight rugby scrum would appear to be an ideal mechanism for producing flexion injury to the cervical spine. The front row and locks have their heads and necks held in a position of slight flexion. When the ball is put into the scrum, the entire scrum pushes forward and, should the front row collapse, the rest of the pack often keep on pushing while the front row players are unable to extricate themselves, Fig. 8. It has been calculated that the force exerted at the point of maximum pressure, that is, the back of the neck of the player in the middle of the scrum can reach a magnitude of 1.5 tons (Stubbs, 1981).

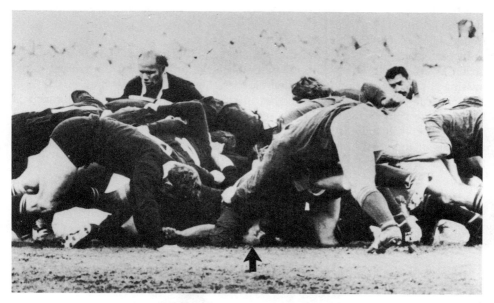

Fig. 8   The head and neck of the prop in the foreground (arrowed) have been forced into acute flexion by the collapsing scrum. (Courtesy South African Medical Journal)

Injury due to crashing of the scrum

Deliberate crashing in an attempt to intimidate or unsettle the opposing pack is a contravention of the rules, as clearly stated in The Laws of the Game of Rugby Football (1981), O'Carrol, Shehan and Gregg (1981). The force or "impact weight" exerted as the packs meet is considerable and, if the front rows are not correctly positioned a dangerous situation may arise. In a study of the kinetics of scrummaging, it was reported (Milburn, 1990) that the forces generated on engagement of the two packs were the greatest of all the forces sustained in the scrum, and that the magnitude of the impulsive, impact force experienced when a scrum engages exceeds the threshold for injury to the spine. This force is related directly to the mass (weight) of the scrum and its speed of engagement.

Tackling injuries

Spinal injuries are sustained by both the tackler because of incorrect technique, and the tackled player, as a consequence of the force of the tackle and the severity of impact on being forced to the ground.

An analysis of the circumstances of and types of injuries sustained reveals three specific mechanisms of injury: injury due to impact of the tackler's head; (2) injury due to the high tackle; and (3 injury due to the double or "sandwich" tackle.

Injury due to impact of the tackler's head
In this group, the player, having launched himself through the air to make a tackle, is brought to a halt abruptly when his head strikes either the ground (after missing his opponent) or the tackled player's thigh.

When the neck is slightly flexed, as in the diving position, normal lordosis is lost and the spine straightens. If severe force is applied to the top of the head when the cervical spine is in straight alignment, this force is transmitted down the long axis of the spine, causing compression fractures of the vertebral bodies, Fig. 9.

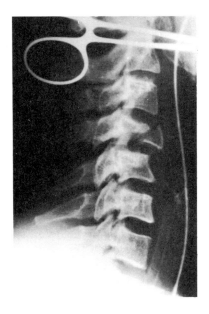

Fig. 9   "Tear-drop", flexion-compression fracture of the vertebral body of C4 sustained after direct impact of the tackler's head into the ground after an unsuccessful dive tackle. (Courtesy South African Medical Journal)

Injuries sustained while being tackled

The high tackle
The spinal injuries sustained by the players subjected to a high tackle varied according to the direction of the tackle. Some players were tackled from behind, the tackler wrapping one arm around his opponent's neck and pulling posteriorly

and downwards. Force applied in this manner would be liable to produce a hyperextension injury to the cervical spine. Because the tackle is made with one arm, the neck tends to become twisted as it is forced into hyperextension, thereby adding rotational stress to the hyperextension force, Fig. 10.

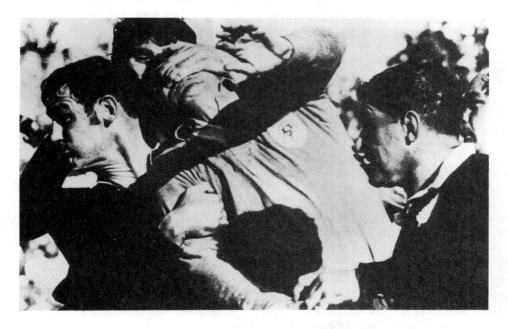

Fig. 10   Extension force applied to the face during a tackle. (Courtesy South African Medical Journal)

Other players were tackled from the side, with the tackler wrapping one arm around the neck and forcing it into hyperflexion, Fig. 11.

Rotational force is also applied to the neck in this type of tackle. All these players sustained flexion-rotation injuries to the spine. It is the rotational stress applied to the cervical spine during a high tackle in particular that makes this type of tackling so dangerous. A player running with the ball or attempting to kick it may have one or both feet off the ground when tackled, Fig. 12. He is then less able to withstand the force being applied to his neck. In addition to being off balance, he is usually unaware of the impending tackle and therefore unable to tense his cervical muscles against the attack.

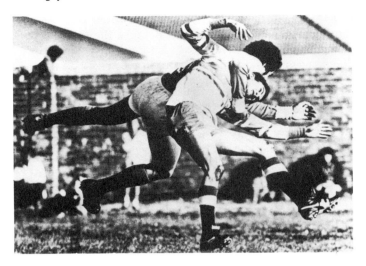

Fig. 11   Tackle around the neck made with one arm. Note that the tackled
player's neck is being both flexed and rotated. (Courtesy South African
Medical Journal)

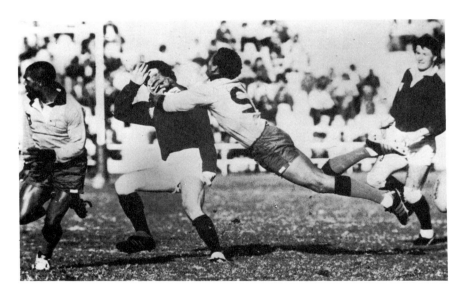

Fig. 12   High tackle of player caught off balance.

The double tackle

This is a rare cause of cervical injury. A double tackle occurs when a player is tackled simultaneously by two opponents. This is also sometimes referred to as a "scissors" or "sandwich" tackle. The double tackle places both the tackled player and tacklers at risk. The tacklers may collide with each other in mid-air, missing their opponent completely. If the double tackle is made successfully, the tackled player is vulnerable to cervical injury for the following reasons.

The tackler nearest to the ball carrier usually tackles low (around the thighs or waist) so that the second tackler is forced to go in high and take the ball carrier around the chest, shoulders or neck, as shown in Fig. 13.

Because the first tackler often tackles fractionally before the second tackler, the tackled player is actually falling forward, allowing the second tackler to tackle from above (see Fig. 5), increasing the force applied to the neck at the moment of impact. Further, because the lower body of the tackled player is firmly held, he is unable to "go" with the momentum of the tackle, and this increases the force dissipated on the cervical spine, particularly as regards rotational stress.

Injuries sustained in rucks and mauls

Ten (20 per cent) of the players in our series were injured in rucks and mauls. These two phases of loose play are not only responsible for spinal injury, but are also an important cause of rugby injuries generally. Illegal play is often generated in rucks and mauls, and 70 percent of the injuries sustained are usually due to kicking and trampling, Fig. 14.

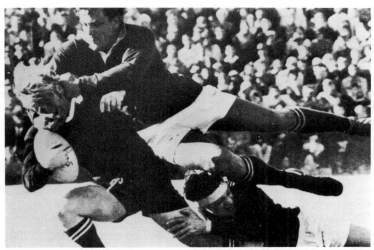

Fig. 13   The tremendous force which can be exerted on the neck of a falling player during a double tackle is well illustrated. (Courtesy South African Medical Journal)

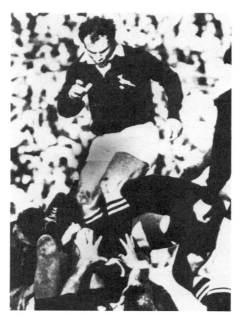

Fig. 14   Deliberate trampling of an opponent. (Courtesy South African Medical Journal)

Spinal injuries as a result of loose play occur in three different ways:

1) forced flexion of the ball carrier's neck, Fig. 15;
2) forced flexion of the neck of the player at the bottom of the ruck; or
3) head and neck injury due to charging into a mass of struggling players.

Discussion of retrospective study findings

The most distinctive characteristics of rugby football in the past 20 years has been the simultaneous and dramatic rise in the annual number of spinal cord injuries reported in all rugby playing countries in which the data have been reported, including England (Hoskins, 1979; Silver, 1984 and 1988), Wales (Williams and McKibbin, 1978 and 1987), New Zealand (Burry and Gowland, 1981; Burry and Calcinai, 1988) Eire and Northern Ireland (O'Carrol, Sheehan and Gregg, 1981; McCoy, Piggot, Macafee, 1984) and Australia (Wiggelsworth, 1987; Taylor and Coolican, 1981). Even countries that have only started playing rugby fairly recently, including Canada (Sovio, Van Petegham and Schweigel, 1984) and the USA (Akpata, 1990) have reported the same phenomenon.

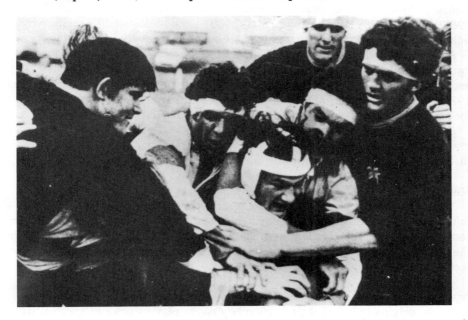

Fig. 15   Twisting of the neck of the ball-carrier in a maul. (Courtesy South African Medical Journal)

For example in England the average number of spinal cord injuries reported each year between 1970 and 1976 was 1.9. This rose suddenly to 6.2 per annum between 1977 and 1982 (Silver, 1984) before falling thereafter (Fig. 5), (Silver, 1984 and 1988). In Australia, 81% of all spinal cord injuries in rugby players and 100% of these injuries in schoolboys have occurred since 1977. In the USA, all but 2 of 42 injuries occurred after 1975. Only in New Zealand was the reported incidence already high as early as 1973; (Burry and Gowland, 1981), nevertheless there was a dramatic increase from an average of 9 injuries per annum to 17 in 1978.

Our study shows that an identical pattern is clearly present in the geographical area of South Africa included in this study. Fig. 1 shows that relatively few (17%) of these injuries occurred before the 1977 season with a progressive increase subsequently.

However, what is even more disturbing is that, uniquely in this geographical area, the number of these injuries has **increased** further in the recent past, whereas in England (Silver, 1988), Australia (Taylor and Coolican, 1987) and New Zealand

(Burry and Calcinai, 1988) the annual number of these injuries has fallen quite remarkably. The failure of the local rugby authorities timeously to adopt specific measures found to be effective in England and Australasia (Taylor and Coolican, 1987; Silver, 1988; Burry and Calcinai, 1988) would adequately explain why the number of these injuries has continued to increase uniquely in this country.

An important finding in this and all similar studies is that the mechanisms of injury previously described are entirely predictable. These injuries are not "freak accidents", as is frequently claimed by influential rugby administrators (Craven, 1989). This study advances these findings by identifying 6 predictable risk factors for spinal cord injuries in rugby players listed in Table IV.

Risk factors for spinal cord injuries in rugby players

Match play

The most obvious risk factor was match play. Ninety-eight per cent of all injuries occurred during match play. This finding is especially significant, since considerably more time is spent in practice than in match play. It would seem that the competitiveness and aggression unleashed in match play must be an important factor contributing to these injuries.

Age

It was originally believed that schoolboy rugby players were at greatest risk of spinal cord injury (Scher, 1979). This and other studies refute this. Sixty-nine per cent of all injuries in this study were sustained by adults. The significance of this is that in most rugby playing countries, except possibly the USA and Canada, far more schoolboys than adults play rugby. In the geographical area of this study, the ratio of schoolboy to adult rugby players may be of the order of 510:1. Thus the more than twofold greater number of spinal cord injuries in adult players could indicate a 10 - 12-fold higher risk for this injury in adults than in schoolboys.

This finding also contradicts statements of the President of the South African Rugby Board (Craven, 1989a and 1989b) to the effect that the rising incidence of spinal cord injuries in this country is due simply to a rising incidence of injury among unfit schoolboys, the so-called "television sissy" or "couch-potato syndrome".

Level of play

The third risk factor is level of play. Injury risk was greatest at the higher levels of play, since 69% of injuries were suffered by players in either first or age-group A teams. Since there are relatively few such players in the total rugby-playing population, this finding suggests that high levels of both skill and physical fitness, far from protecting against these injuries, must actually make injury more likely.

The greater number of injuries in the more skilled players is probably explained

TABLE IV. PERCENTAGE OF INJURIES OCCURRING IN THE DIFFERENT PHASES OF PLAY IN THE DIFFERENT COUNTRIES

| | Scrum | | | Tackle | | | Ruck |
Country	Collapse	Engagement	Total scrum	Tackling	Being tackled	Total tackle&	maul
Wales (1974-1977)[7]	33	22	55	33	11	44	0
Wales (1964-1984)[26]	30	3	40*	10	20	30	30
New Zealand (1973-1984)[12]	-	-	36	-	-	30	34
New Zealand (1980-1984)[31]	-	-	52	-	-	34	14
New Zealand (1985-1986)[31]	0	0	20*	-	-	60	20
N Ireland (1979-1980)[23]	42	0	42	-	-	18	42
Eire (1977-1983)[13]	40	0	40	-	-	60	0
Canada (1975-1982)[21]	-	-	56	-	-	22	22
England (1973-1978)[9]	39	0	39	8	19	27	27
England (1952-1982)[24]	-	-	21	17	20	40	30
England (1983-1987)[30]	21	16	37	-	-	26	32
Australia (1960-1985)[29]	19	40	62*	-	-	22	14
USA (1970-1989)[35]	14	31	62*	22	7	29	9
South Africa (1962-1989) (this study)	-	-	21	21	30	51	18

- indicates that no data exist.
* balance of scrum injuries due to "lifting" or "popping" the scrum.

by their more aggressive approach to the game and their more dangerous style of play (Silver, 1984; Schneider, 1973) both of which might be explained by a "win at all costs" attitude associated with "psyching up" (McCoy et al, 1984; Silver, 1984); Williams and McKibbin, 1987; Taylor and Coolican, 1987; Silver and Gill, 1988). This possibility is further supported by the finding that these injuries occur almost exclusively during matches.

Phase of play

As has repeatedly been shown, four different phases of play contribute the vast majority of these injuries. In this study the tackling phase of the game including tackling (21%) and being tackled (30%) accounted for more than half all injuries (Fig. 3), with the tight scrum (21%) and the ruck and maul (18%) accounting for the majority (39%) of the remaining injuries. Scrum engagement ("crashing the scrum") is a significant contributor to scrum injuries in England, but especially in Australia and the USA in which countries more than 30% of all injuries result from this single mechanism.

Playing position

Backline players suffer most of their injuries in the tackling situation (Silver, 1984) whereas props and hookers are at risk during scrummaging (Barry and Gowland, 1981; Silver, 1984; Taylor and Coolican, 1987; Akpata, 1990). Ruck and maul injuries appear to be more common in forwards (Silver, 1984). It follows that the players at greatest risk will be determined by the specific mechanisms of injury that predominate in any particular country.

In this study the position that carried by far the highest risk was the hooker (Table I). This is a finding common to studies from New Zealand (Burry and Gowland, 1981), Australia (Taylor and Coolican, 1987) and the USA (Akpata, 1990).

Surprisingly, only one previous study has detailed the exact playing positions of injured backline players (Williams and McKibbin, 1987). As in this study, centres and flyhalves were at greatest risk. Virtually all injuries to backline players (85%) occurred during the tackling phase of the game (Table II); the rest occurred in the ruck and maul.

Injuries to forwards, other than the front row, also occur during tackling (54%), the ruck and maul (29%) and scrummaging (11%).

Playing out of position was not a major factor predisposing to injury in this study. The danger of putting an inexperienced player in a high-risk position, such as hooker or prop, is obvious (Silver, 1984; Burry and Calcinai, 1988).

Time of season

As shown in Fig. 2, the period of greatest risk for both adult and schoolboy rugby players was at the start of the season and again after the mid-season break. As repeatedly stated, it is clear that more attention should be paid to pre-season fitness training for rugby players at all levels (Scher, 1979; Akpata, 1990; Nathan, Goedeke and Noakes, 1990; Roux et al, 1987; Clark, Roux and Noakes, 1990).

Other factors

Ground conditions.   Ground conditions seem not to have been a factor, since 60% of injured players indicated that the match was played on a level, well-grassed surface. It has been postulated that wet or soft playing surfaces, particularly in the Western Cape, may cause the scrum in particular to be unstable and therefore more likely to collapse. However, only 3 players (6%) indicated that they were injured while playing on wet surfaces. Thus this study does not provide any evidence that wet playing surfaces, are an important aetiological factor for spinal cord injuries or that this would explain the apparently higher incidence of these injuries in this part of the country.

Foul play.   Only 2 players (3%) reported that they were injured as a result of dirty or foul play. This contrasts with the large proportion of injuries resulting from foul play in England (16%) and Australia (26%) (Taylor and Coolican, 1987).

Players' perception of injury prevention.   Fifty-five per cent of the injured players felt that their injuries could have been avoided either by stricter refereeing, greater awareness of dangerous situation, improved coaching, better first aid and other medical facilities or through rule changes aimed at making the game safer. Specific rule changes were not mentioned.

Review of survey findings

It is evident that the number of catastrophic spinal cord injuries in Cape Province rugby players has increased dramatically since 1977 (Scher, 1989 and 1990a). This increase is not due to any single factor but to an increase in the number of injuries in all phases of play.

It is also important to appreciate that serious spinal cord injuries represent only the "tip of the iceberg" (Taylor and Coolican, 1987) of all rugby neck injuries. Our at present unpublished evidence suggests that for each serious spinal cord injury in rugby players, there may be as many as 10 severe neck injuries without spinal cord involvement. It is clear that rule changes can have a major effect in reducing the incidence of spinal cord injuries. It is therefore particularly disturbing that the Chairman of the Medical Committee of the South African Rugby Board should write (Hugo, 1990) as recently as June 1990 that: "It is obvious that none of the published reports analysed the true mechanisms of (spinal cord) injuries.... It has become essential to obtain a more accurate analysis of these rugby injuries before any constructive recommendation can be proposed to improve the game and to make it a safer one". The evidence presented here directly contradicts that statement.

Spinal cord concussion

During an analysis of rugby players who had sustained cervical spinal cord injury, a group of 9 players were identified who had sustained only transient paralysis and on x-ray revealed no evidence of fracture or dislocation of the cervical spine.

A retrospective analysis of the clinical and radiological findings in this group of rugby players has been made. The cervical spine x-rays were analysed for evidence of spinal stenosis, congenital anomalies and degenerative disc disease. Using the ratio method of assessment for spinal stenosis, spinal canal narrowing maximally at C3 and C4 was found in 5 of the 9 players. In the remaining 4 players, one showed evidence of osteoarthritic change at 2 levels while another had congenital fusion of two vertebral bodies, Fig. 16. In 2 players, no radiological evidence of any abnormality was detected.

Spinal cord concussion is a transient disturbance of spinal cord function, with or without vertebral damage and no demonstrable pathological change, that results from a rapid change in velocity following trauma, and resolves within 48 hours (Del Bigio and Johnson, 1989).

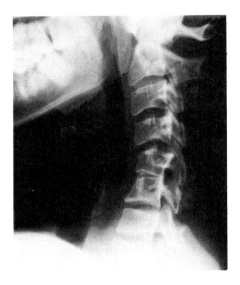

Fig.16.   Congenital fusion of the vertebral bodies of C5 and C6 in the cervical spine of a rugby player who sustained spinal cord concussion.

The association between developmental stenosis of the spinal canal and the development of spinal cord pathology was first commented on in 1957 (Payne and Spillane, 1957). Narrowing of the sagittal diameter of the cervical spine may be as a result of a diffuse developmental condition or an acquired stenosis, usually in association with osteoarthrosis.

It is particularly hyperextension trauma that places patients with developmental or acquired spinal canal narrowing at risk. Hyperextension causes the posterior longitudinal ligament and the ligamentum flavum to thicken, the dural diameter to decrease in size, and the diameter of the spinal cord to increase in size.

Previous reports have shown that in patients with congenital fusion, the remaining free articulations are more susceptible to acute trauma due to the relative inflexibility of the cervical spine (Scher, 1979). These players are particularly prone to hyperextension trauma and in a report on spinal cord concussion in American Football players 5 players who sustained temporary paralysis had congenital fusion of cervical vertebral bodies (Torg et al, 1986).

The question of whether a player who has sustained neurapraxia of the cervical spinal cord should be allowed to continue playing is a controversial one. In a group of 6 American Football players who had suffered episodes of spinal cord concussion and subsequently continued to play football, 3 had second episodes within 2 years of the initial episode.

In view of the above, rugby players with spinal stenosis or vertebral fusion who have escaped the catastrophe of spinal cord injury on one occasion would be well advised to channel their sporting activities into a less dangerous direction.

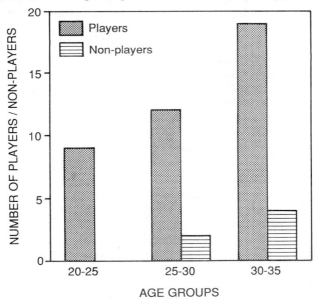

Fig. 17   Radiological changes of degenerative disease of the cervical spine in 150 rugby players and in a control group of 150 non-rugby players of different ages. (Courtesy South African Medical Journal)

Table V.   Playing position in the 40 players showing changes of degeneration

disease

Position   No of players

Front Row and locks 30
Loose Forwards   4
Backs   6

Premature onset of degenerative disease of the cervical spine in rugby players

There have been very few studies on the effect of chronic, recurrent trauma of the cervical spine. Nevertheless, the observation of radiographic changes of severe degenerative disease of the cervical spine seen in rugby players with complaints of cervical and arm pain suggested that players were prone to an earlier onset of degenerative disease. Confirmation of this supposition was therefore investigated by obtaining radiographs of the cervical spine of 150 asymptomatic club rugby players, ranging in age from 20 to 35 years. Similar x-rays of a control group of 150 non-rugby playing men with an identical age spectrum, were also obtained.

The radiographs were assessed for the presence of the following conditions:

1. Degenerative disease of the cervical spine.

   The following criteria were used:
   (i)   disc space narrowing of at least 50%;
   (ii) evidence of sclerosis of the subchondral bone of the   vertebral body in relation to the disc space narrowing;
   (iii) osteophytic spurring, either anterior or posterior;
   (iv) evidence of degenerative disease at the apophyseal joints as demonstrated by osteophyte formation, sclerosis or subluxation.
2.   Any bony deformity suggestive of a previous fracture of the posterior elements or vertebral body.
3. Evidence of congenital or acquired fusion

Results

Incidence of degenerative change
As can be seen from Fig.17, a significantly higher percentage of rugby players showed changes of degenerative disease of the spine, Fig. 18, ccmpared to the control group.

The 40 players showing degenerative changes were then divided according to their playing position. As can be seen from Table V, the highest incidence of degenerative disease was present in the tight forwards (props and locks).

Evidence of previous vertebral fracture
Eight of the 150 players showed evidence of healed fractures; 6 had compression fractures of the vertebral bodies and 2 fractures of the spinous processes.

Presence of congenital or acquired fusion.
Only 1 of the 150 rugby players showed change of congenital fusion.

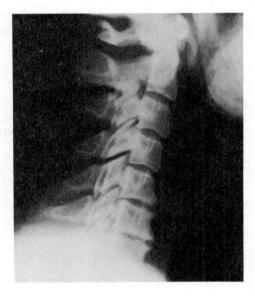

Fig.18.   Marked disc space narrowing and osteophytosis at the C5/C6 and C6/C7 levels in the cervical spine of a 26-year old prop.

Discussion
The findings indicated a higher incidence of degenerative disease of the cervical spine in rugby players in particular those who play as tight forwards than in the general population.
Given the tremendous strain to which the cervical spine and supporting structures are submitted in the tight scrum, it is not surprising that degenerative disease of the cervical spine occurs at an earlier age and with greater severity in front row forwards and locks.
The risk of spinal cord injury is also increased in the presence of degenerative

disease. Under these circumstances, the spinal cord is vulnerable to damage after hyperextension injury to the head or neck, even in the absence of any fracture or dislocation. In view of the above findings and potential dangers, the necessity for routine radiological examination of the cervical spine of all rugby players is evident. It would not be unreasonable to suggest that all rugby players, participating regularly in club or social rugby, undergo radiological examination of the cervical spine at least once during their playing career.

Should any abnormality be present, the radiologist's report will draw the attention of the player to these changes. The player, in consultation with his medical practitioner can then decide whether to continue his active rugby career. If significant changes are present and particularly if his playing position is that of a tight forward, he will be well advised to either cease playing or to change his playing position to one where his cervical spine is less exposed to stress.

References

Akpata T. (1990) Spinal injuries in US rugby: 1970-1990. Rugby, April/May, 14-15.

Burry HC and Calcinai CJ. (1988) The need to make rugby safer. Br Med J, 296, 149-150.

Burry HC and Gowland H. (1981) Cervical injury in rugby football - a New Zealand survey. Br J Sports Med, 15, 56-59.

Clark DR, Roux C and Noakes TD. (1990) A prospective study of the incidence and nature of injuries to adult rugby players. S Afr Med J, 77, 559-562.

Craven DH. (1989) Quoted by McCraken P: "Who is wrecking rugby?" Personality, 7 August, 7, 14.

Craven DH. (1989) Quoted by Partridge T: "Craven is set on ruling out scrums". Sunday Times, Jhbg, June 11.

Del Bigio MR and Johnson GE. (1989) Clinical presentation of Spinal Cord Concussion. Spine, 14, 37-39.

Horan FT. (1984) Injuries to the cervical spine in schoolboys playing rugby football (Editorial). J Bone Jt Surg (Br), 66, 470471.

Hoskins T. (1979) Rugby injuries to the cervical spine in English schoolboys. Practitioner, 223, 365-366.

Hugo EP. (1990) Severe spinal injuries in South African rugby, 1990 - a true perspective. South African Association for Sports Science, Physical Education and Recreation/South African Sports Medicine Association Congress Abstracts, Port Elizabeth, 25-28 June 1990, 13.

Kew T, Noakes TD, Kettles AN, Goedeke RE, Newton DA and Scher AT. (1991) A retrospective study of spinal cord injuries in Cape Province rugby players, 1963-1989. S Afr Med J, 801, 127-133.

McCoy GF, Piggot J, Macafee AL and Adair IV. (1984) Injuries to the cervical spine in schoolboy rugby football. J Bone Joint Surg (Br), 66, 500-503.

Milburn PD. (1990) The kinetics of Rugby Union scrummaging. J Sports Sci, 8, 47-60.

Nathan N, Goedeke R and Noakes TD. (1983) The incidence and nature of rugby injuries experienced at one school during the 1982 rugby season. S Afr Med J, 64, 132-137.

Noakes TD. (1980) For Chris Burger. S Afr Sports Med, 10, 11-13.

O'Carrol PF, Sheehan JM and Gregg TM. (1981) Cervical spine injuries in rugby football. Ir Med J, 74, 377-379.

Payne EE and Spillane JD. (1957) The Cervical Spine: An Anatomico-Pathological Study of 70 Specimens (Using a Special Technique) with particular reference to the problem of

Cervical Spondylosis. Brain, **80**, 571-596.

Roux C, Goedeke R, Visser GR. Van Zyl AW and Noakes TD. (1987) The epidemiology of schoolboy rugby injuries. S Afr Med J, **71**, 307-313.

Scher AT. (1977) Rugby injuries to the cervical spinal cord. Afr Med J, **51**, 473-475.

Scher AT. (1978) The high rugby tackle - an avoidable cause of cervical spinal injury. S Afr Med J, **53**, 1015-1018.

Scher AT. (1979) Rugby injuries to the cervical spinal cord (Correspondence). S Afr Med J, **56**, 205.

Scher AT. (1980) Rugby injuries to the cervical spinal cord (Correspondence). S Afr Med J, **57**, 37.

Scher AT. (1981a) The high rugby tackle - a continuing menace. S Afr Sports Med, **11**, 3-5.

Scher AT. (1981b) Vertex impact and cervical dislocation in rugby players. S Afr Med J, **59**, 227-228.

Scher AT. (1982a) Rugby injuries to the cervical spinal cord sustained during rucks and mauls. S Afr Med J, **64**, 592-594.

Scher AT. (1982b) "Crashing" the scrum - an avoidable cause of cervical spinal injury. S Afr Med J, **64**, 919-920.

Scher AT. (1983a) Rugby injuries of the upper cervical spine. S Afr Med J, **64**, 456-458.

Scher AT. (1983b) The "double tackle" - another cause of cervical
spinal injury in rugby players. S Afr Med J, **64**, 595-596.

Scher AT. (1985) Neck and back injuries. S Afr J Cont Med Educ, 3 Nov, 39-48.

Scher AT. (1987) Rugby injuries of the spine and spinal cord. Clin Sports Med, **6**, 87-99.

Scher AT. (1989) Rugby injuries of the cervical spine and spinal cord - has the situation improved? (Opinion). S Afr Med J, **76**, 46.

Scher AT. (1990a) Rugby injuries of the cervical spine and spinal cord - has the situation improved? S Afr Sports Med, **5**, 9-14.

Scher AT. (1990b) Premature onset of degenerative disease of the cervical spine in rugby players. S Afr Med J, **77**, 557-558.

Scher AT. (1991a) Paralysis due to the high tackle - a black spot in South African rugby. S Afr Med J, **79**, 614-615.

Scher AT. (1991b) Spinal cord concussion in rugby players. Am J Sports Med, Sept/Oct.

Schneider RC. (1973) Head and Neck Injuries in Football. Williams & Wilkins, Baltimore, 3-4.

Silver JR. (1984) Injuries of the spine sustained in rugby. Br Med J, **288**, 37-43.

Silver JR and Gill S. (1988) Injuries of the spine sustained during rugby. Sports Med, **5**, 328-334.

Sovio OM, Van Petegham PK and Schweigel JF. (1984) Cervical spine injuries in rugby players. Can Med Assoc J, **138**, 735-736.

Stubbs DA. (1980) Personal communication.

Taylor TKF and Coolican MRJ. (1987) Spinal-cord injuries in Australian footballers, 1960-1985. Med J Aust, **147**, 109-110.

Tomasin JD, Martin DF and Curl WW. (1989) Recognition and prevention of rugby injuries. Physician Sportsmed, **17**, 114-126.

Torg JS, Pavlov H, Genuario SE, Sennett B, Wisneski RJ, Robie BH and Jahre C. (1986) Neurapraxia of the Cervical Spinal Cord with Transient Quadriplegia. J Bone & Jt Surg, **68-A**, 1354-1370.

Walkden L. (1975) The medical hazards of rugby football. Practitioner, **215**, 201-207.

Wiggelsworth EC. (1987) Spinal injuries and football. Med J Aust, **147**, 109-110.

Williams JPR and McKibbin B. (1978) Cervical spine injuries in Rugby Union football. Br Med J, **2**, 1747.

Williams P and McKibbin B. (1987) Unstable cervical spine injuries in rugby - a 20-year review. Injury, **18**, 329-332.

PART SIX

Closing papers

Introduction   Closing papers

Three papers have been included in the closing section of the Proceedings. Throughout this publication the papers have dealt with sportsmen and women but the spectators also deserve consideration. After a series of tragic accidents the Lord Justice Taylor Report entitled 'Safety in Sports Grounds' set the standards which were incorporated in an Act of Parliament passed by the British Government. The Taylor Report and subsequent Act have been the subject of detailed scrutiny and are of direct relevance to all sports bodies and sports medicine.

The athletes' 'will to win' in competitive sport is such that they are prepared to make enormous personal, family, social and career sacrifices to get to the top. Prevention of burn-out and injury by appropriate team work between the athlete, the coach, the fitness adviser, the doctor, health care professionals and sports scientists is the underlying concept which the International Rugby Football Board hopes will result from the Sports Medicine Congress proceedings in this publication.

D.A.D. Macleod

Medical facilities at stadia: the Taylor report and the Medical Officer

W.S. Hillis

Abstract. Supervision of First Aid Facilities at grounds is an important function of the Sports Medical Officer. This requires supervision of a First Aid Room and equipment and requires the co-ordination of services including Police, First Aid Workers, Ambulance authorities and Stewards within the ground. The Taylor report has provided guidelines and has major implications, not only for major sporting events, but also for clubs with only occasional needs for crowd control and safety provision. (Taylor)

Keywords: Spectators, First Aid Facilities, Crowd Doctor, Order and Security in the Stadia.

Introduction

Sport is for the enjoyment of all, the players, the supportive, technical and medical staff and the spectators. The presence of a large crowd greatly adds to the excitement of all sporting events, but unfortunately in the presence of large crowds problems of safety may occasionally arise. Over the years different problems have been recognised and a general improvement in attitudes to safety have arisen. These problems have been addressed in the aftermath of such disasters as that occurring in Ibrox Stadium in 1970, the Bradford City ground fire, the Heysel Stadium riot and, most recently, the Hillsborough Stadium tragedy of April 1989 when some 95 deaths occurred, and many more spectators were injured. This last disaster focused attention on the provision of medical emergency services and highlighted the problems of co-ordination involving police control, provision and access of emergency vehicles, and the creation and coordination of medical facilities. In view of the problems associated with such provisions, specific recommendations were made following the enquiry and final report from Lord Justice Taylor in January 1990. These recommendations were suggested mainly for introduction at soccer grounds and resulted in responses from the Football Association, the Scottish Football Association, UEFA and FIFA. The guidelines however are applicable to all major sporting events and give new responsibilities to sporting clubs and their medical attendants, even when relatively small crowds are the norm. In Scotland, ground inspection at soccer clubs has been undertaken by the Scottish Football Association and Football League in collaboration with the St Andrew's Ambulance Association (Mr R Scott). In England the problems were addressed by the Football League, and the Gibson report published. Although general recommendations have been made, each club must take account of their own arrangements and decide on the level of overall medical attendance required. A spectrum exists of requirements for the provision of medical cover at large-scale games to a local need for a doctor to look after the primary needs of the players, and to be available to look after the small number of spectators in the event of any illness.

The tragedy at Hillsborough emphasised the problems which can occur within a large crowd, however it was clearly recognised that "It would be unreasonable to expect at all sports stadiums, medical facilities capable of dealing with a major disaster such as occurred. To have in advance at the ground, resuscitators, stretchers, other equipment and medical staff sufficient to deal with over 100 casualties is not practicable". It has however provided the stimulus to organisations to arrange for appropriate facilities. In general, the requirements include the provision of the basic level of first aid, both in terms of the provision of a First Aid Room and attendant trained first aid workers, professional medical attention, and ambulance attendance. In terms of the latter, a system of coordination is required to bring the emergency services to the scene quickly and in appropriate numbers.

Medical role of the crowd doctor

The crowd doctor should provide leadership in terms of co-ordination of services. They should liaise with the police for communication, liaise with the First Aid staff in terms of distribution and communication, with the availability of two-way radios, and, where appropriate help in the co-ordination of stewards if they play a role in first aid provision. The crowd doctor should liaise in the setting up of a First Aid Room and to ensure the appropriate replacement of materials used. Appropriate liaison with ambulance and other emergency personnel should be undertaken, and, where appropriate scenarios should be created so that emergency conditions are simulated to allow appropriate training.

These provisions are appropriate to sporting clubs with relatively small crowds, but who may face the challenge of a large crowd in exceptional circumstances.

First aid facilities

The Taylor Report suggested that the numbers of trained First Aiders should be appropriate to the crowd. This included 1 trained First Aider per 1,000 spectators in general terms. There should be 3 in attendance for up to 1,000, 1 per 1,000 up to 10,000 and in the Gibson Report from the Football League, a suggested 1 additional First Aider for every 2,000 thereafter. An appropriate First Aid Room/s should also be provided - the number, size and equipment specified by the local authority. In terms of providing the large numbers of trained First Aiders required for major sporting events, this may be outwith the resources of the available voluntary organisations, and the training of stewards who have a role in crowd direction and control has been subsequently widely applied. The provision of a heated, comfortable, adequately sized First Aid room with appropriate plumbing facilities has been addressed and recommendations have been made concerning the provision of First Aid equipment. The kits recommended by the St Andrew's Ambulance Association and the equipment suggested as a basic provision in the Gibson Report is contained in Appendix I. Uniformity of provision of such equipment should be undertaken, as has been the case with St Andrew's Ambulance First Aid Workers in Scotland.

Provision of medical practitioners

The Taylor Report recommended that if the crowd was <2,000 a Medical Practitioner should be immediately contactable, and that the arrangements of such an "on-call" system be known by the police. Where a crowd is >2,000 a designated Medical Practitioner trained in advanced first aid should be available at the ground. The Practitioner should be present 1 hour before kick-off and 30 min after the game, and the whereabouts known to the police and they should be immediately contactable. Clear demarcation of duties of the Club Doctor looking after players and the crowd doctor providing first aid facilities should be determined.

Provision of ambulances

If the crowd numbers >5,000, at least 1 fully equipped ambulance should be in attendance. This should be provided by or have the approval of the appropriate ambulance authority. The ambulances should be adequately equipped, with facilities for full cardiopulmonary resuscitation and defibrillation. The total number of ambulances required should be specified by the local authority. If the crowd is >25,000 it is recommended that a major incident vehicle be available. This would follow the design of the Scottish Ambulance group and be equipped for up to 50 casualties. It should provide the storehouse for medical equipment, including at least 50 stretchers, blankets and appropriate medical supplies. This vehicle should be deployed in addition to other ambulances.

International competition

The increase in International competition at club and national level, particularly within Europe, has also provided a major stimulus to the football governing body of Europe (UEFA) to address provision for crowd safety on an International basis. These are particularly important when high risk matches are identified, including all UEFA finals, semi and quarter finals of club competitions and international championships. High risk matches may also be identified by declaration if there have been previous incidents which might threaten safety with supporters of one or both teams. This may also occur if the travelling support is >10% of the stadium capacity, or if >3,000 travelling supporters are admitted. If the crowd is >50,000, all games are deemed high risk, or if the local nation has a large number of emigrants or foreign workers of the same nationality as the visiting team.

The UEFA measures at the ground included guarding of the stadium with police control points at an outer perimeter fence. Entry controls define the appropriate sector for supporters and personal searches should exclude the possession of dangerous objects, and should also exclude known troublemakers. The police responsibility includes adequate security presence before, during and after the game until dispersal of the crowd. It has been suggested that segregation of the different supporters be undertaken by a solid construction and/or police cordon. To prevent ingress of supporters on the field the playing area should he protected by a fence of 2.2 metres or a moat. The appropriate barriers should have police presence to prevent access. An important safety feature is the presence of security gates opening on to the field to allow rapid dispersal of the crowd, if required, as a safety measure. At high risk games, appropriate police presence is required, and prohibition of sale of alcohol, both in the neighbourhood and in the ground, is indicated. Appropriate back-up of police should be available for intervention.

Safety measures at grounds

These have been clearly stated - that emergency exits should be clearly marked, and that corridors and gangway be cleared. There should be no movement of the crowd from section to section within the stadium and adequate stewarding and effective public address system should be available. The ticket allocations for UEFA games are made appropriate to the size of the travelling support and their previous behavioural record, and the circumstances of any previous ties.

In most of the previous problems of crowd control, problems have occurred where the large proportion of the crowd have been in terraced, standing areas. The importance of provision of fully seated stadia has been emphasised by both the Taylor report and subsequent action by UEFA and FIFA. In UEFA competitions, all qualifying matches for 1996 will be played in all-seated stadia, and from season

1993 to '94, all high risk matches will be played before all-seated stadia. Only some 70% of tickets can be sold for terracing at the present time, and there will be a 10% reduction in each subsequent season.

As a result of the Taylor report, the provision of all-seated stadia will occur with appropriate 10% reduction in terracing areas per season, with the final provision of all-seated stadia for major events by the year 2000.

The lessons learned from previous problems are now being widely applied. Hopefully this will have an appropriate influence on safety at all large sporting events, and provide the facilities for treatment if illness or injury should be sustained in the crowd, and provide an environment once more for sport to be enjoyed by all.

References

Gibson Report
Lord Taylor. (1990) The Hillsborough Disaster 15th April, 1989. London, HMSO, CM962.

Appendix I

Medical First Aid Pack For First Aid Room

50 x Gauze swabs 7.5 x 7.5 cm. 12 ply 5 per pack (Sterile)
50 xCotton Wool Balls Hospital Qual. Large - 5 per pack   (Sterile)
50 x Gallipots 60 ml (Sterile)
50 x Sterile Forceps
12 x HIBIDIL Sachets
 3 x Saline for eye irrigation sterile 300 ml
 6 x Crepe bandage 5 cm
 6 x Crepe bandage 7.5 cm
 1 x 100 latex gloves large
 1 x 2.5 cm Hypoallergenic adhesive tape
12 x Eyepads (first aid pack) sterile
24 x W.O.W. bandage 5 cm
24 x W.O.W. bandage 7.5 cm
24 x W.O.W. bandage 10 cm
12 x First Aid Dressings - (12 x 4 sizes)
 1 xTube gauze (suitable for fingers) shortest length available
 1 xTube gauze (suitable for ankles and knees) shortest length available
 2 x Elastic adhesive dressings (composite pack mixed sizes)
 1 x 25 Triangular bandages (not calico, but non-woven   disposable)
 1 x Safety Pins (pack)
 1 x Box Large Paper Tissues

Equipment for Crowd Doctor

Airway Management

Oxygen powered ventilator	1
Bag valve mask and 2 masks - adult/child with oxygen reservoir	
Guedel Airway - 1 of each size 2 - 5	4
Sphygmomanometer	1
Stethoscope	2
Vitalograph aspirator	1
14G suction catheter	2
Smaller gauge suction catheter for children	1
Yankauer suction catheter	1
Nebulizer with independent power (?foot pump variety)	1
Laerdal face mask with oxygen port	2

Intubation

Catheter mount, tubing and appropriate connector	1
KY jelly	1
Magill forceps	1
Spencer Wells 5" forceps	1
1" bandage roll	1
20 ml syringe marked "INTUBATION"	1
Laryngoscope handle LARGE AND STANDARD	1 of each
Adult blade	1
Child blade	1
Batteries and bulbs for the above	2
ET tubes precut 5mm, 6mm, 7mm, 7.5mm, 8mm, 8.5mm, 9mm	7
ET tube 2.5mm in sterile bag	2
Plastic gloves pair	3
Introducer	1
Nasopharyngeal tubes (Portex 100/210)	2

Infusion

Giving sets + 1 with a burette	3
Syringes - 3 x 20ml, 5 x 10ml, 5 x 5ml, 10 x 2ml	23
Hypodermic needles - 10 each 25g, 23g, 21g	30
Intravenous cannulae - e.g. venflon (assorted)	10

Haemaccel 500ml	2
Hartmanns Solution 500ml	2
Armlock splint	1
Adhesive tape - 1 each 1", 2", 3"	3
Blood sample bottles - 2 each cross match + haemoglobin	4
Scissors	1
Antiseptic wipes	6
Sharps min-bin	1
Hepsal 5 mls	2

Chest Drainage

Chest drainage set e.g. Portex Kit	1
Ampules 1% lignocaine 5mls	2
Spencer Wells forceps 5"	2

Drugs should be supplied by Medical Officer

Miscellaneous items

To be provided, as suggested by Gibson Report

Triangular bandages	2
Inflatable/box splints	2
Steri strip dressings	10
Roll of clingfilm	1
Burns sheet	1
Field dressings	2
Multi purpose velcro fastening strap set (6)	1
Cervical collar (stiffneck) pack of 6	6
Tie on labels or triage cards	50
Patient ID bracelets adult/child sizes	6
Red ID bracelets for allergies	6
Melonin/granuflex dressings	6
Mini-trach II tracheostomy set (or cricothyrotomy kit)	1
Monitor/defibrillator OR	1
Semi automatic defibrillator, charger, recorder	1
Box of BM or Dextrostix	1
Oxygen cylinders D size	2
Entonox cylinders D size	2

Closing papers

Tabard "DOCTOR"	1
Tabard "MEDICAL INCIDENT OFFICER"	1
Portable headlamp, e.g. Petzel	1

Prevention is easier than cure

T. Reilly

Abstract. Preventative measures, whether of injury or decrements in performance, rely on empirical principles more than on mathematical certainties about occurrences. Prevention entails a circumspect approach towards fitness for the game, matched to its specific requirements and demands. Muscle strength, aerobic fitness, flexibility training are important as are warm-up pre-competition and the ability to cope with competitive stress. Special considerations are needed in rehabilitation prior to returning to competition, in the use of plyometric training drills, and in the reduction of spinal loading. Biological rhythms should also be taken into account. A team approach towards preventative practices is recommended.

Keywords: Circadian Rhythms, Flexibility, Games, Injuries, Shrinkage, Strength, Warm-Up.

Introduction

That prevention is easier than cure is always true in hindsight when it is possible to trace the events in the causal chain leading to injury. At least those concerned with caring for the injured games player have a definite process to manipulate in treatment or in rehabilitation. Principles of prevention operate on the probability that injuries or other problems that detrimentally affect performance can be predicted. Most scientists recognise that prediction from data points on single human subjects is fraught with uncertainty.

The chain of events dictates that injuries are due to error, some of which cause accidents and some of which in turn lead to trauma. The effects of error differ from sport to sport; in running, for example, about 75% of injuries may be attributed to training error such as improper footwear, abrupt change in mileage, change in running surface, excessive mileage and so on (Garbutt et al, 1990). In contrast the ratio of training to competition injuries in games players is reversed, roughly one-third of injuries occurring in training in soccer (Reilly, 1975) and rugby football (Reilly and Hardiker, 1981; Reilly and Stirling, 1992). A majority of the injuries occur in game-related activities - the tackle, ruck and maul in rugby and in tackling or playing the ball in soccer. The non-contact injuries tend to be correlated with individual predisposing factors which may be identified in fitness and screening tests. Injury predispositions may also render individuals susceptible to damage during physical contact. An ergonomics approach provides a model by which the physical and physiological demands of the game are evaluated and the fitness requirements delineated. The capabilities of players must match these demands and, if not, deficiencies must be remedied by appropriate training.

Demands of the game

The work-rate of soccer players may be represented as distance covered for game and for outfield players averages about 20 km. This of course varies with the positional role, but is reasonably consistent for a particular style of play. The distance is a function of the aerobic power of the individual, as reflected in the correlation between VO_2max and distance covered in a game (Reilly, 1990).

Profiles of activity for the various football games, according to the level and type of activity, have been established (Reilly, 1990). It has also been possible to quantify the additional demands of dribbling a soccer ball, in terms both of the increased blood lactate concentrations and the alterations in stride rate that occur (Reilly and Ball, 1984). It is important that these factors should be considered in the training programme.

Rugby differs from the others in terms of the greater amount of game related activity during a match - e.g. scrums, rucks and mauls. It is not surprising that most injuries occur in these game-related activities. The main contexts are tackling, being tackled, rucks/mauls and scrums. There are few injuries of a serious nature in line-outs or in free-running as occurs in the case of hamstring injuries in sprinters (Reilly and Hardiker, 1981).

Of course the physiological capabilities may deteriorate as the game progresses. This has been observed to occur in the second half in soccer (Reilly, 1990). This fatigue is related to falls in glycogen levels in active muscles. Those players affected simply lower their work-rate. This means that performance is likely to drop before muscle damage occurs in high level rugby.

When errors are related to energy sources it is noteworthy that errors towards the end of exercise lasting 80-90 min can be reduced by provision of fluid. This amelioration can be furthered by provision of energy drinks. Although the research work has been done in experimental conditions (Reilly and Lewis, 1985), it may have relevance in games play.

The time of play that injuries occur was found to happen not when players were exercising most intensely at the start, or in the last quarter where they might be fatigued, but after half-time. This was attributed to cold conditions and a lack of warm-up after half-time (Reilly and Hardiker, 1981).

There is some evidence that lack of warm-up and flexibility are predisposing factors to injury. In one study by Reilly and Stirling (1992) flexibility data on rugby, soccer, hockey and handball players were combined. A total of 25 flexibility measures was reduced by factor analysis and then it was possible to distinguish between the frequently injured and infrequently injured players. The evidence was that:-

a. hip flexibility was related to absence of injury; other flexibility measures were not;

b. warm-up did reduce injury incidence - duration of warm-up was not related to injury proneness.

c. the injured player had paid less attention to jogging, technique work and lower body exercise than did the less frequently injured players.

Additional evidence comes from Ekstrand (1982) who showed a high incidence of muscle tightness in Swedish players, especially those shown to be injury prone. The soccer players were less supple than a reference group in hip abduction, hip extension, knee flexion and ankle dorsiflexion (Ekstrand and Gillquist, 1982). An intervention programme of flexibility exercises did reduce the incidence of injuries in Swedish players over a full season.

Hypermobility is associated with certain types of acute injuries, notably sprains and dislocations. Lysens and colleagues (1991) confirmed that non-traumatic joint laxity or joint instability pre-disposed athletes to sprains and dislocations. High muscle flexibility and joint mobility within the normal range of motion do not seem to constitute a predisposition to injury.

Training

When games players' training profiles are examined, the variety of elements that have to be accommodated can be noted. An example is the typical training components used in professional soccer (Reilly, 1990). The relative contributions of each to the total training programme was: warm-up, 8.1; flexibility, 6.4; running, 10.2; circuit-training, 10.0; skills practice, 15.0; drills, 19.2; games, 23.9; recovery intermissions, 7.2%.

For rugby, very often players are unfit to cope with strenuous training and do not do the requisite training in their own time. Similar trends were observed in soccer players on returning after the off-season when the emphasis is on endurance work. This is at the expense of strength which tends to decrease until the training load and competitive programme are settled (Reilly and Thomas, 1977). Strength gradually returns to pre-season levels whilst aerobic fitness is maintained.

Is strength training relevant to football? Work at Brussels has shown that it is. Strength training was found to improve kick performance using the distance the ball travelled as a criterion (De Proft et al, 1988).

Soccer players spend a lot of their time inactive (Reilly and Thomas, 1979).

Those individuals with extra-curricular training were found to have the higher fitness levels and the fewer injuries (Reilly and Thomas, 1980). A factor analysis of strength measures showed that strength did have a protective value - this agrees with evidence in the literature stating that strength training can reduce the incidence of both knee injuries and cervical injuries in American Football.

The evidence that strength training will protect the spine is supplemented by work on spinal shrinkage - changes in stature are measured with a sensitive stadiometer, the changes being related to compressive loading on the spine with a consequent loss in inter-vertebral disc height. (Reilly et al, 1991). Stature varies with time of day, a loss of about 18 mm occurring between morning and late evening. The shrinkage due to activity does not depend on whether it is continuous or intermittently high.

In response to weight training the disc loses more height in the morning than in the evening. The greater stiffness in the evening is compensated for by the increased muscular strength - this reduces the vulnerability to injury that might otherwise apply (Wilby et al, 1987).

An alternative protective strategy is to unload the spine by resting. Examples are the Fowler posture and gravity inversion. Though effects are only short-lived, evidence from cricket bowlers is that there may be some protective effect (Reilly and Chana, 1991). The implications are mainly for training rather than competition, for activities such as scrummaging and so on. Whilst the concern has been with back-injuries - noting the long disability time players with back injuries incur - it is acknowledged that back pain has been a problem for the medical profession since the time of Hippocrates and will not be solved by 10 minutes hanging upside down.

Stress and behaviour

The level of play also affects the injury rate. For example, higher incidences are seen in First Division soccer compared with A team or reserves (Reilly, 1975).

Teams that stick together have a greater degree of success, implying a relation between injury and performance. This was demonstrated on analysis of the relation between League position and number of players used per season in the English League (Reilly, 1975). When morale is positive players are reluctant to report as injured or acknowledge injuries of a minor nature.

The converse may be related to stress. Anxiety was found to be related to injuries, probably due to a breakdown in skill and lack of commitment in tackling (Thomas and Reilly, 1975). Consequently some emphasis must be placed on injury avoidance and on coaching techniques to reduce stress.

Plyometric exercises

Muscles are injured mainly during an enforced stretch when they are operating in the high force range. This has prompted the use of plyometric training where the muscle operates through its stretch-shortening cycle. Such activities include bounding, drop-jumping and so on. There is some debate about what drop-height is optimal for training. Lees and Fahmi (1992) have shown that the heights used by athletes may be beyond the optimal, indicated either by power output or muscular efficiency.

A more recent study looking at back and lower limb musculature used loaded drop-jumps. This showed variability between individuals in absorbing the impact shocks (Fowler et al, 1992). The suggestion is that some individuals may be unsuited for plyometric training such as repetitive bounding or drop-jumping.

It is not certain that such activities do lead to improved performance in games players. For example, no improvement was found in muscle power measures in Rugby League players introduced to plyometric drills during their season. They did, however, report an enhanced enjoyment of the training (Reilly and Doyle, 1992).

Plyometric training does induce muscle damage as reflected in delayed onset muscle soreness. There may be some protection from pre-stretching in warm-up but there is a repeated bouts effect. Over 4 weeks while this adaptation occurs, the maximum muscle force is depressed (Adams and Reilly, 1987).

There may also be some protection from use of the pendulum technique without the damaging effects on muscle and its connective tissue. This method entails sitting in a specially constructed chair and swinging onto a vertically placed rigid platform from which to rebound with a stretch-shortening cycle of leg muscle action. The body and the swinging part of the pendulum are driven back to be ready for the next swing. The chair can be loaded with additional weights to increase the force of impact with the platform and presumably enhance the training effect.

Re-injury

In the case of muscle injuries, there is obvious pressure to take players back into competition quickly and frequently players return to competition before they are completely rehabilitated. Isokinetic test profiles may help in determining readiness to return. After three surgical operations on a top level soccer player, which included section of part of the tendon of the long head of biceps femoris, he was left with weak hamstrings, assymetry between left and right and a low hamstrings/ quadriceps ratio in the right leg. The final injury had been incurred on back-heeling the ball in the first match after return from a prolonged lay-off. This left his strength-angle curve abnormal. After 3 test periods over 9 weeks of concentric, eccentric and isometric training he was able to resume, by returning first to the "A" team and continuing strength training in field conditions. This case study demonstrates the importance of a graded approach to the return to match-play in such circumstances.

Environmental factors

There are also environmental factors to be taken into consideration. The line-ups of many English League professional soccer teams this year (1991-92) have both an unfamiliar list of names and a lot of corrections on the match programme denoting late changes. Pre-season training was responsible for an unusually large number of injuries. The summer was unique in the hardness of the pitches and the training surfaces on some grounds were rock hard. Pre-season training entailed a host of predisposing factors: abrupt changes in load, inadequate attention to footwear, inattention to surface characteristics, insufficient recovery from hard training, and so on.

Biological rhythms

The body's biological rhythms must also be taken into consideration. One of these is the circadian rhythm in body temperature to which many performance rhythms are related. These include e.g. ventilatory response to exercise, which partly explains why exercising hard in the morning is not advisable. Many football teams travelling abroad ignore the stress placed on the players by desynchronisation of their circadian rhythms. An example was provided by a study of student rugby players performing in New Zealand. Body temperature responds slowly, usually has not adapted prior to the first match abroad (Reilly and Mellor, 1988).

Preventative techniques for coping with jet lag are now validated. One of our successes has been with professional soccer players using exercise to help synchronise their rhythms after coming back from Japan. They were well adjusted when they played their opening League match on the Saturday following arriving home on Sunday morning. Later that afternoon the team had a physical training session at its ground to accelerate the process of resynchronisation.

The concern so far has been with male players. Women's sport is growth fast, particularly participation in soccer and rugby. There is evidence of cyclical changes in mood in female athletes, the fluctuations being closely correlated with alterations in hormonal levels during the menstrual cycle (O'Reilly and Reilly, 1990). There is some evidence that injuries are more likely to occur pre-menses and during menses (Moller-Nielsen and Hammar, 1989) and perhaps medical personnel may help in singling out vulnerable individuals.   This review has attempted to highlight some factors which predispose to injury. Some practices in the training of games players have also been described. Although prediction of injury occurrence is rather imprecise, introduction of injury avoidance elements into training regimens is wise. While research has provided evidence to demonstrate the importance of warm-up, strength and flexibility training and so on in games players, there is still scope for work in characterising the likelihood of injury risk. In this respect the sports scientist has an important future role. The prevention of injury is a team effort that embraces scientist, coach, team physician, physiotherapist and player in preventing the latter from going a bridge too far during training or match-play.

References

Adams C and Reilly T. (1987) Attenuation of delayed muscle soreness with eccentric training. Communication to British Association of Sports Medicine Meeting (Liverpool).

De Proft E,Cabri J, Dufour W and Clarys JP. (1988) Strength training and kick performance in soccer players, in Science and Football (eds T Reilly, A Lees, R Davids, WJ Murphy), E & FN Spon, London, pp. 108-113.

Ekstrand J. (1982) Soccer injuries and their prevention. Medical dissertation No.130 Linkoping University.

Ekstrand J and Gillquist J. (1982) The frequency of muscle tightness and injuries in soccer players. Amer J Sports Med, 10, 75-78.

Fowler NE, Lees A and Reilly T. (1992) Spinal shrinkage in unloaded and loaded drop-jumping. Ergonomics, 35, (in press).

Garbutt G, Boocock MG and Reilly T. (1988) Injuries and training patterns in recreational marathon runners, in Proceedings of the Eighth Middle East Sport Science Symposiuu (ed A Brien). Ministry of Information, Bahrain, pp. 56-62.

Lees A and Fahmi E. (1992) Optimal drop heights for plyometric training. Ergonomics, 35, (in press).

Lysens RJ, de Weert W and Nieuwboer A. (1991) Factors associated with injury proneness. Sports Med, 12, 281-289.

Moller-Nielsen J and Hammar M (1989(Women's soccer injuries in relation to the menstrual cycle and oral contraceptives. Med Sci Sports Exerc, 21, 126-129.

O'Reilly A and Reilly T. (1990) Effects of the menstrual cycle on responses to exercise, in Contemporary Ergonomics 1990 (ed E J Lovesey), Taylor and Francis, London, pp. 149-153.

Reilly T. (1975) An ergonomic evaluation of occupational stress in professional soccer. Unpublished PhD thesis, Liverpool Polytechnic.

Reilly T. (1990) Football, in Physiology of Sports (eds T Reilly, N Secher, P Snell and C Williams). E & FN Spon, London.

Reilly T and Ball D. (1984) The net physiological cost of dribbling a soccer ball. Res Quart Exerc Sport, 55, 267-271.

Reilly T and Chana D. (1991) Spinal shrinkage in fast bowling. J Sports Sci, 9, 347-348.

Reilly T and Doyle M. (1992) Investigation of plyometric training in Rugby League players, in Science and Football II (eds T Reilly, JP Clarys and AB Stibbe). E & FN Spon, London.

Reilly T and Hardiker R. (1981) Somatotype and injuries in adult student rugby football. J Sports Med Phys Fit, 21, 186-191.

Reilly T and Lewis W. (1985) Effect of carbohydrate feeding on mental functions during sustained physical work, in Ergonomics International 85 (eds ID Brown, R Goldsmith, K Coombes and MA Sinclair). Taylor and Francis, London, pp. 700-702.

Reilly T and Mellor S. (1988) Jet lag in Rugby League players following a near maximal time-zone shift, in Science and Football (eds T Reilly, A Lees, K Davids and WJ Murphy). E & FN Spon, London, pp. 245-256.

Reilly T and Stirling A. (1992) Flexibility, warm-up and injuries in mature games players, in Kinanthropometry IV (eds W Duquet and J Borms). E & FN Spon, London.

Reilly T and Thomas V. (1979) Estimated energy expenditures of professional association footballers. Ergonomics, 22, 541-548.

Reilly T and Thomas V. (1980) The stability of fitness factors over a season of professional soccer as indicated by serial factor analysis, in Kinanthropometry II (eds M Ostyn, G Beunen and J Simons), University Park Press, Baltimore, pp. 245-257.

Reilly T, Boocock HG, Garbutt G, Troup JDG and Linge K. (1991) Changes in stature during exercise and sports training. Appl Ergonomics, 22, 308-311.

Thomas V and Reilly T. (1975) The relationship between anxiety variables and injuries in top-class soccer, in Proceedings European Sports Psychology Congress (Edinburgh).

Wilby T, Linge K, Reilly T and Troup JDG. (1987) Spinal shrinkage in females: circadian variation in stature and the effects of circuit weight-training. Ergonomics, 30, 47-54.

The will to win

D.B. Whitaker

Abstract. Enabling players to achieve their best performances as individuals and as a members of a team requires a complex interaction of many varied factors. Fitness, skill and experience must be matched with an attitude of mind and the commitment that is associated with the "Will to Win". Players must be prepared to take personal responsibility for their own performance and the coach acts as a catalyst to promote self and team belief.

Keywords: "The Will to Win", Commitment, Personal Responsibility.

I stand before you not as a sports scientist of any standing or achievement but as a person who has had the privilege of working with performers at all levels, including the Olympic Games, and perhaps had the good fortune to help them promote their undoubted "will to win".

Graf thrives on competition, on hard work on an endless search for a perfection which drives her on to the practice court at sunrise and which, very probably only exists in the recesses of her mind, like an oasis.

The topic is, I believe, the least scientific of the Conference and yet it is one that exercises the minds of everyone involved in developing competitive performance. It may, therefore, be an art in which we are all involved. It is sometimes perceived as an almost magical concept: we all know when it is there but having the skill to instill, promote or sustain it is far more challenging.

I have produced a subtitle for this presentation which, I believe, begins to shed light on the concept of "the Will to Win" and ways of developing it. The subtitle is very simply; .....

"Commitment .... the physical expression of belief".

It is borne out of the desire to get better and better every time you perform. Commitment, like the "will to win", is almost impossible to define in words but easy to see.

I have one simple yet undying cameo of "the Will to Win" from rugby and interestingly it was not from match play. It was the entry of the Scottish team for the Calcutta Cup match at Murrayfield in 1990. They **walked** across that treacherousiy vulnerable area from the safety of the stand to the relative security of the centre of the field and the match. For me that epitomised a group "will to win" even before the game.

So, what is it this "commitment to the cause" or "will to win"? Some people seem to illustrate it in abundance and sometimes you see a whole team exude it. The danger for coaches and managers is that we can begin to believe that we are the source of it! At best this is foolish and a misunderstanding of the complexity of the concept, and at worst sheer arrogance. It can often appear and grow in a player or team **in spite of** the management; in fact I have played in a team when that was so. The tragedy was that our "will to win" could have been even better if the coach/manager had been able to help us promote and direct it even more effectively. That is the challenge for the coach. How do you identify, nurture, direct, massage this crucial element in performance? Well, to be perfectly honest, with a great deal of difficulty!

It is based upon a matrix of interrelated factors and it has to be an integral element in every part of performance because "the will to win" is not enough on its own. Fine words are totally insufficient. The "will to win" must include that physical expression of belief. When it comes to the crunch fitness, skill and experience are not the whole story of performance. The attitude of mind is crucial to performance and "the will to win" or "commitment" and all that goes with it is an attitude of mind.

One method would be to search the highways and byways of our sports for people who both illustrate the appropriate attitudes and match it with their behaviour but this can take enormous amounts of resource which few sports have .... So, what we all have to do is **grow our own.**

What makes up this "will to win"?

Desire? Belief? Dedication? Commitment? Motivation? Single Mindedness? Personal Responsibility? Well, yes all of these things and probably more but how can I get my players to develop more of each? The answer is, I believe, as simple and yet as complex as this.....

<u>"It all hinges on the way you work with them".</u>

Selection can be orientated towards seeking the "will to win" but it is not always easy to get it right by using this as a principal selection criterion. Far better to seek, find and promote the "will to win" in the players.

Desire is promoted by the vision of what they could achieve. Coaches have visions; it is essential that we hold onto them and transmit them to the players. This picture for them must have elements of fulfillment, a sense of achievement if they get there.

Belief is based upon the self esteem and security of the performer and this is promoted by putting them at the centre of the development process. This also values them and involves them which reinforces self esteem and security. Insecurity can be used in the selection process to test desire, belief, etc but I am not a great believer in extending this situation unnecessarily. It is inherent in the process anyway and to enlarge its importance can be counter-productive.

Commitment is based upon the belief that they can achieve the vision and so if the first two are in tune the commitment is likely to be maintained. Coaches must continually check the levels of commitment and enhance it through appropriate interaction with the players.

Motivation is tied in closely with all these factors and is also continually influenced by the coach/performer interaction. The coach has a crucial role to play in promoting motivation in players.

Single mindedness is about appropriate focus not bloody mindedness and can be influenced **greatly by the coach.**

All these factors are influenced by the coach through the interactive process with players and we owe it to the players to get this interaction to the highest quality possible.

Will the autocratic coach promote: belief?
                                       commitment?
                                       motivation?
                                       desire?

Will the **laissez faire** approach develop these qualities to the optimum? Very unlikely.

We all propose a "partnership" approach .... and I propose **even more.** I tried to work so that the players were finding the solutions to problems rather than me giving all the answers. I **asked** them more than I **told** them. The reasons for this approach are simply these:

- They took personal responsibility for their own performance in every part of preparation - training, skill development, psychological match strategies
- Many of the solutions to challenges are wrapped up in the performers
- Ownership of the behaviour had to be **theirs** not **mine**
- They had to become decision makers in the dynamic environment of performance
- They needed to feel that they were controllers of their own destiny
- I needed to empower them and this is impossible without all the other factors above

This approach promoted the crucial factors of self-evaluation, self-regulation and self-motivation. These support the will to win by promoting personal and group responsibility.

It meant that they had met most situations during our development of the team and had learnt from each one.

The transference of these concepts from individua] to team is built over time with trust and respect as the mortar which binds the bricks. The team spirit which this process can evoke enhances the corporate "will to win". Team spirit is crucial yet very difficult to quantify: it is developed through a whole variety of experiences and is something that coaches and managers may not be able to be part of. It is theirs (the players) and it needs to be theirs. We may help develop it yet be excluded from it.

When we are promoting this will to win we are often in that mode of interaction that has as its objective the motivation of the players; and I have learnt some very important lessons in this area: Firstly, motivation is all about their needs as players not yours as coach. Secondly, if one accepts that, then it is vital that coaches say what they need to hear not just what coaches want to say.

Very often their "will to win" needs controlling - how often do we take them beyond optimum arousal? You **want** and **need** the "will to win" yet it is a double edged sword. It is essential we recognise **their** needs.

The "will to win" is more than just behaviour in competition, it is an **approach to the whole process of competition.** It manifests itself in all that a person or team does in their preparation.

Words about the "will to win" are not enough, everyone can talk a good game, it is deeds that matter and that is why it **is a physical expression of belief.**

I had the pleasure of watching a team I coached exemplify that belief and "will to win" in Seoul in 1988. I could not have helped them to do it without scientists such as you but most of all I could not have helped them if they had not wanted to do it themselves.

You cannot make people have a "will to win" but if you shirk the responsibility of enabling people to find and develop their own and corporate "will to win", then I believe you may be robbing them of an opportunity of greatness. Coaches are rarely the source of the "will to win" in a performer for that must come from within but the coach **can be** the catalyst that promotes and develops it, such that it shines for everyone to see in the competitive arena.

INTERNATIONAL POSTER COMPETITION

A Poster Display was held in conjunction with the Congress. The International Rugby Football Board awarded a Commemorative Diploma and Quaich (traditional Scottish drinking bowl designed for whisky) for the winning poster, and two runners-up prizes with an appropriate Diploma and Quaich for a native and non-native English speaker. A total of nineteen posters were displayed.

International Rugby Football Board Winning Poster

Rugby injuries in Canada

B.W.D. Badley
Victoria General Hospital and Dalhousie University, Halifax, Canada

Purpose of the Study

To assess the frequency, type and causes of injury in Canadian Rugby and to consider whether additional law changes might reduce the incidence of injuries.

Definition

An injury was defined as: "An incident that prevented a player from completing a game or practice, or from participating in any future game or practice." This definition differs from others used in comparable studies.

Methods

Rather than the usual "longitudinal" study involving a number of teams throughout a season of play, information on injuries was obtained from all teams playing in Canada during one week of the playing season (a "cross-sectional" or "snapshot" study). The data were recorded on a standardized form in which the majority of responses were predefined and there was a minimum of free text, allowing the results to be readily transferred to a computer program.

Results

On average, a team lost a player to injury once in every 1.4 games. Incidents in the scrummage (mainly whilst engaging or collapsing) were responsible for 13% of injuries. Twenty- three percent of injuries occurred during rucks and mauls, mostly during the drive, with a lesser number occurring as a consequence of collapse or pile-up. Tackling or being tackled was responsible for 43% of injuries.

There were nine fractures of various bones and 34 joint or ligament injuries involving predominantly the shoulder, ankle and knee. Tackling was responsible for seven of the 11 head injuries recorded. There were no significant spinal injuries.

Conclusions

A common definition of injuries should be established.
The patterns and causes of injury in Canadian Rugby are similar to those occurring in other countries.
The findings of a cross-sectional survey are comparable to those of longitudinal studies and may, therefore, be suitable for assessing the results of changes designed to reduce the incidence of injuries.
Stricter compliance with existing laws should reduce the incidence of injury.
Law changes designed to reduce injuries should be applicable to all levels of the game.

International Rugby Football Board Runner-Up (Non-English Speaking) Prize

Muscle strains and isokinetic power profile of the thigh muscles in rugby football players

T. Okuwaki
Tsukuba Medical Center Hospital, Japan

I. Kono and M. Eda
University of Tsukuba, Japan

J. Murakami
Fukuoka University, Japan

The purpose of this study was to survey muscle strains in rugby football players and to assess the isokinetic power profile of their thigh muscles using an isokinetic machine, Biodex. And we also evaluated the usefulness of the isokinetic rehabilitation for players with muscle strains. Seventy rugby football players of the University of Tsukuba were inquired about muscle strains at pre-season medical checkups. Fifteen percentage of the players had suffered muscle strains in the previous season. In the majority of the injured, they had experienced recurrence of the strains at the same portion. The muscle strains occurred more frequently in the knee flexors than in the extensors. On the average, it took 3 weeks to return to the field. However, in some players, it took more than 3 months to recover from the damage. The analysis of the isokinetic power profile were performed at the pre-season medical checkups. It disclosed that the power of the flexors were weaker than the extensors in the players. Players with extreme imbalance seemed to sustain more frequently muscle strains than those without imbalance. Gathering with the high incidence of muscle strains and the remarkable imbalance of the thigh muscle power, we concluded the imbalance might play a major role in the mechanisms of the muscle strains in rugby football players. For the injuries, we designed the treatment and rehabilitation programs using isokinetic exercise as follows: Step 1: Initially injured players were treated with rest, ice, compression and elevation. Step 2: After 48 hours light exercises were started to gain the range of motion. Step 3: After gaining full range of the knee, high speed isokinetic exercises were begun. Step 4: They were allowed to jog when the peak torque of the injured portion reached 70-80% of that of the uninjured at the high speed isokinetic exercise. Step 5: Players could dash, jump, kick and step after gaining 70-80% peak torque in the lower speed isokinetic exercise. Step 6: Finally, they were allowed to return to the game. During all steps hot-pack and stretching of the injured portion were performed before exercises and they were treated with ice-massage after them. We found the rehabilitation program useful for injured players to return, and prevent recurrences of muscle strains in rugby football players.

International Rugby Football Board Runner-Up (English-Speaking) Prize

A pilot study into the effect of physiotherapy interaction on competitive state anxiety

S.J.M. Airth
Queen Margaret College, Edinburgh, Scotland

This pilot study investigated the effect of physiotherapy interaction prior to competitive sport, on the Competitive State Anxiety of participants in rugby, football and athletics.

Each physiotherapy interaction involved the application of a strapping or a massage by a Chartered Physiotherapist during the pre-event period.

Massage and strapping applied before competitive sport events are often regarded as being mainly for psychological benefit. There is also a suggestion that sophisticated stress management techniques may be effective in part because the athlete has contact with an interested therapist before the event. This study, therefore, attempts to look at both these aspects.

The competitive state anxiety of the subjects was measured before and after physiotherapy contact during the pre-event period using the Competitive State Anxiety Inventory (CSAI-2, Martens et al, 1983). The subjects used in this study included rugby players competing at U-21 District level, athletes competing in the Scottish National Indoor Championships, Kelvinhall and professional footballers competing in the Premier League.

The results showed that physiotherapy interaction appeared to have had a positive effect on the state anxiety of competitors in all three sports.

The rugby players who had physiotherapy contact had significantly lower levels of cognitive and somatic anxiety as well as more self confidence than those who had no interaction. This pattern was similar with the results of the athletes.

The physiotherapy interaction appeared to have prevented the footballers' anxiety from rising as high as might be expected during the pre-event period.

These results were confirmed in a second questionnaire, in which 65% of the rugby players reported that they felt "more ready to compete" following physiotherapy interaction. Similarly, 50% also said that they would not have felt as confident in competition if they had had no interaction.

This study outlines the problems of high state anxiety with regards to both performance and the occurrence of injury. Also identified are the problems which may arise if more extensive research was undertaken in this area.

Throughout this study, literature and results have indicated the need and value of further investigation.

Other Posters Submitted

Dr E Brady   IRE Use of Isokinetics to Evaluate Muscle Imbalances in Soccer and Rugby Players

Dr H R Broughton NZ Premature Degeneration of the Cervical Spine in a Rugby Union Player

Mr P A Butlin   UK Making Rugby the Fourth 'R' - Rugby Football Union Cross Curricular Project for Primary Schools

Mr J Clegg	UK	Mouth Protection for the Rugby Football Player
Dr T Durkin	UK	A Survey of Injuries in a First-Class English Rugby Football Club from 1972-1989
Mr R J Fordham Dr G Vanderfield	AUS	Australian Rugby Football Safety Directives
Dr V Ignat	ROM	Study about the Traumatology of the Shoulder
Prof Dr W Kuhn	GER	A Comparative Analysis of Selected Motor Performance Variables in American Football, Rugby Union and Soccer Players
Mr J McKenna	UK	Fitness Testing and Player Development
Prof L Romanini	IT	Consideration on an Epidemiological Study of Rugby Injuries
Mr Y Sagara	JPN	Effect of Restriction on Chest-Wall Movement during Exercise in Young Athletes
Ms S Turl	UK	Rugby Injuries - are the clubs medically prepared?
Dr G Vanderfield	AUS	Concussive Injuries in Rugby and their Management
Dr G Vanderfield	AUS	Heat Problems when Playing Rugby in the Tropics
Dr D VandeVoorde	BEL	Data Collection Injuries 1988-89
Dr F von Bergen	SWE	Sports Injury First-Aid Kit

SPONSORSHIP

The International Rugby Football Board, the Scottish Rugby Union and the Rugby World Cup are delighted to acknowledge the generous financial support the Sports Medicine Congress received from its sponsors.

It would not have been possible to bring together an international faculty of speakers of the quality we secured without the financial security provided by sponsorship.

The four main sponsors for the Congress were:

Lederle Laboratories

Lederle Laboratories are one of the top ten ethical pharmaceutical companies in the UK, with primary interest in antibiotics, anticancer and rheumatology products. Lederle are enthusiastic supporters of Sports Medicine and sponsor the magazine "Sports Medicine and Soft Tissue Trauma". Lederle manufacture the topical NSAID TRAXAM* GEL.

* Registered Trademark

Chattanooga Group Ltd

In Britain, the United States and more than 50 countries of the world the Chattanooga Group strives to meet the needs of Physiotherapy health care professionals.

In addition the Chattanooga Group is supporting research and professional education programmes throughout the world.

Chattecx, a division of the Chattanooga Group, manufactures KIN-COM, the first system with eccentric testing and training capabilities. Using KIN-COM can evaluate and train patients ranging from the frail and elderly to the elite athlete on a single system.

Scottish Life	Established in 1881, The Scottish Life Assurance Company is a leading mutual life office. With assets in excess of £2 billion and reserves of £300 milion, the company is counted among the market leaders, offering a wide range of competitive life, pensions and investment contracts. Scottish Life's award winning range of mortgage products are considered the most innovative and comprehensive available from any life office.
The Carnegie Partnership	The Carnegie Partnership is a Scottish based business management organisation providing strategic and financial management for professional sports-related organisations and individual sportsmen and women. The Carnegie Partnership specialises in tailor-made financing projects, particularly in the area of stadium redevelopment where its most recent success has been the launching of the £36.75 million Murrayfield Debenture scheme.

In addition to acknowledging the financial support received from their sponsors, the Organising Committee of the Congress are most grateful to Mercury Telecommunications plc for providing Congress participants with commemorative folders.

Index

This index uses keywords assigned to the individual chapters as its basis. The numbers are the page numbers of the first page of the relevant chapter.